FEEDING AND CARE OF THE HORSE

Second Edition

LON D. LEWIS, DVM, PhD

Diplomate, American College of Veterinary Nutrition
Topeka, Kansas

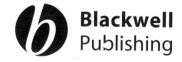
Blackwell Publishing

©2005 Blackwell Publishing, Fifth printing
          All rights reserved
©1996 Lippincott Williams & Wilkins, First, second, third, and fourth printings

Blackwell Publishing Professional
2121 State Avenue, Ames, Iowa 50014, USA

Orders: 1-800-862-6657
Office: 1-515-292-0140
Fax: 1-515-292-3348
Web site: www.blackwellprofessional.com

Blackwell Publishing Ltd
9600 Garsington Road, Oxford OX4 2DQ, UK
Tel.: +44 (0)1865 776868

Blackwell Publishing Asia
550 Swanston Street, Carlton, Victoria 3053, Australia
Tel.: +61 (0)3 8359 1011

First edition, 1982

Library of Congress Cataloging-in-Publication Data

Lewis, Lon D.
          Feeding and care of the horse / Lon D. Lewis.—2nd ed.
                p. cm.
          Includes bibliographical references and index.
          ISBN 0-683-04967-4
          1. Horses—Feeding and feeds. I. Title.
SF285.5.L48   1994
636.1′084—dc20

                                                                    94-18096
                                                                    CIP

The last digit is the print number: 9 8 7 6 5

DEDICATION

Dedicated to the memory of

Two outstanding horsemen:

Everette Corwin Lewis, my father, whom I didn't have the pleasure of knowing and
Lee M. Brunk, my father-in-law, whom I did.

Two great cattlemen:

Del J. and Dorcas M. Bigelow, my grandparents, who taught me much about life

and

Veterinary editor and friend to the profession and those they serve,
Kit (Christian C. Febiger) Spahr, Jr.,
editor of the first edition of this book.

All of whom live on in the memory of those who knew them and/or
have benefited from the many contributions they left us.

PREFACE

There has been an extensive amount of research conducted, as well as experiences and recommendations reported, on all aspects of feeding and caring of the horse. Much of this information is accurate and applicable, however, some is not. Some must be interpreted or combined with other information to be directly applicable and useable. Results with other species of animals are sometimes reported for horses. Often these are found not to be applicable for horses. Some experiences, recommendations, and ''old wives' tales'' are well proven not to be true, or to be true only under certain circumstances, but unfortunately are often repeated by those unaware of studies or experiences refuting them. Occasionally, financial gain rather than scientific validity appears to be the motive behind information and recommendations given. Generally, there is some factual basis for the statements or implications made, but what has been demonstrated is not understood, is misrepresented, is exaggerated, or most often, is extrapolated to circumstances to which they either don't apply or to which there is no evidence that they do. This book is an effort to alleviate these shortcomings in bringing together research results, experiences, and recommendations in as accurate, complete, and as useable a manner as possible for horse owners, who are not veterinarians or nutritionists.

For the veterinarian and nutritionist the referenced textbook **EQUINE CLINICAL NUTRITION: Feeding and Care** is more useful. It provides the details necessary for a more complete understanding, for diagnosing, and for both dietary as well as medical management necessary to most successfully treat nutritional and feeding-related diseases affecting horses. Dietary management of non-feeding related diseases for both sick horses and foals are also described, including fluid and electrolyte therapy, and oral and intravenous feeding. Studies confirming the validity and basis for information and recommendations given are described and referenced so additional details can be found if wanted. **FEEDING AND CARE OF THE HORSE** is an abridgment of this more medically oriented textbook. Research details and references are omitted allowing information to be presented more succinctly. This greatly assists in making the information easier to find, understand and use. There is minimal use of medical and other words not common to non-health professionals. However, at times their use is necessary. In addition, there are some words common to some but not others, and that have different meanings to different people and in different situations. Because of this, a glossary of over 750 words has been added to this book.

The book is divided into three sections. In the first section on ''Nutrition and Feeds for Horses'' emphasis is on the nutrients needed by the horse and their many sources. In the second section on ''Feeding and Care of Horses'' feeding to meet these needs, as well as additional aspects of care, are described. The last section contains the glossary and appendix tables which provide information referred to throughout this book and needed repeatedly in feeding and caring for horses.

The book begins with a listing of chapter titles and their location. Each chapter begins with a detailed table of contents for quickly finding specific topics of interest and items involved with or described under that topic. Most chapters end with a description of additional information recommended on topics covered in that chapter.

Chapters 1, 2, and 3 describe the sources, utilization, and functions of nutrients by the horse, and causes, effects, and treatment of deficiencies and excesses of these nutrients — water and energy-providing nutrients in Chapter 1, and the many minerals and vitamins needed, harmful, and given to horses in Chapters 2 and 3, respectively. The multitude of different feeds, both harvested and pasture, that provide these nutrients are described in Chapters 4 and 5. No topic in feeding horses is of greater concern than that of the various feeds that may be used, or are harmful to horses. These feeds include types, forms and cuttings of hay; the many different cereal grains; high-moisture harvested feeds; vitamins, minerals, protein and fat supplements; commercially available feed mixtures; and various by-product feeds, and feed additives fed to horses. However, for many horses the major and often only feed needed is pasture forage for which its types, planting, management and benefit are described. How to determine the nutrient content of the horse's diet and, therefore, if it is providing inadequate or excessive amounts of each nutrient, and how to mix feeds together so that nutrients low in one feed are balanced by feeding another feed higher in these nutrients, and thus prevent or correct nutrient deficiencies and excesses are described in Chapter 6. How to do this as economically as possible is described in Chapter 7.

The use of the information in Section I on ''Nutrition and Feeds'' to feed and care for the horse is described in Section II. General feeding and management practices for all horses are given in Chapters 8 and 9. This includes needs, methods and frequency of feeding different types of feeds, the description, harm and control of internal and external parasites and infectious diseases, dental, foot and hair coat problems and care, recordkeeping, housing, and fences. Specific feeding and care for each stage of life, activity and environment are given in Chapters 10 through

15. This includes during hot or cold weather, and for idle, working and aged horses, for athletic performance, for breeding stallions, broodmares and growing horses including orphans. Nutrients, training, fitness evaluation, diseases due to and selecting horses for athletic performance are also described in Chapter 11. Chapters 12 and 13 also include breeding evaluation, procedures and problems, including nutritional effects on reproduction and on milk production and composition. Mare and foal care at foaling, including their behavior, and maternal aggression and complications are described in Chapter 14. Following Chapter 15 describing feeding and care of growing horses, the most common problems occurring in fast growing light horse breeds, developmental orthopedic diseases, are described in Chapter 16.

A tremendous thanks to Dr. Tony Knight for the extensive and thorough compilation given in Chapter 18 of all plants growing in North America confirmed to cause poisoning of horses. The plants are presented according to their major detrimental effect on the horse. This presentation greatly assists in knowing which plants, if any, to consider as a cause of abnormalities in horses. Dr. Knight's extensive training, experience and expertise in internal medicine combined with his life-long avocation — botany, have resulted in an extremely useful source of information never before available. For each plant a description for its identification, along with colored pictures, its toxic principle and its effects, clinical signs, diagnosis, treatment, and

means of preventing poisoning of horses are given. Similar information is given in Chapter 19 on feeds which, in contrast to poisonous plants, are intended for horses, but which under certain circumstances may cause poisonings. These include toxins produced by molds including: fescue poisoning, moldy corn disease, and grass staggers. Poisonings due to antibiotics in feeds intended for other species, botulism, lead and blister beetles are also covered. Cottonseed and nitrate poisonings are described because they are often of concern, although they rarely if ever cause poisoning of horses.

Behavioral problems in horses along with their causes, treatment, and prevention are described in Chapter 20. These include a number of escape, oral, and flight or fight vices. Most are caused by feeding and care without consideration of the horse's psychological needs. As described in this chapter, understanding and caring for these needs will prevent or eliminate many of these vices and are as important in maintaining the horse's health, happiness, performance, and enjoyability as is maintaining the horse's physiological well-being as described in the previous chapters of this book.

It is intended and hoped that this book provide an accurate and useful compilation and transmission of the multitude of valid and useful information available on feeding and care of the horse to those providing this care.

Topeka, Kansas   LON D. LEWIS

CONTENTS

SECTION I: NUTRITION AND FEEDS FOR HORSES

Chapter 1.   Water, Energy, Protein, Carbohydrates, and Fats for Horses   3

Chapter 2.   Minerals for Horses   19

Chapter 3.   Vitamins for Horses   42

Chapter 4.   Harvested Feeds for Horses   62

Chapter 5.   Pasture for Horses   103

Chapter 6.   Diet Evaluation, Formulation, and Preparation for Horses   112

Chapter 7.   Minimizing Horse Feeding Costs   138

SECTION II: FEEDING AND CARE OF HORSES

Chapter 8.   General Horse Feeding Practices   147

Chapter 9.   General Horse Care Management Practices   155

Chapter 10.   Feeding Idle and Working Horses   186

Chapter 11.   Feeding and Care of Horses for Athletic Performance   193

Chapter 12.   Breeding Stallion Feeding and Care   224

Chapter 13.   Broodmare Feeding and Care   229

Chapter 14.   Mare and Foal Care at Foaling   242

Chapter 15.   Growing Horse Feeding and Care   264

Chapter 16.   Developmental Orthopedic Diseases in Horses   277

Chapter 17.   Feeding and Care of Horses with Health Problems   289

Chapter 18.   Plant Poisoning of Horses   300
                By: Anthony P. Knight, BVSc, MS, MRCVS, Dipl ACVIM

Chapter 19.   Feed-Related Poisonings of Horses   346

Chapter 20.   Behavioral Problems in Horses   370

GLOSSARY   380

APPENDIX TABLES:
EQUINE NUTRITIONAL REQUIREMENT TABLES

Table 1.   Dietary Energy, Protein, Calcium, and Phosphorus Recommended in Horse's Diet and
            Amount of Feed Consumed   411

Table 2.   Mineral Concentrations Recommended in Horse's Diet Compared to that in Feeds   412

Table 3.   Vitamin Concentrations Recommended in Horse's Diet Compared to that in Feeds   413

Table 4.   Daily Energy, Protein, Calcium, Phosphorus and Vitamin A Recommended for Horses   414
            Table 4–200 Daily Nutrient Requirements of Ponies (440 lb, or 200 kg, mature weight)   415
            Table 4–400 Daily Nutrient Requirements of Horses (880 lb, or 400 kg, mature weight)   415
            Table 4–500 Daily Nutrient Requirements of Horses (1100 lb, or 500 kg, mature weight)   416
            Table 4–600 Daily Nutrient Requirements of Horses (1320 lb, or 600 kg, mature weight)   416
            Table 4–700 Daily Nutrient Requirements of Horses (1540 lb, or 700 kg, mature weight)   417
            Table 4–800 Daily Nutrient Requirements of Horses (1760 lb, or 800 kg, mature weight)   417
            Table 4–900 Daily Nutrient Requirements of Horses (1980 lb, or 900 kg, mature weight)   418

Table 5.   Energy Needs for Physical Activity   418

FEED TABLES

Table 6.   Nutrient Content of Horse Feeds   419

Table 7.   Mineral Supplements Composition   422

Table 8.   Feeds — Weight/Unit Volume   423

CONVERSION TABLES

Table 9.   Conversion Factors   424

Table 10.   Symbols, Weights, and Valences of Common Elements   425

INDEX   427

Section One

NUTRITION AND FEEDS FOR HORSES

Chapter 1

WATER, ENERGY, PROTEIN, CARBOHYDRATES, AND FATS FOR HORSES

Nutrients	3	Protein	12
Water	3	Needs	13
Needs	3	Nonprotein Nitrogen (Urea) for Horses	14
Deficiency	6	Deficiency	14
Quality	7	Excess	15
Dietary Energy	8	Diet-Induced Allergy	15
Sources and Use	8	Carbohydrates	16
Needs	9	Types and Utilization	16
Deficiency	10	Dietary Fiber	17
Excess	11	Fats	18

NUTRIENTS

A nutrient is any feed constituent that is necessary for the support of life. Nutrients accomplish this in the following ways:

1. By serving as constituents of the body.
2. By enhancing or being involved in chemical reactions that occur in the body, i.e., body metabolism.
3. By serving as a source of energy.
4. By transporting substances into, throughout, or out of the body.
5. By assisting in the regulation of body temperature, for both heat production and dissipation.
6. By affecting feed palatability and, therefore, consumption.

There are six basic classes of nutrients: (1) water, (2) proteins, (3) carbohydrates, (4) fats, (5) minerals, and (6) vitamins. Some nutrients fill a number of these life-support functions. For example, water and several minerals are needed for all of the functions, except as sources of energy. Proteins, carbohydrates, and fats may all be used for energy but are also constituents of the body. In contrast, vitamins serve only one function: they are necessary for body metabolism.

The major sources, needs, and functions, and the causes and effects, and diagnoses of inadequate and excessive intake of nutrients by the horse are described in Chapters 1, 2, and 3; for those described in this chapter (water, protein, fiber, fats or fatty acids, and nutrients used for energy), they are summarized in Table 1–1.

Nutrients are, of course, present in feeds, which should be thought of simply as nutrient packages—packages that vary in their appearance and palatability, as well as in the quantity of different nutrients they contain, but little in which nutrients they contain. Except for vitamin and mineral supplements, which may contain only certain specific vitamins or minerals, and oils, which contain only fats, all other feeds contain nearly the entire spectrum of different nutrients. Feeds differ therefore not in which nutrients they contain but in the amount of each nutrient they contain. For example, soybean meal, corn, and hay each con-

tain all the nutrients, but soybean meal contains much more protein and less carbohydrate than corn and hay, and hay contains much more fiber than soybean meal and corn. These, as well as other differences in various feeds for the horse, are described in Chapters 4 and 5.

Regardless of the feed, in order for its nutrients to be utilized, they must be released from the feed that has been ingested, broken down sufficiently by digestion, and absorbed into the body by the digestive tract, as shown in Figure 1–1.

WATER

An adequate supply of good-quality, palatable water is essential for horses. Always ensure that adequate, good-quality, palatable water is readily available for all horses at all times. The only exception is that after exercise, the horse should be cooled down before being allowed to drink as much as it wants. Consumption of excess cold water by a horse that is hot from physical exertion may cause colic or founder. However, just before and during prolonged physical activity, the horse should be allowed to drink as often as practical and as much as it wants.

Water Needs

Voluntary water intake by the horse at rest in a moderate or cool environment, eating dry forage, varies from 0.3 to 0.8 gal/100 lbs body weight/day (25 to 70 ml/kg/day). The amount actually required is near the lower end of this range. At rest water requirement in quarts or liters/day is approximately equal to digestible energy requirement in megacalories/day, which for the horse is given in Appendix Tables 4 and 5.

The amount of water needed varies primarily with the amount of water lost from the body, which is altered by the amount, type, and quality of the feed consumed, the ambient temperature and humidity, and the health, physiological state, and physical activity of the horse. The horse, like all animals, consumes more water than needed if palatable water is readily available. The amount of water consumed, however, will decrease to just meet needs if water is poorly accessible or poorly palatable. The amount of

TABLE 1–1
Water, Energy, Protein, Fiber and Fat: Causes and Effects of Deficiencies and Excesses

Nutrient Imbalance	Causes	Effects
Water deficiency	Unavailable or unpalatable water, or ↓ thirst due to excess loss of salts in sweat	↓ Performance ↓ Feed intake Dehydration
Energy excess	Food intake > needs due to high palatability and/or little exercise	Hyperactivity ("high") and/or excess body fat
Energy deficiency	Inadequate feed: 1) available, 2) caloric density, or 3) eating or utilization ability	Weight loss and/or ↓ growth, performance, or lactation
Protein excess	Diet protein > needs (See App. Ts. 1 and 4)	↑ urine volume and heat production
Protein deficiency	Protein < needs (see App. Ts. 1 & 4). Low protein digestibility or inadequate feed intake	Same as energy deficiency. Rough hair coat and may eat feces
Fiber excess	Diet crude fiber >34–40%, depending on energy needs	"Hay belly" and same as energy deficiency
Fiber deficiency/nonfiber carbohydrate excess	Sudden grain excess or grain >50 to 90% of diet	Diarrhea, colic, and founder
Fat deficiency	Not known to occur in horses	In others, dry, dull hair, scaly skin, hair loss and ↓ reproduction
Fat excess	Adding >20% oil to diet or >30% oil to grain mix	↓ palatability, loose, fatty appearing stools. Long-term it results in excess energy

App. = Appendix; T. = Table; ↑ = increase; ↓ = decrease; > = greater than; < = less than.

water drunk, but not consumed, also decreases with increasing moisture content of the feed. Feed containing 40% or more moisture supplies enough water to meet the idle horse's needs in a moderate environment. Although hay, grain, and nongrowing forage contain less than 15% moisture, growing forage contains from at least 60% to over 80% moisture. Thus, the horse consuming growing forage does not need to drink any water, although most will if it's available and palatable. (Figure 1–2).

The amount of water drunk directly correlates with the amount of feed dry matter consumed. Although horses generally drink 1.5 to 2 quarts of water per lb. (3 to 4 L/kg) of hay or grain only about 1 quart/lb (2 L/kg) are normally needed. Donkeys generally drink 1.2 to 2.6 and Shetland Ponies 2.2 to 2.5 L/kg, which may reflect at least the donkey's desert origin. Water intake decreases with increasing diet digestibility, because increasing diet digestibility decreases the amount of feces and, therefore, the amount of fecal water excreted. Diet digestibility increases, and therefore the amount of water per unit of feed dry matter consumed decreases, with increasing forage digestibility and as the amount of grain in the diet increases.

Water needs and intake also increase with increasing protein and salt intake. Increased protein intake increases nitrogenous waste products excreted in the urine, and this, like increased salt intake, increases urine volume.

Lactating mares have increased water needs to compensate for increased water loss in the milk. Lactation may increase water needs, and also dietary energy needs 1.5 to 1.8 times that required for maintenance. There is also increased water needs during growth and the last trimester of pregnancy. Although a small amount of increased water need for growth is caused by increasing body size and, in pregnancy, placental fluids and the fetus, most of the increased water need during growth, pregnancy, and lactation is due to increased feed intake.

One of the major factors affecting how much water the healthy horse needs is how much water the horse loses through sweat and expired air in order to prevent the body's overheating from physical activity or the environment. The amount of water needed may increase as much as 3 to 4 times with work at high ambient temperatures. Moderate work alone may increase water needs 1.6 to 1.8 times and hard work 2.2 times that needed at rest. At an

Fig. 1–1. Gastrointestinal tract (GIT) of the horse. The stomach of the 1100 lb. (500 kg.) horse holds 2 to 4 gallons (7.5 to 15 liters). Some protein digestion and partial breakdown of the feed occur in the stomach. Liquids pass from the stomach rapidly with 75% gone within 30 minutes after ingestion. Of the feed dry matter ingested, only 25% is gone from the stomach by 30 minutes, and more than 98% by 12 hrs following its ingestion. Although solid particles are partially broken down in the stomach by the acid, and protein by pepsin which it secretes, little digestion occurs in the stomach. In addition, in contrast to most animals, the horse cannot vomit or regurgitate material from the stomach. Most of the feed dry matter ingested passes as particulate matter to the small intestine. The small intestine is 50 to 70 ft (15 to 22 m) long, 3 to 4 inches (7 to 10 cm) in diameter, and holds 10 to 12 gal (40 to 50 L). Much of the fat and protein, and about 50 to 70% of the soluble carbohydrate or nitrogen free extract are digested in the small intestine. These and most of the vitamins and minerals are absorbed from the small intestine. Liquids pass through the small intestine rapidly, and reach the cecum 2 to 8 hours after ingestion. In another 5 hours, most of the liquid that reaches the cecum passes on into the colon. Passage of both liquids and particulate matter through the colon is slow and occurs over a period of about 36 to 48 hours. Nearly all of the crude fiber or cellulose and much (over 50%) of the soluble carbohydrate in feeds passes through the small intestine into the cecum. The cecum is 3 to 4 ft. (0.9 to 1.2 m) long and holds 7 to 8 gal (25 to 30 L). It, like the ascending colon, contains bacteria that digest much of the fiber and about one-half of the soluble carbohydrate (NFE) ingested. After digestion, these nutrients are absorbed from the cecum and colon. Some bacterial protein is also produced, digested and absorbed from the cecum

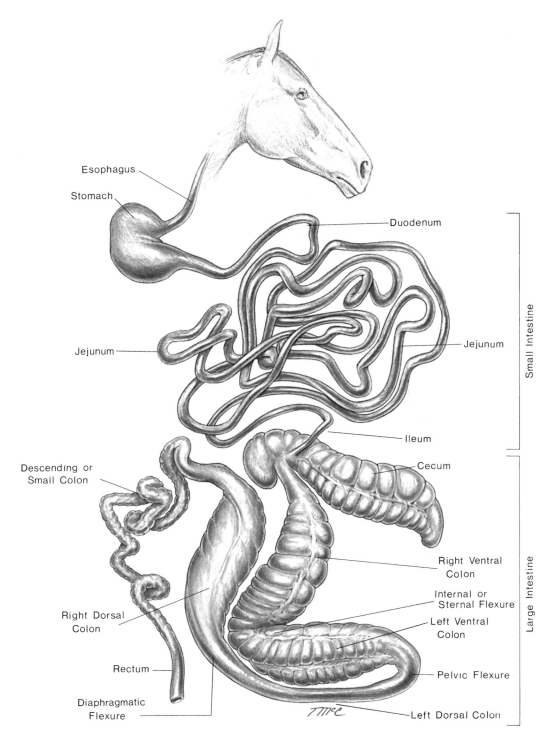

Fig. 1-1 *(Continued)* and colon. The large, or ascending, colon is 10 to 12 ft (3 to 3.7 m) long with an average diameter of 8 to 10 inches (20 to 25 cm) and holds 14 to 16 gal (50 to 60 L). It consists of four portions: (1) the right ventral colon, (2) the sternal flexure to the left ventral colon, (3) the pelvic flexure (where obstruction most commonly occurs) to the left dorsal colon, and (4) the diaphragmatic flexure to the right dorsal colon, which connects to the small colon. The small colon is about 10 ft (3 m) long, 3 to 4 in (7.5 to 10 cm) in diameter, and holds about 5 gal (18 to 19 L). When it enters the pelvic inlet, it is called the rectum, which is about 1 ft (0.3 m) long and opens to the exterior at the anus. The large colon, small colon, and rectum make up the large intestine. The empty GIT constitutes 4.2 to 5.2%, the liver 1.1 to 1.4%, and the pancreas 0.9 to 1.0% of the mature horse's body weight. All decrease with exercise, probably because of blood shunted away from them. All increase when grain is fed, particularly the small intestine. The GIT is smaller and the liver larger in foals, with each constituting 3.5% of body weight at birth and being the same as the adult's at six months of age. The foal's GIT is smaller because of an undeveloped large intestine. Intestinal tract length increases rapidly in the fetus, and foal, from mid-gestation to 1 yr of age, and changes little thereafter. Small intestine length increases rapidly during the first month of life, while large intestine length increases most when forage consumption increases.

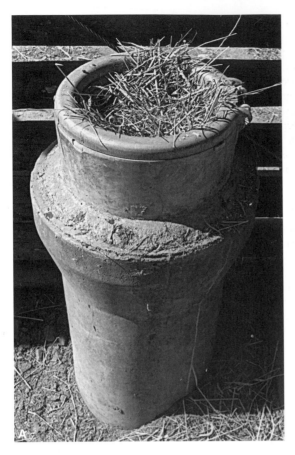

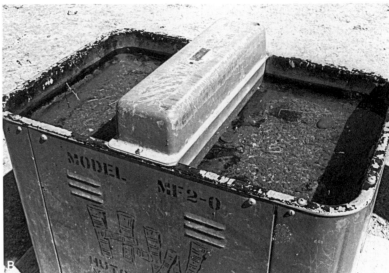

Fig. 1–2(A,B). Waterers that automatically fill when their water level is lowered. They may have a thermostatically controlled heater to prevent the water from freezing during cold weather. Although many automatic waterers' basins hold only 1 to 2 gal (4 to 8 L), they refill rapidly. If horses always have an automatic waterer readily available, one is generally enough for a number of horses, even during hot weather, because regardless of water needs, horses drink a relatively small amount at one time. With increased water needs, horses drink more frequently, not longer nor with more than generally 1 or 2 drinks each drinking bout. This may not be the case, however, if the horses have access to water for only specific short periods of time. Feed and other debris should be removed from water containers daily, and they should be thoroughly cleaned frequently. They should be placed away from the feed-bunk to minimize their contamination with feed (A). A double waterer (B) may be placed between two stalls or two paddocks.

ambient temperature of 0°F (− 18°C), horses consume 1 qt water/lb (2 L/kg) dry feed eaten, whereas at 100°F (38°C) they will consume four times this amount. An increase in temperature from only 55°F (13°C) to 70°F (21°C) increases the horse's water requirements by 15 to 20%.

When water is readily available, increased water consumption occurs as a result of increased drinking frequency, not increased drinking duration or the number of drinks taken during a drinking bout. For example, there is a direct correlation between drinking frequency and ambient temperature, with a large increase in frequency at temperatures above 85°F (30°C). When water is readily available, most horses drink once for only about 30 seconds or less every few hours. However, if water is not readily available such as if there is a long distance between preferred grazing areas and water, more and longer drinks may be taken during a drinking bout.

Water Deficiency

Inadequate water intake is quite detrimental. With the exception of inspired oxygen, a deficiency of water produces death more rapidly than a deficiency of any other substance. The first noticeable effect of inadequate water intake is decreased dry feed intake, followed by decreased physical activity and ability. Inadequate water intake is also believed to increase the risk of intestinal impactions and

colic. Water deprivation for 24, 48, and 72 hours decreased the normal resting horse's body weight 4%, 6.8%, and 9%, respectively, when the ambient temperature was 63–81°F (17–27°C). At an ambient daytime maximum temperature of 104°F (40°C), body weight decreased 11 to 13% after 60 hours, and 14 to 16% after 72 hours of water deprivation. Signs of dehydration, such as dry membranes and mouth and sunken eyes, are not evident until at least a 6% loss of body weight has occurred. Less than one-half this amount of dehydration is likely to decrease physical performance. Thus, the horse's physical performance ability is decreased long before a water deficiency induced dehydration can be detected from the horse's appearance.

Inadequate water intake occurs when water is poorly palatable or accessible. Palatability is best determined by tasting the water and, if there has been a change in the water or its source, comparing its taste to that to which the horse is accustomed. Poor palatability may be due to poor water quality. Water may be poorly accessible for many reasons, such as if electric heaters with wiring problems cause the animal to be shocked when attempting to drink, or if water is frozen over. Ambient temperature-induced variations in water temperature may not alter water intake. Although this situation has not been studied for horses, cattle drink similar amounts of cold or warm water, although individual cattle or horses may have a preference. Cattle, and therefore possibly horses, will consume sufficient snow or crushed ice to meet their water needs if snow or ice is available but water isn't. However, in doing so, the total amount of water and feed consumed will be reduced.

Water Quality

The single most reliable indication of water quality is the amount of total dissolved solids (TDS) in the water. The amount of TDS, as given in Table 1-2, provides a useful overall indication of the suitability of a particular water source for livestock use. Water high in TDS may be undesirable or unfit for consumption. This occurrence is most prevalent in arid areas, such as the western non-coastal part of the United States. A TDS of 6,500 ppm (parts per million or mg/L) is considered the upper safe limit in water for horses.

The amount of TDS is the sum of the concentrations of all substances dissolved in water. The term "salinity" as applied to fresh water is often used synonymously with TDS. Another term used to described water quality is total alkalinity, but this is not as good an indication of water quality as is TDS. Total alkalinity is the sum of the concentrations of alkali metals, which are primarily sodium and potassium, but may also include lithium, rubidium, cesium, and francium. The hydroxides of these metals are alkaline; i.e., in water they neutralize acids. The total alkalinity of water is always less than its TDS, or salinity, since TDS and salinity include the sum of the concentrations of all substances dissolved in water, and total alkalinity includes only the sum of the concentrations of alkali metals. Salinity and TDS should not be confused with hardness. Highly saline waters may contain low levels of the minerals responsible for hardness. Water "hardness" indicates the tendency of water to precipitate soap or to form a scale on heated surfaces. Hardness is generally expressed as the

sum of calcium and magnesium reported in equivalent amounts of calcium carbonate. Other substances, such as strontium, iron, zinc, and manganese, also contribute to hardness.

Sodium, potassium, calcium, magnesium, iron, chloride, and sulfate in water are not toxic, but high concentrations decrease water palatability. In contrast, a number of other substances, which may be present in water, are quite toxic if sufficiently high concentrations are present. Toxic concentrations of water contaminants, excluding pesticides and herbicides, most commonly occur as a result of stagnant or runoff water that contains disease-producing organisms, or from industrial wastes. A list of the recommended upper limits for some potentially toxic substances in drinking water for horses, and those not toxic but which, if present at concentrations above those given, reduce water palatability, is given in Table 1-3. Some potentially toxic substances do not reduce water palatability and, therefore, water intake. Thus, they are potentially even more harmful than those that do decrease palatability. In addition to these contaminants, drinking water containing some bacteria and algae may be harmful.

Some species of blue-green algae, which grow on pond and lake water, may result in poisoning; therefore, water with heavy algae growth should be avoided. Heavy algae growth occurs most commonly during summer and fall in shallow, still water rich in organic nutrients. These nutrients may be increased, and thus algae growth promoted, by runoff of nitrogen or phosphate from slurry lagoons, or of fertilizers applied to fields. Steady prevailing winds may concentrate the algae at one end of the pond or lake, increasing the risk of poisoning. The algae may be visible on the water surface or mixed with the water.

Blue-green algae poisoning in domestic livestock may cause sudden death or else photosensitization, tremors, weakness, bloody diarrhea, and convulsions. Clumps of algae may be found in the gastrointestinal contents of animals that die suddenly. Copper sulfate added to pond water up to a concentration of 1 ppm (1 mg/L) has been used successfully to kill algae blooms, but will probably be harmful to other types of aquatic life.

Water high in bacteria is usually also high in nitrates as a result of surface contamination from manure and barnyard runoff. However, high nitrate water levels may come from other nitrate sources, such as crop fertilizers, and not be high in bacteria. Nitrates may build up in well water by leaching down through the soil. Water nitrate levels may fluctuate widely; they are generally highest following wet periods, and lowest during dry periods of the year. Since nitrates dissolve in water, they cannot be filtered out; however, commercially available anion exchange units remove both nitrates and sulfates. Nitrate toxicosis, however, as described in Chapter 19, is rare in horses, if it occurs at all, and in livestock is most often associated with high nitrate levels in forage, not water. Water sulfate concentrations exceeding 1000 ppm may cause diarrhea, although animals develop a tolerance to a constantly high level of sulfates and can tolerate two to three times this concentration after a period of time. Water with low levels of sulfates, however, may have an odor and reduced palatability.

In most areas and situations, bacteria in water pose a

TABLE 1-2
A Guide to the Suitability of Water for Livestock

TDS (ppm)[a]	Suitability and Effect
1000–3000	Satisfactory for all livestock and poultry. May cause mild and temporary diarrhea in livestock not accustomed to it, but should not affect their health or performance.
3000–5000	Should be satisfactory for livestock, although it might cause temporary diarrhea, or be refused at first by animals not accustomed to it.
5000–7000	Can be used with reasonable safety for livestock. May be advisable to avoid water approaching the higher level of ppm for pregnant or lactating animals.
7000–10,000	Unfit for poultry and swine. Considerable risk may exist in using this water for pregnant, lactating, or young animals, or for any animals subjected to heavy heat stress or water loss. In general, the use of this water should be avoided, although animals other than those listed here may subsist on it for long periods.
Over 10,000	Not recommended for use by any animal under any condition

[a] Total dissolved solids, total soluble salts, or salinity in the water in ppm or mg/L

TABLE 1–3
Recommended Upper Safe Level (USL)
of Water Contaminants

Contaminate	USL[a]
Arsenic	0.2
Cadmium	0.05
Calcium	500[b]
Chloride	3000[b]
Chromium	1
Cobalt	1
Copper	0.5[b]
Cyanide	0.01
Fluoride	2[c]
Hardness	200
Hydrogen Sulfide	0.1
Iron	0.3[b]
Lead	0.1
Magnesium	125[b]
Manganese	0.05
Mercury	0.01
Nickel	1.0
Nitrate (see Ch. 19)	400 ± 10[d]
Nitrate nitrogen	100
Nitrite nitrogen	10
Potassium	1400[b]
Selenium	0.01[e]
Silver	0.05
Sodium	2500[b]
Sulfate	2500[f]
TDS (see Table 1–2)	6500
Vanadium	0.1
Zinc	25[g]

[a] All values given are in parts of contaminate per million parts of water (ppm or mg/L). For conversion to other units, see Appendix Table 9.
[b] These contaminates are not toxic but at concentrations above the amount given may decrease water palatability. In contrast, many of the other contaminates listed may be toxic if water containing concentrations above those given here is the only water consumed.
[c] A higher concentration may be safe for horses, as 2.5 ppm results in mottled enamel during teeth development in calves but no observable effects occur in mature cattle at concentrations of less than 8 ppm, and horses are reported to tolerate fluoride intakes two to three times greater than cattle. A concentration of 4 ppm is probably marginally safe for horses, but water with more than 8 ppm should be avoided.
[d] High nitrate concentrations in water occur most commonly as a result of fecal contamination.
[e] Although chronic selenium toxicosis has been reported as a result of consumption of water containing 0.0005 to 0.002 ppm selenium, concentrations below 0.01 ppm are not generally considered harmful.
[f] Or 833 ppm sulfur. Although sulfate concentrations above 300 to 400 ppm can be tasted, and above 750 ppm can have a laxative effect in people, a concentration below 2500 ppm has no effect on growing or reproducing cattle or swine.[55] The highest no-effect concentration in horses isn't known but is probably similar to that for cattle and swine.
[g] High zinc concentrations may occur where galvanized pipes are connected to copper. This results in electrolysis, releasing zinc from the galvanized pipes into the water.

greater threat than the contaminants previously discussed and listed in Table 1–3. Most infectious diseases can be transmitted from contaminated water to animals. If water nitrate or phosphate concentrations are low, the water probably does not contain excessive bacteria. However, if either is high, bacterial levels may be elevated and should be checked. The accepted criterium for the sanitary quality of water is the absence of coliform bacteria. Although all coliform bacteria are not disease producing, many are, and their presence indicates that other infectious bacteria and viruses may be in the water. The U.S. Public Health Service considers water containing coliform bacteria (M.P.N.) of 9 or more coliforms per 100 ml unsafe for human consumption. In some countries, levels of 50 coliforms/100 ml are acceptable. What amount is safe for horses isn't known but, of course, also depends on which organisms are present.

Salmonella species is generally the bacterial contaminant in water most likely to cause disease in farm animals. Giardia is the most common cause of water-related illness in people, partly because it survives chlorination. Although giardiasis is rare in farm animals, it can cause diarrhea in young animals. The most common method of destroying bacteria in a water supply is chlorination, although iodine, ozone, exposure to ultraviolet rays or ultrasonics, or filters may be used. Objectionable chlorine taste and odor can be removed from water by an activated carbon filter.

In summary, flowing surface water is most likely to have bacterial contamination, pond or lake water is most likely to contain blue-green algae, and well water, particularly in arid areas, is most likely to have high mineral concentrations. Coliform counts and measures of total dissolved solids are the main indications of water quality.

DIETARY ENERGY

Energy Sources and Use

As described by the first law of thermodynamics, energy can be changed from one form to another but can be neither created nor destroyed. The source of all energy for all living things is sunlight. This energy is captured by plants, which use it via photosynthesis to change carbon dioxide, present in the air, and water to oxygen and the carbon compounds that make up the plant. These carbon, or organic, compounds in plants are carbohydrates, fats, and, along with nitrogen, protein. Nitrogen, like the small amount of minerals needed by plants, is taken up from the soil but is originally from the air. Carbohydrates, fats, and proteins are stored sources of energy.

Animals eat plants, or tissues of others that have eaten plants. The stored sources of energy, carbohydrates, fats, and proteins in the plants are digested, absorbed, and transported to the animal's body cells. Some are used to make up the structural components of the cell and thus the animal; but, if needed in the future, along with oxygen from the air, they can be converted by chemical reaction to carbon dioxide and water, in the process producing energy. Animals use the energy to produce heat and adenosine triphosphate, or ATP, which cells then use to function. Thus, plants and animals have a mutually sustaining relationship in which plants produce carbon compounds (C-cpds)—organic matter and oxygen (O_2)—that support animals, and animals produce the carbon dioxide (CO_2) and water (H_2O) that support plants. Thus, the horse, like us, plants, and all living things on earth, are products of the air and the soil, and function solely as the result of solar energy.

Energy has no measurable dimension or mass, but it can be converted to heat, which can be measured. Oxidation, or burning, converts stored energy (carbohydrates, fats,

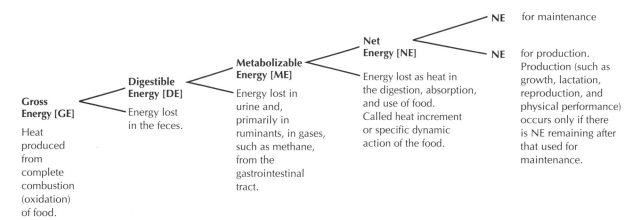

Fig. 1–3. Dietary Energy Partition.

and proteins) to heat, carbon dioxide, water, and a nitrogen compound. These are returned to the air and soil, where they originated, available to begin the cycle again. When a substance is completely oxidized, the heat produced, called the heat of combustion, is the total or gross amount of energy stored in, and thus available from, that substance. However, as shown in Figure 1-3, the animal cannot use all of the gross energy present in a feed. Some of the stored energy in a feed is not digested and is lost in the feces. Of the remainder, called digestible energy, some is lost in the urine as urea and in the gastrointestinal tract as gases (primarily methane), leaving metabolizable energy, of which some is used in metabolizing feed. What remains is the net energy available for maintenance, growth or fattening, milk production, and physical activity. Most of the total dietary energy needs are for maintenance. Even during heavy lactation or physical activity over 50% of dietary energy is needed for maintenance, and for young horses, 60 to 95% of dietary energy needs are for maintenance, leaving 5 to 40% for their growth.

The amount of heat produced by oxidation (burning) that raises the temperature of one gram of water 1°C is defined as one calorie. This is also known as the small, gram, or standard calorie. However, it is not used in nutrition for animals or people. The calorie used in nutrition is the amount of heat required to raise one kilogram of water 1°C. It is called the large calorie, Calorie, or kilocalorie (kcal) since it is equal to 1000 small calories. In nutrition, the word calorie always refers to kilocalorie, even if it is not capitalized and neither the kilo- or k- prefix is used. For large animals, such as horses, megacalorie (Mcal), therm, or total digestible nutrients (TDN) are usually used. One megacalorie equals one therm, and both equal 1000 kilocalories. Occasionally, primarily in England, instead of calorie, the joule, or, in the physical sciences, the British Thermal Unit (BTU) is used. One megacalorie equals 4.1855 megajoules and 3968 BTU. TDN is a measure of digestible energy expressed in units of weight or percent, with 1 lb TDN equal to about 2.0 Mcal DE (1 kg TDN = 4.4 Mcal). TDN is the sum of digestible carbohydrates, plus digestible protein, plus digestible fats times 2.25, because

fats provide about 2.25 times more energy than an equal weight of carbohydrates or proteins. Starch equivalent, or SE, is occasionally used as an energy term by comparing the energy provided by a feed to that provided by starch, which is assigned a value of 100%. Although occasionally used for ruminants, SE is unsuitable for horses because of their different digestive process.

When calculating energy intake, or the amount of feed needed to provide a certain amount of energy, such as that necessary to meet the animal's energy requirements, any of the various energy terms may be used. Of course, the same units must be used for both the energy content of the feed and the animal's energy needs. Net energy is the most accurate, followed by metabolizable energy (Fig. 1-3). However, they are the most difficult to determine and, as a result, are not routinely available for most horse feeds. Digestible energy values (or TDN) are generally available for most horse feeds and therefore are the most commonly used energy terms. Energy available from forages is usually 5 to 15% higher for cattle than for horses because of ruminants' more efficient utilization of fiber. Therefore, if the energy content of forages for cattle, or other ruminants, is used to determine the amount of these feeds needed by horses, the amount determined generally will be erroneously low.

Energy Needs

Numerous factors can influence the energy requirements of the horse. These include environmental conditions, the horse's functions and activity (including intensity and duration of work, weight and ability of the rider, and conditions of the traveling surface), and its physical condition and degree of fatigue. Even when all of these factors are identical, individual horses vary in their energy needs. The average amount of energy needed, as given in Appendix Tables 1, 4, and 5, should therefore be considered only a general guideline—an amount that will be relatively close for a group of horses but either inadequate or excessive for some individuals.

The amount of digestible energy (DE) needed for maintenance (i.e., for no weight change by the mature, idle nonreproducing horse at moderate environmental conditions) by the average horse weighing 1320 lbs (600 kg) or less can be calculated from the following equation.

$$\text{Mcal DE/day} = 1.4 + 0.03 \times (\text{kg body wt or lbs} \div 2.2)$$

However, energy needs are lower per unit of body size in horses weighing over 1320 lbs (600 kg) and can be calculated from the following equation.

$$\text{Mcal DE/day} = 1.82 + (0.0383 \times \text{kg body wt or lbs} \div 2.2)$$
$$- [0.000015 \times (\text{kg body wt or lbs} \div 2.2)^2]$$

Estimates of energy requirements for physical activity or work depend primarily on the total weight carried (horse, intestinal fill, rider, and tack) times the distance moved, but increase with decreasing ability of the rider and physical condition of the horse, difficulty of the terrain and surface covered, and other factors. For ponies and light horses, the Mcal DE/day for light, medium, and intense work has been estimated to be respectively 1.25, 1.50, and 2.0 times that needed for maintenance (Appendix Table 4); with light work being activities such as Western and English pleasure, bridle path, hack, and equitation; medium work being ranch work, roping, cutting, barrel racing, and jumping; and intense work being race training, endurance racing, and polo. Digestible energy needs greater than those required at rest have also been estimated in Mcal/hr/100 kg (220 lbs) total weight carried to be 0.17 for a slow walk; 0.25 for a fast walk; 0.6 for a slow trot; 1.0 for a medium trot or slow lope; 1.3 for a fast trot; 2.0 for cantering, galloping or jumping; and 3.9 for a fast gallop (Appendix Table 5).

For draft horses, energy needs depend on factors such as the size of the load pulled and the type of work. Increasing maintenance energy needs by 10%/hr of field work is a reasonable estimate.

For pregnant mares, energy needs do not increase greatly until the last 3 months of gestation, which is when the greatest development of the fetus occurs. Energy requirements for the ninth, tenth, and eleventh months of pregnancy average, respectively, 1.11, 1.13, and 1.20 times that needed for maintenance (Appendix Table 4). During the first 3 months of lactation, energy needs average 1.8 times, and from 3 months until weaning, averages 1.5 times that needed for maintenance (Appendix Table 4). For young horses, energy needs increase with increasing growth rate and size, but per unit of body weight decreases as the horse gets older and bigger, and growth rate slows (Appendix Table 4).

Guidelines on the amount of feed needed to meet the horse's energy requirements are given in the feeding programs described throughout this book. How to calculate the amount of energy and feed needed by the horse is described in Chapter 6.

Energy Deficiency

After an animal's initial adjustment to the palatability of the feeds in its diet, the average amount consumed by the healthy animal will be an amount adequate to meet its energy needs if the feed is available and its gastrointestinal tract will hold that amount. The maximum daily amount of air dry feed that a horse can consume is equal to 3 to 3.5% of its body weight. If this amount of feed does not meet the horse's energy needs, the energy concentration of the diet must be increased. For the horse, this is accomplished by feeding more grain, adding fat to the diet or feeding a more digestible, better-quality forage.

There are four reasons the horse may not consume enough dietary energy to meet its needs: (1) a sufficient amount of feed is not available, (2) its gastrointestinal tract won't hold enough of the available feed because the digestible energy density of the feed is too low, (3) it can't consume enough because of a physical problem (e.g., injury or bad teeth), or (4) it doesn't want to consume enough because of illness, stress, inadequate water intake, or poorly palatable feed. Regardless of the reason for inadequate feed intake, the first and most noticeable effect is lassitude. This is because horses need 80 to 90% of all the feed ingested for energy, 8 to 14.5% for protein, 2 to 3% for minerals, and less than 1% for vitamins. With inadequate feed intake, the greatest deficit will be dietary energy, followed by protein. Unless there is a disease-related increase in the loss of minerals or vitamins, signs and effects of deficiencies of these nutrients, during periods of inadequate feed intake, occur much later, to a lesser degree, and are masked by signs of energy and protein deficiency.

Inadequate feed and, therefore energy, intake causes hormonal changes that decrease the body's energy utilization by reducing physical activity, milk production, and growth rate. The hormonal changes increase utilization of the body's stored and structural sources of energy (carbohydrates, fats, and proteins) resulting in weight loss. The utilization, or deposition, of excess body fat and protein alter the horse's appearance, as described in Table 1–4.

The horse's small stores of carbohydrates are depleted within the first few days of total food deprivation. Within 1 week, the body adapts by increasing body fat utilization, thus conserving body protein. Because the principal function of body fat is as a storage source of energy, its loss during starvation does not impair critical body functions. For this reason, loss of body fat does not seriously threaten survival, unless peripheral body fat stores are mobilized very rapidly, resulting in hyperlipidemia, i.e., excessive lipids in the blood. This generally occurs in ponies, particularly if they are obese, and in ponies and horses when there is both a decrease in feed intake and an increase in stress, such as transit, systemic illness, pregnancy, or lactation. Depression, weakness, decreased food intake, incoordination, recumbency, and death may occur. In most cases of inadequate feed intake, however, hyperlipemia doesn't occur sufficiently to cause these effects.

Once body fat stores near depletion, utilization of the body's only remaining source of energy, protein, accelerates. Body protein use is not random. Proteins providing structural support in the form of bones, ligaments, tendons, and cartilage are used after those in the blood, intestines, and muscle. During feed deprivation, a loss of function occurs earlier in the tissues and organs whose protein is used first. The order of occurrence of decreased organ function either as a result of feed and, therefore, energy

TABLE 1–4
Horse's Appearance Associated with Dietary
Energy Intake[a]

Body Score	Description
1 Poor	Animal extremely emaciated; spinous processes, ribs, tailhead, tuber coxae, and ischii project prominently; bone structure of withers, shoulders, and neck easily noticeable; no fatty tissue can be felt.
2 Very thin	Animal emaciated; slight fat covers base of spinous processes; transverse processes of lumbar vertebrae feel rounded; spinous processes, ribs, tailhead, tuber coxae, and ischii prominent; withers, shoulders, and neck structure faintly discernible.
3 Thin	Fat buildup about halfway on spinous processes; transverse processes cannot be felt; slight fat cover over ribs; spinous processes and ribs easily discernible, tailhead prominent, but individual vertebrae cannot be identified visually; tuber coxae appear rounded but easily discernible; tuber ischii not distinguishable; withers, shoulders, and neck not obviously thin.
4 Moderately thin	Slight ridge along back; faint outline of ribs discernible; tailhead prominence depends on conformation, but fat can be felt around it; tuber coxae not discernible; withers, shoulders, and neck not obviously thin.
5 Moderate	Back is flat (no crease or ridge); ribs not visually distinguishable but easily felt; fat around tailhead beginning to feel spongy; withers appear rounded over spinous processes; shoulders and neck blend smoothly into body.
6 Moderately fleshy	May have slight crease down back; fat over ribs spongy, fat around tailhead soft; fat beginning to be deposited along the side of withers, behind shoulders, and along the sides of neck.
7 Fleshy	May have crease down back; individual ribs can be felt, but there is noticeable filling between ribs with fat; fat around tailhead soft; fat deposited along withers, behind shoulders, and along neck.
8 Fat	Crease down back; difficult to feel ribs; fat around tailhead very soft; area along withers filled with fat; area behind shoulders filled with fat; noticeable thickening of neck; fat deposited along inner thighs.
9 Extremely fat	Obvious crease down back; patchy fat appearing over ribs; bulging fat around tailhead, along withers, behind shoulders, and along neck; fat along inner thighs may rub together; flank filled with fat.

[a] A body condition score of 5 indicates the proper amount of dietary energy intake, 3 or less inadequate energy intake, and 7 or greater indicates excess energy intake.
(From Ott EA, Chairman, Subcommittee on Horse Nutrition: Nutrient Requirements of Horses. 5th ed. National Academy Press, Washington, DC (1989).)

deprivation or as a result of protein deprivation is as follows.

1. Liver and plasma proteins decrease. If sufficiently severe, the decrease allows fluid to leave the plasma, resulting in edema and stocking.
2. Gastrointestinal tract degeneration. With prolonged feed deprivation, intestinal mass, absorptive surface area, and enzyme activity decrease, which impairs nutrient digestion and absorption.
3. Diminished defense against infectious organisms making the individual more susceptible to the occurrence and severity of infectious disease.
4. Impaired respiratory and cardiac function.

5. Skeletal muscle degeneration, which decreases muscle mass and strength. This change occurs more slowly than the changes previously described.

By the time muscle wasting or weakness is evident, feed-deprivation-induced alterations of other body functions are well underway. To prevent and correct these alterations, the causes for inadequate feed intake should be corrected, if possible, and adequate dietary calories and protein given to meet the horse's needs and correct the deficits present.

The thin, weak horse should be fed a good quality forage and up to an equal weight of grain, or, instead of forage and grain separately, a complete feed containing both. Water and salt should be easily available at all times or several ounces (60 to 120 g) of salt may be added to the grain to encourage water intake to decrease the risk of feed impaction. The amount of feed fed weak, thin horses (with a body condition score of 3 or less, as described in Table 1–4) should be increased gradually to prevent diarrhea, colic, feed impactions, other gastrointestinal disturbances, or founder. Begin by feeding one-third of the amount the idle mature horse would need if it were at its optimum (not current) body weight. This would be about 0.5 lb of total feed per 100 lbs of optimum body weight per day (0.5 kg/100 kg day). Divide the amount fed into at least four feedings daily. If a problem occurs, feed smaller amounts more frequently. If no problem occurs, gradually increase the amount fed over the following 1 to 2 weeks, up to twice that needed for maintenance. This is about 3 lbs of total feed per 100 lbs body weight per day (3 kg/100 kg/day). At this time, or initially for horses that are only moderately thin (Table 1–4), the forage or complete feed may be available at all times for the horse to eat as much as it likes. When this is done, unless there is some reason the horse will not or cannot eat normally, it will consume daily an amount close to 3% of its body weight and gain about 2 lbs (0.9 kg) per day. If the thin, malnourished horse does not eat and gain these amounts, it should be thoroughly examined, the reason determined, and this reason corrected. Is the horse unable to eat normally because of a physical problem or pain, or is it unwilling because it is sick? See also Chapter 17.

Energy Excess

Just as the first and major effect of inadequate feed intake is inadequate energy, the only clinically significant effect of *excess* feed intake is a surplus of dietary energy. If the feed excess is large and occurs at a single feeding—such as the horse suddenly having access to a large amount of a palatable, high-energy dense feed, such as a cereal grain—it may result in diarrhea, colic, or acute laminitis. However, if excess energy intake occurs over a more prolonged period, most of the surplus is stored in the body as fat. Some of the excess energy is given off as heat and used for increased physical activity. Increased body-heat production is used by many species of animals, including people, to compensate for excess dietary energy intake. The horse is unique in that it also compensates by increasing its physical activity. As a result, the horse that receives excess dietary energy is more apt to be excessively high spirited and buck, shy, and run away. Conversely, one way to calm a horse is to reduce its dietary energy intake. In addition to increased body fat deposition, heat production, and physical activity, excess dietary energy intake by the growing horse increases its growth rate and is thought to be a factor contributing to the occurrence of developmental orthopedic diseases, as described in Chapter 16.

The horse, like people and other animals, will eat the amount of feed needed to meet its energy needs if it is physically capable of doing so and the feed is available. But, if the feed is sufficiently palatable and high in energy density, some horses, like some individuals of nearly all species, will eat more than is needed. Although the excess over time averages only slightly above what is needed, if it continues, it will result in obesity and the appearance described in Table 1-4 for a horse with a high body score.

Being overweight, like being underweight, is detrimental to health and performance ability. One of the first noticeable effects of excess body fat in the horse is decreased physical performance ability and increased sweating with physical activity. Sweating is due primarily to a decreased ability to cool the body because excess fat provides increased insulation. Twenty minutes of trotting by a horse that cannot cool itself properly produces sufficient heat to cause hyperthermia-induced fatigue and even death, as discussed in Chapter 11. Respiratory difficulties probably also contribute to decreased physical activity and performance in the overweight horse. Obesity increases respiratory difficulties because excess body mass increases oxygen needs, but decreases oxygen intake ability. The additional mass against the chest wall increases respiratory effort, reduces respiratory efficiency, and may lead to alveolar hypoventilation. These effects are reversed by weight loss.

Being either overweight or underweight is known to increase joint and locomotion problems in dogs; it may in horses. These problems are due to carrying excessive weight or, in the underweight animal, having decreased muscle mass. Obesity in other species is known to increase heart, circulatory, digestive and skin diseases, and cancer, to decrease resistance to infectious disease, and, as a result, shorten life span. Mortality at any age is 9, 25, 65, 230, and 1200% higher in people that are 15, 25, 40, 55, or 100% overweight, respectively. Whether obesity causes these effects in horses isn't known, but it probably does to varying degrees. The effect of being overweight or underweight on the mare's reproductive ability, the foal, and milk production is discussed in Chapter 13.

There is only one way to correct obesity: dietary energy intake must be less than energy utilization. There are two ways to produce a body energy deficit: decrease feed intake or increase exercise. The use of both together is best.

Exercise in conjunction with reduced caloric intake has been shown in other species to be beneficial for weight reduction for many reasons, including:

1. Increased energy expenditure.
2. Prevention of a decrease in resting energy expendi-

ture that would otherwise occur when caloric intake is reduced.
3. Reduction in appetite, which may occur with a moderate increase in exercise by the relatively inactive individual.
4. Prevention of muscle and bone mineral losses that occur when caloric intake is reduced without increased physical activity.

The following exercise is recommended: walk, then trot, the horse long enough to make the horse begin sweating; then walk to cool down. Do this once and preferably twice daily.

Decreasing the horse's caloric intake sufficiently to cause it to lose weight requires that the horse be confined to a dry lot or paddock, or to a stall without straw bedding. Coarse, high-fiber, low-calorie, long-stem hay free of dust, mold, and weeds is preferred. The amount of hay recommended is that which provides 50 to 75% of the horse's caloric needs at rest and at optimum body weight (Appendix Table 1-4). For example:

A horse's obese weight is 1100 lbs (500 kg) and it is estimated that it should weigh about 880 lbs (400 kg). As shown in Appendix Table 5-400, the 880-lb horse for maintenance needs 13.4 Mcal daily, and therefore for weight reduction needs (50 to 75%) × 13.4, or 6.7 to 10 Mcal daily. As shown in Appendix Table 6, most mature grass hay provides 0.7 to 0.9 Mcal/lb. For weight reduction, you would feed the horse about 6.7 to 10 Mcal/day ÷ 0.7 to 0.9 Mcal/lb of hay, or about 8 to 14 lbs of hay daily. Ideally, divide the amount fed into at least two feedings daily. Water and salt should be always available, and no grain or protein supplement containing feed should be offered. The amount of hay fed should be adjusted as needed for each individual horse to obtain the decrease in body weight desired.

Weight reduction should be continued until the horse has a body condition score of 5 to 6 (Table 1-4), at which time the amount fed should be increased sufficiently to maintain that weight. Following weight reduction, the horse may be able to be put on pasture without regaining excessively if exercise is continued, but if ample pasture forage is available, or if exercise is discontinued regain will occur.

PROTEIN

Protein consists of many amino acids bonded together. Different types of proteins consist of different combinations and numbers of amino acids. As an analogy, if amino acids were letters in the alphabet, proteins would be words. Just as different words consist of different numbers and combinations of letters, different proteins consist of different numbers and combinations of amino acids.

Amino acids, like carbohydrates and fats, contain many carbon molecules linked together, with hydrogen and oxygen attached to the carbon. However, they also contain nitrogen, and some contain sulfur. Most proteins contain 16 ± 2% nitrogen; therefore, the protein content of a feed is estimated by determining its nitrogen content and dividing this amount by 0.16 (or multiplying by 1 ÷ 0.16, or 6.25). The value obtained is the crude protein (CP) content of the feed. Thus, a feed containing 1.6% nitrogen would contain about 10% crude protein (1.6% ÷ 0.16). This calculation does not indicate a feed's protein content if that feed contains any nonprotein nitrogen, such as urea.

Proteins are composed of 22 different amino acids. Although all of them are needed for synthesis of body protein, some can be produced in body tissues and do not need to be supplied in the feed or absorbed from the intestine. These are referred to as nonessential or dispensable amino acids, while those that must be provided in the diet, or synthesized by micro-organisms in the intestinal tract, are called essential or indispensable amino acids. Essential and nonessential, therefore, indicate whether the amino acid must be absorbed from the intestinal tract. Proteins composed of a high proportion of essential amino acids are referred to as high-quality proteins. Those containing a high proportion of nonessential amino acids are low- or poor-quality proteins.

Feeds commonly fed to horses, in conjunction with microbial synthesis of amino acids in the cecum and colon, and the possible absorption of some of these amino acids, contain a sufficient amount of each amino acid to meet the mature horse's needs for all amino acids, provided the feed meets the horse's dietary protein needs. Because of this, it doesn't matter which amino acids, or type of protein, are consumed by mature horses. However, the amount and digestibility of dietary protein does matter.

Protein Needs

The amount of crude protein needed in the diet depends on: (1) the amount of that diet consumed, (2) the digestibility of the protein in that diet, (3) that individual animal's need for protein, and (4) for the growing horse, but not the mature horse consuming feeds commonly fed to horses, the amino acid content or quality of the protein consumed.

The lower the digestibility of the protein ingested, the greater the amount needed in the diet. Protein digestibility varies with the source of the protein, the amount of protein and fiber in the diet, and the amount of heat produced in feed processing and storage. Horses are able to digest 45 to 85% of the protein in most commonly fed feeds, being on the upper end of this range for cereal grains and the lower end for mature grass forage. These values are considered in the indicated amount of crude protein needed. Protein digestibility does not, therefore, need to be considered unless it is reduced to below normal levels. This may occur if the feed has undergone excessive heating, as may occur with improper feed processing, or during storage because of inadequate drying prior to storage.

In addition to digestibility, the amount of a nutrient needed in a diet depends on the amount of that diet consumed. The amount of a diet consumed depends on the animal's dietary energy needs and the energy content of the diet. The higher the energy content of the diet, the less of that diet the animal needs and will consume to meet its energy needs, and, therefore, the higher the concentration of all nutrients in that diet must be so that the animal will receive enough of them to meet its needs. Thus, as shown in Appendix Table 1, a diet with an energy density of 0.9 Mcal/lb (2.0 Mcal/kg), as recommended for maintenance, should contain 8% protein, whereas one providing 1.3 Mcal/lb (2.85 Mcal/kg), as recommended for intense work, should contain 11.4% protein.

Although previously it was believed that physical activity had little or no effect on the horse's protein needs, several studies indicate that the amount of protein needed increases with increased physical activity. The increased amount of protein is needed for: (1) increased muscle development and mass with increased physical condition, (2) perhaps increased muscle protein content, and (3) nitrogen lost in sweat. However, the increase in protein needed for physical activity is less than the increase in energy needed.

Besides water, the nutrient for which need increases the most as a result of physical activity is dietary energy, which the horse will consume if sufficient feed is available. As a result of the increased feed intake, more protein is consumed. This increase in protein consumption is more than that required to provide the additional protein needed for physical activity. Thus, although more protein is needed for physical activity, an increase in the protein percentage in the diet is not needed, unless the energy or caloric density of the diet is increased. In fact, if the energy density of the diet is not increased, the protein percentage in the diet can be decreased. However, most diets fed and those preferred for physical activity are higher in energy density than those fed the idle horse. This higher energy density is beneficial because it allows the physically active horse to obtain the increased energy needed without too large an increase in the amount of feed consumed. As a result of the lower feed intake because of the diet's increased energy density, however, the additional protein needed for physical activity may not be consumed unless there is an equivalent increase in the percent protein in the diet. These are the reasons a higher percentage of protein, as well as a higher energy density, are recommended in the diet of the working horse and also of the stallion during breeding season (Appendix Table 1).

During pregnancy, the mare's protein and energy requirements are not increased until the last 3 months. As shown in Appendix Table 1, a diet with an energy density of 1.0 to 1.1 (2.2 to 2.4 Mcal/kg), as recommended for the ninth month of pregnancy until foaling, should contain 10 to 11% crude protein.

During the first 3 months of lactation, both milk protein content and the amount of milk produced are at a peak. As a result, the amount of protein needed is greatest during this period. A diet with an energy density of 1.2 Mcal/lb (2.6 Mcal/kg), as recommended for the first 3 months of lactation, should contain 13% crude protein, and a diet with an energy density of 1.1 Mcal/lb (2.45 Mcal/kg), as recommended for lactation after the first 3 months, should contain 11% crude protein (Appendix Table 1).

For growth, both the amount of protein and its quality or amino acid content are important. An energy density of 1.3 Mcal/lb (2.9 Mcal/kg), as recommended for weanlings, should contain 14.5% crude protein, and a diet with an energy density of 1.25 Mcal/lb (2.8 Mcal/kg), as recommended for yearlings, should contain 12.5% crude protein (Appendix Table 1).

TABLE 1–5
Effect of Dietary Lysine Content on Horse's Growth

	SBM[a]	CSM[a]	CSM + Lysine
Lysine (%)	0.65	0.49	0.65
Initial wt (lbs)	580	580	580
Gain (lbs/day)	1.23	1.01	1.23
Feed efficiency (lbs feed/lb of gain)	12.2	15.5	12.3

[a] Soybean meal (SBM) or cottonseed meal (CSM) used in the diet. All three diets contained the same total protein content.

A greater amount of the essential amino acid lysine is needed by the young horse for growth than is available from microorganisms in its intestinal tract and than is present in many feeds. Two other essential amino acids, methionine and tryptophan, are also present in low quantities in cereal grains. However, the most, and generally only, limiting amino acid in the growing horse's diet is lysine, although if the forage consumed is grass, threonine intake may also be marginal. The diet should provide at least 0.65% lysine and 0.50% threonine in its dry matter. The effects of inadequate lysine are well illustrated by the study results shown in Table 1–5 in which soybean meal, cottonseed meal, and cottonseed meal fortified with lysine were used as the protein supplements in the diet. Although all three diets had an identical protein content, when cottonseed meal without added lysine was fed, growth was slower and more feed was required.

To provide the amount of lysine needed by the horse for growth, all of the additional protein above that provided by the grain and forage consumed that is needed to meet the growing horse's protein requirements should be provided by a protein supplement in which the protein contains at least 5 to 6% lysine, such as canola, soybean, fish or meat meals, or milk products (Table 4–7). These protein supplements, when used to provide sufficient protein to meet the growing horse's protein needs, will also provide adequate lysine. They are also relatively high in other essential amino acids needed by the horse for growth. If other protein supplements are used, i.e., those that do not contain at least 5 to 6% lysine in their protein, more of them than is needed to meet the horse's protein requirements must be fed to provide adequate lysine. If not, growth rate and feed efficiency will be reduced (Table 1–5).

Nonprotein Nitrogen (Urea) for Horses

Microbial organisms present in the rumen of cattle, sheep, and other ruminants, and in the cecum and colon of the horse, are able to utilize the nitrogen in urea or other nonprotein nitrogen-containing substances to synthesize protein, providing the animal consumes sufficient nonfiber sources of dietary energy. In ruminants, the protein produced by these organisms passes from the rumen to the stomach and small intestine, where it is digested and absorbed. Thus, a nonprotein source of nitrogen, such as urea, may be fed to ruminants to provide them with protein. If all of the urea ingested is converted to protein, one unit of urea would provide 2.81 units of protein, since most feed-grade urea used currently contains 45% nitro-

gen, and protein contains 16% nitrogen (45% ÷ 0.16 = 281%). However, feeding urea or nonprotein nitrogen is of little value in providing protein to the horse. Most of the nonprotein nitrogen fed to the horse is absorbed from the small intestine and excreted in the urine before it reaches the cecum and colon, where it may be used for protein synthesis. Although that which reaches the cecum and colon may be used for protein synthesis, little of it is digested and absorbed from the cecum or large intestine. Thus, although some of the nonprotein nitrogen fed to the horse may be used for protein synthesis, much of that protein is unavailable to the horse and, therefore, is excreted in the feces.

By U.S. law, feeds containing nonprotein nitrogen must state on the feed tag the amount of protein from nonprotein nitrogen. It is important to realize that the feed will provide this amount of protein only if all of the nonprotein nitrogen it contains is converted to protein and is utilized by the animal. Since little of it is utilized by the horse, this amount should be subtracted from the feed's protein content to determine how much protein that feed will provide the horse. For example: a feed tag states that the feed contains 26% crude protein with 10% protein equivalents from urea. This feed, therefore, provides only 26% − 10%, or 16%, crude protein for the horse. The 10% protein equivalent from the urea is of no benefit (or harm) to the horse.

Excessive intake of nonprotein nitrogen is toxic. Before microorganisms use nonprotein nitrogen to synthesize protein, the nonprotein nitrogen is converted to ammonia. If an excessive amount of nonprotein nitrogen is ingested, toxic quantities of ammonia are absorbed. Initially, affected animals wander aimlessly and are incoordinated. Following this, they may press their heads against fixed objects, become recumbent, then comatose, convulse, and die. Although ponies succumb to single doses of 0.5 kg (1.1 lbs) of urea, intakes of feed containing up to 5% urea (14% protein equivalents from urea) as the total diet, and providing as much as 0.25 kg (0.55 lb) of urea daily, do not have any detrimental effects on mature horses. This is several times greater than the amounts that are toxic to cattle or sheep. Therefore, diets made for cattle or sheep that contain urea, or other nonprotein nitrogen sources, may be fed to the horse. Even though the nonprotein nitrogen compound is of little benefit to the horse, it is not harmful in the amounts present in these diets.

Protein Deficiency

The most obvious manifestations of a protein deficiency are reduced growth in young animals, and weight loss and reduced performance ability, endurance, and production (such as reduced milk production during lactation) in mature horses. Hair growth and shedding are slowed resulting in a rough, coarse, unkempt appearance (Figure 1–4). Hoof growth is slowed, which may result in increased hoof splitting and cracking. A protein deficiency in the horse may also cause appetite depravity and eating feces, which are alleviated within 5 to 7 days after correcting the deficiency. A protein deficiency may decrease food intake, which not only worsens the protein deficiency but causes

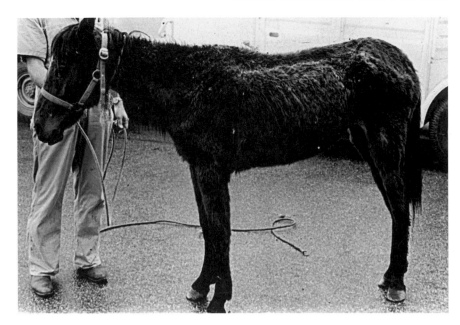

Fig. 1–4. Horse with a long, scruffy-looking hair coat, primarily the result of a protein deficiency. A vitamin A deficiency or excess, if sufficiently severe and prolonged, may have a similar effect but with less severe body weight loss. The horse was also suffering from a dietary energy deficiency as a result of inadequate feed intake, which would worsen the protein deficiency since what protein was ingested would be used primarily for energy needs, rather than protein needs.

an energy deficiency. An energy deficiency contributes to the clinical signs and further worsens the protein deficiency, because most of the protein that is consumed will then be used to assist in meeting energy, not protein, needs. The results of either a protein or energy deficiency are those described previously in the section on Energy Deficiency.

Protein deficiencies are caused by the following factors:

1. Inadequate protein in the diet, such as may happen with any horse eating certain mature grass forages, many of which contain 10 to 40% less protein than needed for maintenance.
2. Poorly digestible dietary protein, such as heat-damaged protein.
3. Inadequate feed intake, in which case the major effect is due to an energy deficiency.

If there is inadequate intake of the other two sources of energy—carbohydrates and fats—protein is used for energy and not for the animal's protein needs, thus resulting in a protein deficiency. It is futile to provide protein for the animal's protein needs if energy needs are not being met. Always ensure adequate energy intake before trying to meet protein needs.

Protein Excess

If more protein is ingested than needed, nitrogen, in the form of ammonia, is removed from the amino acids that make up the protein. The remainder of the amino acid is used for energy, or, if energy is not needed at that time, it is stored as fat or glycogen for later use as energy. The ammonia that is removed from the amino acids is converted by the liver to urea. This increases the plasma or blood urea nitrogen concentration (BUN) which is directly related to dietary protein intake. The increased amount of urea produced is excreted in the urine. This increases

urine volume and water requirements. It also increases the ammonia smell in the urine which can be noticed in poorly ventilated stables when horses are fed higher-protein-containing feeds such as alfalfa.

The more protein eaten above the animal's needs, the greater the blood flow through the kidney. Prolonged renal hyperperfusion from chronic excessive protein intake is known to decrease renal function in people and some species of animals. Currently there appear to be no studies of whether this occurs in horses. Even if it does, it is doubtful that it would be a problem in any practical situation. However, if the horse, like other animals and people, has a decrease in hepatic function, there is a decreased ability to convert ammonia to urea; or, if there is a decrease in renal function, there is a decreased ability to excrete urea, and the amount of ammonia or urea in the body increases. Limiting protein intake to that just sufficient to meet needs is, therefore, beneficial in the management of an animal with liver or kidney disease.

The utilization of protein for energy produces three to six times more heat than the utilization of carbohydrates or fats. This may be beneficial in a cold environment, but may contribute to excessive sweating and heat exhaustion during physical activity, particularly in a warm environment. Although some have claimed that high-protein diets for horses impair endurance performance, others are unable to find any beneficial or detrimental effects. Excessive protein intake may, however, contribute to developmental orthopedic diseases, as described in Chapter 16.

Diet-Induced Allergy

Occasionally, allergies to a specific protein may occur. This may result in the rapid development of round elevated areas on the skin surface over all or small portions of the body (Fig. 1–5). These are referred to as urticaria, wheals, plaques, or protein bumps. They may or may not itch, and they may persist for a few hours to several days, disappearing as rapidly as they developed. Numerous factors other

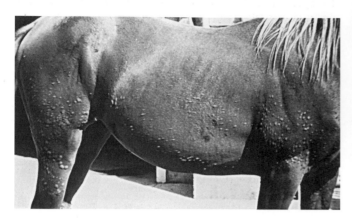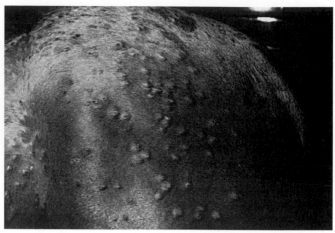

Fig. 1–5. Urticaria, wheals, plaques, hives, or protein bumps. These welts or bumps appear and disappear suddenly. There may be only a few or there may be many all over the head and body. They may or may not itch and may persist for a few hours to several days. They are caused by an allergic response to a specific protein in, e.g., feed, insect bites, drugs, insecticides, inhaled pollens or chemicals, internal parasites, or vaccines.

than dietary protein may be responsible, including insect bites, inhalation of chemicals or pollens, internal parasites, vaccines, and reactions following administration of drugs such as penicillins, streptomycin, and tetracyclines. When caused by the diet, the allergy is due to a specific protein in the diet, not to the amount of protein in the diet, and is frequently associated with itching. Severe tail rubbing may occur. Feeds reported to most frequently cause allergic reactions in horses include potatoes and their by-products, distillery wastes, beet pulp, buckwheat, clover, St. John's wort, wheat, oats, barley, bran, tonic, and chicory. Corticosteroid administration usually results in recovery within 24 hours.

Less commonly, an allergy to an ingested protein, such as clover pasture in bloom or fish meals, may result in the sudden occurrence of subcutaneous edema, which gravitates ventrally. The head is the most commonly affected site. Eyelids may be edematous, the third eyelid may swell and protrude, and profuse lacrimation may occur. Although the condition may be caused by a feed allergy or snakebite, drugs are most often implicated. Spontaneous recovery is common. Treatment consists of emptying the gastrointestinal tract to prevent further absorption of an ingested allergen, and administering corticosteroids, antihistamines, and epinephrine. If the condition is believed to be due to the diet, feed forage only. If it recurs following reintroduction of a particular feed, that feed most likely contains the protein causing the allergy.

CARBOHYDRATES

Carbohydrate Types and Utilization

Carbohydrates are composed of simple sugars, or monosaccharides, such as glucose (dextrose), fructose, galactose, and xylose. Many glucose molecules attached together by alpha bonds form the polysaccharides starch, present in plants, and glycogen, present in animals. These are called nonstructural, soluble, or nonfiber carbohydrates; they are also called nitrogen-free-extract (NFE) be-

cause of the way in which their amount in a feed is determined (as shown in Figure 6–3). Nonfiber carbohydrates are readily utilized and provide much of the horse's dietary energy. However, other forms of carbohydrates in feeds also provide a substantial amount of dietary energy for the horse.

If glucose molecules are attached together by beta, instead of alpha, bonds, they form the structural polysaccharide, or insoluble fiber, cellulose. Cellulose is a hollow fibril that is analogous to the reinforcing rod in the concrete of the plant's cell wall, the concrete being the structural polysaccharide or insoluble fiber hemicellulose, which is many molecules of the monosaccharide xylose attached together by beta bonds. Since monosaccharides are the only form of carbohydrate that is absorbed from the intestinal tract, the alpha and beta bonds between monosaccharides must be broken for carbohydrates to be utilized directly by animals.

The alpha bonds in starch, glycogen, and other soluble carbohydrates are broken by the digestive enzyme amylase. Amylase is secreted by all animals primarily from the pancreas into the small intestine. Amylase digestion breaks starch and glycogen down to the disaccharide maltose. Maltose, like the disaccharides sucrose (table sugar) and lactose (milk sugar), are split into their two monosaccharide units by the disaccharidase enzymes maltase, sucrase, and lactase, which are a part of the intestinal brush border. If this brush border is damaged or missing, such as with enteritis, carbohydrate utilization is impaired and a high amount of it remains in the intestinal tract, which may cause diarrhea. Animals past nursing age lose lactase and, therefore, the ability to digest and absorb the milk sugar lactose. Horses over 3 years old have little lactase. As a consequence, sudden introduction of lactose-containing milk products into a mature horse's diet may induce diarrhea.

Absorbed monosaccharides are used for energy. If dietary energy isn't needed at that time, they are stored as glycogen. If glycogen storage depots in the liver, kidney, and muscle are full, the monosaccharides are converted to and stored as fat. Glycogen and fat can be utilized for energy when needed.

Dietary Fiber

In contrast to the primarily nonstructural, nonfiber carbohydrates whose monosaccharides are linked by alpha bonds which animals are able to digest, no animal produces the digestive enzymes necessary to break the beta bond linking the monosaccharides that make up fibers. Only bacteria have the enzymes necessary to break these beta bonds and, therefore, digest and utilize fiber directly. However, by having these bacteria in their gastrointestinal tracts, and by being able to utilize the products of bacterial digestion of fiber, animals are able to utilize plant fiber with varying degrees of efficiency. In using plant fiber for their own functions, bacteria convert the fiber to short-chain, or volatile, fatty acids (acetic, propionic, lactic, isobutyric, butyric, isovaleric, and valeric). These volatile fatty acids, or VFAs, are absorbed and provide 30 to 70% of the horse's, and 70 to 80% of the ruminant's, total digestible energy needs, with the amount provided being at the upper end of these ranges on high-fiber (high-forage) diets, and the lower end of these ranges on high-nonfiber carbohydrate or starch (high-grain) diets. Bacterial fermentation of fiber occurs primarily in the rumen of ruminant herbivores, such as cattle and sheep; the cecum and colon of nonruminant herbivores, such as horses, rabbits, and rats; and in the large intestine of omnivores, such as people, pigs, and dogs, and carnivores, such as cats.

What is analyzed in a feed as dietary fiber consists of not only polysaccharides composed of monosaccharides linked by beta bonds, but also lignin and, in overheated feeds, starch that has been rendered undigestible because of heat damage. Lignin is completely resistant to digestion and fermentation by both animals and bacteria. The beta-bond polysaccharides or fiber consist of the insoluble plant structural fibers cellulose and hemicellulose, and of soluble fibers. Soluble fibers are the parenchymatous portions and secretions of plants, such as sap, resin, gums, pectin, and mucilages present primarily in fruits, vegetables, cereal grains, beans, and lentils. Insoluble fibers, on the other hand, are highest in nonseed and nonfruit portions of plants, such as the leaves, stems, hulls, and wood.

Total dietary fiber, therefore, is the sum of soluble and insoluble fiber, plus small amounts of lignin and, in heat-damaged feed, undigestible starch. Although the amount of each in a feed can be determined by enzymatic procedures, this is unnecessary for feeding purposes and is rarely done. Nonenzymatic fiber analysis excludes soluble fibers, which are, therefore, included with the calculated amount of nonfiber carbohydrates, or NFC, in the feed. This is of little consequence because in feeds commonly fed the horse, the amount of soluble fiber is small compared to the amount of nonfiber carbohydrate, and because both are fairly equally utilized and provide the same amount of dietary energy. In contrast, insoluble fiber is the most poorly utilized potential source of dietary energy. Thus, the higher the insoluble fiber content of feed, the lower

the amount of usable dietary energy that feed will provide. Undigested feed, which for most feeds is primarily undigested insoluble fiber, helps maintain normal gastrointestinal motility and function, and helps prevent too rapid an intake of the readily digested nonfiber carbohydrates. Excessive intake of readily digested nonfiber carbohydrates at one feeding may result in diarrhea, colic, and laminitis or founder.

All animals use nearly all of the soluble fiber ingested. However, for ingested insoluble fiber, the sooner its beta bonds are broken, the greater the percent digested and utilized by the animal. Thus, insoluble fiber utilization is greatest for ruminants, less but still quite high for horses, and least but still significant for nonherbivores. People, for example, are able to utilize 30 to 85% of the insoluble fiber in commonly eaten foods. Horses and cattle are equally effective in digesting low-fiber feeds. But cattle are better able to digest high-fiber feeds. Fiber digestion by horses is only 65 to 75% of that by cattle and sheep, whereas it is 115 to 120% for llamas, 65 to 75% for elephants, 50 to 55% for swine, and 40 to 45% for rabbits and hamsters. In all species, however, as the fiber content of the diet increases, the digestibility of diet organic matter generally decreases, but the reduction in digestibility is greater for horses than it is for cattle. The horse compensates for the lower energy content and energy digestibility in diets higher in fiber content through greater consumption of that diet. Donkeys can eat more and tend to digest fiber the most effectively; they therefore can get by better on high-fiber diets than can ponies and horses.

There are several methods used for determining the amount of insoluble fiber in feed. The crude fiber method, as determined in the approximate analysis procedure shown in Figure 6-3, is the oldest and most commonly used method. It is the only fiber value available for many feeds for the horse and is, therefore, used in this book. Unfortunately, crude fiber analysis is quite inaccurate; as much as 85% of the hemicellulose and 50% of the cellulose may be lost, resulting in an unpredictable underestimation of the fiber content of the feed and, therefore, as shown in Figure 6-3, an overestimation of the nonfiber carbohydrate content of the feed. Since nonfiber carbohydrate is more digestible and utilizable than fiber, overestimating a feed's nonfiber carbohydrate content may result in an overestimation of its caloric content and, therefore, its feeding value. Other fiber analyses occasionally used are neutral and acid detergent fiber (NDF and ADF) methods. Although NDF includes nearly all cellulose and over 50% of the hemicellulose, it also erroneously includes a high amount of amylase digestible starch. Although acid treatment removes the starch, it also removes most of the hemicellulose.

Because most of the hemicellulose is utilizable by the horse, its loss in the ADF analysis results in an underestimation of that feed's insoluble fiber content and, therefore, overestimation of the feed's energy content and feeding value. However, ADF is the most accurate indication of a feed's poorly utilizable fiber content that is generally available. Although amylase treatment of NDF is a more accurate indication of a feed's insoluble fiber content than is ADF, because amylase removes only digestible starch, its amount in feeds for horses is available even less frequently than is ADF content.

FATS

Fats are triglycerides which are composed of one molecule of glycerol and three long-chain fatty-acid molecules, which may be the same or different. In contrast to the short-chain or volatile fatty acids produced by bacterial fermentation of ingested carbohydrates, which contain only two to five carbon atoms, most long-chain fatty acids in fat contain 16 to 20 carbon atoms. The more unsaturated the long-chain fatty acids (i.e., the greater the number of double bonds between its carbon atoms) and the shorter their chain length (i.e., the fewer carbon atoms they consist of), the lower the melting point of the triglyceride. When the melting point is less than room temperature, the triglyceride is referred to as an oil; when it is greater than room temperature, it is referred to as a fat. Triglycerides, like other lipids (phospholipids, sphingolipids, glycolipids, steroids, and waxes), are soluble in organic solvents such as ether. Other nonmineral constituents of plant and animal tissues are water soluble and are relatively insoluble in organic solvents. This difference is the basis for extracting and determining the amount of lipid in a sample, as shown in Figure 6–3, and the reason lipids are referred to as ether extracts, which in horse feeds is almost entirely fats and oils.

Fats or oils are needed in the horse's diet for the absorption of the fat-soluble vitamins A, D, E, and K, and as a source of the unsaturated fatty acid linoleic acid. Linoleic acid is essential in the diet of all animals. The amount needed by horses hasn't been determined, although at least 0.5% linoleic acid in the diet dry matter is recommended for all horses, the requirement is probably much lower than this. The horse can synthesize in sufficient quantities all other fatty acids needed, including linolenic and arachidonic acids, which are also often referred to as essential fatty acids. Therefore, fatty acids other than linoleic acid are not needed in the horse's diet.

Unsaturated fatty acids such as linoleic acid become oxidized (rancid) with increasing time, temperature, and humidity if sufficient antioxidants aren't present. Rancid fats don't provide the animal's linoleic acid needs. Fat rancidity also impairs the utilization of vitamins A, D, and E, as well as several B vitamins, and decreases the fat's palatability so that the horse may refuse to eat feed containing it. Rancidity may occur: (1) if unsaturated fatty acids that do not contain sufficient antioxidants, such as Vitamin E, are added to the diet, and (2) with prolonged storage of cereal grains, with or without added fat or oil. The time required for rancidity to occur decreases with increasing temperature and humidity, both of which may increase sufficiently for rancidity, as well as mold growth, to occur if cereal grains contain more than 12 to 15% moisture when stored.

An essential fatty acid deficiency in most species causes a dry, lusterless hair coat and scaly skin, and may predispose to skin infection. If the deficiency persists, hair loss, edema, and exudation from localized areas of the skin, resulting in moist inflammation, may ensue. Reproductive efficiency may be impaired. If pregnancy occurs, there may be neonatal abnormalities and death. However, in the horse, an essential fatty acid or linoleic acid deficiency is not known to occur. No clinical symptoms, visual indications of skin or hair coat alteration, or decreases in plasma concentrations of triglycerides or free fatty acids, including linoleic acid, occurred in ponies fed extremely low-fat diets for 7 months. However, at the lowest fat intake (0.05% in the diet), tissue and plasma vitamin E concentrations fell significantly, perhaps indicating inadequate absorption of this fat-soluble vitamin. Common horse feeds contain 2 to 6% fat, i.e., many times more than that present in the diets used in this study. The fats present in common horse feeds are also high in linoleic acid; e.g., corn oil is 55% and safflower oil 73% linoleic acid. In contrast, coconut, palm, and olive oils are 1 to 2%, butter fat 2.5%, beef fat 4%, linseed or flax seed oil 14%, pork fat 18%, and poultry fat 22% linoleic acid. Thus, a dry, lusterless hair coat in the horse is unlikely to be due to a fatty acid deficiency. Instead, it is more likely to be due to a dietary protein, energy, or Vitamin A deficiency.

Ingested fats are used primarily as a source of dietary energy, although if a diet contains adequate available carbohydrate and protein, fats are not needed as a source of energy. Digested fats provide over 2.25 times more utilizable energy than an equal weight of digested carbohydrate or protein. Because of their high energy density, as described in the section "Fat and Oil Supplements for Horses" in Chapter 4, these feeds may be added to a horse's diet to increase its dietary energy intake in an effort to increase its growth rate, milk production, reproductive efficiency, or physical performance.

MINERALS FOR HORSES

Calcium and Phosphorus	20
Functions, Utilization, and Needs	20
Calcium Deficiency/Phosphorus Excess	22
Causes	22
Effects	23
Treatment	23
Calcium Excess	24
Effects	24
Causes	25
Phosphorus Deficiency	25
Sodium Chloride Salt	25
Utilization, Needs, and Feeding	25
Excess	26
Deficiency	27
Potassium	27
Magnesium	27
Sulfur	28
Selenium and Vitamin E	28
Functions and Utilization	28
Selenium Needs and Sources	29
Vitamin E Needs and Sources	30
Selenium and Vitamin E Deficiencies	31
Equine Degenerative Myeloencephalopathy (EDM)	32
Vitamin E and Reproduction	33
Iodine	33

Utilization, Needs, and Sources	33
Deficiencies and Excesses	33
Causes	33
Effects	34
Diagnosis	35
Treatment	35
Copper	35
Molybdenum	36
Zinc	36
Utilization	36
Needs and Deficiency	37
Excess	37
Manganese	37
Iron	38
Utilization, Needs, and Sources	38
Deficiency	38
Excess	38
Deficiency and Excess Diagnosis	39
Cobalt	39
Fluoride	39
Utilization, Needs, and Sources	39
Fluorosis	40
Causes	40
Effects	40
Diagnosis	40
Treatment	41

Although important for a variety of functions, inorganic elements or minerals constitute only a small fraction of the body weight and of the amount of nutrients needed in the diet. On a weight basis, the horse's body consists of approximately 60 to 65% water; 30 to 35% of the energy source nutrients protein, fats and carbohydrates; and 4% minerals. Most of the body's minerals are the major, or macro, minerals: calcium, phosphorus, sodium, chlorine, potassium, magnesium, and sulfur. Macrominerals are minerals for which the amount needed in the diet are best expressed as parts per hundred (percent). Trace, or micro-minerals, are those for which dietary requirements are best expressed as parts per million (ppm or mg/kg)—units 10,000 times smaller than those used for macrominerals. Trace minerals needed in the diet include selenium, iodine, copper, zinc, manganese, iron, and cobalt.

Macrominerals are needed for body structure, for maintaining the body's acid-base and fluid balance, and for nerve conduction, and muscle contraction. Most trace minerals are needed as components of enzymes that are involved in controlling numerous diverse biologic reactions. Iodine is a necessary constituent of thyroid hormone, iron of blood hemoglobin and muscle myoglobin, and cobalt of vitamin B_{12}.

Trace minerals needed in the diet but for which deficiencies outside the laboratory have not been verified in animals, include: vanadium, nickel, chromium, tin, silicon, and arsenic. Whether the trace mineral fluoride is needed in the diet is unknown. The term heavy metal in science refers not to rock music but to minerals which, even when consumed in relatively small amounts, cause adverse ef-

fects. Heavy metals include: lead, nickel, mercury, arsenic, aluminum, and cadmium. However, all minerals, like all other nutrients, can have an adverse effect if sufficiently high levels are consumed, as shown in Figure 2-1.

The width of the curve in Figure 2-1 (i.e., the intakes which are deficient or toxic, marginal and optimal) varies for each nutrient and situation. The amount given as that required in the diet for most nutrients is toward the lower intake side of the range at which animal health and performance are optimal. This amount reduces feeding costs while still maintaining optimal health and performance. However, as Figure 2-1 illustrates, feeding more of a nutrient than that required does not improve health or performance, and impairs them if a sufficient excess is fed. This is an important concept often ignored by those selling or administering nutrient supplements, or trying to maximize an animal's health or performance by nutritional supplementation in the feed or by their direct administration. It is particularly important for all minerals, and for vitamins A and D, for which excesses in the diet can be quite harmful.

Dietarily, minerals should be regarded as a group rather than individually. As the intake of a mineral increases above that needed, the amount absorbed and/or excreted in the urine and/or feces also increases. An excess amount absorbed may be harmful. That not absorbed may bind other minerals, decreasing their absorption and possibly resulting in a deficiency of these minerals.

It is the balanced amount of all minerals in the diet that is important. Indiscriminately adding one or even several minerals to the diet is likely to be more harmful than beneficial. Minerals, therefore, should not be added to the diet

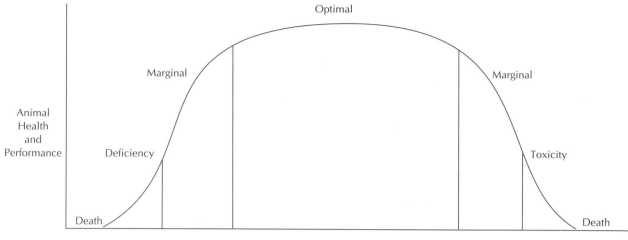

Fig. 2–1. Effects of amount of nutrient consumed on animal health and performance. Marginal intake of a nutrient impairs health and performance, cannot be detected clinically, but for some nutrients can be detected by laboratory tests. Clinical signs occur only at an intake below or above that which is deficient or toxic, respectively. The nutrient level required or toxic is near the lower or upper end of the range, respectively, at which health and performance are optimal. The intake range between requirement and toxic levels differs for different nutrients, e.g., from a fewfold for fluoride to 20-fold for selenium, to no toxic level known for some nutrients such as many of the B vitamins.

unless it is known which ones and how much are needed. Knowledge of which minerals are needed, when, and in what amounts can be obtained from the information given for each feeding situation throughout this book; the amount present in a feed or the total diet can be determined as described in Chapter 6.

The mineral contents of feeds and mineral supplements commonly fed to horses are given in Appendix Tables 2, 6, and 7. The recommended minimum and maximum concentrations of each mineral needed by the horses are given in Appendix Tables 1, 2, and 4. These recommended amounts represent the total, not the available, mineral amounts that are either needed or toxic, based on the low or high, respectively, average availability of that mineral from feeds that commonly make up the horse's diet. For example, calcium and phosphorus requirements given assume that 50% of the calcium and 35% of the phosphorus (45% for lactating mares and growing horses because their diets are typically supplemented with phosphorus-containing minerals, which are more available than the phosphorus in feeds) consumed will be absorbed. Since absorption of the calcium and phosphorus from feeds for horses is generally near this amount or higher (50 to 80% for calcium, 30 to 55% for phosphorus, and both higher in mineral supplements), absorption does not usually need to be considered in ensuring that the horse receives adequate calcium, phosphorus, or other minerals. However, as described for each mineral, numerous factors may decrease their efficiency of absorption. Only if one or more of these factors are present does the availability of that mineral need to be considered.

The only minerals generally of concern in feeding horses are calcium, phosphorus, salt (sodium chloride), in some geographical areas selenium, and for growth copper and zinc. Other minerals are unlikely to be present in inade-

quate or excessive amounts in feeds commonly fed, unless mineral supplements are given, the feed is contaminated by industrial waste, or the horse ingests selenium-accumulating plants (Table 18-9). If this is not the case, these minerals are the only ones whose intake needs to be evaluated. Although other mineral deficiencies and toxicoses are rare as described in this chapter and summarized in Table 2-1, they do occur and, therefore, should be evaluated if a threatening situation is present.

CALCIUM AND PHOSPHORUS

Functions, Utilization, and Needs

Calcium and phosphorus comprise about 70% of the mineral content of the body and from 30 to 50% of the minerals in milk. About 99% of the calcium and over 80% of the phosphorus in the body are in the bones and teeth. However, both calcium and phosphorus play a critical role in numerous other body functions. Phosphorus is necessary as a buffer, for energy metabolism, and for numerous other cellular functions. Calcium is necessary for blood coagulation, cell membrane function, glandular secretion, temperature regulation, the regulation of the activity of many enzymes, and mitochondrial and neuromuscular functions. If the plasma calcium concentration is significantly increased or decreased, it has the opposite effect on muscle membrane excitability; i.e., hypercalcemia decreases muscle tone and hypocalcemia increases muscle tone (see "Hypocalcemic Tetany" in Chapter 11).

Dietary calcium and phosphorus deficiencies or excesses result in excess mobilization or deposition of these minerals in bone, causing skeletal disease. These effects, however, maintain plasma concentrations and, therefore, nonskeletal functions are maintained. Thus, skeletal diseases are the major effect of a dietary deficiency or excess

TABLE 2–1
Mineral Deficiencies and Excesses: Causes and Effects in Horses

Mineral Imbalance	Causes	Effects
Calcium deficiency	Diet Ca < needs (Appx T-1) (e.g., high grain-low legume), diet Ca:P < 0.6:1, or Ca:oxalate < 0.5:1 & oxalate > 0.5%	DOD, ↓ bone density, stiff, lame, ↓ movement, big-head, lose wt & condition; fractures
Phosphorus excess	Bran as majority of diet or excess P added to diet	Calcium deficiency
Calcium excess	Ca:P > 6–10:1 adult diet or 3:1 weanling diet due to excess added Ca	DOD, P def., ↓ abs of Zn, Mn or Fe unknown, ↑ to normal bone density
Phosphorus deficiency	Diet P < needs (Appx T-1), no added P for growth, excess Ca or > 0.15% Aluminum	Same as Ca deficiency. If long & severe, ↓ bone density
Sodium deficiency	No salt available or in feed	↓ sweating & performance, ↓ food & water intake, wt. loss, weak, dehydration, excess licking & ± ↓ appetite & constipation
Sodium excess	Salt in only water, or feeding salt without adequate water available	Colic, diarrhea, polyuria, weak, staggering, posterior paralysis, recumbency
Potassium deficiency	Excess sweating especially when on a high-grain (low-potassium) diet, diuretics, or diarrheic	Fatigue, weak, lethargy, ↓ feed and water intake & wt loss
Potassium excess	Doesn't occur clinically except in horses with potassium-induced periodic paralysis (see Chapter 17)	
Magnesium deficiency	↓ Mg_p & Ca_p may rarely occur with transit	Muscle tremors, staggering, collapse, sweating, convulsions
Magnesium excess	Doesn't occur clinically	
Sulfur imbalance	Doesn't occur clinically	
Selenium deficiency	In foals due to < 0.05 ppm Se in mare's diet	↓ immunity & growth. Stiff, listless, difficult nursing and respiration, lung edema, ↑ HR, RR & salivation, "white muscle disease." Adult stiff.
Vitamin E deficiency	Se & vit. E deficiency	Progressive emaciation & without appetite loss, painful SC swelling, rough haircoat, ventral SC edema, yellow gritty fat, "wobblers," stiff gait
Selenium excess	Diet Se > 2–5 ppm from high-Se plants (Ch. 18) or mixing errors	"Blind staggers" or wt loss, listless, anemia, hair rough & loss from mane or tail, dark-fluid feces, stiff, feet painful, abnormal hoof growth & rings
Iodine deficiency	Diet I < 0.1 ppm	Most often in newborn. Stillborn or weak, DOD. Hypothyroidism & goiter with I excess & occasionally deficiency. Hair rough & loss, & myxedema rarely.
Iodine excess	Diet I > 5 ppm or 0.08 mg/kg bw/d due to I supplements, kelp, EDDI, or iodized salt in feed	
Copper excess	Adding 800 to 2800 ppm Cu to diet	Acute hemolytic anemia & icterus, lethargy & death. Hepatic & renal damage.
Copper deficiency	Diet Cu adult < 5 & weanling < 25 ppm Diet zinc > 700 ppm or Cu:Mo of 1:8 but not at < 1:4	DOD. Uterine artery rupture in aged parturient mares. Anemia & ↓ hair color in ruminants but not horses.
Molybdenum excess	Contaminated or alkaline soils. Diet Cu:Mo of 1:8 but not at < 1:4	Cu deficiency
Molybdenum deficiency	Never reported	
Zinc deficiency	< 15 ppm in adult & < 40 ppm in weanling diets	DOD, ↓ feed intake, ↓ growth, flaky skin, and hair loss
Zinc excess	Diet Zn > 700 ppm and If > 3600 ppm	DOD, stiff & lame. Also get anemia & ↓ growth.
Manganese deficiency	Diet Mn < 200 ppm, especially on limed soils	Possibly bone abnormalities in newborn
Manganese excess	Never reported	
Iron deficiency	Chronic or severe blood loss—Rarely due to deficiency in diet	↓ performance ability followed by anemia
Iron excess	Excess administered, esp. if vit. E def & foals. Rarely diet	Death of neonate. ↓ bacterial resistance
Cobalt deficiency or excess	Neither ever induced or reported	Vit. B_{12} deficiency
Fluoride deficiency	Never induced or reported	
Fluoride excess	Fluoride in phosphorus minerals, or industrial contamination. Diet F > 50–200 ppm or water > 8 ppm	Teeth slow coming in, mottled & pitted causing ↓ feed & water intake & chronic debilitation. Stiff, lame, ↑ bone density.

Abbreviations used are: Ca:P or Cu:Mo ratio of amount of calcium to phosphorus, or copper to molybdenum, in the diet; DOD = developmental orthopedic diseases as described in Chapter 16; ↑ = increased; ↓ = decreased; NC = no significant change; > = greater than; < = less than; SC = subcutaneous or under the skin; HR = heart rate; and RR = respiratory rate.

TABLE 2-2
Calcium and Phosphorus Needed by the Horse as
Compared to Amount in Feeds

	% in Total Diet Dry Matter	
	Calcium	Phosphorus
Recommended for:		
Maintenance	0.3	0.2
Pregnancy (last 3 mo) and lactation	0.5	0.3
Growth at ages:		
1–4 mo	0.8	0.5
6–12 mo	0.7	0.4
12–18 mo	0.5	0.3
18 mo–mature	0.4	0.25
Present in:		
Grains	0.05–0.09	0.3–0.4
Bran	0.1	1.3
Grass hay	0.3–0.5	0.1–0.3
Legume hay (e.g., alfalfa)	0.8–2.0	0.1–0.3

of either calcium or phosphorus. Horses are more likely to suffer from a lack of calcium or phosphorus, and as a result skeletal diseases, than from a lack of any other minerals. The amounts of calcium and phosphorus recommended in the horse's daily diet are given in Appendix Tables 1 and 4.

As is the case with all nutrients, to meet an animal's needs not only must the diet contain adequate amounts of appropriate nutrients but, in addition, the animal must be able to absorb and utilize them. A number of substances in the diet may decrease either calcium or phosphorus absorption.

Excess dietary phosphorus in any form binds calcium, preventing its absorption. In contrast, excess dietary calcium has little effect on phosphorus absorption. This is because, in the horse, calcium is absorbed in the small intestine, whereas phosphorus absorption occurs farther back in the large intestine. Most excess calcium ingested is absorbed from the small intestine and excreted in the urine; it is, therefore, not available to decrease phosphorus absorption from the large intestine. Thus, excess dietary calcium is much less detrimental than excess phosphorus. If quantities of both calcium and phosphorus in the diet are adequate to meet the animal's requirements, as given in Table 2-2, the amount of calcium with respect to phosphorus, or the Ca:P ratio, in the diet of the mature horse probably can vary from 0.8:1 to 8:1, and in the growing horse from 0.8:1 to 3:1, without resulting in problems. However, as a safety margin and because of the variation in the content and availability of calcium and phosphorus in feeds, a ratio of less than 1:1 is not recommended for any horse, and a ratio of greater than 6:1 is not recommended for the mature horse. The Ca:P ratio, however, is of secondary importance. Of primary importance is sufficient amounts of both calcium and phosphorus in the diet to meet the animal's requirements. Unless the diet contains inadequate amounts of both calcium and phosphorus, their ratio is of little importance. If the amount of dietary calcium or phosphorus is insufficient to meet the horse's requirement, or if the amount of one mineral with respect

to the other is outside of these ratios, skeletal alterations may occur.

Calcium Deficiency/Phosphorus Excess

Calcium Deficiency/Phosphorus Excess Causes

Excess phosphorus in the horse's diet occurs only if bran constitutes the majority of the diet, or if excess phosphorus-containing mineral supplements are fed. In contrast to what is occasionally stated, a high cereal grain diet does not cause a harmful phosphorus excess. As shown in Table 2-2, cereal grains contain about twice as much phosphorus as needed for maintenance and less than that needed for rapid growth, but they contain only $\frac{1}{10}$ to $\frac{1}{3}$ as much calcium as needed. Thus, the problem with a high cereal grain diet is not excess phosphorus, it's inadequate calcium.

The only clinically important role of excess dietary phosphorus for the horse is that the excess phosphorus binds calcium, decreasing its absorption. This effect becomes more detrimental the lower the calcium content of the diet. A sufficiently high phosphorus and low calcium content in the diet (a Ca:P ratio of less than 1:1) causes a calcium deficiency.

Excess oxalates, like excess phosphorus, bind calcium, decreasing its absorption. Therefore, if the diet contains sufficient oxalates with respect to calcium (i.e., has a sufficiently low calcium:oxalate ratio), it will cause a calcium deficiency. This is likely to occur when horses consume a diet with a total oxalate content over 0.5% in its dry matter, and with a calcium:oxalate ratio of less than 0.5:1. Plants that may have these characteristics are listed in Table 2-3. Oxalate content may increase and calcium decrease in pasture grass during the summer. This is unlikely to cause a problem in mature horses but may in young, growing horses. In any age, horse consumption of high amounts of halogeton, greasewood, or Oxalis species, which may be very high in oxalate, may cause acute oxalate poisoning, which generally results in gastroenteritis and diarrhea (Table 2-3).

A calcium deficiency from grazing plants high in oxalates and with a low calcium:oxalate ratio occurs in horses of all ages, but the incidence and severity are highest in lactating mares and weanlings because of their high calcium requirements and high feed and, therefore, oxalate intake. The prevalence of visible effects in herds grazing pastures containing these types of grasses varies widely. Up to 100% may be affected, with the onset of clinical signs varying from 2 to 8 months after being on the pastures. Cattle grazing these pastures may remain healthy.

There has been concern as to the amount of oxalate in, and therefore calcium availability from, alfalfa. Several studies have reported that calcium availability for ruminants is low from alfalfa, which is high in oxalates. However, this does not appear to be the case for horses, at least up to the lowest Ca:oxalate ratio found in alfalfa in the United States. Even in high-oxalate alfalfa, calcium availability does not need to be considered in ensuring that the horse's requirements are met. It has been suggested that an acidifying type diet (one with low cation:anion balance) may increase urinary calcium excretion suffi-

TABLE 2–3
Plants Containing Potentially Harmful Amounts of Oxalate[a]

Common Name	Scientific Name
Five hooked bassia	*Bassia hyssopifolia*
Halogeton[b]	*Halogeton glomeratus*
Greasewood[b]	*Sarcobatus vermiculatus*
Shamrock, soursob, sorrel[b]	*Oxalis* spp.
Red-rooted pigweed	*Amaranthus* spp.
Purslane	*Portulaca oleraceae*
Russian thistle, tumbleweed	*Salsola* spp.
Sorrel, dock	*Rumex* spp.
Rhubarb	*Rheum rhaponticum*
Sugar beet	*Beta vulgaris*
Lambsquarter	*Chenopodium* spp.
Bristle, foxtail grass	*Setaria* spp.
Panic grasses	*Panicum* spp.
Paspalum, Argentine & Dallis grasses	*Paspalum* spp.
—	*Sporobolus* spp.
Buffel grass	*Cenchrus ciliaris*
Signal grass, para grass	*Brachiaria* spp.
Pangola grass	*Digitaria recumbens*
Napier, mission grass	*Pennisetum* spp.
Kikuyu grass	*Pennisetum clandistinum*
Setaria grass	*Setaria sphacelata*
Foxtail millet	*Setaria italica*

[a] When total diet dry matter contains over 0.5% oxalate and the calcium:oxalate ratio is less than 0.5:1.

[b] Most commonly responsible for causing acute oxalate poisoning, which generally results in gastroenteritis and diarrhea. Other plants contain lower oxalate levels, which with prolonged consumption cause a calcium deficiency, resulting in lameness, bone and joint tenderness, and may result in "big head" (Fig. 2–2), loose teeth, emaciation, and respiratory noise.

ciently to cause a net loss of calcium from the body and bone dimineralization. Adding enough acidifying salts to this diet to decrease dietary cation:anion balance ($[Na^+ + K^+] - Cl^-$) from a normal of about 230 meq/kg diet dry matter to less than 30 (1% added $CaCl_2$ plus NH_4Cl), but not to 130, increased urinary calcium, and fecal phosphorus, magnesium and potassium excretions sufficiently to decrease but not to cause a negative balance of any of these minerals. Thus, it appears unlikely that common horsefeeds will be sufficiently acidic to cause a problem. Increased grain intake has been shown to increase fecal and urine acidity and to increase the renal clearance ratios of phosphorus and of calcium slightly independent of dietary cation-anion balance. However, the effect on mineral excretion in the feces and, therefore, net mineral balance, was not determined.

Calcium Deficiency/Phosphorus Excess Effects

Regardless of the cause, inadequate calcium absorption decreases the plasma calcium concentration. This decrease, although not sufficient to be of benefit in diagnosing the deficiency, is sufficient to inhibit calcitonin and stimulate excessive parathyroid hormone (PTH) secretion, i.e., to induce hyperparathyroidism. Hyperparathyroidism decreases urinary calcium and increases urinary phosphorus excretion; and stimulates calcium and phosphorus mobilization from the bone. These effects maintain a near

normal plasma calcium concentration and result in a normal or decreased plasma phosphorus concentration. As bone minerals are mobilized, they are replaced by fibrous connective tissue, increasing the size of the bone. Although all of the skeletal system is affected, in growing horses the effect is most noticeable in the growth plates of the legs and cervical vertebrae, resulting in developmental skeletal disease, as described in Chapter 16. In young mature horses this condition, called osteodystrophia fibrosa, is frequently most noticeable as an enlargement of the facial bones. This is frequently the most notable effect giving rise to the name "big-head" for this condition (Fig. 2–2); in older mature horses little or no facial bone enlargement may occur. The condition has also been called Miller's disease and bran disease, because it occurs on diets high in bran due to bran's high phosphorus (1.2%) and low calcium (0.1%) content.

Other clinical signs of extensive bone demineralization may occur prior to an observable enlargement of the facial bones or the growing horse's bone growth plates of the legs. An insidious, shifting leg lameness and generalized bone and joint tenderness occur. Severely affected horses may have a gait similar to that of a hopping rabbit, and a reluctance to move. The lameness may be started or worsened by exercise. Horses that appear to be normal may collapse suddenly when ridden. Affected horses tend to lose weight and may become emaciated. Lameness may be present for several months before radiographic changes are evident. A cardboard sound may be heard on percussion of the facial sinuses. Later, firm enlargements of facial bones occur above and behind the facial crests on each side of the skull. The mandibles become irregularly thickened. The nasal passages may become obstructed, resulting in upper airway noise. Cases have been observed in which the upper airway noise at exercise was the only thing noticed, and lameness or other abnormal physical findings were not evident. Resorption of dental alveoli may occur, causing the teeth to become loose or fall out, which results in abnormal chewing and decreased feed intake. Fractures of long bones of the legs and compression fractures of the vertebrae may occur.

Much of the lameness, tendinitis, and spontaneous fractures in racing Thoroughbreds in Australia has been speculated to be due to inadequate dietary calcium. Most of these horses' diet during racing and training consists of over 75% cereal grains, which contain less than 0.1% calcium and more than 0.3% phosphorus. Based on elevated renal clearance ratios of phosphorus, it was concluded that 40% of these horses were receiving inadequate calcium.

Calcium Deficiency/Phosphorus Excess Treatment

Treatment of a dietary calcium deficiency or phosphorus excess is to correct the diet by increasing calcium and/or decreasing phosphorus. For the first 2 to 3 months they should be twice that needed to meet the horse's requirements, after which they should be decreased to that required (Table 2–2). Ensure that the total diet Ca:P ratio is 1:1 to 3:1. Prolonged excessive calcium intake (greater than 5 times maintenance requirements) should be avoided: during recovery it may result in excessive bone density and inadequate bone remodeling, which may pre-

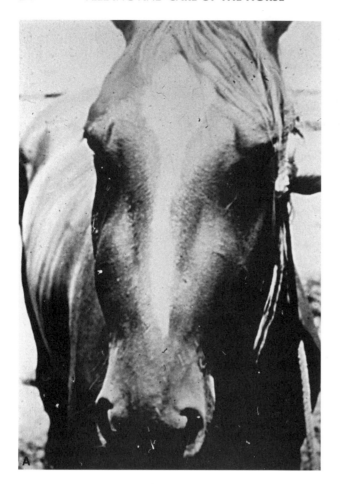

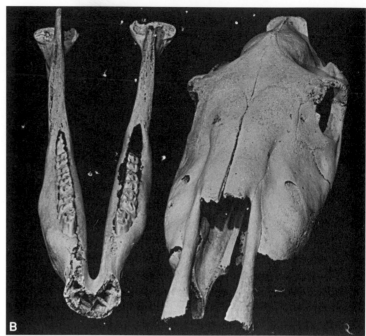

Fig. 2–2(A,B). Calcium deficiency due to either inadequate dietary calcium or excess phosphorus or oxalate, which decrease calciums absorption, causes nutritional secondary hyperparathyroidism. The increase in parathyroid hormone causes calcium and phosphorus mobilization from the bone and increases urinary phosphorus excretion. Bone minerals are replaced by fibrous tissue, which increases the size of the bone. In mature young horses, as shown in A, the increased size is often most noticeable on each side of the nose and on the lower jaw, giving rise to the common name for the condition "big-head." The skull of an affected horse (B) shows these enlargements. (Courtesy of JR Joyce, Texas A&M University.)

vent bone strength from returning to normal upon recovery. Affected animals should be confined for the first several months of the disease until radiographic density of the affected areas has returned to normal. Anti-inflammatory drugs may be indicated if pain is excessive, but should be used with caution. Reduced pain may result in increased physical activity, leading to fractures or more subtle complications. Lameness may disappear within 4 to 6 weeks after the diet has been corrected, but may not resolve in some cases, depending on the duration and severity of the condition. In many cases there is little regression of enlarged facial bones. Disappearance of the lameness and return of radiographic density doesn't indicate complete recovery. Nine to 12 months may be necessary for full recovery of normal bone strength.

When the calcium deficiency is due to excess oxalate intake, the preferred treatment is to decrease oxalate intake by not feeding high-oxalate-containing feeds, and, for the first 2 to 3 months, to feed a diet that provides twice the calcium and phosphorus required (Table 2–2) at a ratio of 1:1 to 3:1. After this time, ensure that the diet meets the horse's calcium and phosphorus requirement (Table 2–2). However, sometimes decreasing oxalate intake is not practical because low-oxalate feeds are not readily available. If lower-oxalate feeds are not fed, both calcium and phosphorus intakes must be increased to above normal

requirements, to prevent a net calcium and phosphorus loss from the body. This may be accomplished by making available to each horse once weekly 2.2 lbs. (1 kg) of a mixture of 60% molasses and 40% of a mineral containing 25 to 35% calcium and 12 to 18% phosphorus (Appendix Table 7). The additional calcium and phosphorus needed may also be provided by feeding a grain mix to which these minerals have been added; e.g., for a 1000-lb (450 kg) horse, adding 1 oz. (30 g) of a mineral containing 25% calcium and at least 12.5% phosphorus to a sweet feed daily.

Calcium Excess

Calcium Excess Effects

A sufficient excess of dietary calcium results in excess secretion of the thyroid hormone calcitonin. Calcitonin inhibits the conversion of cartilage to bone and the resorption of calcium from bone. This may result in bone and cartilage inflammation (osteochondrosis) predisposing affected horses to fractures. In addition, excess calcium is known to decrease some species' absorption of zinc, manganese, and iron, and may contribute to causing a deficiency if the diet contains only marginal amounts of these minerals. Whether this occurs in horses isn't known. Excessive, like inadequate, calcium does not result in changes in the plasma calcium or phosphorus concentrations sufficient to be of diagnostic benefit.

Calcium Excess Causes

Horses have been fed calcium at more than 5 times that required without detrimental effect, provided the level of phosphorus is adequate, if it is not, the problem is a phosphorus deficiency, not a calcium excess. However, greater than 2% calcium in the horse's diet dry matter, or more than 6 to 10 times that required, if fed continually over a long period of time, may be harmful. The major, if not only, way this occurs is if excess calcium-containing minerals are added to the diet. It is generally believed that a dietary calcium excess sufficient to be harmful to the horse does not occur from natural feeds commonly available, including high-calcium legumes, such as alfalfa.

Phosphorus Deficiency

As shown in Table 2–2, forage obtained from low phosphorus soils may contain less phosphorus than that needed by the mature horse for maintenance, and all feeds, except bran, contain considerably less phosphorus than needed by the young horse for rapid growth. The phosphorus content of forages, however, is higher in early than in late stages of plant growth. For example, the phosphorus content of smooth brome and orchardgrass early in their growth is 2 to 3 times what the horse needs for maintenance, whereas late in plant growth it may be less than that needed. Even when it is less than that needed, it causes little problem for mature horses on pasture all year because they are able to make up their phosphorus deficit in the spring, and generally in the fall, when they consume growing plants that are higher in phosphorus content.

The low phosphorus content of mature forages also causes little problem for the young horse receiving only pasture forage. Because of mature forage's low energy and protein, as well as low phosphorus, content, the horse's growth rate is slowed, decreasing its phosphorus needs. If the low intake of these nutrients is sufficient and sufficiently prolonged, the horse's mature size is decreased. Wild horses' smaller size is an example of this. Problems, however, arise if a faster growth rate and maximum mature body size are wanted, as is the case for most domestically raised horses. These goals are obtained by feeding grain and protein supplements. However, if the diet does not contain sufficient phosphorus, or other minerals, to support a faster growth rate, developmental orthopedic diseases may occur, as described in Chapter 16. Unfortunately, most mineral deficiencies don't slow growth rate significantly. Growth continues but without adequate minerals for skeletal development; as a result, skeletal problems occur.

Inadequate dietary phosphorus may be caused not only by inadequate amounts in the diet, but also by excessive amounts of substances that bind it, preventing its absorption. Excess calcium in a diet having a Ca: P ratio of greater than 6 to 10:1, or in the growing horse 3:1, may have this effect. Greater than 1500 ppm (mg/kg) of aluminum in the horse's diet also decreases phosphorus absorption to the extent that it may cause a negative phosphorus balance;

i.e., more phosphorus may be lost from the body than is consumed. On high-aluminum-containing acidic soils, forage may contain as much as 2500 ppm aluminum. Magnesium, zinc, iron, and copper utilizations by the horse are not affected by dietary aluminum levels as high as 4500 ppm. This amount of aluminum also doesn't decrease calcium absorption but, due to its inducement of a negative phosphorus balance, does result in increased urinary calcium excretion because enough phosphorus isn't available for calcium utilization in bone formation.

A dietary phosphorus deficiency results in bone demineralization and inadequate bone mineralization and, as a result, an increase in urinary and calcium excretion. Feed intake may decrease, resulting in weight loss, poor condition, and a rough hair coat. If sufficiently prolonged and severe, there may be shifting leg lameness and spontaneous fractures. The plasma phosphorus concentration is usually decreased, although the decrease may not be sufficient to be diagnostically significant. A phosphorus-deficiency-induced bone demineralization may not only increase urinary excretion of calcium but also of phosphorus. The increase in urinary phosphorus excretion, therefore, is the opposite of the nutritional imbalance that induced it, so is quite misleading. As with other dietary calcium and phosphorus imbalances, the only way to confirm their presence or absence, and the only way to ensure that the imbalance if present is adequately, but not over-corrected is to evaluate and correct the diet as described in Chapter 6.

SODIUM CHLORIDE SALT

Salt Utilization, Needs, and Feeding

Both sodium and chloride are needed in the diet for regulation of all body fluids, maintenance of the acid-base balance, and generation of the membrane potential and conduction of electrical impulses in nerves and muscles. For maintenance, the horse's diet dry matter should contain at least 0.1% sodium (i.e., 0.25% common salt, which is 39% sodium and 61% chloride); for work resulting in sweating, 0.3% (0.75% common salt). The chloride requirements for the horse have not been established, but they are thought to be met when sodium requirements are met with sodium chloride.

Many feeds contain less than 0.1% sodium, and thus less than that needed even for unexercised horses (Appendix Table 2). In addition, increased salt intake in the additional feed consumed as a result of exercise is not sufficient to compensate for increased sodium losses that may occur with exercise. Exercise increases salt requirements proportional to the amount that it increases sweating, as sweat contains a significant amount of both sodium and chloride.

To ensure that both sodium and chloride needs are met, 0.5 to 1% salt should be added to the grain mix fed, or instead, salt should be available at all times for free-choice consumption by all horses. In feeding horses, this is the only thing that needs to be done, since if salt is available, horses will consume enough to meet their needs. Sodium is the only mineral for which a clearly defined appetite exists and, therefore, if available, will be consumed by horses in an amount sufficient to meet their needs. Horses' salt needs can be met by providing either block or loose salt, although consumption of the loose form is generally greater.

Trace-mineralized salt is recommended to assist in providing some of the trace minerals needed. The additional cost of trace-mineralized salt is small and can be considered low-cost assistance in ensuring adequate intake of these minerals. Common trace-mineralized salt generally contains sodium chloride (98%), zinc (0.1 to 0.35%), manganese (0.20 to 0.28%), iron (0.15 to 0.35%), copper (0.02 to 0.04%), cobalt (0.05 to 0.007%), and iodine (0.007%). Trace-mineralized salt containing high levels of copper (0.25%), zinc (0.75%), and/or selenium (0.0025%) is also available. As 0.5% of the diet, it will meet lactating mares' and growing foals' requirements for these minerals, as well as for sodium, chloride, and iodine. Salt containing up to 0.009 and 0.012% (90 and 120 ppm or mg/kg) selenium is approved in the United States for sheep and cattle, respectively, and, therefore, is available. As 0.5% of the diet, this salt provides 0.45 and 0.6 ppm, respectively, in the diet, as compared to the 0.1 to 0.2 needed and the 2 to 5 upper safe level (Appendix Table 2). About one-third ounce (10 g) of this salt would provide the horse's selenium needs. Iodized salt contains 0.007% (70 ppm) iodine without any other trace minerals. Plain salt does not contain any iodine or other minerals. In contrast to what some people mistakenly believe or assume, none of these salts contain any calcium or phosphorus. Feeding common trace-mineralized salt for free-choice consumption or in a grain mix does not supply adequate minerals for the growing horse or the mare during late pregnancy or lactation. Trace-mineralized salt is generally blue-grey or dark reddish-brown in color: iodized salt, a lighter red; and plain salt, white (Fig. 2–3). However, the colors may vary, so don't rely on them. Look at the labels.

Although horses will consume sufficient salt to meet their needs if it is available, much of the salt they consume is based on preference or habit. There is a wide variation in the amount of salt consumed by horses under similar conditions. In one study, voluntary intake of salt from a block by mature unexercised horses averaged 53 g/horse/day (0.8 lbs/week), but varied from 9 to 143 g/day between horses, and from 5 to over 200 g by the same horse on

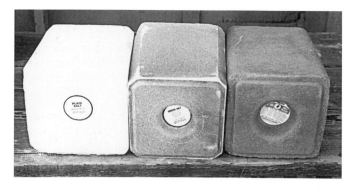

Fig. 2–3. Plain salt, iodized salt, and trace-mineralized salt. Trace-mineralized salt, available for free-choice consumption, is recommended.

different days. Voluntary salt intake by horses being fed hay and grain wasn't influenced by the season of the year. However, if horses are worked, salt intake increases, particularly during hot, humid weather. In addition, horses on pasture may consume more salt during periods of plant growth, as has been shown to occur in pastured ruminants. The variation in salt intake also, of course, greatly affects the intake of substances mixed with the salt.

Salt is occasionally mixed with various substances, such as calcium and/or phosphorus, as well as trace minerals, to increase the consumption of these minerals. Dry molasses and/or protein supplements may also be mixed with salt and other minerals to increase the intake of these minerals. While these procedures are generally effective in increasing the intake of substances mixed with salt and/or dried molasses, the variability in salt and therefore their intake may not ensure that the proper amount is consumed by each individual.

Although horses voluntarily consume more salt than needed, most prefer a grain mix without added sodium. Salt is sometimes used to limit feed intake, especially of grain or protein supplements, although this is not generally as effective in horses as in ruminants. The addition of at least 10% salt may be required to limit sufficiently the horse's intake of a grain mix.

A sufficient increase in salt intake above a threshold level increases water intake and urine excretion. Stalled horses allowed free access to salt may, because of boredom, consume excessive amounts of it, resulting in excess water consumption, and a wet stall. If this occurs, efforts should be made to relieve boredom, as described in Chapter 20. If the excess salt consumption cannot be alleviated, add an ounce (30 g or 2 tablespoons) of salt daily to the grain fed, and do not allow free access to salt.

From 75 to 95% of sodium and chloride ingested are absorbed, and excesses are excreted in the urine. As a result, urine sodium and chloride excretion vary directly with their consumption, whereas their fecal excretion is not affected by excess intake.

Sodium Chloride Salt Excess

Horses tolerate high levels of salt intake providing they have access to sufficient nonsaline-containing water. Salt toxicosis occurs as a result of: (1) horses' drinking salt brine (probably 1% or greater in sodium concentration) because other water is unavailable, (2) feeding salt to salt-hungry horses, or (3) including 2% or more salt in the diet without having adequate water available. Clinical signs of salt toxicosis include colic, diarrhea, frequent urination, weakness, staggering, paralysis of the hind limbs, recumbency, and death. Treatment is nonsaline-containing water provided in small amounts at frequent intervals; ideally, the first day 1 to 2 qts (or liters) every hour, then gradually increasing the amount given and decreasing the frequency. If too much nonsaline water is drunk too rapidly, excess water moves into the cells, causing cellular swelling. This is particularly harmful to the brain, where there is limited room for expansion. As a result, intracranial pressure increases, which decreases cerebral blood flow. Symptoms of central nervous system distress, such as blindness, head pressing, convulsions, coma, recumbency, and death, may occur.

Sodium Chloride Salt Deficiency

Horses consume salt in excess of their needs if it is available. As a result, a salt deficiency occurs only if the horse doesn't have access to salt. The time required for a deficiency to occur is shorter the greater the sodium and chloride losses are from the body. Thus, a deficiency is more likely to occur during lactation and increased sweating. A lack of sodium decreases milk production and sweating. Decreased sweating results in an increased body temperature and decreased performance.

If a sodium chloride deficiency occurs quite rapidly, muscle contraction and chewing become uncoordinated, gait becomes unsteady, and the plasma concentrations of sodium and chloride are decreased while potassium is increased. Generally, however, the deficiency develops over a longer period of time. The first effect of either a sodium or a chloride deficiency is a tendency for affected animals to develop an abnormal appetite and to lick objects that might have salt on them. If the deficiency isn't corrected, there is a decrease in the rate and the amount of food and water consumed. This results in weight loss, weakness, and dehydration. Constipation, increased water intake, and urination occur.

A chloride deficiency without a sodium deficiency, although not reported in horses, may occur, as it has in lactating cows, if sufficient sodium without chloride is provided, such as feeding sodium bicarbonate. In dairy cattle, clinical signs similar to those resulting from a sodium deficiency occur, and the plasma concentration progressively decreases for chloride and increases for bicarbonate. This decrease is one of the earliest and most diagnostic indications of a chloride deficiency in lactating cows.

POTASSIUM

Forages contain 1 to 4% potassium; cereal grains may contain 0.2 to 0.7 potassium, but usually have 0.3 to 0.5%, as compared to 0.4% recommended in the horse's diet (Appendix Table 2). Although 0.25% potassium may be adequate in the idle horse's diet, more than 0.6% may be needed for the horse in training or with frequent physical activity sufficient to result in substantial sweating. Thus, even during these periods, the horse's potassium requirements are met by most practical diets consisting of commonly used feeds. Excess potassium intake is not harmful, unless renal excretion is decreased, as excesses are readily excreted in the urine. If adequate water is not available, or renal function is sufficiently impaired to decrease potassium excretion, the horse won't eat; so even then, excess dietary potassium is not a problem, except in horses with potassium induced periodic paralysis, which is a genetic disease uncommon except in certain lines of Quarter Horses as described in Chapter 17. Thus, excess potassium intake is rarely a problem. In contrast, a potassium deficiency may occur and is quite detrimental.

Sweating increases potassium loss both in the sweat and in the urine. Sweating-induced water and sodium losses result in increased aldosterone secretion. Aldosterone increases renal reabsorption of sodium and excretion of potassium. Increases in urinary potassium losses are aggravated by the use of diuretics, such as furosemide (Lasix), which is commonly administered to try to decrease exercise-induced pulmonary hemorrhage (bleeders), as described in Chapter 11. The probability of a potassium deficit occurring as a result of these increases in potassium losses is more likely if a low-potassium diet, such as a high-grain low-forage diet, is fed. In one study, a net loss of body potassium occurred in horses exercised daily and fed a diet consisting of $\frac{1}{3}$ grass hay and $\frac{2}{3}$ oats—a diet typical of that often fed horses in training and use. Increased potassium losses also occur in horses with many diarrheal diseases who, in addition, may have a reduced potassium intake because they don't feel well and decrease their feed intake. Prolonged or frequent physical activity, such as endurance racing or training, particularly in a warm and/or humid environment, may also result in a potassium deficit, which may be a major factor responsible for causing post-exercise fatigue as described in Chapter 11.

Fatigue, muscle weakness, lethargy, exercise intolerance, and decreased water and feed intake are the major effects of a potassium deficit. Increased restlessness and timidity to noise have also been reported. Foals fed an experimental potassium-deficient diet gradually decreased their feed and, as a result, their potassium intake. They consequently lost weight and became unthrifty in their appearance.

Treatment of a potassium deficit includes increasing potassium intake and doing whatever is necessary or possible to decrease body potassium losses. Since one of the major effects of a potassium deficit is decreased appetite and, as a result, decreased feed intake, increasing potassium intake generally requires that potassium be administered. This is usually best accomplished by giving 2 to 3 gal (8 to 12 L) of an oral nutrient-electrolyte fluid high in potassium (e.g., Life-Guard, Norden Labs, Lincoln, NE 68501) every 4 to 8 hours until the horse is rehydrated and begins eating. When the horse is eating, potassium intake may be increased by adding several ounces (50 to 100 g) of "lite" or "low sodium" salt to the grain at each feeding. "Lite" or "low-sodium salt" is one-half sodium chloride, or common salt, and one-half potassium chloride, and contains 26% potassium. It can be purchased in most grocery stores, and is preferred to the more unpalatable "sodium-free" salt, which is entirely potassium chloride. This same procedure should be used to prevent a potassium deficit when potassium losses are increased, particularly if dietary potassium may be low, such as with a high-grain diet.

MAGNESIUM

The magnesium content of feeds commonly consumed by horses is 0.1 to 0.3%, as compared to the 0.1% needed in the horse's diet (Appendix Table 2). Thus, the horse's magnesium requirements are met by most diets consisting of commonly used feeds.

Although neither a magnesium deficiency or an excess has been reported in horses fed natural feeds, a low blood magnesium induced tetany responsive to magnesium and calcium administration has been reported in lactating mares and in horses during stress and fasting of transit. Both blood magnesium and calcium concentrations are generally reduced. This occurs most commonly in lactating cows and rarely in other cattle feeding on lush, green pasture. It may also occur: (1) in cattle during the stress and fasting of transit, (2) in cattle when poor-quality roughage is the only feed available during the winter, and (3) in calves receiving a total milk diet. In each situation there is decreased magnesium absorption and often increased magnesium losses from the body. Green rapidly growing grasses are low in magnesium and high in potassium, which decreases magnesium absorption and increases magnesium excretion in milk. Although this condition—called grass, transit, winter, or lactation tetany—has been reported in lactating mares, it is rare. Pastures conducive to causing tetany and death in ruminants do not affect horses similarly. This is probably because the horse absorbs magnesium much more efficiently than do ruminants. Ruminants absorb only 7 to 35% of the magnesium ingested, as compared to 40 to 60% absorption by horses.

When the blood magnesium falls, it results in nervousness, muscle tremors, and staggering, followed by collapse, increased respiratory rate, sweating, convulsions, and paddling. It is most frequently misdiagnosed as colic.

Death will occur within a few hours if magnesium-containing solutions are not given. Generally, solutions containing both magnesium and calcium are given intravenously.

In areas where low magnesium induced tetany tends to occur, its incidence may be decreased in both horses and cattle by feeding 1 to 2 oz (30 to 60 g) of magnesium oxide daily. Potassium magnesium sulfate (langbeinite) and magnesium sulfate (epsom salts or kieserite) are not recommended. Both are much lower in magnesium content (Appendix Table 7) than magnesium oxide, and the high potassium content (18.5%) of potassium magnesium sulfate makes it unsuitable because excess potassium is thought to be a causative factor (Appendix Table 7). Magnesium sulfate is also poorly palatable, although magnesium oxide is also fairly unpalatable. Although for cattle it is best to add magnesium oxide to a grain, or a mixture of 70% salt, 20% magnesium oxide, and 10% soybean meal or dry molasses, adding as little as 5% magnesium oxide to the salt may be effective in preventing grass tetany in horses, if it is the only salt available. Magnesium intake should be increased several weeks before and continued throughout the time of year when grass tetany is expected to occur. Excessive magnesium intake by the horse is not known to be harmful.

SULFUR

Sulfur is needed as a constituent of several amino acids (methionine, cystine, and cysteine) and vitamins (biotin and thiamin), as well as a number of other body constituents (e.g., coenzyme A, heparin, insulin, glutathione, lipoic acid, taurine, and chondroitin sulfate a component of cartilage, bone, tendons, and blood vessels). The concentration of sulfur-containing amino acids, and therefore sulfur, is highest in hoof and hair, which contain the protein keratin which is 4% sulfur. Sulfur concentration in water and feed may be reported as sulfate, sulfur, or sulfate sulfur. Concentrations reported as sulfur and as sulfate sulfur are the same. Sulfate is one-third sulfur; therefore, divide the sulfate concentration by three to obtain the sulfur concentration.

Sulfur requirements for the horse have not been determined. Most horse feeds contain at least 0.15% nonmineral or organic sulfur, which appears to be adequate to meet the horse's sulfur requirement. Most of the sulfur in plants, as well as animals, is organic sulfur present in the amino acids making up their protein. This is the only form of sulfur readily utilized by the horse.

A sulfur deficiency has not been reported in the horse. In other species it decreases appetite, growth, hair or wool growth, and milk production, and in the mature animal results in weight loss. Chronic excess dietary sulfur (greater than 0.3% in diet dry matter) in swine and ruminants decreases copper absorption, but there is no evidence that this occurs in horses. No detrimental effect from excess sulfur intake from high sulfur-containing feeds has been reported in horses. Excess sulfur is excreted in feces and urine. Fecal sulfur intake is closely correlated to sulfur intake. However mature horses accidentally fed 200 and 400 g of nearly pure inorganic sulfur (flowers of sulfur) became lethargic within 12 hours, followed by colic. There was a yellow frothy discharge from the nose, icterus, and labored breathing. Two of the 12 developed an expiratory snort, cyanosis, and convulsions, and died despite treatment.

SELENIUM AND VITAMIN E

Functions and Utilization

Selenium and vitamin E function jointly in protecting body tissue—particularly cell membranes, enzymes, and other intracellular substances—from oxidation-induced damage. Oxidation is the metabolic process by which fats, carbohydrates, and proteins are converted to carbon dioxide, water, and energy, i.e., burned to produce the energy needed for body functions. However, oxidation of the body's structural and functional components is harmful. Although not entirely accurate, a simple analogy is that gasoline is burned to provide the energy to run a car, but we don't want to burn up the car. The body must have an antioxidant defense mechanism to protect it from oxidation-induced damage. Selenium and vitamin E function as major components of this defense mechanism.

In the process of oxidizing organic or carbon-containing nutrients for energy, oxygen is used and carbon dioxide and water are produced. In the process of reducing oxygen to water, free radicals are produced. These free radicals are powerful oxidizing agents which, if they aren't destroyed, damage living cells, notably their proteins and lipids. Unsaturated fatty acids, which are the major component of all cell membranes, are particularly susceptible. Their oxidation is quite damaging to cell function. Vitamin E helps prevent this from occurring by blocking free radical attacks on lipids and thus the formation of lipid peroxides. Even with adequate vitamin E, some lipid peroxides form, but without adequate vitamin E, even more form.

Selenium functions as an integral part of the intracellular

enzyme glutathione peroxidase, which helps prevent the formation of free radicals and destroys lipid peroxides that form and are released into the cell. Thus, the occurrence and extent of oxidation-induced damage depends on: (1) the antioxidant protective mechanisms of the lipid-soluble vitamin E that is present in the cell membrane and decreases the formation of lipid peroxides, and (2) the water-soluble selenium-containing glutathione peroxidase in the aqueous intracellular fluid that removes those lipid peroxides that do form. Inadequate amounts of either result in increased oxidation-induced damage and, therefore, similar effects; giving either tends to treat or alleviate these effects. In addition, the amount of either needed by the animal depends on the amount of the other available. If there is inadequate vitamin E, more peroxides are formed and, therefore, more selenium is needed; conversely, if there is inadequate selenium, fewer peroxides can be removed and, therefore, more vitamin E is needed to prevent their formation. Optimum amounts of both, however, are necessary to minimize oxidation-induced tissue damage. These optimum amounts appear to be higher than the amounts needed to prevent clinically apparent disease. Thus, both selenium and vitamin E should be considered together, both in regard to the animal's requirements and in regard to the effects and treatment of a deficiency of either. However, some effects are more prominent as a result of a deficiency of one than the other, and are more responsive to the administration of that one.

A number of additional substances also have antioxidant activity and, therefore, can decrease vitamin E and selenium needs when their intake is high, but increase vitamin E and selenium needs when their intake is low. These include the sulfur-containing amino acids cystine and methionine, vitamin C, and the synthetic antioxidant ethoxyquin, which is commonly added to commercially prepared feeds. Ethoxyquin is readily absorbed and excreted, whereas vitamin E has a slower buildup but is maintained for a longer period. In addition, ethoxyquin can't replace vitamin E in some organs, such as the adrenals, which is one reason vitamin E in the diet can't be replaced entirely by synthetic antioxidants. In addition, vitamin E serves a number of other functions: it enhances the immune system; is essential for cellular respiration; is involved in DNA synthesis; acts as a cofactor in the synthesis of vitamin C; reduces signs of zinc deficiency; has a protective function against the harmful effects of lead, mercury and silver; decreases platelet aggregation; and enhances vitamin A absorption and storage. Ingestion of excess vitamin A, like excess unsaturated fatty acids, increases the amount of vitamin E needed, whereas ingestion of excess vitamin E decreases vitamin A reserves. These interactions are the reason most commercial preparations containing vitamins A and E contain both (and also vitamin D) at an optimum ratio for maximum absorption of each vitamin which is 5 IU of E and 150 IU of D per 1000 IU of A for the horse, whereas (2 to 3 of E and 100 of D is considered optimum for ruminants and swine).

Selenium Needs and Sources

The selenium requirement of the horse is estimated to be 0.1 ppm (mg/kg) of diet dry matter. Blood selenium

concentration is reduced at levels of 0.08 mg/kg, and signs of a deficiency occur at levels of 0.05 or less, while levels above 0.14 don't increase idle mature horses' plasma selenium concentration and, therefore, don't appear to be of any benefit to them. However, 0.2 ppm is recommended and may be of benefit for the horse in use or training and during the last trimester of pregnancy during lactation, and during growth. However it should not exceed 2 ppm, as excess selenium is quite toxic to all animals, particularly the horse. The minimum lethal dose for the horse is 3.3 mg/kg body weight (equivalent to 150 to 200 ppm of diet dry matter) as compared to 10 for cattle and 17 for pigs.

Feeds commonly consumed by horses may contain from 0.01 to 10 ppm of dry matter, but most contain from 0.05 to 0.3 (Appendix Table 2). Although some plants may contain from 50 to 10,000 ppm (Table 18-9) and thus cause acute selenium toxicosis, as described in the section "Selenium Toxicosis" in Chapter 18, horses rarely eat these plants even when they are available because of their poor palatability. Cases of acute toxicosis attributable to accidental oversupplementation with injections and feed supplements are reported more frequently than are those attributable to feeds having a naturally occurring high-selenium content. However, the amount of selenium present in feeds that are commonly consumed by horses may result in either a deficiency or, much less commonly, a chronic toxicosis.

Forages grown in most areas around the Great Lakes, in the eastern and western part of the United States, and in all of Canada (except the lower half of Manitoba, Saskatchewan, and Alberta) tend to be low in selenium (Fig. 2-4). Selenium deficiency is an important problem in all states except the four not reporting deficiencies (Del., R.I., W. Va., and Wyo.) and the nine reporting only mild or moderate deficiencies (Conn., Ga., La., Miss., N. Car., N. Hamp., S. Car., Tenn., and Texas). Selenium deficiency is a widespread problem throughout most of the United States. In a recent survey of state veterinarians and diagnostic laboratories, selenium deficiency was reported to be an important livestock problem in regions of 37 states, with mild or moderate deficiencies in 9 additional states. Selenium deficiency problems were not observed in only four states. In contrast, pasture forage grown in some areas of the Rocky Mountain and Great Plains states may contain toxic levels of selenium. Selenium toxicosis attributable to native plants was reported in eight states (Ca., Col., Idaho, Mont., Ore., S. Dak., Utah, and Wyo.). In all of these states, except Wyoming, selenium deficiency was also reported to be an important problem.

Forage selenium content varies from field to field and even in the same field. Soil selenium content and alkalinity are the major factors that influence the selenium content of plants. Selenium is taken up by plants more readily if the soil is alkaline, which is most common in areas of low rainfall (under 20 inches or 50 cm/yr). Selenium toxicosis is unlikely to occur from plants grown on acidic soils. Selenium deficiency from plants grown on humus, acidic soils is due to the formation of only slightly soluble selenium complexes with iron, as well as leaching losses. Liming acidic soils, as well as adding selenium and phosphorus to fertilizers, have been used successfully to increase forage

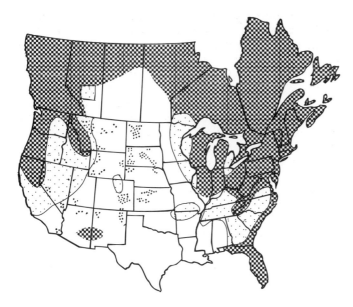

Fig. 2-4. Regional distribution of forage and grain selenium content in the United States and Canada.

▦ Low-approximately 80% of all forage and grain contain < .05 ppm of selenium.

▨ Variable-approximately 50% contains > .1 ppm.

▢ Adequate-80% of all forages and grain contain > .1 ppm of selenium

● Local areas where selenium accumulator plants contain >50 ppm.

selenium content and to prevent deficiencies in low-selenium areas. Properly done, these procedures also increase plant production and thus the amount of forage available.

Vitamin E Needs and Sources

Although there are eight forms of naturally occurring vitamin E that vary greatly in their biologic activity, d-alpha-tocopherol is the major and most active form in feeds and the only significant form in the horse's body. To function effectively as an antioxidant, vitamin E must be easily oxidized; as a consequence, naturally occurring forms and synthetic alcohol forms (tocopherols) are relatively unstable. Commercial synthetic forms that have been esterified, such as the tocopheryl acetates or acid succinates, do not have antioxidant activity until their ester linkage is broken in the digestive tract. As a result, tocopheryl esters are quite stable. Dl-alpha tocopheryl acetate is the form most widely used commercially. Moisture in stored feeds sufficient for fermentation and mold growth to occur (over 13%), as well as grinding, storage, and heat, all greatly decrease the vitamin E content of a feed. Nearly all vitamin E activity is lost in high-moisture feeds such as ensilage, haylage, and acid-treated grains.

Green growing forage contains 50 to 200 (100 to 450), average quality grass or legume hays 5 to 25 (10 to 60), dehydrated alfalfa pellets 10 to 35 (20 to 80) and cereal grains 2 to 15 (5 to 30) IU of vitamin E/kg dry matter. The amount in forages decreases with plant maturity: by 70 to 90% from early growth to maturity in grasses, and 35 to 65% in alfalfa from bud to post-flowering. Whole oilseeds are good sources of vitamin E, but most vitamin E has been removed from oilseed meals. From 30 to 80% of vitamin E activity is lost between cutting to baling hay; another 50 to 75% loss occurred in alfalfa hay stored at 97°F (33°C) for 12 weeks. A survey of 40 hays from various states showed that over 50% had a vitamin E content of less than 23 IU/lb (50/kg) while 15% had over 35 IU/lb (80/kg). Although no ill effects are observed in idle mature horses consuming less than 7 IU/lb (15/kg) diet dry matter, higher amounts appear to be beneficial and are recommended. Forty five IU/lb (100/kg) diet dry matter are needed to maintain maximum liver and muscle vitamin E levels.

Higher tissue vitamin E levels give greater antioxidant protection against tissue damage. This may be beneficial when nutrient oxidation increases in order to satisfy energy needs that occur with exercise or exertion. This benefit was demonstrated by the absence of muscle soreness and lameness of horses and zebras following their capture and restraint when their diets contained 100 IU vitamin E/kg; soreness and lameness occurred when their diet contained only 50 IU/kg. The lower vitamin E diet also resulted in lower plasma alpha-tocopherol concentrations. Lower tissue vitamin E levels not only increased the risk of exercise-induced muscle damage but may also decrease performance. Although not demonstrated in horses, exercise endurance of vitamin E-deficient rats has been found to be reduced by 40%.

In addition, although again not known for horses, dietary vitamin E requirement for optimum immune response in rats exceeds 23 IU/lb (50/kg) of diet and are thought to be as high as 45 (100). For these reasons, the National Research Council recommends 23 IU vitamin E/lb (50 kg) of diet dry matter for the idle mature horse and 35 to 45 (80 to 100) for foals, pregnant and lactating mares, and working horses. These recommendations seem appropriate, but they require vitamin E supplementation for all horses except those on adequate pasture during plant growth, since other horse feeds generally contain only 2 to 25 IU/lb (5 to 60/kg) of diet dry matter.

Supplemental vitamin E (usually at 6 to 20 times that recommended in the diet of the healthy animal) has been shown to enhance immunity in many different species of animals. As a result, when a herd or flock is infected with an infectious pathogen, vitamin E supplementation appears to lessen clinical signs of the disease, and the administration of vitamin E as an adjuvant to vaccination may improve efficacy of the vaccine.

In a number of species of animals, vitamin E needs are known to increase with increased intake of polyunsaturated fatty acids, which are high in vegetable oils. Adding vegetable oil to the horse's diet does not, however, appear to increase the horse's vitamin E needs.

Unlike the other fat-soluble vitamins, A and D, there are few available or mobilizable vitamin E stores in the body. The vitamin E concentration in the plasma and liver falls to pre-supplemented levels within 3 and 7 weeks, respectively, of stopping the supplementation. The drop takes slightly longer in the muscle and body fat. Thus optimum body vitamin E status decreases over the winter, or for more than a few weeks at the most of inadequate intake. If there is inadequate vitamin E in the horse's diet, then daily, or at a maximum weekly, supplementation is needed to correct it. A periodic vitamin E injection is not sufficient.

Also, unlike the other fat-soluble vitamins, A and D, excess vitamin E is relatively nontoxic. Signs or detrimental effects of vitamin E toxicosis have not been reported or produced in horses. Dietary levels of at least 500 to 900 IU/lb (1000 to 2000 kg) of diet dry matter can apparently be fed for prolonged periods without harm to rats and chicks. However, because very high intakes of vitamin E may interfere with utilization of other fat-soluble vitamins, and even induce a blood coagulation disorder in the mildly vitamin K-deficient dog, a conservative maximum tolerable level of 450 IU/lb (1000/kg) diet dry matter is recommended.

Selenium and Vitamin E Deficiencies

There are six general types of selenium/vitamin E deficiencies according to the organ system or tissues most affected. They differ in different species. These are:

1. Vascular disorders causing capillary leakage or loss of red blood cell integrity: e.g., exudative diathesis in chicks.
2. Nutritional myopathies that cause degeneration of smooth, cardiac, or skeletal muscle: e.g., white muscle disease in foals, calves, and lambs, mulberry heart disease in swine, and brown gut syndrome in dogs.
3. Encephalopathies: e.g., crazy chick disease and degenerative myeloencephalopathy in several species and possibly horses.
4. Vital organ damage that causes liver, kidney, or pancreatic damage: e.g., hepatosis dietetica in swine.
5. Reproductive disorders that involve spermatogenesis, sperm or ovarian function, or uterus or fetal development: e.g., infertility and retained placenta in cattle and sheep.
6. Adipose tissue inflammation and insoluble pigment accumulation that cause steatitis or yellow-fat disease in foals, calves, lambs, dogs, and cats. Steatitis is primarily affected by vitamin E rather than selenium.

These categories are not mutually exclusive, as varying degrees of two or more occur together in many cases, although one type will generally predominate. Nutritional myopathy, often accompanied by vascular disorders, particularly in newborn foals, and steatitis are the predominant forms occurring in horses.

Most horse feeds are relatively low in selenium (Fig. 2-4): they commonly contain less than the 0.1 ppm (mg/kg) needed by the horse and sometimes less than 0.05, at which signs of a deficiency may occur. Except for green forage, horse feeds are also relatively low in vitamin E, compounding the problems that occur with low levels of selenium.

Clinically apparent selenium or vitamin E deficiencies, however, are uncommon in horses other than foals from birth to 1 month of age, but may occur up to 8 months of age. They occur as a result of inadequate selenium intake by the dam during pregnancy or inadequate selenium and/or vitamin E intake during lactation. Selenium, but not vitamin E, is transferred across the placenta, and both are secreted into the milk, being particularly high in the colostrum. However, the amount of each transferred depends on how much of that nutrient is consumed by the mare.

The only observable effect of a mild deficiency of either selenium or vitamin E may be a decrease in the animal's immune response to infectious diseases, and with selenium slower growth. A decreased immune response increases the animal's susceptibility to, and the severity and duration of, infectious diseases, and decreases response to vaccinations. Although not confirmed in foals, immune response depression is well documented as an important predisposing cause of diarrhea in neonatal calves in selenium-deficient areas. Typically this diarrhea does not respond to routine therapy, but it will respond, and can be prevented, by giving the calf selenium injections at birth. Additional selenium-responsive disorders that quite likely occur much more commonly than do specific selenium-deficiency symptoms include: (1) decreased growth rate, (2) decreased efficiency of feed utilization, (3) decreased viability and motility of spermatozoa, (4) increased retained placentas, (5) decreased female fertility, (6) increased embryonic mortality, and (7) reduced milk production.

More severe deficiencies of selenium, vitamin E, or both, in foals, cause myopathies (muscle damage), steatitis (fat inflammation), or varying severities of both. Foals in which muscle damage is the major effect (which is the most common syndrome) may be stillborn, alive but affected at birth, or appear normal at birth but during the first weeks of life become stiff, weak, and listless, develop a stilted hopping gait in the rear legs, and have muscle pain. The tongue may be involved, resulting in difficulty in nursing and swallowing; this must be differentiated from botulism or shaker foal syndrome and lead toxicosis (Table 19-1). The tongue involvement and difficulty in swallowing may result in aspiration pneumonia. In severe deficiency cases, myoglobin that is lost from damaged muscles is excreted in the urine, giving it a pink to coffee-colored appearance. Both the skeletal and heart muscles may be affected. Young foals exhibit more heart, diaphragmatic, and respiratory muscle involvement. These foals develop heart failure, difficult respiration, and lung edema, and frequently die within a few hours to two days after the onset of clinical symptoms. Older foals may become recumbent and have a normal temperature, increased heart and respiratory rate, excess salivation, painful swellings under the mane, and loss of the surface layer of the tongue. Muscular exertion may initiate the onset of symptoms. Although uncommon, selenium and vitamin E deficiencies may occur in the mature horse, affecting the muscles of mastication, or those of the legs, resulting in a stiff, stilted gait.

Generalized fat inflammation, instead of muscle damage, may be the predominant effect of primarily a vitamin E, but also a selenium, deficiency, although this is uncommon. This situation occurs particularly in older foals up to several months of age, and may manifest as progressive emaciation and debilitation in spite of a good appetite.

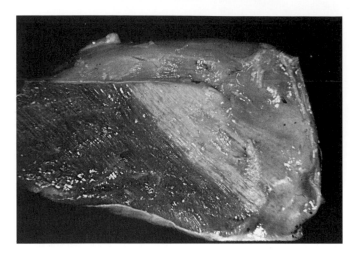

Fig. 2–5. White muscle disease induced by a selenium/vitamin E deficiency. A cross-section of muscle from an affected animal showing white areas of ischemic degeneration and calcification that give this disease this name.

Affected horses have multiple hard swellings composed of mineralized and dead fatty tissue and ligaments under the mane. Fluid may accumulate under the skin of the underline and legs due to capillary leakage. A rough, shaggy haircoat may also be present. There may be extensive or minimal skeletal muscle involvement.

When this inflammation occurs, fat deposits throughout the body are yellowish brown because of insoluble pigment accumulation, giving rise to the name "yellow fat disease." The fat has firm nodules and a gritty feel. Necropsy lesions evident in foals with muscle involvement include excess fluid under the skin and a white appearance of affected heart and skeletal muscles, particularly those of the hind legs, neck, and tongue (Fig. 2–5). Because of this, the condition is often referred to as "white muscle disease." Affected muscle fibers feel gritty when cut.

Selenium and vitamin E deficiencies, like most nutrient imbalances, are best diagnosed by determining the amount of these nutrients currently in the diet as compared to the amount required, as described in Chapter 6. Blood, serum, and/or tissue, but not urine, concentrations, are helpful or may be used instead of diet evaluation. Hair selenium content is indicative of selenium toxicosis but may be affected by intake of other minerals and environmental contamination.

A selenium deficiency should be treated by giving a preparation containing selenium and vitamin E intramuscularly, and either allowing free access to selenium-containing salt as the only salt available or adding additional selenium and vitamin E to the diet. In the United States, salt containing up to 90 ppm selenium (90 mg/kg) for sheep and 120 ppm (90 mg/kg) for cattle is allowed by the FDA. Either potency may be used for horses in selenium-deficient areas to assist in preventing a deficiency. Each additional 0.1% in the diet of these high selenium-containing salts increases the diet's selenium content 0.09 and 0.12 ppm (mg/kg). Thus, if the diet consisted of one-third grain mix, adding 0.5% of these salts to it adds 0.15 and 0.20 ppm selenium to the total diet (0.5% × 0.12 ppm/ 0.1% × ⅓ grain = 0.20 ppm). Instead of adding these salts to the diet, they may be fed as the only salt available. Consumption of 0.3 to 0.5 oz (10 to 15 g) per day would provide the selenium needed by the horse. Nearly 1 lb (454 g) daily would need to be consumed to cause selenium toxicosis, but this quantity is considerably more than the horse will voluntarily eat. In areas where selenium deficiency is a problem in foals, in addition to providing supplemental selenium for their dams, the foals should be given a selenium and vitamin E injection at birth. It may not be necessary to repeat this injection, providing their creep and weanling diets contain adequate amounts of selenium and vitamin E. Although not known in horses, the selenium blood level in cattle in selenium-deficient areas is still significantly above pre-injection concentration 6 months after its administration. Although parenteral administration of selenium and vitamin E to the mare in the last trimester of pregnancy and during lactation may be helpful, it may not prevent a deficiency in their foals. There is a relatively poor correlation between selenium levels in the mare's blood, her milk, and her foal's blood. Care must be taken, however, not to add excess selenium to the diet, as more than 2 to 5 ppm is toxic.

Selenium toxicosis may be acute or chronic, depending on the amount of selenium ingested. The most common causes of toxicosis are dosage errors made in selenium injections and in mixing feeds; less often, it results from ingestion of plants containing toxic amounts of selenium. These plants and selenium toxicosis are discussed in Chapter 18.

Equine Degenerative Myeloencephalopathy (EDM)

A vitamin E, but not selenium, deficiency also results in brain tissue degeneration, without muscle or fat involvement, in many species of animals, and it may occur in horses. Vitamin E deficiency is known to cause encephalomalacia in chicks and degenerative myeloencephalopathy in rats, dogs, monkeys, and people. Degenerative myeloencephalopathy is a diffuse, degenerative disease of the spinal cord and brain stem. In horses, it occurs in both sexes and many different breeds. It most commonly affects foals 1 to 14 months old. Although it may not become apparent until the horse is 2 to 4 years old, signs usually develop at less than 1 year and often at less than 6 months of age. However, EDM may occur in horses from 12 to 20 years of age. The disease develops insidiously as a symmetric spasticity, staggering, and paresis. The onset of gait abnormalities may occur abruptly or, more commonly, progress slowly and stabilize for long periods. Degenerative myeloencephalopathy involves all four legs, although the hind legs commonly are affected more profoundly. Severely affected horses may fall while running. Because of these symptoms, the condition caused by EDM, along with other causes of spinal cord disease in the horse, may be referred to as "wobblers syndrome." There are several causes of "wobblers syndrome," as described in Chapter 16, EDM being one of the most common.

Although the cause of EDM is not known, there appears to be a genetic predisposition. Use of insecticides (mostly pyrethrins) on foals and pregnant mares, exposure to wood preservations/sealers (mostly creosote and oil based) on stables and fences, and frequent periods outside on dirt were also found to increase the risk of EDM, whereas being outside on green pasture decreased the risk. Although a copper deficiency may cause neurologic disease, horses with EDM have been found to have normal blood and liver copper concentrations. Several factors suggest, however, that a vitamin E deficiency is a risk or predisposing causative factor.

Many horses with EDM have a low plasma vitamin E concentration. In addition, vitamin E supplementation decreases the incidence of EDM; long-term vitamin E supplementation (6,000 IU/day) results in clinical improvement in horses with EDM, especially when treated at the onset of symptoms; and a vitamin E deficiency is known to be the cause of EDM in several other species. In one study of 56 cases, however, neither vitamin E nor selenium administration had a significant effect on the risk of EDM. Thus, it appears that EDM occurs in genetically predisposed foals, but what additional factors are necessary for it to occur are unknown. Vitamin E supplementation at 2,000 IU per horse daily for prevention and 6000 IU per horse daily for treatment may be beneficial.

Vitamin E and Reproduction

A vitamin E deficiency is known to impair reproduction in both males and females of many species of animals. The impairments include repeat breeding, early embryonic death, abortion, retained placenta, and degenerative changes in the testes. Although these effects have not been reported in horses, and, as the National Research Council reports, there is no substantial evidence to indicate that vitamin E supplementation helps resolve reproductive problems in horses, vitamin E occasionally is recommended and given to horses to improve reproductive efficiency. Numerous studies, however, have failed to confirm any benefit of vitamin E supplementation in regard to the stallion's or mare's reproductive performance or libido.

IODINE

Utilization, Needs, and Sources

The thyroid gland, lactating mammary gland, and placenta can concentrate iodine from the blood for thyroid gland use, in the milk for their nursing young, and in the amnionic fluid for their fetus, respectively. The ability of these body organs to concentrate iodine from the blood helps protect that animal, the nursing young, and the fetus against a deficiency when dietary iodine is low, but contributes to toxicosis in the fetus or young when the mother's iodine intake is high.

The only known function of iodine in the body, and the reason for its necessity in the diet, is synthesis of the iodine-containing thyroid hormones. An increase in thyroid hormones results in a decrease in thyroid-stimulating hormone (TSH) secretion, an increase in metabolic rate, and consequent oxygen utilization and heat production. A decrease in thyroid hormones, or an increase in TSH, causes a similar change in the production and secretion of thyroid hormones, thus completing a classic negative feedback loop so common in body function.

The iodine content of most horse feeds is 0.05 to 0.2 ppm in its dry matter, but may vary from 0 to 2 ppm, as compared to the horse's estimated requirement of 0.1 ppm (1 to 2 mg/horse/day), with 5 ppm (40 mg/horse/day) being harmful (Appendix Table 2). Thus, an iodine deficiency, but not toxicosis, may occur in the horse fed common horse feeds. A deficiency can be prevented, however, by adding 0.5 to 1%, or as little 0.5 oz (14 g)/horse/day, of iodized or trace-mineralized salt, which contains 70 ppm iodine, to the grain mix fed. Having an iodine-containing salt as the only salt available at all times for free-choice consumption, although generally adequate to prevent iodine deficiency, may not suffice for some mares during pregnancy and lactation because of the wide variability in the amount of salt consumed. Some may consume adequate salt and, therefore, iodine, while others may not. As a result, an iodine deficiency may occur in some foals while not in others in the same herd, even though an iodine-containing salt is readily available for them and their dams.

Deficiencies and Excesses

Iodine Deficiency and Excess Causes

Iodine-deficient areas are known to occur on every continent. In North America, iodine levels below those needed to meet the horse's requirement are most likely to occur in feeds grown in areas adjacent to the Great Lakes and scattered areas of western United States and Canada. Although soils low in iodine tend to produce iodine-deficient plants, there is sometimes little relationship between iodine levels in the soil and in the plant. Soils in areas of recent glaciation, in areas distant from the sea, and in areas of low annual rainfall are most likely to be iodine deficient. Climate, soil type, fertilizer application, and many other factors are known to influence the iodine content of plants. Even in iodine-deficient areas, however, an iodine deficiency will not occur if the procedures given previously are followed.

Horses, particularly during late pregnancy and lactation, appear to be less tolerant of excessive iodine intake than are other species of domestic animals. In recent years, iodine toxicosis in horses has been much more frequently reported than iodine deficiency. Iodine toxicosis may occur as a result of any one of the following situations:

1. Adding more than 4 to 8% iodized or trace-mineralized salt to the total diet. Even though voluntary salt consumption by the horse is quite variable, no cases of iodine toxicosis have been reported in horses as a result of having these iodine-containing salts available for free-choice consumption. For them to cause iodine toxicosis, the mare would have to consume over 1 lb (454 g) daily.
2. Feeding seaweed (kelp), or a sufficient amount of products containing it. Seaweed may contain as much as 1850 ppm of iodine, at which level more than 0.7 oz (20 g) of it/horse/day would be harmful.
3. Feeding an excessive amount, or several, iodine-containing compounds or commercial supplements con-

taining them; e.g., potassium or sodium iodates or iodides, which are 59, 76, 64, and 84% iodine, respectively.

4. Feeding more than 40 to 50 mg/horse/day of an organic iodine, such as EDDI (ethylene diaminedihydroiodide, which is 82% iodine). EDDI is occasionally added to the horse's (more commonly cattle's and sheep's) diet to treat or try to prevent respiratory disease, ringworm, chiggers, or other diseases caused by organisms thought to be inhibited or killed by sufficiently high levels of iodine.

Iodine Deficiency and Excess Effects

Either an iodine deficiency or toxicosis may result in hypothyroidism and thyroid gland hypertrophy or goiter (Fig. 2-6). With iodine deficiency, an insufficient amount of iodide is available to synthesize an adequate amount of iodine-containing thyroid hormones. With iodine toxicosis, on the other hand, excess iodide inhibits thyroid hormone synthesis and/or release by its direct effect on the thyroid gland. In either case, the reduced level of thyroid hormones results in increased TSH secretion. TSH stimulates thyroid gland enlargement in an attempt to increase thyroid hormone secretion and thus correct the hypothyroidism.

Hypothyroidism and goiter may be caused not only by either a deficiency or excess of iodine, but also by the ingestion of large amounts of goitrogenic plants or the administration of antithyroid substances. Goitrogenic plants, such as kale, white clover, rutabaga, turnips, and other plants of the Brassicaceae family, are high in perchlorates, nitrates, or thiocyanates, which interfere with iodide accumulation in the thyroid gland. This effect can be overcome by increased iodine intake. The antithyroid substances, such as thiouracil-, thiourea- and methimazole-containing drugs, do not inhibit iodide uptake but interfere with thyroid hormone synthesis; their effect, therefore, cannot be overcome by increased iodine intake. Although

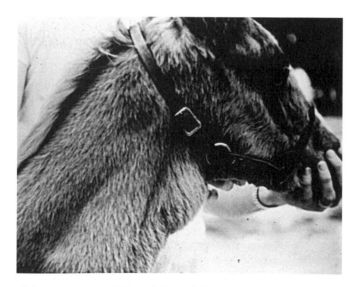

Fig. 2-6. Goiter. Enlarged thyroid glands, which may occur as a result of either a deficiency or excess of iodine.

these plants and antithyroid substances probably have the same effects in horses as they do in other species, I am not aware of any reports of hypothyroidism or goiter due to either occurring clinically in the horse.

Even though iodide is concentrated by the placenta and in the milk, the effects of an iodine deficiency, as well as toxicosis, in horses most commonly occurs or is recognized in newborn foals as a result of inadequate or excessive iodine intake by their dams. Because both an iodine deficiency and toxicosis cause hypothyroidism, their effects are similar. Affected foals are born dead or, if alive, are weak, have difficulty in standing, have a weak or poor suckle response, generally have persistent hypothermia (rectal temperature less than 100°F or 37.8°C), and may have noticeably enlarged thyroid glands (Fig. 2-6). Affected foals may also have respiratory distress due to impaired or incomplete surfactant development. Thyroid hormones have a central role in the development and maturation of several organ systems, including the pulmonary system and its synthesis of lung surfactant. Because of either respiratory or central nervous system disorders that result in weakness and abnormal suckling, most affected foals die within the first few days of life. Affected foals may also have angular leg deformities present at birth or occurring within the first few days of life as a result of the collapse of inadequately ossified carpal or tarsal bones of the knee and back. This may also occur as a result of premature birth of the nonhypothyroid foal.

In full-term normal foals, ossification of carpal and tarsal bones occurs rapidly during the last few weeks of pregnancy and continues less rapidly during the first month of life. This is delayed by hypothyroidism. Hypothyroidism also delays closure of bone growth plates and in affected foals may result in osteochondritis dissecans, subchondral bone cysts, foreleg contracture, extensor tendon rupture, mandibular prognathism, and/or scolioses. These developmental orthopedic diseases of foals, as discussed in Chapter 16, may be caused by a number of other nutritional and non-nutritional factors. In addition, these effects, like thyroid gland enlargement, may occur as a result of either an iodine deficiency or toxicosis. With an iodine deficiency, affected foals may, but frequently do not, have an enlarged thyroid gland (Fig. 2-6), but it is abnormal microscopically. Dams of affected foals may exhibit abnormal estrous cycles but usually do not have thyroid gland enlargement or show other signs of iodine deficiency. However, in mares given 350 mg of potassium iodide (76% iodine) daily for about one year 17 of 39 aborted, and some mares had goiter. One stillborn foal and three that were very weak at birth had large goiters, whereas the remainder had weak fetlocks but no goiter. When iodine supplementation was stopped, foals born 6 to 8 weeks later seemed to be normal.

Other effects of either an iodine deficiency or toxicosis include the following:

1. A dry, lusterless haircoat and hair loss. An iodine deficiency is one of the few things that will cause the birth of hairless (or woolless) young, although this has not been reported in foals. In contrast, diffuse hair loss and dry skin scaliness over the entire trunk

has been reported in a horse given 90 g of EDDI daily for 18 days. This would provide 74 g/day of iodine, or over 1500 times the amount that, when fed to mares, may be harmful to her fetus or nursing foal.

2. Occasionally a thickened skin due to accumulation of mucinous material under the skin referred to as myxedema, particularly in the distal limbs of iodine-deficient foals.
3. In the fetus or young animals, decreased growth and decreased bone calcification resulting, in severe cases, in skeletal deformities leading to coarse heavy extremities and a short body, which is referred to as cretinism. This is not known to occur in horses.
4. Lethargy, dullness, drowsiness, and timidity.
5. Inappetence.
6. Cold intolerance and persistent hypothermia.

An iodine toxicosis may also increase susceptibility to infectious diseases and decrease response to treatment for them. An iodine toxicosis may in the horse, as has been reported in cattle, result in what appears to be a chronic respiratory disease, with coughing, low-grade fever, excessive lacrimation, and nasal discharge that respond poorly to treatment for an infectious condition.

Iodine Deficiency and Excess Diagnosis

Although with hypothyroidism from any cause plasma T_3 and T_4 concentrations are reduced, their resting levels in the foal are quite variable and are not helpful in diagnosis. In one study, plasma total T_3 concentrations ranged from 26 to 733 ng/dl and total T_4 concentrations from 4.4 to 25.1 ng/dl in 10 normal 1-day-old foals. These concentrations are higher than in older foals, adults, and other newborn animals. Plasma T_3 concentrations were found to increase from 24 to 48 hours after birth then decline during the following two weeks. The increase in plasma T_3 concentration in response to TSH administration can be used, however, to determine if hypothyroidism is present. Normal foals the first few days of life respond to the administration of either TSH (5 IU given IV) or TRF (500 µg IM) with a doubling or greater of plasma total and free T_3 concentrations within 1 to 3 hours, and a 16% or greater increase in total T_4 concentration within 3 to 6 hours.

In mature horses, thyroid hormone levels decrease with advancing age and excess dietary protein. In one study it was found that serum free and total T_4 concentrations decreased 0.01 µg/dl for each percent increase in dietary protein above that recommended (Appendix Table 1). The T_4 concentrations were also low in horses eating diets containing excess zinc and copper, but were high in horses eating diets high in manganese and magnesium. In contrast, serum T_3 concentrations were not affected in any specific way by the diet.

With iodine toxicosis, the mare's plasma protein-bound iodine concentration may be increased above the normal of 16 to 27 µg/L. However, the foal may be affected by iodine toxicosis even when the mare's plasma protein-bound iodine concentration is normal.

Iodine Deficiency and Excess Treatment

Treatment for iodine deficiency or toxicosis is to correct the dietary imbalance present. However, since both may cause hypothyroidism and similar symptoms, it is important to determine whether the horses have consumed too little or too much iodine. The best and surest way to do this is to evaluate the diet as described in Chapter 6. If no supplemental sources of iodine (iodine-containing salt or supplements, or organic iodine) or seaweed are being fed, the problem is probably a deficiency, whereas if any of these substances are being consumed, a deficiency is unlikely. It is important to realize, however, that an iodine deficiency may occur in some mares, and as a result, affect their foals, while it may not occur in other mares in that same herd, even when iodine-containing salt is available for free-choice consumption. Once symptoms due to an iodine deficiency occur, treatment is not generally very effective. The nursing foal with iodine toxicosis must be fed an alternate source of milk low in iodine since its dam's milk contains excess iodine. Oral administration of thyroid hormone as well as supportive care may be indicated for affected foals.

COPPER

Copper is involved in bone collagen stabilization, elastin synthesis, the mobilization of body iron stores, and synthesis of the body pigment melanin. Impairment of the latter two functions causes anemia and a loss of hair color in copper-deficient ruminants, but neither of these effects occurs in copper-deficient horses. However, impairment of the first two functions does occur in horses as a result of a copper deficiency, and may result in developmental orthopedic diseases in young horses as described in Chapter 16, and in aorta or uterine artery rupture, particularly in aged foaling mares.

The liver regulates copper metabolism by storing it, incorporating it into the protein ceruloplasmin for vascular transport to the rest of the body, or excreting it in bile. Urine excretion is minimal. Copper is absorbed from all areas of the gastrointestinal tract except the rumen and large intestine. The percent absorbed decreases with increasing intake. Although copper absorption is decreased if there is more than 0.3% sulfur, or 1 to 3 ppm molybdenum (or a dietary Cu:Mo ratio of less than 2:1) in the diet dry matter of ruminants, even much higher levels of either mineral do not have this effect in horses. Even molybdenum levels several times higher than generally present in horse feeds, and a Cu:Mo ratio of 1:4 in the diet, did not appear to interfere with the horse's copper utilization. Copper absorption and retention by horses were reduced, however, when molybdenum was 107 and copper 13 ppm of diet. Excess zinc, like molybdenum and sulfur, decreases ruminants' copper absorption but doesn't have this effect in horses. However, greater than 700 ppm zinc in horses' diets appears to interfere with copper utilization other than by decreasing its absorption, resulting in a decreased plasma copper concentration and developmental orthopedic diseases.

The copper content of horse feeds ranges from 0.5 to 35, but most commonly is 3 to 20 ppm (Appendix Table

2). Plants low in copper content usually grow on either sandy soils that are heavily weathered, or peat or muck soils that may have previously been swampy. The amount of copper needed in the horse's diet is not clearly defined. A copper deficiency rarely occurs in mature horses even though horse feeds commonly contain less than the 10 ppm recommended by the National Research Council. However, 50 ppm copper in the dry matter is recommended in creep feeds and 25 in weanlings' total diet (i.e., for horses from 2 to 12 months of age), after which time one-third this level is probably adequate. Although these amounts may be more than needed, as discussed in Chapter 16, they may help decrease the risk of developmental orthopedic diseases (DOD), and do so at little additional feeding cost and without risk of harm.

Inadequate copper intake doesn't slow the foal's growth rate, rapid growth continues but without adequate copper for normal bone and cartilage development, resulting in decreased bone density and DOD. As discussed in Chapter 16, there are a number of nutritional as well as non-nutritional factors besides a copper deficiency that may cause or predispose to the occurrence of DOD. A correlation between the occurrence of these diseases and reduced concentrations of calcium, phosphorus, zinc, and copper, but not the amount of other nutrients, in weanlings' diets has been noted. The incidence of these diseases decreased significantly when the amount of these minerals, particularly copper, in the diet were increased.

Foals weaned at 1 day of age and fed an experimental low-copper milk replacer developed an intermittent but nondebilitating diarrhea at the onset of a decrease in their plasma copper concentration. Lameness was evident 2 to 6 weeks later. They had a stilted gait and walked on their toes in a manner similar to foals with flexure deformities. Soluble collagen in the articular cartilage and aorta increased, and osteochondritis dissecans was present in many of their joints. However, their growth rate wasn't reduced and, in contrast to copper-deficient ruminants, neither anemia nor a decrease in hair color occurred.

Horses are quite resistant to excess copper intake. Ponies have been reported to tolerate dietary copper as high as 791 ppm (a level that killed lambs within 3 months) for 6 months with no adverse effects, except for an increase in their liver and kidney copper content. One of the ponies had a normal foal about 4 months after being fed this high amount of copper. Feeding horses a diet containing 2800 ppm copper for 2 months caused increased blood copper concentration, hepatic and renal damage, and the death of horses by 6 months. The horse's high tolerance to excess copper ingestion may be in part because copper absorption by the horse decreases with increasing copper intake. Thus, copper toxicosis does not occur at 791 but does at 2800 ppm.

MOLYBDENUM

Molybdenum is an essential component of various enzymes involved in purine metabolism, particularly their degradation to uric acid. Purines are a component of nucleic acids, such as in DNA and RNA. Excess nitrogen in birds is excreted as uric acid, whereas in most mammals, including horses, excess nitrogen is excreted as urea. Thus, birds require considerably more molybdenum than do mammals. The major effect of inadequate molybdenum in both birds and mammals is decreased growth rate.

Common horse feeds contain 0.1 to 10, but more commonly 0.3 to 8, ppm molybdenum in dry matter (Appendix Table 2). However, plants growing on soils industrially contaminated with or naturally high in molybdenum may contain over 200 ppm. Soils of shale and granite origin are likely to be high in molybdenum. Plants grown on these or poorly drained soils, or soils with a neutral to alkaline pH, are likely to be high in molybdenum.

The amount of molybdenum needed or toxic to horses hasn't been determined but appears to be well within the range of that commonly present in horse feeds, since neither a confirmed molybdenum deficiency nor a toxicosis has ever been reported in horses. In fact, a confirmed molybdenum deficiency, natural or experimental, has never been reported in any animal. However, additional molybdenum given to lambs on a very low molybdenum diet has been shown to increase their growth rate. The requirement for beef cattle is only 0.01 ppm or less in diet dry matter. Thus, it appears that the horse's molybdenum requirement is probably considerably less than the lowest amount generally found in common horse feeds: 0.1 mg/kg dry matter.

The major concern in regard to molybdenum is excess, not deficiency, because molybdenum interferes with copper utilization. Although ruminants' copper absorption is decreased by as little as 1 to 3 ppm molybdenum in diet matter, or a Cu:Mo ratio of less than 2:1, even much higher amounts of molybdenum don't appear to have any detrimental effect in horses. High molybdenum pastures, which result in severe disease in cattle, do not affect horses grazing these pastures. Molybdenum levels of 20 ppm in diet dry matter and a Cu:Mo ratio of 1:4 did not decrease horses' plasma copper concentration or appear to interfere with their utilization of copper. Much of the excess molybdenum ingested by horses is absorbed and rapidly excreted in the urine. The excess molybdenum ingested, therefore, doesn't remain in the intestinal tract to interfere with the absorption of other minerals. A persistent protein-bound thiomolybdate, which forms in ruminants consuming excess molybdenum and is thought to be responsible for causing the decrease in their copper utilization, doesn't appear to form in horses consuming excess molybdenum. However, a Cu:Mo ratio of 1:8 with 107 ppm molybdenum in diet dry matter (over 10 times that commonly present in horse feeds but less than half that which has been found in forages) did decrease horses copper absorption and retention.

ZINC

Utilization

Zinc's major function in the body is to act as a component of many enzymes involved in protein and carbohydrate metabolism. Its absorption is regulated by the animal's needs and may vary from 5 to 90%. Its urine excretion is small and does not differ with dietary zinc intake in excess of that needed. It isn't known whether phytate or excess calcium decrease zinc absorption in horses, as they are known to do in several other species. If they do, it's not sufficient, at least with the amount of phytate in common horse feeds or calcium in practical diets, to cause a recognized problem.

Zinc Needs and Deficiency

Forty ppm zinc in diet dry matter has been recommended as the amount needed for all horses. Foals fed an experimental synthetic diet containing 4 ppm but not 40 ppm zinc had clinical signs similar to those reported in other species as a result of a zinc deficiency. These included decreased feed intake and growth rate. Only if the zinc deficiency is sufficiently severe do additional effects occur, which include parakeratoses (especially of the lower legs) ranging from small patches of dry rough skin to severe acne. Hair loss, lethargy, diarrhea, decreased serum and tissue zinc concentrations, and decreased plasma alkaline phosphatase and lactic dehydrogenase activities (zinc-containing metalloenzymes) may also occur. Studies have shown that 18 ppm zinc in diet dry matter during pregnancy and lactation is adequate.

Feeds commonly fed horses often contain as low as 15 ppm zinc (Appendix Table 2). Yet a naturally occurring zinc deficiency, detrimental effects from inadequate zinc intake, or, conversely, any beneficial effects for the mature horse of adding additional zinc to the diet, have not to my knowledge been reported. Because of this, it appears that 15 ppm in diet dry matter is adequate for mature horses. However, even the 40 ppm that has been recommended by the NRC for all horses may not be adequate to minimize the risk and incidence of developmental orthopedic diseases (DOD) in young horses.

Bone density was significantly higher in Thoroughbred yearlings fed for 5 months a diet supplemented to contain zinc 60, copper 9.5, manganese 57, and iron 127 ppm than in those fed the same diet unsupplemented, which contained zinc 32, copper 6.5, manganese 48, and iron 100 ppm. Based on a farm survey, the incidence of DOD was found to be lower in young horses fed diets higher in zinc, copper, and calcium. Three-month-old foals fed a diet containing 152 ppm zinc had fewer cartilage defects at 6 months of age than those fed a diet containing 42 ppm, and a similar number of defects to those fed diets containing 80 ppm. All of these diets contained 35 ppm copper.

Although 40 ppm zinc in diet dry matter, or even less, may be adequate for the rapidly growing horse, as these studies suggest, higher amounts may be of benefit. Because of this, the minimal increased feeding cost for additional zinc as compared to the loss of not adding it if higher levels are of benefit, and because of no known risk from the higher levels recommended, at least 60 ppm zinc in of total diet dry matter is recommended for foals, and 40 for yearlings.

Zinc Excess

The horse is quite resistant to high zinc intake. Although excess zinc decreases copper absorption by ruminants, as high as 1200 ppm zinc in diet dry matter did not decrease copper absorption by the horse. However, greater than 700 ppm appears to interfere with copper utilization by means other than decreasing its absorption, resulting in DOD. DOD has been a consistent manifestation of excessive zinc intake in young horses, swine, cattle, and rats. Hock effusions, bone growth plate enlargements, and chronic swelling, followed by joint cartilage detachment from underlying bone, radiographic lesions similar to those with osteochondritis dissecans, and flexure deformities, have been reported in young horses as a result of excessive dietary zinc. Initially there are enlargements of the growth plates of long bones without apparent pain. This is followed by lameness with a stiff gait or reluctance to move. Severely affected foals will often stand with their head held low, have an arched back, and resist curving the spine laterally when turned to the side. Decreased growth rate, poor condition, and progressive anemia may also occur. Foals fed 3600 ppm zinc in their diet dry matter developed anemia and had decreased growth, enlarged growth plates of the long bones of the legs, stiffness, lameness, and increased blood and tissue zinc concentrations.

Most clinical cases of zinc toxicosis have been due to pastures contaminated by airborne pollution from zinc smelters or mines, brass foundries, and other industries, such as galvanized iron manufacturing plants. Other causes include zinc oxide top-dressing of pastures, excess zinc in grain mixes due to mixing errors, and excess zinc in water. Zinc may be released into the water by electrolysis when galvanized and copper pipes are joined.

MANGANESE

Manganese is essential for carbohydrate and lipid metabolism and for the synthesis of chondroitin sulfate necessary for cartilage formation. These are functions involved primarily in growth and reproduction; a manganese deficiency will therefore affect primarily these functions. Manganese is also a superoxide scavenger decreasing free-radical damage, which includes lipid peroxidation, membrane rupture, and cell death in a wide variety of normal and disease conditions, including ischemia and inflammatory conditions.

In ruminants, manganese absorption is decreased by excessive ingestion of calcium, phosphorus, and iron; conversely, excessive manganese decreases the absorption of these minerals. Whether these effects occur in horses isn't known. Excess manganese is stored in the liver and kidney and is excreted in the bile.

The amount of manganese needed by the horse is not known. Based on other species, 40 ppm in diet dry matter has been recommended for all classes of horses. This amount appears to be more than needed. Although common horse feeds contain from 3 to 170 ppm (Appendix Table 2), total diets containing less than 20 are not uncommon, particularly in areas such as the northwestern United States, where manganese deficiencies are a problem in ruminants. However, the only known case or report of a suspected manganese deficiency in the horse was thought to have occurred as a result of excessive lime added to the soil. Thus, it would seem that 20 ppm diet dry matter or less is adequate for horses.

A manganese deficiency in ruminants, swine, and poultry manifests primarily in the newborn and in impaired reproductive performance. Its effects include sterility, decreased libido, delayed estrus, decreased conception, poor growth, and abortion or stillbirths. Manganese deficiency also results in birth of weak young that may show incoordination or have leg deformities such as enlarged joints, knuckled-over pasterns, twisted forelegs, and bones that are weak, thickened, well calcified, brittle, and shortened, resulting in lameness, stiffness, joint pain, bowed legs, and a reluctance to move. A manganese deficiency has been implicated, but not confirmed, as a cause of similar skeletal afflictions in newborn foals. The suspected manganese deficiency was thought to have occurred as a result of a greatly reduced manganese availability caused by extensive liming of the soil required to offset acidic effects of smelter effluent.

Although excessive manganese intake is known to be harmful to other species, harmful levels are not known for the horse. Manganese toxicosis does not appear to occur naturally in the horse, even with the ingestion of large amounts over a long period of time.

IRON

Utilization, Needs, and Sources

Iron is essential as a constituent in molecules and enzymes involved in oxygen transport and use. It is distributed primarily in blood hemoglobin (60% of the body's iron), muscle myoglobin (20%), storage forms (bound to ferritin and hemosiderin), and transport forms (bound to transferrin). Iron absorption increases with increasing need and decreases with excessive intake of cadmium, cobalt, copper, manganese, and zinc.

The horse's dietary requirement is estimated to be 50 ppm in diet dry matter for growth, pregnancy, and lactation, and 40 for other classes of horses. Forages contain 50 to 400 ppm iron, but usually 100 to 250, and cereal grains 30 to 90 (Appendix Table 2). Thus, common feedstuffs provide adequate iron for the horse.

It has been speculated that iron needs increase with increased physical exertion due to iron loss in sweat and increased red blood cell breakdown. Increased red blood cell breakdown, however, doesn't increase dietary iron needs, as the iron from these cells is reutilized for the synthesis of new red blood cells. In addition, physical exertion increases dietary energy needs; more feed and, as a result, iron are therefore consumed. As a result, if iron needs do increase with increased physical exertion, the increase is not sufficient to cause an iron deficiency, and there is no benefit from iron administration or supplementation.

Iron Deficiency

The foal, like nursing young of other species, is the most susceptible to an iron deficiency because milk is low in iron and because of the foal's rapid growth rate. Increased blood volume and muscle mass require a higher iron intake. Mares' milk contains 12 to 28 ppm iron dry matter at foaling, and decreases to 5 at 4 months after foaling. A clinically recognized iron deficiency rarely occurs in either foals or mature horses at any performance level.

An iron deficiency occurs in horses only if there is chronic or severe blood loss. The blood loss may be inapparent, such as that due to severe lice infestation or intestinal parasitism. The initial effect of an iron deficiency is a decrease in iron storage in the liver, spleen, and bone marrow, paralleled by a decrease in the plasma ferritin concentration. The decrease in iron required for enzymes decreases exercise capacity. This occurs before anemia, and the iron-deficient anemic animal responds to iron administration with an increase in endurance capacity before there is any significant increase in blood hemoglobin concentration. The final stage or effect of an iron deficiency is anemia. The anemia causes a further decrease in the iron-deficient animal's endurance capacity.

Treatment of an iron deficiency is twofold: (1) correct the cause of the blood loss that resulted in the iron deficiency, and (2) give the nutrients necessary for increased red blood cell synthesis. The only nutrient the non-malnourished animal generally needs in increased amounts is iron, which in the anemic animal is usually injected. For this purpose, iron dextran, although alright for other species, may be harmful to horses. Iron in any form should not be given to the horse unless a confirmed anemia and/or iron deficiency is present.

Iron Excess

Because the horse's performance is impaired by an iron deficiency, preparations containing iron are often given orally or intramuscularly to improve performance. Their administration will improve performance only if an iron deficiency is present. If not, iron administration will either have no effect or be harmful. It will not be beneficial. Iron toxicosis due to iron administration is much more common in horses than is iron deficiency.

Excessive iron is stored in various tissues, particularly the liver, which may cause damage. Foals are particularly susceptible to iron toxicosis their first few days of life. At birth, foals have a high plasma iron concentration and transferrin saturation, and absorption of iron is considerably higher in neonates than adults. These decrease rapidly in the first few days of life so that foals are less susceptible to toxicosis by 2 to 3 days of age. A vitamin E and/or selenium deficiency may increase the foal's susceptibility to acute iron toxicosis. Iron-toxicosis-induced liver failure and death of foals has occurred as a result of the oral administration of a digestive inoculum containing iron. Prior to death, the foals exhibited depression, diarrhea, icterus, dehydration, and coma. Morphologic changes included erosion of intestinal villi, pulmonary hemorrhage, massive iron deposits in the liver, and liver degeneration. Iron toxicosis has also been reported in mature horses, but the toxic dose of iron for the mature horse is as much as 25 times greater than that for the neonatal foal.

Iron administration, even in much smaller amounts than those necessary to induce iron toxicosis, increases the animal's susceptibility to bacterial infections. Iron is required for the growth of nearly all living organisms, including bacteria. When bacteria invade mammals, one determinant of their success or failure to establish an infection is the availability of the iron they need for their multiplication.

Most mammals are able to decrease their body's accessible iron as a mechanism of defense against bacterial infections. During a bacteria-induced inflammatory response, neutrophils release lactoferrin, which binds available iron. The lactoferrin is then phagocytized, thus decreasing iron's availability for bacterial use. Excess available iron in the animal's body decreases the efficacy of this protective mechanism, increasing the animal's susceptibility to bacterial infection. Excess available iron may be caused by the administration of either corticosteroids or iron. This is one mechanism by which corticosteroids increase susceptibility to bacterial infection. Excess available iron is most often induced by injecting iron rather than giving it orally.

The body has no means of excreting excess iron. The only means of protection against excess iron is decreased absorption. Injected iron, therefore, bypasses the body's only means of protection against iron toxicosis. Thus, even a much smaller amount of iron given by injection is more likely to cause toxicosis than an amount given orally. Because of the body's ability to decrease iron absorption, iron toxicosis as a result of an excess in the diet is uncommon in horses. It can occur, however, as previously described in neonatal foals given the iron-containing inoculum orally. Excess dietary iron intake may decrease the absorption of other minerals, perhaps resulting in deficiencies of those minerals. Very high amounts of iron in the diet are required to cause this effect in horses.

As high as 1400 ppm iron in the of total diet dry matter for 3 months has been shown to have no effect on weanling or yearling horses' feed intake, growth rate, red blood cell count, hematocrit; serum, liver, kidney, or spleen iron, calcium, phosphorus, copper, zinc, or manganese concentrations; serum unbound-iron-binding capacity; or total iron-binding capacity. These high iron levels also did not affect calcium or phosphorus absorption or bone mineral content, breaking strength, or size.

Iron Deficiency and Excess Diagnosis

A low body-iron status is routinely due to prolonged excessive blood loss, not inadequate iron in the diet. A harmful excess of iron in the body may be due to an excessive amount in the diet, but more often is due to the administration of iron directly to the horse. Thus, means other than evaluating the diet are necessary to determine the presence of either an inadequate or excessive iron status.

The hematocrit and blood hemoglobin concentration are commonly used to evaluate the horse's iron status; however, they are quite insensitive. Neither decreases until a severe anemia is present and thus a severe iron deficiency has been in existence for a prolonged period. The horse has large stores of red blood cells in the spleen and, when excited or during exertion, it contracts the spleen, which can increase the hematocrit and hemoglobin concentration by more than 50%, thus masking an iron-deficiency-induced decrease, or any cause for a decrease, in their concentration. When a blood sample is taken, varying degrees of splenic contracture occur, resulting in spurious hematocrit and hemoglobin concentration values.

In contrast, the serum concentration of ferritin, the storage form of iron, is an accurate measure of the horse's iron status. Its decrease is the earliest sign of inadequate body iron, and its increase is an early indication of excess iron. It is not affected by stress, excitement, or exertion. If the horse's serum ferritin concentration is low (less than 30 ng/ml), chronic blood loss should be suspected and the horse should be evaluated to determine the cause and treated accordingly. Iron administration may be of benefit. If the ferrition concentration is high (over 250 to 300 ng/ml), however, a search for a source of excess iron should be made and, if found, alleviated.

COBALT

Cobalt's only known function is as an integral part of vitamin B_{12}. Cecal and colonic microflora of horses, like ruminal microflora, use dietary cobalt to synthesize vitamin B_{12}. Therefore, a cobalt deficiency results in a vitamin B_{12} deficiency. Neither a deficiency nor an excess of either cobalt or vitamin B_{12} has been reported or induced experimentally in the horse. The amount of cobalt needed or toxic in diets for horses has not been determined. At least 0.1 ppm cobalt in diet dry matter has been recommended for horses. This recommendation is based on the occurrence of deficiency symptoms (a starvation appearance) in cattle and sheep at levels of less than 0.04 to 0.07 ppm in diet dry matter. However, the horse's requirement is probably considerably less than this, as horses have remained in good health while grazing pastures so low in cobalt that ruminants confined to these pastures died. An upper safe level of 10 ppm cobalt in diet dry matter for the horse has been recommended. This amount is based on what is recommended for cattle. However, it is reported that cattle tolerate up to 26 ppm cobalt in their diet, sheep 70, and swine 200. Thus, a cobalt deficiency or toxicosis are unlikely to occur in horses at levels of less than 0.05 or greater than 25 ppm cobalt in diet dry matter, as compared to 0.05 to 0.6 in all common horse feeds (Appendix Table 2). Therefore, neither a cobalt deficiency nor toxicosis are likely to occur naturally in the horse.

FLUORIDE

Utilization, Needs, and Sources

Fluoride is incorporated into teeth and bone increasing their crystalinity and hardness and decreasing their solubility, thus impairing osteolysis and dental caries. Adding 1 to 2 ppm fluoride to the drinking water decreases dental caries in people of all ages by an average of 60%, particularly in the young. Whether fluoride is needed in the diet is unknown since a confirmed deficiency has not been reported or produced experimentally.

Uncontaminated forages and cereal grains contain 2 to 16 and 1 to 3 ppm fluoride in dry matter, respectively. The tea plant and camellia are exceptions, with fluoride concentrations of 100 ppm or more. Water seldom contains over 1 ppm fluoride unless it is contaminated by high-fluoride-containing dust or is from deep wells in phosphate rock formations in endemic fluorosis areas. In the latter case it may contain 3 to 5 ppm fluoride. Thus, inadequate fluoride intake doesn't occur; excess of flouride resulting in fluorosis does, however.

Fluorosis

Fluorosis Causes

One of the most common sources of excess dietary fluoride is phosphorus supplements such as rock phosphates, phosphatic limestone, or fertilizer-grade phosphates that have not been adequately defluorinated. Prior to defluorination, they may contain 2 to 5% fluoride and, therefore, each 1% of these phosphate minerals added to the diet will increase the diet's fluoride content by 200 to 500 ppm. Bone ash normally contains less than 1500 ppm, but from animals grazing fluoride-contaminated pastures, it may contain over 10,000 ppm (1%). Thus, phosphorus supplements vary greatly in fluoride content depending on origin and manufacturing process. When processed sufficiently to qualify as defluorinated, feedgrade phosphates must contain no more than 1 part fluoride per 100 parts phosphorus.

Another cause of fluorosis is forage and water contaminated by effluent from manufacturing plants or mining operations processing minerals containing fluoride (such as cryolite or aluminum, fluorspar, fluorapatite, and rock phosphate), and steel processing plants that release large amounts of fluoride into the air. Fluoride is used as flux in electroplating aluminum and is driven off during the firing of iron and phosphate ores. In areas where these facilities are located, contaminated forage is the most common cause of fluorosis. Forages and cereal grains are seldom a cause of chronic fluorosis unless they are contaminated by fluoride-bearing dusts, fumes, or water.

Animals are most commonly affected by fluorosis during growth, although the adult and the fetus may also be affected. Fluoride is transported across the placenta, therefore excessive intake by the mare during pregnancy may result in mottling of the deciduous teeth of the fetus and a decrease in birth weight. However, excess fluoride intake has minimal effect on the fluoride content of the milk, so the nursing animal is not affected.

Greater than 2 to 5 ppm fluoride in calves' drinking water will result in mottled enamel during teeth development, but no other effects are observed in cattle at levels of less than 8 ppm. For cattle, greater than 30 ppm fluoride in diet dry matter may cause problems during growth and lactation, and greater than 50 may cause problems during maintenance. Horses are known to tolerate 50 ppm of diet for extended periods without detrimental effects. Lifetime intakes in ppm in diet dry matter considered safe for dairy cows is 30, beef cows 40, sheep 50, swine 70, horses 90, turkeys 100, and chickens 180. Although horses are reported to tolerate fluoride intakes two to three times greater than cattle, water and feed concentrations above the amounts that may cause problems in cattle should be avoided if possible. However at less than 200 ppm in the of diet, harmful effects may not occur in mature horses for several years.

Fluorosis Effects

Fluorosis is characterized almost entirely by signs involving bone and teeth. It is very insidious and may be confused with any chronic debilitating disease. Fluoride accumulates in the bone and teeth throughout life, and an excess therefore is a cumulative poison. In young animals, teeth generally show the first signs of fluorosis. There may be delayed eruption of permanent teeth, oblique eruption, and incomplete or defective teeth development. During (but not after) the period of calcification, the teeth enamel becomes mottled. Affected teeth are initially chalky white in color and progress to having yellowish-brown to black mottling that cannot be removed by scraping. In severe cases the teeth become pitted, worn, and eroded to the extent that nerves may be exposed. As a result of these changes, eating and drinking cold water may be extremely painful. Feed and water intake is decreased, resulting in decreased growth and weight loss. Feed may be held in the mouth. The central portion of the cheek teeth may be lost, allowing feed particles to be forced into the pulp cavity. As a result, abscesses in the lower jaw may occur. Infected areas are often 2 to 3 inches (4–7 cm) in diameter and can include a fistulous tract that drains from the ventral aspect of the jaw. Teeth that have erupted are not affected adversely by subsequent fluoride ingestion and, therefore, horses that are more than 4 to 5 years of age do not develop typical fluorosis-induced dental lesions.

Horses with moderate to marked fluorosis appear unthrifty even when ample amounts of good-quality feed are available. They may stand with an arched or humped back, their hair coat becomes rough and dry, and shedding the winter coat occurs slowly in the spring. As the fluorosis becomes more severe, a nonspecific generalized stiffness and lameness occurs. Enlargement, roughening, and thickening of the bone occurs. Frequently this is first noticeable on the inside surfaces of the upper one-third of the rear cannon bones. As the condition progresses, the lower jaw, front cannon bones, and ribs become involved. The phalanges below the fetlocks may have abnormal, rough textured enlargements, particularly at tendon insertions. Enlargement of the coffin bone increases pressure within the hoof, leading to a founder-like syndrome. Intra-articular structures in the joints are not generally involved, which helps differentiate fluorosis from osteoarthritis, in which bony changes are initially in the joints, with marginal lipping in advanced cases. With fluorosis, the bones become chalky white instead of ivory, are larger in diameter and heavier than normal, and may have a roughened irregular surface.

Fluorosis Diagnosis

Diagnosis of fluorosis is difficult because there may be an extended interval of time between ingestion of excessive fluoride and the appearance of toxic signs. Diagnosis is based on the clinical signs, a history of feed or water fluoride concentrations greater than the values given, or the discovery of excessive fluoride in rib and tail bones.

In addition to being deposited in bone and teeth, excess fluoride is excreted in the urine. Although an increase in urine fluoride concentration occurs only after extensive fluoride deposition in bone, it may occur before clinical signs are evident. However, urine fluoride concentrations reflect only current, not past, fluoride intake. The fluoride concentration in plasma, like urine, changes rapidly with intake. The fluoride content of milk, hair, hooves, and soft tissues is low and only minimally affected by dietary fluoride intake.

Fluorosis Treatment

Treatment of fluorosis starts with the determination and alleviation of the cause of excess fluoride intake. The effects of fluoride toxicosis are not reversible. In addition, no substance will completely prevent the toxic effects of excess fluoride intake. However, aluminum sulfate, aluminum chloride, aluminum acetate (but not aluminum oxide, calcium aluminate, calcium carbonate or limestone), and defluorinated phosphate will decrease fluoride absorption. One of the salts that decreases fluoride absorption should be added at levels of 2 to 4% in the total diet, or mixed with equal parts of salt for free-choice consumption as the only salt available. The toxic effects of fluoride can also be counteracted to some extent with green forage and liberal grain feedings.

Chapter 3

VITAMINS FOR HORSES

Vitamin A	45	
Utilization and Functions	45	
Sources	46	
Requirement	46	
Beta-Carotene's Effect on Mare Reproduction	46	
Imbalances	47	
Occurrence	47	
Effects	47	
Prevention and Treatment	48	
Vitamin D	48	
Forms and Sources	48	
Functions	49	
Requirement	49	
Administration for Skeletal Diseases	49	
Deficiency	49	
Toxicosis	49	
Occurrence	49	
Effects	50	
Treatment	50	
Vitamin E	Ch. 2	
Vitamin K	50	
Forms, Sources, Metabolism, and Functions	50	
Dietary Requirement	51	
Deficiency (Sweetclover Poisoning)	51	
Clinical Usage	51	
Toxicosis	52	
Thiamin (Vitamin B_1)	52	
Forms, Sources, Metabolism, and Functions	52	
Dietary Requirement and Clinical Usage	52	
Deficiency	53	
Toxicosis	53	
Riboflavin (Vitamin B_2)	54	

Sources, Metabolism, and Functions	54	
Dietary Requirement and Imbalances	54	
Niacin	54	
Sources, Metabolism, and Functions	54	
Dietary Requirement and Imbalances	54	
Pantothenic Acid	55	
Sources, Metabolism, and Functions	55	
Dietary Requirement and Imbalances	55	
Pyridoxine (Vitamin B_6)	55	
Sources, Metabolism, and Functions	55	
Dietary Requirement and Imbalances	55	
Biotin	56	
Sources, Metabolism, and Functions	56	
Dietary Requirement and Imbalances	56	
Folacin	56	
Sources, Metabolism, and Functions	56	
Dietary Requirement and Imbalances	57	
Cobalamin (Vitamin B_{12})	57	
Sources, Metabolism and Functions	57	
Dietary Requirement and Imbalances	58	
Choline	58	
Sources, Metabolism and Functions	58	
Requirements	58	
Deficiency	59	
Clinical Usage	59	
Toxicosis	59	
Vitamin C (Ascorbic Acid)	59	
Sources and Metabolism	59	
Functions	59	
Deficiency	59	
Requirement and Clinical Usage	60	
Administration	60	
Toxicosis	61	

Vitamins are organic (i.e., carbon-containing) compounds required in trace amounts to promote and regulate a multitude of body functions. They are classified as fat or water soluble, a property that affects how they are absorbed, stored and excreted (Table 3-1). The fat-soluble vitamins are A, D, E, and K; the water-soluble vitamins are the B vitamins and vitamin C. All but vitamins A and E are produced in the body. Vitamins D, C, and the B vitamin niacin are produced by the horse; all the B vitamins and vitamin K are produced by microbes in the horse's cecum and large intestine. Most are also conserved in the body by efficient recycling mechanisms. Although experimental studies in horses indicate that their large intestinal synthesis and absorption are inadequate to maintain tissue levels of most B vitamins except pyridoxine, vitamin B and K deficiencies occur only if there is interference with their production or utilization. When this occurs, generally there is a deficiency of several, not just one, of the B vitamins. Since many of the B vitamins assist in regulating energy metabolism, and all are involved in many biochemical reactions, their deficiencies produce similar clinical signs, including decreased feed intake and, as a result, unthriftiness, poor growth or loss of weight, poor performance, and poor hair coat.

Since fats, and therefore substances soluble in them, are poorly excreted from the body, excess intake of fat-soluble vitamins A and D is detrimental. In contrast, since water and, therefore, water-soluble substances are readily excreted from the body, excessive intake of water-soluble vitamins is rarely detrimental.

Since vitamins A and E are not produced in the body, they must be supplied entirely by the diet. Green forages (pasture or hay) are good sources of these vitamins as well as of vitamins K, B_1, B_2 and folacin. Sun-cured forages are good sources of vitamin D. The causes, effects, and diagnosis of vitamin deficiencies and excesses in the horse as described in this chapter are summarized in Table 3-2. Under normal feeding situations, vitamin deficiencies or excesses sufficient to cause clinically apparent detrimental effects in the horse are unlikely. However, normal diets for the horse may not contain a sufficient amount of certain vitamins for maximum beneficial health effects. For example, symptoms of a vitamin E deficiency do not occur unless vitamin E is less than 10 to 15 IU/kg of dry diet, an amount exceeded by most feeds. On the other hand, 50 to 100 IU/kg, which is more than that present in most feeds, increases tissue levels and appears to increase resistance to infectious diseases and exertion-induced muscle damage.

TABLE 3–1
Characteristics and Functions of Vitamins

Vitamins	A, D, E, and K	B and C
Absorbed with	Fat (their absorption decreases if fat absorption decreases)	Water (their losses increase if water losses increase)
Required in diet of healthy horses	Yes, the vitamins or their precursors, except vitamin K, since sufficient K_2 (menaquinones) produced by intestinal bacteria is utilized by the horse	No or minimal amounts needed because all B vitamins are produced by intestinal bacteria, and an adequate amount of vitamin C is produced by the liver
Major diet source	Green forage, and vitamin D in sun-cured forages	B vitamins high in brewer's yeast. Vitamin C high in fruits and vegetables.
Form in plants	• Beta-carotene is activated by intestine to vitamin A • D_2, like D_3, produced in skin, are activated by liver and kidney • Alpha-tocopherol, is most active form of vitamin E • K_1, like K_2 and K_3 (synthetic form), is activated in liver	• B_1 is activated in liver and kidney • B_6 is activated in the body • All other B vitamins and vitamin C are present in their active form in plant source feeds
Body storage	A and D, 3 to 6-month supply in liver. E and K less than 1 to 3-week useable supply.	Less than a few weeks, except B_{12}, for which many months to years supply is stored.
Deficiency symptoms	A = Decreased feed intake, increased respiratory and intestinal disease, slow growth, wt loss, poor fertility, dull hair, anemia, tearing, and night blindness. D = Decreased feed intake and growth, enlarged bone growth plates, and bone demineralization E = Muscle damage and/or inflammation of body fat, and impaired immunity K = Decreased blood clotting and hemorrhage	B vitamins = Decreased feed intake, unthriftiness, and poor growth or weight loss. Biotin = Hoof wall crumbling & tender soles. Folic Acid, B_6 and B_{12} = Anemia but deficiencies not reported in horses. C = Decreased wound healing and capillary fragility resulting in bleeding and scurvy, but a deficiency hasn't been reported in horses
Toxicosis symptoms	A = Decreased feed intake and growth, dull hair, anemia, and increased bone size D = Reduced feed intake, performance or growth, weight loss, recumbency, debilitation. E = Doesn't occur clinically. K_1 & K_2 = not toxic; K_3 = acute renal failure, depression, colic, bloody urine	Toxicosis from ingestion of vitamins B and C doesn't occur or is rare as excesses are readily excreted.
Clinical usage	Beta-carotene = Improve reproductive efficiency in mares not getting green forage—may help A = Prevent deficiency in horses not on green forage. D = Skeletal diseases and horses not getting sun or sun-cured feed—rarely indicated E = Exertion-induced muscle damage, a deficiency, and to enhance immunity or reproduction—may help reproduction when not on green forage K = Deficiency due to spoiled sweetclover, warfarin, oral antibacterials, or impaired fat absorption resulting in slow blood clotting. No benefit for bleeders (exertion-induced pulmonary hemorrhage).	B_1 = Increase appetite and decrease tying-up and anxiety—of questionable benefit. B_2, niacin & pantothenic acid = Rarely used. B_6 = Anemia—rarely beneficial. Biotin = Improve hoofs—helps some cases Folacin = Ensure optimal performance of stabled horses during racing & training—questionable benefit B_{12} = Anemia, enhance performance and increase appetite—doubtful benefit Choline = Fatty liver and heaves—questionable benefit C = Bleeders and muscle damage, and enhance performance, fertility, and skeletal development—questionable benefit for all of these uses

For each vitamin, the minimum amount necessary for optimum health and performance, as well as the upper safe levels for prolonged continuous consumption, as compared to the amount generally present in common horse feeds, are given in Appendix Table 3. The amounts recommended are, for many vitamins, more than the amount needed to prevent clinical signs of a deficiency yet considerably less than that which produces toxicosis. As indicated in this table, unless growing forage constitutes a majority of the horse's diet, adding additional vitamins A and E to the horse's diet may be beneficial, although rarely is this necessary to prevent a clinically apparent deficiency.

The majority of commercial grain mixes for the horse contain vitamins added at a level high enough to meet or exceed optimum levels of vitamin intake when the amount of grain mix recommended is fed. However, the amount of grain mix recommended may be more than you want to feed because it may unnecessarily increase feeding costs, or because it may provide more dietary energy than needed. Situations in which vitamin supplementation may be needed or beneficial are:

1. In horses receiving or having received prolonged antimicrobial drug therapy orally. These drugs may inhibit cecal and intestinal bacteria and their production of B vitamins and vitamin K. In this situation, additional amounts of B vitamins particularly may be beneficial and can be provided by giving a sufficient amount of a B-vitamin supplement to provide 50 to 75 mg of thiamine (B_1) and 20 to 40 mg of riboflavin (B_2)/horse/day. A commercial supplement, feeding nearly 1 lb (454 g)/day of brewer's yeast or 0.5 to 1 oz/day of a vitamin supplement similar to that given in Table 3–5 may be used. Brewer's yeast is quite high in all of the B vitamins except B_{12}, which doesn't appear to be needed in the horse's diet.

TABLE 3–2
Vitamin Deficiencies and Excesses: Causes and Effects[a]

Vitamin Imbalance	Causes	Effects
A deficiency[b]	< 225 IU/lb diet DM or < 5 IU/lb bw for > 6 mo, e.g., when green forage is < ½ of diet	↓ Feed intake & growth, anemia, poor hair, ↑ respiratory disease & diarrhea, ↓ conception, weakness, ↑ tearing, night blindness, ↑ skin & cornea keratin, and convulsions
A excess	Giving vitamin A > 9,000 IU/lb diet DM or > 180 IU/lb bw	↓ Feed intake & growth, poor hair & hair loss, anemia, depression, weak, incoordination, ↑ blood clotting
D deficiency	No sun exposure & feed stored > 1–2 yrs	↓ Feed intake, growth & bone ash. Enlarged bone growth plates, emaciation, & recumbency.
D excess	Excess vitamin D given or added to diet or ingestion of plants containing vitamin D (Table 18–8)	↓ Performance, feed intake & growth, weight loss, stiff, ↑ resting HR, ↑ urination, recumbency, seizures
E deficiency	See Table 2–1	
K deficiency	Dicoumarol (moldy sweetclover) or warfarin intake.	Hemorrhage and, if sufficient blood loss its effects
K excess	Excess K$_1$ (plant form)	None
	Excess K$_3$ (menadione) IM or IV	Renal failure, depression, colic, painful urination, bloody urine
Thiamin (B$_1$) deficiency	< 3 ppm in diet DM from long storage & ↓ intestinal flora production, or thiamine antagonist intake	↓ Growth, ↓ grain appetite, incoordination, muscle tremors, stiff, cold extremities, general congestion & hemorrhage, pulmonary edema

[a] The absence of a description of a vitamin deficiency or excess indicates that such a vitamin imbalance is not known to occur in the horse. Abbreviations: bw = body weight; DM = dry matter; ↑ = increase; ↓ = decrease; < = less than; > = greater than; HR = heart rate; IM = intramuscular; IV = intravenous.

2. When feeding a high grain and, therefore, a low forage diet, or
3. When feeding poor-quality hay or hay stored for more than one season.

In both situations 2 and 3, giving vitamins A and E may be beneficial. The amount given should be sufficient to supply the horse's requirements as given in Appendix Table 3. Although this can be accomplished for vitamin A by giving an injection every 2 to 4 months, there is little body storage of vitamin E, and therefore it is best to feed it daily.

Vitamin activity is decreased by external factors such as sunlight, feed grinding, heat, and exposure to air, and by a number of internal factors that occur particularly in vitamin supplements. Losses during storage are greatest for vitamins A, D, K, and B$_1$ (thiamin) Table 3–3. However, since vitamin A is the only one of these vitamins that the horse obtains only from the diet, it is the only one whose loss during storage is generally a problem. The factor that has the greatest effect on the loss of vitamin A activity during storage is moisture. For example, after 3 months of storage, vitamin A retention in a feed was 88% when both temperature and moisture were low, 86% when only temperature was high, but only 2% when both were high. Vitamin activity is also lost during feed processing (Table 3-4).

Additional situations in which vitamin supplementation may be beneficial are:

1. Horses under stress, such as frequent traveling or showing, or those at the track or on the show circuit.
2. Nervous or hyperactive horses.
3. Horses in training or frequent or prolonged physical activity.

4. Horses not eating well for any reason, such as illness, following surgery, strange surroundings, etc.
5. Anemic horses who, in addition to vitamin-B complex supplementation, should be treated for the cause of the anemia. Although iron and copper, as well as several B vitamins, are necessary for the increased production of red blood cells necessary to correct anemia, rarely is the administration of these

TABLE 3–3
Vitamin Stability in Feeds

Vitamin	% loss/ month	% of Initial Activity Remaining after Normal Storage Conditions for				
		6 mo	9 mo	12 mo	18 mo	24 mo
A (beadlet)	9.5	55	40	30	16	9
D$_3$ (beadlet)	7.5	62	50	39	25	15
E acetate	2.0	88	83	78	70	62
K (MSDC)[a]	17	33	17	10	3	1
K (MDPB)[a]	15	38	23	14	5	2
B$_1$ HCl	11	50	35	25	12	6
B$_1$ Mononitrate	5	74	63	54	40	29
B$_2$ (riboflavin)	3	83	76	69	60	48
Niacin	4.6	75	65	57	43	32
Ca Pantothenate	2.4	86	80	75	65	56
B$_6$ (pyridoxine)	4	78	69	61	48	38
Biotin	4.4	76	67	58	44	34
Folic Acid	5	74	63	54	40	29
B$_{12}$	1.4	92	88	84	78	71
C (ascorbic acid)						
Uncoated	30	12	4	1	0	0
Coated[b]	7	65	52	42	27	17
Choline	1	94	91	89	83	78

[a] Menadione sodium bisulfite complex and menadione dimethyl pyrimidinol bisulfite
[b] Coated with ethylcellulose

TABLE 3–4
Vitamin Stability During Feed Pelleting
and Extrusion

Vitamins	% Vitamin Retention During	
	Pelleting[a]	Extrusion[a]
A (650 beadlet)	85–95	75–93
D_3 (beadlet)	80–95	60–95
E (acetate)	95–99	94–98
E (alcohol)	30–75	10–65
K_3	55–80	25–70
B_{12} & Choline	95–99	93–98
Other B vitamins	80–95	70–95
C	40–75	20–65

[a] At 140 to 220°F (60 to 105°C) for pelleting, and 230 to 350°F (110 to 175°C) for extrusion, for 0.5 to 3 minutes. Retention is highest the lower the temperature and conditioning time.

trace minerals or vitamin B_{12} needed or of benefit, as most diets provide ample quantities of them for maximum red blood cell synthesis.

In all of these situations, a balanced supplement providing additional quantities of all vitamins, without excessive amounts of any specific vitamin, as given in Table 3–5, is best.

Many of the vitamins, when added to a feed that is not for immediate consumption, must be protected to maintain their activity and efficacy. Commercial vitamin suppliers accomplish this by coating the vitamins with things like gelatin, wax, ethylcellulose, or sugar. Many vitamins in an unprotected form are incompatible with other vitamins and minerals. For example, B_1 is incompatible with

B_2, both are incompatible with B_{12} in the presence of light, and most vitamins are prone to oxidative destruction by iron, copper, sulfates, sulfides, phosphates, and carbonates. It is difficult to prevent these destructive interactions in liquid vitamin preparations such as liquid hematinics, or "blood builders or tonics," that contain iron, copper, or incompatible vitamins. Convincing evidence of biological activity of the vitamins in these products should be provided by the company selling them; if not, they are not recommended.

VITAMIN A

Utilization and Functions

Horses derive their vitamin A naturally and entirely from dietary carotenoid pigments present in plants, the major pigment being beta-carotene. Beta-carotene in the wall of the small intestine is cleaved by intestinal enzymes, with varying degrees of efficiency by different species, to yield two moles of vitamin A per mole of beta-carotene. Rats and chicks do this most efficiently, horses relatively inefficiently, and cats and mink not at all, deriving 1667, 400, and 0 IU of vitamin A activity per milligram of beta-carotene, respectively. One IU or USP unit of vitamin A is equal to 0.3 μg of retinol.

Until recently, it was believed that the only function of beta-carotene was as a source of vitamin A and, therefore, it could be replaced entirely by vitamin A. However, some of the beta-carotene that is not cleaved into its molecules of vitamin A is absorbed intact and transported to a number of body tissues and organs, including the fat, skin, and ovary for use and storage. Storage in the ovary is primarily in the corpus luteum. Absorbed beta-carotene and other carotene pigments in plants are responsible for the yellow coloration of fat, milk, skin, and egg yolks in animals and birds consuming feeds high in carotene, such as green

TABLE 3–5
Vitamin Supplements for Horses[a]

Vitamin—Units	Amount of Vitamin per Ounce (30g) of Supplement	Amount Provided When Recommended Amount of Supplement is Fed[b]	Amount Recommended
		Amount/Kilogram[c] of Total Diet Dry Matter	
A—IU	40,000	2500–5000	2000–3000
D—IU	4,000	250–500	300–800
E—IU	1,000	70–130	50–100
K—mg	20	1.3–2.7	
Thiamin (B_1)—mg	75	5–10	5
Riboflavin (B_2)—mg	40	25–50	2
Niacin—mg	120	8–16	
Pantothenic acid—mg	48	3–6	
Pyridoxine (B_6)—mg	12	0.8–1.6	
Biotin—mg	1.5	0.1–0.2	
Folacin—mg	20	1.3–2.7	
Cobalamine (B_{12})—μg	120	8–16	
Choline—mg	600	40–80	

[a] Recommended for growing, reproducing, show, athletic performance, nervous, and hyperactive horses, and those not eating well. The recommended amount of vitamin supplement is 1 oz (30g)/1000 to 1100 lb horse/day and the amount for foals/day is: ⅛ oz (3.5g) from birth to 2 mo, ¼ oz (7g) 2 mo to weaning, ½ oz (15g) weaning to yearling, and 1 oz (30g) to 1- to 2-years old. Adjust accordingly for horses whose mature weight differs significantly from this.
[b] Based on horses consuming an amount of air-dried feed equal to 1.5 to 3% of their body weight daily.
[c] For amount/lb, divide amount/kg by 2.2.

grass. In the ovary, beta-carotene, rather than vitamin E or A, serves as an antioxidant and is used to assist in maintaining plasma vitamin A concentration. Beta-carotene in the corpus luteum is also involved in the control of progesterone secretion and, as a result, the control of ovulation, embryo implantation, and pregnancy maintenance. These activities are therefore impaired by inadequate amounts of beta-carotene and cannot be corrected by vitamin A.

Upon absorption, vitamin A is transported to the liver for storage, rather than to the ovary for storage as is beta-carotene. Vitamin A is either released from the liver into the blood for transport to the tissue for use, or excreted in the bile; that which is not reabsorbed is excreted in the feces. Small amounts of the vitamin A and its metabolites may also be excreted in the urine.

In the retina, vitamin A metabolites combine with the protein opsin to form rhodopsin (known as visual purple), which is necessary for vision, particularly at night. Vitamin A is also needed for bone and muscle growth, reproduction, and maintenance of healthy skin. It is thought that its mode of action in these activities is as a participant in the synthesis of glycoproteins that control cell differentiation and gene expression. A deficiency or excess of vitamin A affects and manifests by alterations in these functions.

Vitamin A Sources

Since vitamin A is not produced in the body, except from its precursors, it or its precursors, primarily beta-carotene, must be consumed in the diet. The concentration of vitamin A precursors in the vegetative portions of plants varies widely. Most grains are almost devoid of them, the exception being yellow corn (maize), which has a small amount (2 to 4 mg/kg). Beta-carotene is present in its highest concentration in green forage leaves and yellow vegetables. Carotenes in growing pasture grass and alfalfa (lucerne) may reach 300 to 600 mg/kg of dry matter (equivalent to 120,000 to 240,000 IU of vitamin A for the horse/kg), whereas carotenes in high-quality hay (U.S. No. 1) are 20 to 40 mg (8,000 to 16,000 IU) and in poor-quality hay (U.S. No. 3) are only 4 to 5 mg (1,600 to 2,000 IU)/kg of dry matter. This is compared to the 2,000 to 3,000 IU/kg recommended in the horse's total diet dry matter recommended (Appendix Table 3). If cut forage is rained on and the period of field drying is extended, appreciable leaf loss may occur prior to storage and feeding, resulting in a serious decrease in the hay's carotene as well as vitamin E, protein, and dietary energy content.

Regardless of the type of forage, hay or pasture, if it contains any significant amount of green color and constitutes the majority of the horse's diet, it will provide an adequate amount of beta-carotene, and also alpha-tocopherol (vitamin E), for optimum benefit for the horse, and therefore, additional amounts of either vitamin are unlikely to be of any benefit. Although carotenes are a yellow-orange pigment, the amount of green color present in forage gives a rough approximation of the amount of beta-carotene and alpha-tocopherol it contains.

Because carotenes are destroyed gradually by light and heat, even with optimum harvesting the carotene concentration (on a dry matter basis) in sun-cured forage or hay is lower than in green forage. During protected dry storage, vitamin A activity in feeds decreases an average of 9.5% per month and, therefore, less than one-half, one-third, and one-tenth would remain after 7, 12, and 24 months, respectively (Table 3–3). This is probably a good estimate of the rate of decrease in carotene concentration in feeds. Carotene concentration will decrease much more rapidly if moisture content or temperature during storage are high. Carotene content is also much lower in moldy feed.

Vitamin A Requirement

Expressed in IU of vitamin A per kg of total diet dry matter (and per kg body weight/day) (divide amount/kg by 2.2 to obtain the amount/lb), in horses 300 to 500 (9 to 11) IU is reported to prevent clinical signs of a deficiency and 900 (17 to 19) IU to be sufficient for production of maximum semen quality and quantity and stallion libido. However, 2,000 to 6,000 (60 to 200) IU was needed by foals for optimum growth and maintenance of blood parameters, biochemical parameters, and tissue vitamin A concentrations. As a result, a minimum of 2,000 (30) IU is recommended for maintenance and 3,000 (60 to 80) IU for all other horses. No benefit from additional vitamin A has been demonstrated. However, beta-carotene, in addition to its benefit as a source of vitamin A, may enhance reproductive efficiency, as described below.

The young horse's growth rate is substantially decreased at a preformed vitamin A intake of 184,000 IU/kg of feed dry matter (4,000 IU/kg body wt/day), and begins to decrease at intakes of greater than 20,000 (400) IU. Although clinical signs due to excessive vitamin A intake are unlikely in mature horses at intakes less than 100 times that recommended, 16,000 IU of preformed vitamin A/kg of total diet dry matter is recommended as the upper safe level for continuous prolonged consumption. When administered for long periods, this amount would be expected to substantially increase liver stores but not saturate liver storage capacity and, therefore, not result in above-normal increases in plasma vitamin A concentrations.

Beta-Carotene's Effect on Mare Reproduction

Beta-carotene, because of its role as an antioxidant and in controlling progesterone secretion by the corpus luteum, may impair the mare's reproductive ability, if deficient. Although beta-carotene in hay may be sufficient to provide adequate vitamin A, it may not be sufficient to maintain high plasma beta-carotene concentration and ovarian storage, and to maximize reproductive ability. Horses on green pasture have plasma beta-carotene concentrations 8 to 13 times higher than those fed hay and grain.

Beta-carotene supplementation to both cows and mares not grazing green grass has been reported by some to improve ovarian activity, produce earlier and stronger periods of estrus, improve conception rates, and reduce embryonic mortality; others report no benefit for either mares or cows. However, beta-carotene given orally would be expected to be of little benefit since much of what is ingested is split into vitamin A upon absorption. Beta-carotene availability is also low in conventional beta-carotene preparations because apparently it is present in large-droplet form. Beta-carotene's bioavailability is greatly enhanced in emulsified products (such as Equate, BASF Corp, Parsippany, NJ 07054).

A significant benefit of injecting mares and sows with an emulsified preparation of beta-carotene has been reported. In one study, conception rates in 155 randomly selected Thoroughbred mares on 6 farms near Ocala, Florida, injected intramuscularly with beta-carotene (10 ml) on the second or third day of estrus, and again 2 to 3 days later, during April was 91.6% versus 67.6% in 108 mares on the same farms not injected. No localized swelling or adverse reactions to the injections were observed. The administration of a highly bioavailable beta-carotene preparation may, therefore, be of significant benefit, particularly for mares receiving forage with little or no green color. However, it may be of much less or no benefit for mares on green pasture forage or consuming hay containing a significant amount of green color and, therefore, high amounts of beta-carotene.

Vitamin A Imbalances

Vitamin A Occurrence

If the mature horse consumes fresh green forage for a period of 4 to 6 weeks, it will saturate its liver-storage capacity for vitamin A and thus will have sufficient vitamin A to meet its needs for 3 to 6 months, although it usually takes at least a year before mature adults' vitamin A reserves become depleted. However, a longer period of time without green forage or supplemental vitamin A may result in a vitamin A deficiency, sufficient to cause a clinical effect.

The effects of a vitamin A deficiency most commonly occur in the foal. Vitamin A, like all fat-soluble vitamins, is poorly transported across the placenta. As a result, regardless of the amount of these vitamins consumed by the mare, the foal is deficient in them at birth. Colostrum contains high quantities of vitamins A, D, and E, providing the mare has adequate quantities of these vitamins available. If she does not, or if the foal doesn't receive adequate quantities of colostrum or has enteritis, which may decrease vitamin A absorption, the deficiency persists.

Excess, like inadequate, vitamin A is harmful. However, just as vitamin A deficiency and its effects don't occur until hepatic storage is depleted, vitamin A toxicosis and its effects don't occur until hepatic storage is exceeded. Nor does vitamin A toxicosis occur as a result of excess carotene intake, probably at least in part because carotene's conversion to vitamin A decreases with increasing carotene intake. Thus, since plant source feeds don't contain preformed vitamin A, vitamin A toxicosis occurs only as a result of vitamin A supplementation sufficient to exceed hepatic storage capacity.

Vitamin A Imbalance Effects

A vitamin A deficiency is characterized and suggested by excessive tearing and night blindness (Fig. 3–1). The only other known cause of night blindness in horses is a non-nutritionally related night blindness present from

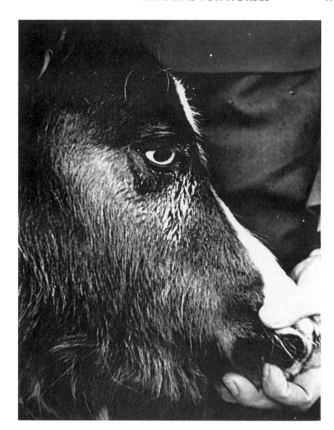

Fig. 3–1. Excessive tearing caused by vitamin A deficiency. (From Evans, J. W., Borton, A., Hintz, H. F., and Van Vleck, L. D.: The Horse. W.H. Freeman and Company, 1977.)

birth that occasionally occurs primarily in Appaloosas. These horses show apprehension to darkness and seek light; other signs of vitamin A deficiency are not present. Their eyes are free of ophthalmic lesions, whereas with vitamin A deficiency, the corneas may appear cloudy. In addition, although night blindness may develop, it is not present at birth in the vitamin A-deficient foal.

Although these eye abnormalities are characteristic of a vitamin A deficiency, they are observed only if the deficiency is sufficiently prolonged and severe. Earlier, and generally more commonly observed although less diagnostic, signs include reduced feed intake and growth rate; a rough, dry, dull, brittle, and long hair coat; and in foals an increased incidence and severity of respiratory and diarrheal diseases. Additional clinical signs in foaling mares include reduced fertility, abortion, and endometritis. The same hair coat changes occur with vitamin A toxicosis and protein deficiency as well as with inadequate feed and, therefore, inadequate protein, calorie, and vitamin A intake. Vitamin A-deficient stallions may have decreased libido and soft, flabby testicles. Foals born to vitamin A-deficient mares may be weak at birth. Although similar statistics aren't available for foals, the effect of vitamin A deficiency on respiratory and diarrheal diseases has been well documented in children. In one study, mortality was increased fourfold, and these diseases were threefold higher in children with a mild vitamin A deficiency than in those not deficient. Supplementing these children with vitamin A reduced childhood mortality by more than 30%.

Additional effects of a vitamin A deficiency include: sublingual salivary gland abscesses, impaired conception, convulsive seizures, progressive weakness, and declines in plasma, liver, and kidney vitamin A concentrations.

A vitamin A deficiency has not been identified as a clinical cause of skeletal problems in horses. However, in other species, a severe vitamin A deficiency increases bone growth and cause abnormal bone remolding, resulting in a reduced medullary cavity. Bony foramina fail to enlarge to accommodate the spinal cord, optic nerve, and cranial nerves which pass through them. This causes compression of these nerves, which may result in posterior incoordination, convulsions or paralysis, deafness, and blindness. Vitamin A deficiency is reported to be the major cause of blindness in children throughout the world, and, after protein and calorie deficiencies, to be the next most common nutritional disease (excluding obesity) occurring in people worldwide.

Some of the effects of a vitamin A deficiency also occur as a result of vitamin A toxicosis. Ponies 4 to 9 months old fed diets providing either less than 22 or greater than 4,000 IU of vitamin A/kg of body weight daily (800 or 130,000 IU per kg of total diet dry matter, respectively) gained 20 to 30% less weight, grew 43% less in height, and had duller hair coats and lower hematocrits, number of red blood cells and plasma albumin, cholesterol and iron concentrations than those receiving 40 IU of vitamin A/kg of body weight daily (1,450 IU/kg of total diet dry matter).

Prolonged feeding of excess vitamin A may also cause bone fragility, increased bone size, scaly skin, teratogenesis, and decreased blood clotting, which may result in internal hemorrhage. Severe toxicosis (40,000 IU/kg of body wt/day) produces decreased feed intake and unthriftiness by 15 weeks and, shortly thereafter, rough hair coats, poor muscle tone, and depression. By week 20, there is a loss of large areas of hair and the outer layer of skin, periodic incoordination, and severe depression, with much time spent lying on their sides, with a failure to respond to external stimuli, and death shortly thereafter. Degeneration, fatty infiltration, and reduced hepatic and renal function also typically occur as a result of vitamin A toxicosis. Vitamin A toxicosis also causes microphthalmia, crooked legs, and cleft palates.

In the growing horse a low red blood cell count and low plasma albumin and cholesterol concentrations are characteristic of both a mild vitamin A deficiency and excess sufficient to decrease growth rate, often without causing other clinical signs. If either an inadequate or excessive vitamin A intake is suspected, or if the values for these three parameters are reduced, procedures should be taken to evaluate vitamin A intake.

A total vitamin A concentration of less than 10 µg/dl indicates vitamin A deficiency and greater than 40 to 60 µg/dl an excess, although clinical signs of vitamin A toxicosis are unlikely to occur until concentrations exceed 100 µg/dl. However, plasma vitamin A concentrations in the normal range are poorly correlated with either intake or liver stores.

Like other effects of a vitamin A imbalance, substantial changes in the plasma vitamin A concentration do not occur until liver storage capacity is either nearing depletion or being exceeded.

Since the liver can store sufficient vitamin A to meet all of the horse's vitamin A needs for 3 to 6 months, a horse would need to continually consume a diet providing inadequate, or excessive, vitamin A for many months to years before its vitamin A storage capacity would be depleted, or exceeded, and, therefore, its plasma vitamin A concentration would move outside the normal range.

Vitamin A Imbalance Prevention and Treatment

If a forage, hay or pasture, without a significant amount of green color is being consumed for more than a few months, it is best to give a balanced vitamin supplement such as that given in Table 3–5. An inadequate intake of both vitamins A and E is likely. A sufficient amount of vitamin supplement should be given to the growing, pregnant, or lactating horse to provide 60 IU of vitamin A/kg body wt/day or 3,000 IU/kg of total diet dry matter (27 or 1,365/lb), and for other horses 30 and 2,000 IU, respectively (14 and 900 lb).

Instead of adding vitamin A to the diet, a water-soluble emulsion of vitamin A may be given intramuscularly or subcutaneously at a dosage of 6,000 to 7,000 IU/kg (2,700 to 3,200 IU/lb). This amount will saturate the liver's storage capacity and, therefore, does not need to be repeated for at least 3 months. Injecting more than four times this amount, or prolonged feeding of more than 5 to 10 times the amount recommended, may be harmful.

Vitamin A toxicosis is prevented by not giving more than the recommended amounts of vitamin A, and is treated by removal of excess vitamin A from the diet. If death is avoided, recovery from vitamin A toxicosis occurs rapidly. However, there may not be complete resolution of some changes.

VITAMIN D

Forms and Sources

Ultraviolet rays from sunlight convert 7-dehydrocholesterol, which is synthesized in the body, to vitamin D_3 (cholecalciferol) in the skin, and in the dead leaves of plants, they convert ergosterol to vitamin D_2 (ergocalciferol). This occurs, although more slowly, even during cloudy, overcast days, but not if the sunlight passes through glass. Glass blocks ultraviolet rays. Chlorophyll in living plants also blocks out ultraviolet rays. Thus, vitamin D_2 is present in plants after they have been cut and exposed to sunlight, and in the dead leaves of living, insolated plants. One IU of vitamin D (absence of a subscript indicates either vitamin D_2 or D_3) is equal to 0.025 µg of crystalline vitamin D.

The "sunshine vitamin," either ingested or produced in the skin, is stored and converted to 25-hydroxy vitamin D (25-OH-D) in the liver. This compound is transported to the kidney, where it is further hydroxylated to either the most active form—1,25 dihydroxy vitamin D (1,25 $(OH)_2D)$—or calcitrol if needed; or if not needed, it is converted to the more inactive form $24,25(OH)_2D$. The

25-OH-D$_3$ form is 2 to 5 times, and the 1,25(OH)$_2$ D$_3$ is 5 to 10 times, more potent than vitamins D$_2$ or D$_3$. Vitamin D$_3$ is reported to be more potent and absorbed preferentially to vitamin D$_2$ by horses as well as by cattle and swine.

Functions of Vitamin D

The only function of vitamin D is to assist in maintaining the plasma calcium concentration ([Ca]$_p$). It accomplishes this by interacting with parathyroid hormone (PTH) and calcitonin.

While 1,25(OH)$_2$D is the primary "effector" in this system, PTH is the primary "controller," with calcitonin playing an assisting role. For adequate control of calcium and phosphorus metabolism, adequate amounts of all elements in the system must be present. This includes calcium, phosphorus, vitamin D, PTH, and calcitonin. When there are deficiencies or excesses of any of these substances, skeletal diseases occur.

Vitamin D Requirement

If the horse receives sun-cured hay not stored for more than one season, or dormant sun-cured pasture forage, or is outside unshaded for an average of several hours daily, its vitamin D needs will be met. In this case, supplemental vitamin D is not needed, is not of any known benefit, and is not recommended. However, stabled horses not allowed access to direct sunlight for periods in excess of several months should have in their total diet dry matter 800 IU of vitamin D/kg during growth, pregnancy, and lactation, and 300 IU/kg during all other periods (365 or 135 IU/lb, respectively). In IU/kg (or/lb) of body weight, these amounts are equivalent to 24(11) for rapid growth and early lactation, 16(7) for late pregnancy, and 6(3) for maintenance. Sun-cured hay initially contains 2,000 IU of vitamin D$_2$/kg dry matter (or 900/lb; Appendix Table 3). However, the activity of vitamin D, like other vitamins, decreases during storage. During protected dry-feed storage, vitamin D activity decreases an average of 7.5%/month; therefore, only 39% and 15% would remain after 1 and 2 years, respectively (Table 3–3). Thus, hay stored for more than one season may contain inadequate vitamin D to meet the horse's requirements, which is of no consequence for the horse that receives an average of a few hours or more of sunlight daily. However, for those that don't, the amount of vitamin D recommended above should be given. Vitamin D may be preferably added to the diet or it may be given as an injection. Vitamin D$_2$ and D$_3$ have a 6 to 18-week effect, versus 4 to 12 weeks for 25-OH-D$_3$ and 1 to 6 days for 1,25(OH)$_2$D. Thus, if vitamin D is injected, it should not be given any more frequently than every 6 to 18 weeks, and then only if needed.

Vitamin D Administration for Skeletal Diseases

Since vitamin D increases intestinal calcium and phosphorus absorption and bone mineralization, it is occasionally given to growing horses to assist in the treatment or prevention of skeletal disease. Skeletal disease in the growing horse, as discussed in Chapter 16, is associated with numerous nutritional imbalances, most commonly either calcium or phosphorus deficiencies or both, but not vitamin D deficiency. Although high amounts of vitamin D can to some extent compensate for low dietary calcium and phosphorus by increasing their intestinal absorption, unless the situation described above, in which giving vitamin D is recommended, is present, vitamin D administration is unlikely to be of more than minimal, if any, benefit. No amount of vitamin D will compensate to any significant degree for inadequate calcium or phosphorus, or an improper Ca:P ratio, in the diet. Dietary calcium and phosphorus imbalances can be treated and prevented only by ensuring that the diet contains the proper amount of these minerals by evaluating and formulating an adequate diet as described in Chapter 6.

Vitamin D Deficiency

A vitamin D deficiency in most species results in rickets in the young and inadequate bone mineralization in the adult. A highly stable bone-cartilage matrix that is uncalcified and difficult to resorb is produced. This results in cartilage cells not degenerating, and a buildup of large cartilage cells, which produce more nonresorbable bone matrix. A palpable and observable broadening of the bone growth plates because of to the presence of uncalcified cartilage and bone matrix occurs. In severe or chronic cases, affected animals are reluctant to stand and do so with difficulty and pain. The bones become soft and flexible, resulting in bowed legs. However, often the most striking feature of the condition is emaciation. If the condition is treated early, all effects are readily reversed.

The skeletal effects of vitamin D deficiency, either naturally occurring or experimentally induced, have not been reported in horses. Ponies 3 months and 9 months of age deprived of all sunlight for 5 months and with no vitamin D added to the diet did not develop any of the clinical signs of rickets. However, there was a decrease in appetite, feed intake, growth, bone ash content, bone cortical area, and bone breaking strength. No difference in feed efficiency or in plasma calcium, phosphorus, or magnesium concentrations were observed as compared with ponies deprived of sunlight and given vitamin D daily or those that were outside with no vitamin D added to the diet. In addition, bone growth plates were irregular, widened, and poorly defined on radiographs, and were late in closing in the ponies deprived of sunlight and not given vitamin D. There was no difference in any of these parameters between ponies deprived of sunlight and given vitamin D, and those outside but not given vitamin D.

Vitamin D Toxicosis

Occurrence of Vitamin D Toxicosis

Vitamin D toxicosis is the most common of all vitamin toxicoses. It occurs as a result of improperly formulated vitamin D-supplemented feeds, administration of excessive oral or injected vitamin D, or the ingestion of plants containing vitamin D glycosides (Table 18–8), which are found primarily in subtropical areas of the world but also Florida, Texas, and southern California. Most commercially available vitamin D, both injectable and for oral administration, is synthetic vitamin D_3. Vitamin D_3 is used preferentially and, therefore, is more active and toxic than vitamin D_2 for horses, as it is for most animal species evaluated.

Excess vitamin D is cumulative. It may take several weeks or longer for its effect to become evident. A maximum upper safe level of 2,200 IU of vitamin D_3/kg (1,000/lb) of total diet dry matter is recommended for continual long-term consumption. This is equivalent to 40 to 60 IU/kg (18 to 27 IU/lb) of body wt daily. This amount would not be expected to increase plasma 25-OH-D_3 levels above normal, which is a sensitive indicator of vitamin D_3 excess. A vitamin D_2 intake of more than 10 times this level is probably safe. In addition, greater than 10 times this amount of vitamin D_3 is probably not harmful for periods of less than 60 days.

Vitamin D Toxicosis Effects

Vitamin D in excess performs its normal functions in the body, but does so in excess, thus stimulating excessive calcium and phosphorus absorption and calcium deposition. Calcium deposition occurs in various soft tissues, especially heart walls and valves, walls of large blood vessels (e.g., pulmonary arteries and aorta), and also the kidney, gastric mucosa, salivary glands, and diaphragm.

Vitamin D toxicosis results in the following clinical signs and alterations given in the order of their occurrence.

1. Decreased exercise tolerance and performance.
2. Increased blood phosphorus concentration, which is an early, consistent, and persistent alteration in affected horses.
3. Weight loss or decreased growth rate.
4. Stiffness and decreased spontaneous activity. Flexor tendons and suspensory ligaments may be sensitive to palpation.
5. Decreased feed intake.
6. Increased resting heart rate (to 55 to 80 beats/min).
7. Decreased renal function, resulting in increased urination, which increases drinking.
8. Gradual deterioration resulting in recumbency for increasingly longer periods. Generalized seizures and thumps or synchronous diaphragmatic flutter have been reported.
9. A normal to high plasma calcium concentration throughout. It may be above normal late in the course of vitamin D toxicosis, but frequently in the horse it isn't elevated except in toxicosis due to ingestion of plants high in vitamin D activity.

Vitamin D toxicosis is confirmed by an elevated plasma concentration of vitamin D or 25-OH-D of the form of the vitamin responsible (D_2 or D_3), which is normally below 5 ng/ml. These concentrations begin increasing the first day of excessive vitamin D consumption.

Vitamin D Toxicosis Treatment

Treatment of vitamin D toxicosis should include removal of all supplemental vitamin D, calcium, and phosphorus, and utilization of feeds as low as possible in these nutrients: i.e., a high-grain diet. For this purpose, grains' low vitamin D and calcium content more than offsets their

generally higher phosphorus content than that present in most forages. In addition, a high-grain diet helps increase feed and dietary energy intake by the horse that frequently has a poor appetite and is below optimum body weight due to excessive vitamin D intake. A diet consisting of an equal weight of grain and a grass forage is recommended. To accomplish this, the amount of grain fed may be safely increased up to 1 lb/100 lbs body wt (1 kg/100 kg)/day. Green grass and grass hay stored for a prolonged period are preferred over more recently sun-cured hay as they are lower in vitamin D. Grass, not a legume, should be fed, as it is much lower in calcium. In addition, the horse's exposure to sunlight should be minimized to decrease the production of vitamin D_3 in the skin. A calcium chelator such as sodium phytate may be of benefit in decreasing intestinal calcium absorption.

In addition to minimizing calcium and phosphorus intake, urinary excretion should be enhanced by having drinking water always easily available, and by initially giving noncalcium- and phosphorus-containing fluids both by stomach tube and intravenously. Fluid therapy is particularly justified for debilitated animals that are recumbent and unable or unwilling to drink. If no dehydration is present, diuretics may be of benefit.

Strenuous exercise should be prevented for several weeks after evidence of cardiac insufficiency (murmurs and increased heart rate) has disappeared, as it may induce sudden death.

Complete recovery from vitamin D toxicosis may require several months.

VITAMIN K

Forms, Sources, Metabolism, and Functions

There are several forms of vitamin K. The natural forms include vitamin K_1 (phylloquinone), which is high in green leafy plants, fresh or dried; and vitamins K_2 (menaquinones), which are produced by bacteria in the gastrointestinal tract of all animals in varying amounts. They, and the synthetic naphthoquinone, vitamin K_3 (menadione), are converted to hydroquinone, the active form, in the liver. Vitamins K_1 and K_3 are available commercially, both in injectable and oral forms. Because of its lower cost, water-soluble forms of vitamin K_3 are the predominant form used for oral administration. The two most common forms of vitamin K_3 and their stability in feeds are given in Table 3–3.

The natural forms of vitamin K, like other fat-soluble vitamins, are absorbed from the intestine with fats. Impaired fat absorption greatly decreases the absorption of the natural forms of vitamin K, but would not be expected to decrease the absorption of water-soluble forms of vitamin K_3. In species of animals studied, not including the horse, vitamin K_3 is rapidly metabolized to conjugates for urinary excretion, whereas vitamin K_1 is excreted in the feces.

Vitamin K is an essential for the activation of several blood clotting factors. A number of other proteins also require vitamin K for their activation.

Vitamin K Dietary Requirement

Dietary adequacy of vitamin K is often defined as the amount needed to maintain normal levels of vitamin K-dependent clotting factors. The amount needed by the horse has not been determined. Ruminants, because of the large amount produced by ruminal bacteria, don't appear to need any vitamin K in their diet. The amount of vitamin K produced by cecal and colonic bacteria in the horse is probably less than that produced in ruminants, but more than the amount produced in people and pigs. Therefore, the horse's dietary requirement, if not zero like that of ruminants, is probably less than the 0.5 to 1.5 µg/kg (0.23 to 0.7/lb) of body wt/day recommended for people, or the 0.5 mg/kg (0.23/lb) of total diet dry matter recommended for pigs. Vitamin K_1 in forage, pasture or most hay, and vitamin K_2 produced by bacteria, presumably meet the horse's requirements in all but the most unusual circumstances.

Vitamin K Deficiency (Sweetclover Poisoning)

Because little vitamin K is stored in the body, a deficiency may develop 1 to 3 weeks after cessation of intake or bacterial synthesis. Vitamin K deficiency can result from decreased dietary intake, decreased bacterial synthesis, impaired intestinal absorption, or decreased hepatic utilization. Compromised intake, absorption, or synthesis can occur with enteritis, colitis, extensive intestinal resection, anything that impairs fat absorption, or disruption of normal gastrointestinal flora by antibacterial drugs. Chronic liver disease, cirrhosis, and other hepatic dysfunctions can decrease hepatic synthesis of vitamin K-dependent clotting factors. Neonates tend to be vitamin K deficient due to minimal body stores at birth, limited dietary intake, and lack of established intestinal flora. Because of this, vitamin K is routinely administered to newborn infants to prevent hemorrhagic disease. A vitamin K deficiency secondary to each of the conditions listed above has been reported in people but has not been documented in the horse. The only documented cause of a vitamin K deficiency in horses is ingestion of vitamin K antagonist dicoumarol or administration of warfarin.

Dicoumarol and its derivatives (warfarin, pindone, diaphacinone, and brodifacoum), which are present in some rodent poisons (D-Con, Prolin, etc.) and blood anticoagulants, and the anti-coccidial drug sulfaquinoxaline, inhibit hepatic synthesis of vitamin K-dependent clotting factors, thus decreasing blood clotting ability. Dicoumarol often occurs in moldy, high-coumarin-containing sweetclover, (Melilotus spp.) hay or haylage. It is formed by some species of Penicillium molds' conversion of coumarin, which prior to its conversion to dicoumarol is not a vitamin K antagonist or harmful. Thus, sweetclover hay or haylage not containing mold-produced dicoumarol is not harmful. Sweetclover is a drought- and cold-winter-resistant legume which prior to maturity is a good feed, providing it doesn't contain dicoumarol. Generally, dicoumarol-containing sweetclover hay or haylage must be ingested for several weeks to cause a vitamin K deficiency. The problem occurs most commonly in cattle, but horses and sheep are also affected. Generally, only a few in a herd will be affected, but if untreated, mortality is high. Fetuses and newborn calves are most commonly affected, often with no clinical effects in the cow. This may also occur in pregnant mares consuming dicoumarol-containing sweetclover hay or haylage. To prevent the risk of dicoumarol-induced vitamin K deficiency, sweetclover hay or haylage should not be fed for at least 2 to 3 weeks before foaling or elective surgery.

Warfarin is given occasionally for the treatment of navicular disease. The degree of depression of blood clotting by warfarin is proportional to the dosage. Warfarin toxicosis, and therefore a vitamin K deficiency, can be potentiated by concurrent administration of phenylbutazone, salicylates, or any highly protein-bound drugs that can displace the highly protein-bound warfarin. Warfarin should not be given during pregnancy or lactation as it crosses the placenta and enters the milk in people and therefore may in horses.

Vitamin K deficiency from any cause decreases blood coagulation and thus increases susceptibility to hemorrhage. There is increased bleeding following trauma or surgery. Bleeding from the nose is frequently one of the first signs in horses. Hematomas under the skin of the neck, ventral chest and abdominal walls, and muscles of the hind limbs, bleeding into knee and hock joints, the gastrointestinal and/or urinary tracts, and/or internal hemorrhage may occur. If sufficient blood is lost, pale membranes, anemia, depression, weakness, a rapid irregular heart rate, a rapid respiratory rate, difficult respiration if there is blood in the thoracic cavity, and death may occur. Hemorrhage in the brain may occur and result in neurologic signs, including blindness and paresis.

A vitamin K deficiency should be suspected if these clinical signs occur, the horse is consuming sweetclover or is being given warfarin, or if blood clotting factors are abnormal.

If blood loss is severe, a blood transfusion is necessary to immediately restore blood clotting ability and blood volume. Vitamin K should also be administered. Although transfusions of whole blood or plasma will stop bleeding, the transfused clotting factors are soon exhausted and bleeding will resume. Additional intravenously administered fluids may be indicated for severe cases. Removal of blood from the thoracic cavity is indicated if respiratory difficulties occur. In less severe cases, eliminating the vitamin K antagonist by not feeding sweetclover or administering warfarin, and giving vitamin K, is sufficient.

Vitamin K Clinical Usage

Therapeutic administration of vitamin K in horses is indicated for dicoumarol- or warfarin-induced vitamin K deficiency and may be beneficial for horses with malnutrition, alterations in intestinal bacterial flora (as from prolonged antibacterial therapy), and gastrointestinal, hepatic, or pancreatic disorders such as enteritis, colitis, extensive intestinal resection, or any cause of impaired fat absorption. The presence of these conditions, along with prolonged blood clotting, serves as a rational indication for vitamin K administration.

Administering vitamin K orally may be more efficacious

than injecting it. Add 3 to 5 mg of vitamin K_1/kg body wt/day (1.4 to 2.3 mg/lb/day) to a grain mix for 7 days for the treatment of warfarin toxicosis, whereas for newer anticoagulant rodent poisons, such as diaphacinone or brodifacoum, continue adding it to the feed for 3 to 4 weeks. For a more rapid effect, vitamin K may be injected. When vitamin K is injected, vitamin K_1 injectable preparations at a dosage of 0.5 to 1 mg/lb (1 to 2 mg/kg) in divided doses, should be used. If poisoning was due to one of the anticoagulant rodent poisons, and vitamin K is not given orally, it may need to be injected for 2 to 3 weeks. Vitamin K_1 is preferred to vitamin K_3 because injected vitamin K_3 may be ineffective and quite toxic to horses. Some vitamin K_1 preparations are recommended only for intramuscular use. Although pain and swelling occasionally occur at the site of intramuscular injections, intravenous administration may cause severe hypersensitivity or allergic reactions.

Intravenous vitamin K_1 administration controls hemorrhage due to a vitamin K deficiency in 3 to 6 hours. If vitamin K_3 is injected, therapeutic benefits are reported to occur within 1 to 2 days; the dosage should be less than 2, and probably not more than 0.5 mg/lb (1 mg/kg) body weight. Injecting greater than 4.4 mg/lb (2 mg/kg) is toxic to most horses.

Vitamin K is sometimes administered in an attempt to treat undiagnosed causes of hemorrhage and to prevent exercise-induced pulmonary hemorrhage (EIPH) or bleeders, which, if sufficiently severe, results in a bloody nose. However, it is not effective in the treatment of prevention of EIPH, which, as described in Chapter 11, is due to exertion-induced rupture of blood vessels and not a decrease in blood clotting ability. Vitamin K should not be given for hemorrhage of undiagnosed cause or known causes other than vitamin K deficiency. No amount of vitamin K will enhance blood coagulation in the animal that is not vitamin K deficient. The anticoagulation effect of heparin is not counteracted by vitamin K.

Vitamins K Toxicosis

Excess ingestion of vitamin K_1 (plant form) appears to be innocuous. Vitamins K_2 and K_3 in the diet also have low toxicity. However, as low as 2 mg/kg (0.45 mg/lb) body wt of vitamin K_3 (menadione sodium bisulfite with 2.2 to 11 mg/kg recommended by the manufacturers) injected intramuscularly or intravenously may cause acute renal damage and death. Clinical signs, which begin 4 to 12 hours after injection and occur in the following order, include:

1. Depression.
2. Renal colic manifested by an arched stance, looking at their flank, and lying down and getting up frequently but not rolling.
3. Repeated backing into a corner and rubbing their perineum and tailhead on the stall or fence, which may be induced by colic.
4. Painful urination.
5. Bloody urine.
6. Decreased feed intake.

Laminitis or founder, ventral edema, and chronic renal failure, resulting in increased urination, drinking, and weight loss, may also occur.

Treatment of horses with vitamin K_3 toxicosis is directed at management of renal failure. Intravenous fluid therapy is indicated to correct volume deficits and electrolyte abnormalities, and to promote diuresis.

In patients unable to urinate, diuretics, may be needed. Generally, if diuresis can be achieved, the prognosis is good. If the horse will not eat or drink, an oral nutrient/electrolyte fluid (such as Life-Guard, Norden Labs, Lincoln, NE) and a pelleted, low-protein gruel given by stomach tube may be beneficial.

THIAMIN (VITAMIN B_1)

Forms, Sources, Metabolism, and Functions

Thiamin, or vitamin B_1, has in the past also been referred to as vitamin F and aneurine. Yeast, green leaves (fresh or dried), and cereal grain germ contain high levels of thiamin. However, it is removed from cereal grains by milling, therefore accounting for the deficiency resulting in beriberi that occurred in people eating little other than milled or polished rice. Thiamin, like all B vitamins and vitamin K, is produced in varying amounts by bacteria in the gastrointestinal tract of all animals. Thiamin hydrochloride and thiamin mononitrate are synthesized for commercial use in animal feeds. Although they have equal activity, the mononitrate form is more stable and, therefore, more commonly used. However, both forms, as well as plant- and bacteria-produced thiamin, are fairly heat labile so that feed pelleting, and particularly extrusion, decreases the amount in these feeds. Feed thiamin levels also decrease during storage at an average rate of 5% and 11%/month for the mononitrate and hydrochloride forms, respectively. One IU or USP unit of thiamin is equal to 3 µg of thiamin hydrochloride.

Thiamin, like riboflavin and vitamin C, is rapidly absorbed with decreasing efficiency with increasing amounts ingested, and excess amounts absorbed are rapidly excreted in the urine. Both of these mechanisms provide protection against thiamin toxicosis. It is converted to its active form, particularly in the liver and kidney. It is one of the vitamins least stored in the body. Body stores, except in pigs, can be exhausted within 1 to 2 weeks, although it takes about 4 months before clinical signs occur in horses on a purified thiamin-free diet.

Thiamin plays an important role in carbohydrate metabolism and in nerve transmission and/or excitation. The major effect of a deficiency is on carbohydrate metabolism, and of a toxicosis on nerve function.

Thiamin Dietary Requirement and Clinical Usage

It has been thought that, like other B vitamins and vitamin K, thiamin production by bacteria in the gastrointestinal tract is ample to meet herbivores needs, and therefore none is needed in the diet. Although this appears to be true for ruminants, it does not appear to be true for the horse. A diet containing less than 3 mg thiamin/kg (1.35 mg/lb) of dry matter decreases growth rate, and less than 5 mg/kg (2.3 mg/lb) may not be adequate for exercising horses. Five mg/kg (2.3 mg/lb) is the minimum amount recommended in the exercising and growing horse's diet, and 3 mg/kg (1.35 mg/lb) is the minimum recommended for all other horses (Appendix Table 3). Greater thiamin intake is recommended for older people because they may use it less efficiently than younger adults. Whether this also occurs in older horses or other animals is not known.

Thiamin administration is reported to stimulate appetite, assist in preventing tying-up (discussed in Chapter 11), and decrease anxiety in nervous horses. There is little evidence to support reports of these effects.

Thiamin Deficiency

Average or better-quality forage (grass or legume hay or pasture) contains 3 to 4 (1.4 to 1.8) and cereal grains 4 to 7 (1.8 to 3.2) mg of thiamin/kg (/ lb) of dry matter (Appendix Table 3), and thus just meets the horse's dietary requirement of 3 to 5 mg/kg (1.35 to 2.3 mg/lb). However, thiamin activity decreases during feed storage at a rate probably similar to that of thiamin hydrochloride, which is 11%/month. As a result, feed thiamin levels would decrease to 50, 25, and 5% of initial levels by 6, 12, and 24 months of storage, respectively (Table 3–3). Higher than normal storage temperatures or moisture would result in an even more rapid decline in thiamin levels. There have been reports of low plasma thiamin concentrations in some stabled horses not receiving supplemental thiamin. Thus, a dietary thiamin deficiency may occur in horses, although:

1. The deficiency would be minimal since most of the horse's thiamin needs are supplied by cecal and intestinal bacterial synthesis.
2. Its effects would rarely be more than a mildly reduced growth rate and perhaps performance ability, which are unlikely to be detected.

As a result, a thiamin deficiency rarely occurs or is recognized unless the deficiency was worsened by any one or more of the following.

1. Disruption of intestinal flora by prolonged oral antimicrobial therapy.
2. Decreased intake or absorption, or increased loss, as might occur with decreased feed intake, colonic disease, or increased urination, respectively.
3. Intestinal parasitism, as strongyles and coccidia are reported to compete for available thiamin.
4. The ingestion of thiamin antagonists such as amprolium, or thiaminase- or caffeic-acid-containing plants, such as bracken fern (Pteridium aquilinum), horsetail (Equisetum spp.) or yellow star thistle (Centaurea solstitialis), (Table 18–7).

Amprolium is an anti-coccidial drug used in poultry and cattle diets. At high doses (400 mg/kg (182 mg/lb) of body wt in horses) it causes thiamin deficiency by interfering with thiamin absorption and activation. A thiamin deficiency also occurs in ruminants secondary to excessive grain-in-take-induced clinical or subclinical ruminal acidosis. Abnormal ruminal flora resulting from the acidosis produce thiaminase. Thiaminase is also present in certain uncooked fish (especially carp and herring), whose ingestion may induce thiamin deficiency. Excessive cooking of foods destroys thiamin and may also cause a thiamin deficiency.

A sufficiently severe thiamin deficiency in horses causes decreased feed intake, incoordination, muscle twitching, tremors or stiffness, and periodic decrease in the temperature of the extremities. In one study in which amprolium was given to induce a thiamin deficiency, these signs occurred in all horses. A decreased appetite for grain, but not hay, occurred 5 to 7 days before other clinical signs. Affected horses' ears, muzzles, and hooves were cold to the touch for periods of 6 to 12 hours. They then warmed for a time before reverting to cold, after which incoordination occurred. Backing resulted in overflexion of the hindlegs, extension of the forelegs, and elevation of the head. If the head was forcibly elevated, it caused dog-sitting. There was little spontaneous movement and no head pressing, as occurs in thiamin-deficient ruminants. These same effects have been reported with plant-thiaminase-induced thiamin deficiency. Additional clinical signs in some affected horses include decreased heart rate, missed heart beats, weight loss, temporary blindness, either diarrhea or constipation, and convulsions. On necropsy, generalized congestion, pulmonary edema, dilated and enlarged heart, and serosal and mucosal hemorrhage may be noted in affected horses.

In treatment of thiamin deficiency, in addition to eliminating any causative factors, if possible, and providing supportive therapy as indicated, thiamin should be given early and repeatedly: 4 times the first 24 hrs, then once daily until 1 to 2 days after improvement of clinical signs ceases. From 0.3 to 0.4 mg of thiamin/kg (0.15 to 0.2 mg/lb) injected, or 2 to 3 times this amount orally, may be the maximum dosage likely to be of benefit. Animals treated early may recover completely. In others, irreversible changes such as neuron cell death may have occurred, and little improvement is seen. Although excess injected thiamin may be harmful, the amount required for toxicosis is many times greater than the dosages recommended.

Thiamin Toxicosis

Thiamin toxicosis due to oral intake is unlikely. Injecting thiamin may be the only way toxicosis can be produced. Laboratory animals fed several hundred times their normal requirement daily for three generations showed no adverse effects. No effect on reproductive performance or teratogenesis occurred. However, 100 mg of thiamin/kg (45 mg/lb) of body wt/day has been reported to inhibit thyroid function in rats without causing thyroid gland enlargement. From 50 to 400 mg of thiamin hydrochloride/kg (23 to 182 mg/lb) of body wt fed to dogs, mice, and rabbits blocks nerve transmission, producing curare-like signs. These include restlessness, convulsions, cyanosis, and labored breathing. Death results from respiratory paralysis, usually accompanied by cardiac failure.

Up to 2000 mg/kg (900 mg/lb) has been given to horses orally, and 5 mg of thiamin hydrochloride/kg (2.3 mg/lb) of body wt intravenously, with no observable effect. However, it is reported that, occasionally, horses injected with high doses show transient signs of excitement.

RIBOFLAVIN (VITAMIN B₂)

Sources, Metabolism, and Functions

Riboflavin historically has been referred to as vitamin G. It is high in yeast and fresh forage, but is low in cereal grains, where it is complexed with proteins. It is synthesized in varying amounts by microbes in the gastrointestinal tract in all animals, thus decreasing their dietary needs. In feeds it is fairly resistant to moisture, oxidation, and heat. Feed riboflavin levels decrease during storage at a rate of about 3%/month. As a result, nearly 70% remains after 1 year, and 50% after 2 years of storage (Table 3–3).

Riboflavin, like thiamin and vitamin C, is absorbed with decreasing efficiency with increasing amounts ingested; excess is rapidly excreted in the urine, and there is little storage in the body. It functions in two coenzymes necessary for oxidative energy metabolism. As a result, a riboflavin deficiency impairs the efficiency of oxidative energy production with the greatest effect being on tissues with the highest oxygen utilization.

Riboflavin Dietary Requirement and Imbalances

The horse's dietary requirement for riboflavin is probably less than 2 mg/kg (0.9 mg/lb) of diet dry matter. No signs of deficiency were noted in horses fed diets providing as low as 0.4 mg/kg (0.2 mg/lb) of diet. Fresh forage contains from 5 to 20 (2.3 to 9) and cereal grains 1 to 3 (0.45 to 1.35) mg of riboflavin/kg(lb) of dry matter (Appendix Table 3). Thus, a riboflavin deficiency is unlikely to occur and has never been documented in horses. However, unsupplemented soy-based, but not milk or milk-based, milk replacers are deficient in riboflavin.

Signs of a riboflavin deficiency in animals in which it has been induced include decreased feed utilization and growth rate; rough, dry, dull hair coat; decrease in skin thickness, hair follicles, and skin glands; scaly skin; a stiff gait and rear end muscular weakness; anemia; inflammation of the lips and tongue; colon ulcers and diarrhea; anestrus and early embryonic death; decreased, testicular size; fatty liver; and eye changes. Eye effects include appearance of corneal blood vessels; inflammation of tissues around the eye, increased sensitivity to light, and tearing. Some years ago, it was suggested that moon blindness (periodic ophthalmia or recurrent uveitis) in horses was due to riboflavin deficiency. However, this appears unlikely. Invasion of the cornea by leptospira or microfilaria of the parasite onchocerca cervicalis, or immunological response to disease, appear to be more likely causes.

High levels of ingested riboflavin appear to be relatively nontoxic. Levels between 10 and 20 times the dietary requirement (possibly 100 times) are known to be tolerated safely by rats and quite likely, by horses.

NIACIN

Sources, Metabolism, and Functions

Niacin, historically referred to as vitamin PP, is nicotinic acid and its amide, nicotinamide. They have equal vitamin activity. Nicotinamide occurs naturally in all living tissue. Cereal grains, animal byproducts, and leafy forages contain substantial amounts of niacin, although that in cereal grains and unprocessed soybeans, but not soybean meal, occurs in a bound form and is essentially unavailable at least for species studied and, therefore, probably also for the horse. Niacin is fairly resistant to all forms of stress (moisture, oxidation, reduction, heat, light, and pH alterations). Its activity in feeds decreases about 4.6%/month during normal storage conditions and therefore would be decreased to 57% of initial levels in 1 year (Table 3–3). It, like all B vitamins, is quite high in yeast and is produced by microbes in the horse's gastrointestinal tract. It is also produced in the body from the amino acid tryptophan by most animals, including the horse. The efficiency of this conversion is a primary determinant of an animal's niacin requirement. Tryptophan-niacin conversion tends to be high at low levels of tryptophan intake and decreases with increasing levels of intake. Other factors, including intake of leucine, total protein, and the vitamin pyridoxine, also decrease this conversion. Many cereal grains and other feeds contain relative excesses of the amino acid leucine and thus decrease tryptophan conversion to niacin. The efficiency of conversion also varies considerably among species, with little or none occurring in cats.

Nicotinic acid is absorbed slower than nicotinamide and is converted to nicotinamide in the intestinal mucosa. Nicotinamide, absorbed or produced from tryptophan, is taken up by tissues and incorporated into substances, which like riboflavin are necessary for oxidative energy metabolism. Nicotinamide plays a critical role in the metabolism of carbohydrates, lipids, and amino acids. Little niacin is stored or retained in the body. Most is excreted in the urine, with 75 to 90% of a high dose being excreted within 24 hours.

Niacin Dietary Requirement and Imbalances

A dietary requirement for niacin has not been established for the horse. The requirement for most animals, excluding the cat, is 5 to 10 mg/kg (2.3 to 4.5 mg/lb) of diet. Supplemental niacin for horses is probably of little or no benefit, although in some circumstances it may increase growth rate and feed efficiency of cattle and swine. Swine diets are usually supplemented with niacin, particularly when they are fed a high-corn diet because it is low in both tryptophan and niacin, and like other cereal grains, its niacin is bound and poorly available.

Niacin deficiency has not been described in the horse. The first signs of niacin deficiency in most species are loss of appetite, reduced growth, generalized muscular weakness, a rough hair coat, vomiting, and diarrhea (which may become bloody, with necrotic lesions in the cecum and colon). A scaly skin, anemia, posterior paralysis, irritability, and emaciation follow these signs. This condition is referred to as black tongue disease in dogs, and pellagra in people and pigs. The niacin-deficient chick also has abnormal leg development called perosis. Whether some of these effects would occur in the horse is not known.

Effects of niacin excess, like a deficiency, have not been described in the horse but have in other species. People consuming 3 g/d have been reported to have blood vessel dilation, itching, sensations of heat, nausea, vomiting, headaches, increased uric acid excretion in the urine, occasional skin lesions, and, at dosages of 3 to 9 g/d, liver toxicity. These doses have a beneficial effect on plasma lipid levels, which is the basis for niacin use when they are elevated. A level of 350 mg nicotinamide/kg of body wt (160 mg/lb), daily is presumed safe for most species of animals for chronic intake. Nicotinic acid may be tolerated at intakes as great as four times this level. Because niacin is well absorbed, limits of safe exposure are expected to be similar for oral and injected administration. Whether any of these effects occur, or levels of intake apply to the horse is unknown.

PANTOTHENIC ACID

Sources, Metabolism, and Functions

Pantothenic acid, previously referred to as vitamin B_3, is widely distributed in plant and animal tissues and, therefore, in feeds. The salt, calcium pantothenate, is the form used in the supplementation of animal feeds. It is fairly resistant to most stress factors, except moisture and acid. Its activity in feeds decreases 2.4%/month during normal storage conditions and, therefore, would be decreased to 75% of initial levels in 1 year (Table 3–3). In addition to being present in feed, pantothenic acid is produced by microbes in the horse's intestinal tract.

Microbe-produced and feed pantothenic acid are absorbed and in excess are excreted in the urine. Pantothenic acid is required for carbohydrate, fat, and protein metabolism.

Pantothenic Acid Dietary Requirement and Imbalances

A dietary requirement for pantothenic acid has not been established for the horse. The amount required for the pig, 15 mg/kg (7 mg/lb) of feed dry matter, has been used for the horse. However, no signs of pantothenic acid deficiency were observed in mature horses consuming diets containing less than 0.2 mg pantothenic acid/kg of dry matter, or in growing ponies on diets containing about 3.5 mg/kg of dry matter.

A pantothenic acid deficiency has not been reported in the horse or ruminants but can be readily induced in swine and most laboratory animals. Signs of a deficiency vary in different species but routinely include slowed growth, scaly skin, a rough hair coat, graying of the hair, nerve inflammation, and gastrointestinal inflammation and ulceration causing vomiting and diarrhea. Affected growing pigs may goose-step with their hind legs and stand on one hind leg while kicking rhythmically with the other due to degenerative changes in the peripheral motor nerves. In mature swine, poor reproductive performance is the main effect of a pantothenic acid deficiency. Decreased immune function may also occur. Affected birds exhibit a feathering disorder, fatty livers, and inflammation at the corners of the mouth. To ensure against decreased growth rate and reproductive performance, most swine diets, particularly when corn based, are supplemented with pantothenic acid. There appears to be little reason for supplementing horses' diets.

Pantothenic acid is generally regarded as nontoxic. No adverse reactions have been reported in any species following the ingestion of high levels in the diet. Rats fed 20 g of calcium pantothenate/kg of diet showed no adverse effects on growth or gross pathology. However, liver damage occurred in rats following the intramuscular injection of 80 mg of sodium pantothenate/kg of body wt, and 1 g/kg of body wt causes death in injected rats.

PYRIDOXINE (VITAMIN B_6)

Sources, Metabolism, and Functions

Vitamin B_6 includes three forms of pyridoxine (pyridoxine, pyridoxal, and pyridoxamine) that have equal vitamin activity on a molar basis. The synthetic form of pyridoxine used for dietary supplementation is generally pyridoxine hydrochloride. Vitamin B_6 in feeds is fairly resistant to most stress factors, except light and alkalinity. Its activity in feeds decreases 4%/month during normal storage conditions and therefore would be decreased to 69% of initial values by 1 year (Table 3–3).

Although pyridoxine appears to be synthesized by microorganisms primarily in the horse's cecum and colon, it is not absorbed in appreciable amounts from the colon. Absorption occurs primarily in the small intestine. Little is stored in the body. Excess is readily excreted in the urine. All forms of vitamin B_6 are converted in the body to the active pyridoxal phosphate forms. This conversion requires adequate quantities of niacin- and riboflavin-containing compounds (NAD and FAD) and, therefore, is decreased by a deficiency of either of these two vitamins. Conversely, pyridoxal phosphate functions in the synthesis of niacin from tryptophan. In vitamin B_6 deficiency, the diminution of this reaction results in the formation of xanthurenic acid, which is excreted in the urine. Urinary xanthurenic acid is therefore a sensitive indicator of vitamin B_6 deficiency.

The active forms of pyridoxine are involved in most reactions of amino acid metabolism. They are also involved in porphyrin biosynthesis, glycogen utilization, lipid and gama-aminobutyric acid (GABA) metabolism, and the synthesis of epinephrine and norepinephrine.

Pyridoxine Dietary Requirement and Imbalances

A dietary requirement for pyridoxine has not been established for the horse. Most nonruminant animals need 1 to 9 mg/kg (0.5 to 4 mg/lb) of diet dry matter, as compared to 3 to 9 (1.4 to 4) in most average-quality forages and cereal grains, and 30 to 50 (14 to 23) in brewer's yeast (Appendix Table 3). Neither a pyridoxine deficiency nor toxicosis have been described in the horse.

Signs of a pyridoxine deficiency in other species include reduced growth rate, muscular weakness, scaly skin, hair loss, anemia, impaired immune function, acrodynia, and neurological abnormalities resembling epilepsy.

Signs of pyridoxine toxicosis in dogs and rats include decreased appetite, incoordination and convulsions due to peripheral sensory neuropathy and degeneration. Maximum dietary tolerated levels for dogs for less than 60 days' consumption is 1000 mg pyridoxine/kg (454 mg/lb) of diet and for more than 60 days is 500 mg/kg (227 mg/lb); for rats it is one-half these levels. Oral doses of 2 to 6 g/day given to adult people over a several-month period have been associated with sensory nervous system dysfunctions and disablement. Dietary levels of at least 50 times nutritional requirements of 1 to 9 mg/kg (0.5 to 4 mg/lb) of diet are considered safe for most species, although probably more than 1,000 times nutritional requirements would have to be included in diets of species studied in order to produce signs of toxicosis. What amount of excess pyridoxine may be harmful to the horse, and whether effects would be similar to those described in other species, are unknown.

BIOTIN

Sources, Metabolism, and Functions

Biotin historically has been referred to as vitamin H. It is a sulfur-containing vitamin distributed widely in plant and animal tissues, much of it bound to protein. The biological availability of protein-bound biotin, which is referred to as biocytin, depends upon the digestibility of the proteins to which it is bound. Particularly rich sources of biotin are yeast, soybeans, cow peas, cauliflower, egg yolk, and liver. D-biotin produced synthetically is used for supplementing animal feeds. In feeds, biotin is fairly resistant to stress factors, although it is somewhat sensitive to heat and to a lesser extent, acid. Its activity in feeds decreases 4.4%/month during normal storage conditions and therefore would be decreased to 58% of initial values by 1 year (Table 3–3).

In adult horses biotin appears to be synthesized by microorganisms primarily in the colon. How well biotin is absorbed from the horse's colon and its availability to the horse in different feeds are unknown. At least some biotin produced by bacteria in the large intestine is absorbed, even by people. It is absorbed well from the small intestine of most species, although protein-bound forms in some feeds are less available, at least for poultry and swine. Little biotin is stored in the body. Its excretion in the urine, like that of most water-soluble vitamins, is closely related to intake. Biotin functions as a coenzyme in carboxylation-decarboxylation reactions. The most important reactions are those involved in gluconeogenesis and the synthesis of glycerol for triglycerides or body fats, the neurotransmitter acetylcholine, RNA, and DNA.

Biotin Dietary Requirement and Imbalances

Dietary requirements for biotin have not been determined for the horse or ruminants. The amount needed by swine (0.08 mg/kg of diet dry matter for growth and 0.2 for sow reproduction or 0.036 and 0.09 mg/lb, respectively) has been suggested as a basis for supplementing the horse's diet. However, it is doubtful that a dietary source of biotin is needed by herbivores, as long as they have normal gastrointestinal flora. Forages and cereal grains generally contain from 0.1 to 0.7 mg/kg (0.045 to 0.3 mg/lb); growing forages have over 0.4 mg/kg (0.18 mg/lb) of highly available biotin; in most cereal grains, however, it is poorly available (Appendix Table 3). To induce a biotin deficiency

in mammals, it is typically necessary to inhibit biotin synthesis and absorption by giving a poorly absorbed antibacterial drug and/or by including raw egg whites, spray-dried egg whites, or avidin in the diet. Avidin is a protein of egg white. It binds biotin, preventing its absorption. Cooking egg white prevents this effect. Fat rancidity in feeds destroys biotin. Thus, the ingestion of rancid and/or moldy feed, uncooked egg white, and antimicrobial drugs increases the risk of a biotin deficiency. In herds of affected sows, only 20% or less may show signs of a biotin deficiency, and many of the experimentally induced clinical signs may not be observed.

Experimentally induced biotin deficiency has been produced in numerous species, including people, but not horses. Deficiency effects that occur include the following:

1. Decreased growth rate.
2. Scruffy skin and scaly non-itching skin inflammation. A scaly greasy skin inflammation which, in advanced cases, may affect the lips, neck, thorax, abdomen, and extremities may occur. Hair loss, beginning on the face, may occur in some species. In fur-bearing animals, depigmentation of the hair around the eyes leads to a condition known as "spectacle eye." Dried saliva and excess eye and nasal secretions may be evident.
3. Weakness, depression or increased sensitivity to noise, and movement.
4. Decreased reproductive performance, including an increased time from weaning to first estrus, and reduced litter size in pigs.
5. Diarrhea, which may be bloody.
6. Decreased appetite and weight loss.
7. Progressive paralysis or spasticity of the hind legs.
8. Soft friable hooves; cracks on the bottom surface and, less commonly, the side-wall of pigs' feet, which may or may not cause lameness.
9. Anemia and increased blood cholesterol.
10. Decreased urine and/or plasma biotin concentration, which is diagnostic for a biotin deficiency.

Which of these effects of a biotin deficiency may occur in the horse is unknown. No unequivocal evidence of either a biotin deficiency or excess in the horse has been published or is known to occur.

Studies with poultry and swine indicate that these species can safely tolerate dietary levels of 4 to 10 times their nutritional requirements of biotin, but because this vitamin is not well retained, the maximum tolerable level may be much higher.

As described in Chapter 17 (see section on "Hoof Defects"), biotin supplementation may have a beneficial effect on horses' hoofs. Biotin supplementation has also been shown to increase litter size about 5%, and to decrease the time from weaning to first estrous by several days in sows. However, biotin supplementation hasn't been shown to affect the mare's reproductive ability.

FOLACIN

Sources, Metabolism, and Functions

Folacin has been referred to as vitamin B_c and, like biotin, as vitamin H. Folacin is the term for all compounds that have the biological activity of folic acid or folate. Metabolism of absorbed, folate produces various one-carbon or methyl derivatives. These one-carbon units carried on folate coenzymes are used to synthesize methionine and purine rings, which are present in DNA and, therefore, are necessary for cell formation. The folate coenzymes, S-adenosyl methionine and vitamin B_{12}, are responsible for the movement of one-carbon units in metabolic pathways. Adequate dietary methionine partially overcomes the effects of a folate deficiency, whereas the effects of a folate deficiency are worsened by a pyridoxine (vitamin B_6) deficiency. Both folate and vitamin B_{12} are needed for red blood cell synthesis. As a result, a deficiency of either results in anemia.

The majority of body folate is, in most species of animals, stored in the liver. In contrast to most B vitamins, which are excreted primarily in the urine, both free folate and folate degradation products are excreted primarily in the bile, and that not resorbed is lost in the feces. But, like other B vitamins, folacin appears to be synthesized in and absorbed from the horse's intestinal tract, with microbial synthesis occurring primarily in the cecum and colon.

Folacin is normally present in relatively large amounts in fresh forage and other greens, and is considerably lower in hay and grains, particularly those that have undergone any stress factors or prolonged storage. Folacin activity in feeds is somewhat sensitive to most stress factors, particularly acidic conditions. During average storage conditions, its activity in feeds decreases about 5%/month so that by one year it is reduced by nearly one-half (Table 3–3).

Folacin Dietary Requirement and Imbalances

Dietary requirements for folacin have not been established for the horse. Adult swine need 0.35 mg/kg (0.16 mg/lb) of diet dry matter. Growing forages contain 1.5 to 5 mg/kg (0.7 to 2.3 mg/lb) of dry matter, hay 0.5 to 1 (0.23 to 0.45 mg/lb), and cereal grains 0.2 to 0.6 mg/kg (0.1 to 0.3 mg/lb) (Appendix Table 3). It has generally been thought that no folacin is needed in the diet of herbivores, unless microbial synthesis in their gastrointestinal tract is inhibited. Ingestion of poorly absorbed antimicrobial drugs, particularly sulfonamides, may have this effect. Sulfonamides' antibacterial action is based on their inhibition of bacterial synthesis of folic acid from para-aminobenzoic acid. Moldy feeds have also been shown to increase pigs' folacin requirements, and, therefore, may increase horses' requirements. However, several studies have suggested that even with normal microbial folacin synthesis and non-moldy feeds, some folacin is needed, or is at least of benefit, in the horse's diet.

Although a folacin deficiency has not been described in the horse, a number of studies have found that horses on low-folate diets have plasma folate concentrations of less than 5 ng/ml, levels that would be considered indicative of a borderline deficiency in people.

In a number of species, and probably in horses, the first stage of inadequate folate intake is a decrease in serum folate followed by a decrease in red blood cell folate concentration. With tissue depletion, DNA and therefore cell synthesis in that tissue are impaired. This occurs first in bone marrow cells, followed by peripheral blood lymphocytes, which become hypersegmented. A decrease in white blood cells follows. The development of macrocytic anemia is the final stage in the progression of folate deficiency and is the stage in which clinical signs of folate depletion occur. These include decreased growth rate and diarrhea. These effects reflect the folate requirement for DNA synthesis in continuously dividing cells necessary for growth, red and white blood cell synthesis, and intestinal epithelial cell synthesis.

Folate intake and serum folate levels have been found to be lower in stabled than in pastured horses, and to decrease further with race training and use. Based on these findings and the effects of inadequate folate intake in other species, supplementation with 20 mg of folacin/day has been recommended for horses during training and racing that are not grazing green grass. This, or lower amounts, may be warranted to ensure that performance is not impaired due to inadequate folacin intake and because there is little or no risk of harm. Because, like most B vitamins, there is little stored in the body, oral supplementation daily may be preferred. Intramuscular injections increase serum or red blood cell folate concentrations for less than 24 hours.

Adverse effects following the ingestion of high amounts of folic acid by animals have not been observed. The vitamin is generally considered nontoxic. Injections of 25 mg of folic acid/kg (11 mg/lb) of body wt have, however, been reported to cause an epileptic response and renal enlargement in rats. This dose is about 1,000 times their dietary requirement.

COBALAMIN (VITAMIN B_{12})

Sources, Metabolism, and Functions

Vitamin B_{12} is unique among vitamins in that it is synthesized in nature only by microorganisms. Sources of the vitamin for all animals, therefore, are microbial contamination (e.g., manure) of substances ingested, microbial production in the gastrointestinal tract, and amounts given or added to the diet. Cobalt is a necessary constituent and is therefore required for microbial synthesis of vitamin B_{12}. Cyanocobalamin is the usual form of the vitamin used to supplement feeds or give to animals. It contains a cyanide group as an artifact of the commercial preparation process. Little, if any, of this form is believed to occur naturally. Naturally occurring forms found commonly in feeds are methylcobalamin and 5'-deoxyadenosylcobalamin. All of the above-mentioned forms have similar vitamin B_{12} activity. Although the amount of vitamin B_{12} is quite low in cereal grains, and in contrast to other B vitamins in brewer's yeast, it is relatively high in forages as compared to most animals' requirements (Appendix Table 3). In feeds it is one of the most stable vitamins. Its activity decreases only about 1.4%/mo, or to 84% of its initial value after 1 year of normal storage conditions (Table 3–3).

Vitamin B_{12} is synthesized primarily in, and appears to be absorbed from, the horse's colon. In contrast, in some species, including people, it is absorbed mainly or exclusively from the ileum, which is the basis for the Schilling's test for ileal dysfunction and vitamin B_{12} status in people.

A serum concentration decrease in vitamin B_{12} and increase in folate are also used in some species as an indication of bacterial overgrowth in the small intestine. These changes occur because intestinal bacteria produce folate and bind vitamin B_{12}. In people, intrinsic factor produced by the gastric mucosa is necessary for vitamin B_{12} absorption. Because of this, people without a stomach due to gastrectomy must be given vitamin B_{12} injections. Whether intrinsic factor is necessary for vitamin B_{12} absorption by the horse is unknown. Excess vitamin B_{12} and its metabolites are excreted in the bile and the urine. In contrast to other B vitamins, large amounts of vitamin B_{12} are stored in the liver, with lower concentrations in the kidney, heart, spleen, and brain. In people, tissue storage and reabsorption of that excreted in the bile are so great that signs of a vitamin B_{12} deficiency may not appear after many years of consuming a deficient diet and months to years after the vitamin has stopped being excreted in urine and bile.

Vitamin B_{12} is required for methionine synthesis and folate entry into cells, and is necessary for DNA synthesis. The resulting defect in DNA synthesis, characteristic of folate deficiency, also is produced by a vitamin B_{12} deficiency. This defect is responsible for the anemia that occurs with a deficiency of either of these two vitamins. In addition, vitamin B_{12} is required for the utilization of propionate, a major source of energy derived from bacterial fermentation of ingested carbohydrates. This is a major reason that with a vitamin B_{12} deficiency growth rate decreases and ketosis in ruminants occurs. Because vitamin B_{12} is required in propionate utilization for its conversion from methylmalonyl CoA to succinate, deficient animals excrete methylmalonic acid in the urine, which is used in the diagnosis of a vitamin B_{12} deficiency.

Vitamin B_{12} Dietary Requirement and Imbalances

It does not appear that the horse requires a dietary source of vitamin B_{12}. Horses consuming a purified diet containing about one tenth of that normally present in forage for 11 months showed no evidence of a vitamin B_{12} deficiency. Although their serum vitamin B_{12} concentration decreased from 6.7 to 1.0 μg/ml by 5 months, they continued to excrete more of the vitamin in the urine and feces than was consumed.

A vitamin B_{12} deficiency has not been described or known to occur in the horse. In a survey of 88 horses in various states of physiology and training, no evidence of vitamin B_{12} deficiency was found, based on serum vitamin B_{12} concentrations or blood parameters. In other species, a vitamin B_{12} deficiency results in anemia, and neuropathies causing posterior incoordination, reproductive failures, decreased appetite, reduced growth rate, a rough hair coat, dermatitis, and methylmalonic acid in the serum and urine.

Vitamin B_{12} is frequently given to horses, particularly race horses in training and use, to treat or prevent anemia, to enhance performance, and/or to stimulate or maintain appetite. There is no evidence that giving vitamin B_{12} does any of these things or is of any benefit. It has been reported that severely debilitated, anemic, heavily parasitized horses appear to respond to vitamin B_{12} injections. For such a horse, treating the parasitism and ensuring that an adequate amount of a good-quality diet is fed will be of much greater benefit than giving vitamin B_{12}. Vitamin B_{12} injections to the horse increase plasma levels for only a short period of time and greatly increase urine excretion of the vitamin.

No unequivocal evidence of adverse effects of excess vitamin B_{12} administered by any route in any species has been published. No adverse effects on growth or survival occurred in mice given several hundred times their dietary requirement.

CHOLINE

Sources, Metabolism, and Functions

Choline, although frequently listed as one of the B-complex vitamins, is not a vitamin in that it can be synthesized in adequate amounts in the body by all mammals and, therefore, does not need to be either in the diet or produced by gastrointestinal microorganisms. It is synthesized in the liver from the amino acid methionine. Choline is also present in feeds as the free form and as a component of lecithin, acetylcholine, and other phospholipids. The form most commonly used for supplementation of diets is choline hydrochloride. Commonly used horse feeds contain 0.5 to 2 g of choline/kg (Appendix Table 3). Choline in feeds is quite sensitive to moisture but resistant to other stress factors. Its content in feeds decreases only about 1%/month under normal storage conditions (Table 3–3).

Choline has three important functions in the body. These are as a component of: (1) the neurotransmitter acetylcholine, (2) lecithin, and (3) betaine. Betaine is necessary for the formation of methionine and creatine. Lecithin is an important component in cell membranes, in lipoproteins for tissue lipid mobilization and utilization, and in lung surfactants. These functions are responsible for the effects of a choline deficiency and the basis for its use clinically.

Lecithins are best known as a "health food" consumed by people to reduce blood cholesterol and improve mental function, i.e., as a "brain food." Lecithins are produced as a by-product in the production of oils from seed, such as soy, cottonseed, and linseed. Feeding lecithin to horses has been purported to make them more manageable, improve athletic performance and to enhance dietary fat use. There are no studies known to support these claims. Feeding lecithin to eight 2- and 3-year old horses did tend to decrease insignificantly their reactivity to visual and auditory stimuli, but had no effect on voluntary activity and decreased feed palatability.

Choline Requirements

The choline requirement for the horse has not been determined. However, none is needed if the diet contains an adequate amount of the amino acid methionine for synthesis of sufficient choline in the liver. Choline in the diet will decrease the amount of, but not the need for, methionine in the diet, whereas sufficient dietary methionine does alleviate the need for choline in the diet. If the horse's protein requirements are met using feeds commonly fed, the diet will contain sufficient methionine so that no choline is needed in the diet. If the horse's protein requirements are not met, although there may be inadequate dietary methionine and/or choline, the effect is a protein, not a choline, deficiency.

Choline Deficiency

A choline deficiency occurs primarily in rapidly growing young animals fed diets deficient in methionine and/or choline. The most characteristic effect of a choline deficiency is the development of a fatty liver, which if continued for a sufficient time may lead to cirrhosis. An experimentally induced deficiency in calves caused weakness with a failure to stand and labored breathing. A chronic choline deficiency in dogs has been reported to cause duodenal ulcers, liver damage, anemia, and edema. Other effects of a choline deficiency include reduced plasma choline concentration, degeneration of the thymus, decreased growth rate, impaired reproduction, and hemorrhagic renal lesions. In birds, "slipped tendon" may occur as a result of abnormal development of the hock joint, allowing slipping of the Achilles tendon from the articular condyle. Which of these effects may occur in the horse is unknown, as a choline deficiency has not been described or known to occur in the horse.

Choline Clinical Usage

Because of choline's functions and the effects of a choline deficiency, this vitamin is occasionally given to try to treat or prevent similar dysfunctions or conditions, although a choline deficiency is not known to be present. The most common clinical usage of choline is to try to treat or prevent hepatic dysfunctions, particularly fatty liver, although there is little data to confirm its benefit. Choline has also been reported, but not confirmed, to be of benefit in treating horses with chronic obstructive pulmonary disease, or heaves. A dosage of 6 to 8 g (0.4 to 0.5 oz) of choline chloride/horse/day is added to the diet for this purpose.

Choline Toxicosis

Care must be taken in giving choline, as detrimental effects of excess choline have been demonstrated in most species studied, which does not include the horse. Pigs appear to have a high tolerance for excess choline, whereas for chicks a dietary level greater than twice that required decreases growth and interferes with vitamin B_6 utilization. In dogs, 8 mg of choline chloride/kg of body wt ingested daily by 10 days caused anemia. This is only about 3 times their apparent choline requirement. Studies in mice and rats indicate that much lower amounts of choline are harmful when injected than when given orally, and that choline chloride is more toxic than cytidine diphosphate choline.

VITAMIN C (ASCORBIC ACID)
Sources and Metabolism of Vitamin C

Vitamin C is available as ascorbic acid, ascorbate-2-sulphate, ascorbyl palmitate, sodium ascorbate, and potassium ascorbate. Ascorbic acid, which is the reduced form, may also be present in the oxidized form, dehydroascorbic acid. For most animals, but not fish, that require a dietary source of vitamin C, only ascorbic acid has significant biological activity. Ascorbic acid is widely distributed in fresh vegetables and fruits; cereal grains contain almost none. Ascorbic acid, either naturally present or added to foods, is readily destroyed by oxidation. Heat, light, alkalinity, and particularly minerals, when it is exposed to air, hasten its oxidation. Ascorbic acid activity in feeds decreases 30%/month. However, coating vitamin C with ethylcellulose decreases its rate of activity loss to only 7%/month (Table 3-3).

Ascorbic acid is synthesized from the simple sugar glucose in the liver of all animals studied except people, several other primates, the Indian fruit bat, guinea pigs, and a few birds, fish, and invertebrates. These species lack the enzyme needed for its synthesis. For other species, ascorbic acid is not an essential dietary nutrient; however, it is physiologically essential for all species. Body storage of ascorbic acid is minimal, as clinical signs in people occur between 60 and 90 days after the beginning of inadequate intake, which means the body is depleted much before this occurs. Excess ascorbic acid and its metabolites are excreted in the urine by most species, whereas in some species, such as guinea pigs and rats, they are metabolized to carbon dioxide and exhaled.

Functions of Vitamin C

The function of ascorbic acid appears to be the same in all species. It is an antioxidant and, therefore, protects lipids, proteins, and membranes from free-radical-induced oxidative damage. Ascorbic acid scavenges oxygen radicals in aqueous solutions, while vitamin E scavenges free radicals within cell membranes. Vitamin C enhances the formation of bone matrix and tooth dentin. It aids in the utilization of folic acid, vitamin B_{12}, a number of the other B vitamins, cholesterol and glucose, and enhances intestinal absorption of iron and immune functions. It is necessary for the synthesis for norepinephrine, tyrosine, carnitine, and steroids. One of ascorbic acid's major functions is hydroxylation of several amino acids: tryptophan, lysine, and proline. Hydroxyproline is a major constituent of collagen. Many of the signs of vitamin C deficiency reflect a lack of normal collagen.

Vitamin C Deficiency

The following effects of a vitamin C deficiency may occur in species that need vitamin C in their diet, but not in those such as the horse that do not need vitamin C in their diet. These effects of a vitamin C deficiency include impaired wound healing, weak brittle bones, and hemorrhage, all of which occur due to a lack of normal collagen, whose production requires adequate vitamin C. The hemorrhaging that occurs includes bleeding between bone and its periosteal covering, and into the heart sac, the peritoneal cavity, the adrenals, and the joints. The gums become swollen and bleed easily; the teeth become loose. A form of arthritis accompanied by effusions into the joints may also occur in adults. In the young, bone formation is impaired and dentition disrupted. Profound fatigue, weakness, and lethargy develop, and pitting edema of the extremities may occur. Death may occur within a relatively short period of time, especially in the young.

This condition due to a vitamin C deficiency is called scurvy. The name scurvy comes from a contraction of the phrase "scourge of the navy," which it was before the 19th century. Sailors on long sea voyages without fresh fruits or vegetables, and therefore adequate vitamin C, frequently became afflicted before it became widely known that it could be prevented with these food items. The nickname "limey" was given to British sailors who sucked on limes to prevent it.

Vitamin C Requirement and Clinical Usage

Horses do not need vitamin C in their diet. Horses fed a semipurified ascorbic-acid-free diet for 6 months had only a 15 to 30% decrease in their plasma ascorbic acid concentration; but their urine excretion remained unchanged compared to those receiving the same diet with ascorbic acid added and it was 4 times greater than it was from horses on fall grass pasture who had plasma ascorbic acid concentrations similar to those fed the semipurified diet with added ascorbic acid. However, the plasma ascorbic acid concentration is decreased in a number of infectious diseases, and studies in pigs, rabbits, and poultry have suggested to some that stressful conditions might increase the requirement for ascorbic acid beyond the animals' ability to synthesize it. This has also been suggested for horses.

Horses over 20 years old, ill, or stressed, may have plasma ascorbic acid concentrations below the normal of 2 to 4 µg/ml (110 to 220 µmol/L). It has been reported, but without confirmatory data, that low plasma ascorbic acid concentrations in horses may be associated with wound infections, bleeding from the nose, strangles, rhinopneumonitis, and decreased performance.

Because a vitamin C deficiency results in hemorrhaging in species that need vitamin C in their diet, it has been given to horses to try to treat and prevent bleeders (exercise-induced pulmonary hemorrhage as described in Chapter 11). However, it appears to be of no benefit for this purpose. Citrus bioflavonoids, a source of ascorbic acid, have been found to be of no benefit.

It is also thought by some that because of vitamin C's antioxidant properties, like vitamin E and selenium, giving it may help protect cell membranes and thus muscles from exertion-induced damage. Although there is no data confirming or refuting its effect for this purpose, it is believed that it is unlikely to be of benefit. Even in species, such as people, that require vitamin C in their diet, a number of good controlled studies have failed to show any benefit in human athletes' physical performance or health as a result of the administration of large doses of vitamin C.

Vitamin C has also been given to treat impaired fertility or to enhance fertility of mares and stallions. There have been anecdotal reports, without confirmatory data, that feeding of vitamin C may help get hard-to-breed mares to conceive. Supplementation of infertile men with ascorbic acid has been reported to improve the viability and motility of spermatozoa. It has been reported that a stallion that had reduced semen motility was successfully treated by giving ascorbic acid. However, giving 10 g of ascorbic acid/horse/day orally for 70 days to five stallions who had less than 25% spermatozoal progressive motility did not increase motility, although it did increase their plasma ascorbic acid concentrations 40 to 140% and decreased spermatozoal tail abnormalities 20 to 58%.

Because vitamin C is necessary for normal skeletal development, it has been suggested that during rapid growth inadequate vitamin C due to insufficient synthesis may cause, or be at least one predisposing factor in the occurrence of, developmental orthopedic diseases such as hip dysplasia in dogs. As a result of suggestions such as this, and the hope that supplemental vitamin C may enhance optimum skeletal development, decrease the risk of developmental orthopedic diseases, and at least not be harmful, vitamin C is occasionally given to young rapidly growing animals. However, there have been no controlled studies that confirm a role for vitamin C in the cause, treatment, or prevention of developmental orthopedic diseases in foals, or any other species that don't require vitamin C in their diet. In a well-controlled study in young rapidly growing Great Dane dogs, vitamin C supplementation appeared to increase, rather than decrease, the occurrence of skeletal disease.

Because vitamin C is excreted in the urine of most species and is an acid (ascorbic acid), it has been used widely in many species to acidify the urine, primarily to assist in the treatment and prevention of urinary calculi or stones due to struvite (magnesium-ammonium-phosphate) whose solubility increases in an acid urine. However, it is poorly effective for this purpose, and its administration may be harmful for urinary caculi due to cysteine and urate, which form best in an acid urine, and for calcium oxalate calculi because it may increase urine oxalate excretion. Calcium carbonate and phosphate, the most common types of urinary calculi occurring in horses, are not known to be affected by vitamin C intake.

For the many reasons described, and others, vitamin C is occasionally given to horses. Conditions under which giving vitamin C has been suggested to be most likely beneficial are: (1) during hot weather, (2) under stress of any type, (3) during rapid growth, (4) during high-level performance, and (5) when something interferes with vitamin C synthesis, such as a dietary energy deficiency, which may result in inadequate glucose for synthesis of sufficient vitamin C. It has also been suggested that, based on studies in species other than horses, not all animals will respond to vitamin C supplementation and, therefore, individual response, not group averages or response, should be observed to determine if giving vitamin C is of benefit. However, remember that vitamin C supplementation to the horse under any condition has not been shown, even in an individual animal, to be of benefit, and that although some studies in other species under certain circumstances suggest a benefit, other studies suggest harm from vitamin C supplementation.

Vitamin C Administration

Because vitamin C given orally has been shown to be poorly absorbed by the horse, and injections to result in marked local irritation, intravenous administration has been recommended. However, following the intravenous administration of even a relatively large dose, the plasma ascorbic acid concentration returns to near pre-injection levels within 4 hours. Although ascorbic acid following a single oral dose doesn't greatly increase the plasma ascorbic acid concentration, its continuous ingestion does, with the maximum increase in its plasma concentration occurring at a dosage of 4.5 g/horse/day.

Although ascorbyl palmitate has been reported to be biologically inactive for most animal species, its oral administration increases the horse's plasma ascorbic acid concentration. This would suggest that it is biologically active for the horse. It appears to be the preferred ascorbic acid oral supplement for the horse. No apparent absorption of ascorbic acid or ascorbyl stearate occurs in some horses, whereas all horses appear to absorb ascorbyl palmitate. It is also the most palatable. Since it is 42.5% ascorbic acid, 2.35 times (1 ÷ 0425 = 2.35) more of it must be given than ascorbic acid to provide a similar amount of ascorbic acid.

Toxicosis of Vitamin C

There appears to be little danger, and no reports, of harm from excessive vitamin C administration to the horse. Effects of excessive vitamin C administration have been reported in other species. Harmful effects reported in people and laboratory animals include increased oxalate and uric acid excretion in the urine, low blood sugar, excessive iron absorption, diarrhea, allergic responses, destruction of vitamin B_{12}, and interference with liver function. However, some of these abnormalities were incidental and were noted in uncontrolled studies, or are controversial. In contrast to other species, mink seem to be quite sensitive to excess ascorbic acid, developing a pronounced anemia and a reduced number and birth weight of kits. A dietary ascorbic acid concentration of 1 g/kg (0.45 g/lb.) of body wt appears to pose no hazard to chickens, pigs, dogs, cats, or horses.

HARVESTED FEEDS FOR HORSES

Hays for Horses	63
Hay Types	63
Hay Forms	65
Hay Cubes (wafers) and Pellets (dehy)	66
Hay Cuttings	67
Hay Quality	68
Cereal Grains for Horses	70
Grain Types	72
Oats	73
Corn	74
Barley	75
Sorghum (Milo)	75
Wheat	75
Rye	76
Rice	76
Millet, Emmer, Spelt and Triticale	76
Grain Processing	76
Grain Quality	77
Grain Storage	78
High-Moisture Feeds for Horses	79
Haylage, Silage, and High-Moisture Grains	79
Acid-Treated Feeds	80
Vitamin-Mineral Supplements for Horses	81
Protein Supplements for Horses	82
Oilseeds and Oilseed Meals	82
Soybeans	83
Cottonseeds	83
Linseed (Flaxseed) Meal	85
Peanut Meal	86
Sunflower Seed Meal	86
Rapeseed (Canola)	86
Grain Protein Supplements	87
Brewers' Grains and Yeast	87
Distillers' Grains	87
Gluten	87
Beans and Peas (Pulse Proteins)	87
Animal-Source Protein Supplements	88
Dried Milk Products	88
Fish Meals	89
Dried Poultry Manure	89
Single-Cell Proteins	89
Fat and Oil Supplements for Horses	89
Grain Mixes and Complete Feeds for Horses	91
Pelleted and Extruded Grain Mixes and Complete Feeds . .	92
Slowing Feed Consumption	94
By-Product Feeds for Horses	94
Bran	94
Straw and Stover	95
Hulls	96
Soybean Hulls	97
Sunflower Hulls	97
Almond Hulls	98
Molasses	98
Condensed Molasses Solubles	98
Sugar Beet Pulp	98
Fruit or Citrus Pulp	99
Fresh Fruits and Vegetables	99
Potatoes	99
Lawn Grass Clippings	99
Feed Additives for Horses	99
Zeolite	99
Flavoring Agents	100
Digestion Enhancers	100
Probiotics (Yeast-Cultures)	100
Antibiotic Feed Additives	101
Mold Inhibitors	101
Antioxidants	102
Bioflavonoids	102

Feeds fed to horses may be classified in a number of ways. In this book they are classified as forages, cereal grains, high-moisture feeds, supplements, concentrate or grain mixes, complete feeds, and by-product feeds. Forages are the leaves, stems, and stalks of plants, while cereal grains are plant seeds. Generally, both when harvested are fed dry, although both may be stored and fed to horses at a high-moisture content. Forages frequently are defined as feeds that contain above some arbitrarily set and relatively high crude-fiber content (usually 18%) or low dietary energy content. However, when defined in this manner, the fiber content of early stages of some rapidly growing forages may be lower, and their dietary energy content higher, than the fiber and energy content of some cereal grains.

Forages may be fed harvested or unharvested. Unharvested forages include pasture and crop residues. Crop residues are that part of plants which remain following harvesting, such as cereal grain stubble and corn and sorghum stalks. Only harvested forages and crop residues are covered in this chapter. Pastures for horses are discussed in Chapter 5.

Supplements are feeds high in one or more nutrients fed to increase the diet's concentration, or horse's intake, of that nutrient. The most common supplements needed and fed to horses are vitamin, mineral, and protein supplements. Supplements mixed with cereal grains, referred to as grain or concentrate mixes, may be home, custom, or commercially prepared. Forages may also be combined with a grain mix to make a complete feed, or total diet, for the horse. Grain mixes and complete feeds that are commercially prepared may be sold as a loose mixture or as a pelleted or extruded feed. In the United Kingdom, feed pellets or cubes may be referred to as "nuts," a compound nut being a grain mix and forage pellet, often a complete pelleted feed; dehydrated forage pellets are referred to as dried grass nuts in the United Kingdom and as dehy or alfalfa pellets in North America, where they routinely consist of alfalfa and, therefore, are also referred to as alfalfa pellets.

Commercial grain mixes and complete feeds may contain additives to increase feed utilization or storage stability, and numerous by-product feeds, such as molasses, bran, straw, hulls, or beet, fruit or citrus pulp. Many by-product feeds are a good source of certain nutrients and make good feeds for the horse, sometimes at a very economical price.

HAYS FOR HORSES

The heads, leaves, and stems or stalks of plants immediately following cutting may be chopped and either fed that day green as green chop or soilage, or stored in an oxygen-limiting facility or silo and fed as haylage upon removal from the silo. However, most often, especially for horses, the forage following cutting is allowed to dry in the field, stored, and fed as hay. Forage, unharvested or harvested and fed in any of these forms, is the most natural, safest, and frequently least expensive feed for the horse. The type, quality, and amount of forage fed determines if, what type, and how much other feeds should be fed. Forages, therefore, should always be the basis for all horse feeding programs.

Forages are extremely important feeds for herbivores, such as the horse, not only for the nutrients they provide, but also for the stimulatory effects of forages on the muscle tone and activity of the gastrointestinal tract. Without adequate forage intake, colic, founder, and often an increase in stable vices will occur. Despite its many advantages as a feed for horses, forage has several shortcomings. Forages vary more in nutrient content and palatability, and more forage and its nutrients are lost in harvesting, storage, and feeding than any other feed for horses. Forages have the following general characteristics with respect to other horse feeds. They are:

1. Bulky, with a low weight per unit of volume. For example, the density in lbs/cubic feet (kg/dl) of cereal grains is 25 to 48 (40 to 77), and baled hay is 5 to 10 (8 to 16), although cubed hay is about 30 (48) (Appendix Table 8).
2. High in fiber and low in digestible energy. Average-quality forage contains 28 to 38% crude fiber and 0.9 to 1.1 Mcal/lb (2.0 to 2.2 Mcal/kg) in its dry matter, whereas cereal grains contain 2 to 12% crude fiber and 1.5 to 1.7 Mcal/lb (3.3 to 3.7 Mcal/kg) (Appendix Table 6).
3. Higher in calcium and potassium but lower in phosphorus. Forages versus cereal grains contain as a percent in their dry matter: potassium >1 versus <0.7, calcium >0.3 versus <0.1, and phosphorus 0.1 to 0.3 versus 0.3 to 0.4 (Appendix Table 2).
4. Higher in vitamins A, E and K and, if sun cured, higher in vitamin D (Appendix Table 3).
5. Variable in protein content. Legumes may contain over 20% and grasses less than 4% protein, as compared to 8 to 14% in cereal grains and more than 20 to 25% in protein supplements (Appendix Table 6).

Hay Types

There are three major types of hay: legumes, grasses, and cereal grain hay (Figs. 4–1, 4–2, 4–3). The major legume harvested is alfalfa (lucerne or *Medicago sativa*). More than one-half of the hay harvested in the United States is

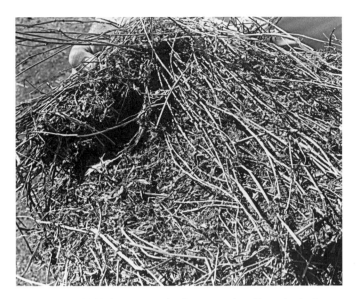

Fig. 4–1. Alfalfa hay. Note the leaves and stalks, which distinguish it from grass hay.

alfalfa or an alfalfa-grass mixture. Other legumes less widely available include clovers (e.g., Alsike, crimson, red, ladino, and sweet), birdsfoot trefoil, lespedeza, soybeans, cowpeas, vetch, and rhizomal peanut forages. A variety of grasses is commonly fed and includes timothy, brome, orchard grass, Bermuda grass, bluegrass, bluegramma, bluestem, fescue, wheatgrass, reed canarygrass, ryegrass, Sudan grass, and many others. Cereal grains, while still green and in which the grain has not been harvested, may be cut and used for hay. The more grain they contain, the greater their nutritional value. They make the most nutritious hay when cut while the grain is in the soft dough stage, but still make good hay when more mature as long

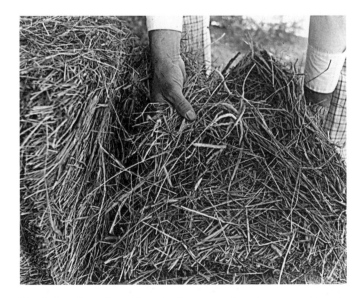

Fig. 4–2. Grass hay. Note the fine stems, long leaves, and heads (below and to the right of the thumb), which distinguish it from legumes.

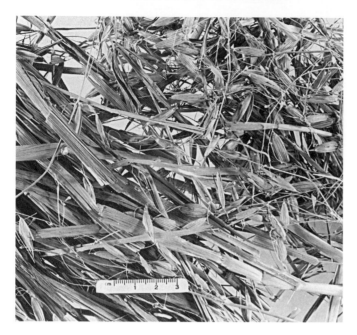

Fig. 4–3. Oat hay. Note the heads which contain the grain.

as the plant is still green. Cereal grain hays are nutritionally similar to grass hays. If the heads or grain are lost, only straw remains, which is a good bedding but, like poor-quality grass hay, is a poor feed.

Legume hays are higher in nutritional value than grass and cereal grain hays, generally containing 2 to 3 times more protein and calcium, and more soluble or nonfiber carbohydrates (often referred to as nitrogen-free extract, or NFE), vitamin A precursor or beta-carotene, and vitamin E (Table 4–1). Because of the greater amount of these nutrients in legumes, and the increased need for these nutrients during growth, lactation, and the last three months of pregnancy (Appendix Tables 1 and 3), legumes are preferred by many during these periods, if it is good quality and available at a reasonable cost as compared to equal-quality grass or cereal grain hay. If a good legume hay is not available at a reasonable cost, grass or cereal grain hay may be fed, and additional nutrients if needed may be added to a grain mix as described in Chapter 6.

In contrast to what is occasionally stated or believed by some, any of the three major types of hay may be safely fed as the only forage for the horse, or the only feed for the horse if a grain mix is not needed to provide additional amounts of certain nutrients. Some individuals recommend against feeding alfalfa, or other legumes, as the only hay. This recommendation is probably based on any one or more of a number of factors, including:

1. Not being familiar with feeding it.
2. Because it is known that green growing alfalfa may induce bloat in ruminants (but it does not cause bloat in horses).
3. Previous experience with or knowledge of detrimental effects, such as:
   a. respiratory problems because it is dusty or moldy
   b. toxicosis because it contained blister beetles or mycotoxins
   c. colic because of excessive consumption of lush green alfalfa
   d. developmental orthopedic diseases when alfalfa is fed because of its high nutrient content which allows for rapid growth and orthopedic diseases to occur if the minerals needed (such as phosphorus) are not provided, as discussed in Chapter 16
   However, it does not cause any of these problems if it is of good quality and fed properly, i.e., the above situations are avoided.
4. Because of the myth that it may be hard on the kidneys or cause renal damage. This myth may have developed because horses fed alfalfa urinate more than horses fed grass. This occurs because of alfalfa's higher protein content. However, there is no evidence that this higher protein level in alfalfa, or alfalfa for any reason, causes, increases the risk of, or predisposes to renal disease in horses or any other species of animal.

Most horses will generally consume more legume than grass hay, even if the legume hay is of poorer quality. Within the same type of hay, the amount consumed is directly related to hay quality, i.e., the higher the hay quality (the lower it is in weeds, dust, and mold; the higher its protein and energy; the lower its fiber content; and

TABLE 4–1
Hay Nutrient Content for Horses

| Hay Type | Maturity | Mcal Dig. Energy/ lb (kg) DM | % in Hay Dry Matter (DM) | | | | Vit. A[c] IU/kg DM × 1000 | Vit. E mg/kg DM |
			Crude Protein	Crude Fiber	Calcium	Phosphorus		
Legumes	Early bloom	1.1 (2.4)	17–20[a]	30[b]	1–1.8	0.1–0.3	50–85	20–40
	Full bloom	0.95 (2.1)	15–18	32	1–1.8	0.1–0.3	10–30	10–20
Grass	Early bloom	0.95 (2.1)	11–14	30–34	0.3–0.5	0.1–0.3	15–25	10–30
	Mature	0.8 (1.8)	6–10	32–36	0.3–0.5	0.1–0.3	5–15	
Cereal grain	Cut green	0.87 (1.9)	9	29	0.15–0.35	0.1–0.3	10–35	

[a] about 11% in lespediza.
[b] 21 to 23% in alfalfa and ladino clover.
[c] mg beta-carotene times 400.

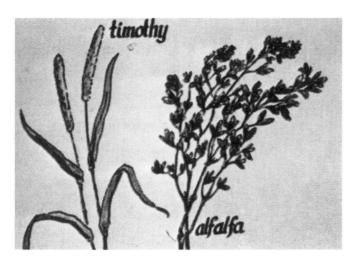

Fig. 4–4. Illustration depicting the differences in appearance between a grass, such as timothy, and a legume, such as alfalfa. In the grass, note the long leaves, their attachment, fine stems, and heads. The stalks of the legume are much coarser, and the leaves less firmly attached. (Courtesy of Dr. R. Seaney, Cornell University.)

the higher its digestibility), the more of it the horse will consume. For equal quality hays, consumption of timothy by horses tends to be greater, and fescue and Bermuda grass lower, than for brome grass, canary grass, and orchard grass. Orchard grass tends to be preferred by horses over flaccid grass and Bahia grass. Bahia grass is not recommended for horses as it is sufficiently unpalatable that many will not eat enough to maintain their weight. Most grains are preferred by most horses over any forage.

The leaves are less firmly attached to the stem in legumes than in grasses. This can result in a greater loss of leaves from legumes if they are not cut at the proper stage of maturity, handled properly after cutting, or fed in a feeder that prevents their loss. Since leaves contain two-thirds of the energy, three-fourths of the protein, and most of the other nutrients present in forages, the loss of leaves greatly decreases the nutritional value and therefore the quality of the hay. The firmer attachment of the leaves and the differences in their size and shape in grass hay makes leaf loss less of a problem with grass hay (Fig 4–4). This permits more latitude in the cutting and processing of grass hays without greatly decreasing their nutritional value. Grass hays also are usually less dusty, making them cleaner to feed and resulting in less coughing and chronic obstructive pulmonary disease or heaves. In addition, grass hays don't contain blister beetles, whereas legume hays may when harvested in areas where, and during the season when, they occur (as discussed in Chapter 19).

The most important factor to consider in selecting the hay to feed is not the type of hay, or the form that it is in, but its quality, availability, and cost.

Hay Forms

There are five major ways that forages may be harvested and fed. These are: grazing, dried, green chop or soilage, haylage or silage, and acid treated. Hay dried to less than

20% moisture content prior to baling, stacking, or storage is by far the most common harvested forage fed to horses. If the moisture is much higher, molding and heating that decreases protein utilization occurs. Stored hay with excess moisture may even undergo spontaneous combustion. However, if hay is allowed to dry (less than 12% moisture prior to baling and storage), there is a greater loss of leaves, particularly with legumes. Drying may be done artificially but generally is accomplished by sun curing. This may be hastened by conditioning (crushing or crimping the plants) and adding drying agents as it is cut. Drying agents (usually a solution of sodium and potassium carbonate or potassium hydroxide) are sprayed on the forage during mowing and conditioning, and can decrease drying time by more than one-half. They are effective only on legumes during favorable drying conditions. The presence of the drying agent on the hay has no effect on animals consuming it. The faster drying occurs, the lower the amount and risk of weather damage to the hay. Hay that is mowed and then rained on before harvest may lose 40 to 50% or more of its nutritional value.

Once sufficiently dried, the hay may be stacked, baled, chopped or, compressed into cubes, wafers, or pellets for storage and feeding. Most forage available commercially and fed to horses is in cubes, pellets, or most commonly long-stem hay in small square bales (45 to 100 lbs or 20 to 50 kg) versus large round or square bales weighing from 500 to 2000 lbs (227 to 909 kg) depending on the equipment used.

Large round bales and stacks of hay are sometimes fed by leaving them in the field and allowing animals free access to them. Doing this alleviates the need for daily feeding. However, this results in storage and feeding losses of 30 to 38% as compared to 8 to 9% loss from bales (4% from cubes and pellets) stored inside and fed in a feed rack (Table 4–2). However, storage losses from large bales may be greatly decreased by wrapping them in plastic, which is done as the hay is baled; a new procedure found to be quite effective is to spray the bale with melted tallow or

TABLE 4–2
Losses in Storage and Feeding of Different Forms of Hay

| | | | % Losses Expected | | |
Hay Form	How Stored	How Fed	Storage	Feeding[a]	Total
Small square bales	Inside	Feed rack	4	5	9
Large round bales	Inside, or outside covered on tires	Feed rack	4	4	8
	Outside uncovered on ground	From bale on ground	16	14–22	30–38
Stack (3-ton)	Outside	Feed rack	9	4	13
	Outside	On ground	9	28	37
Cubes or Pellets	Inside	Feed rack	2	2	4

[a] Losses measured for cattle, which may be a good estimate for horses. Feeding losses from all feeding methods increase greatly if animals are fed more than they need.

animal fat. The tallow is sprayed on at a temperature sufficient to keep it liquid (usually about 120°F [49°C]). It congeals on the hay, providing a water-repellant covering that sheds rain, resulting in almost no loss due to weather spoilage. It takes about 2 gallons (7.6 L) of melted tallow for most large round bales at a current cost of $1.50 to $3.00/bale, as compared to $4.00/bale for plastic wrap. The fat on the hay not only protects it but also increases its dietary energy content and feeding value as described in the section "Fat and Oil Supplements for Horses" later in this chapter.

In contrast to ruminants, in which pelleting roughages decreases crude fiber digestibility, for horses the form in which hay is fed doesn't appear to affect its digestibility. Chopping hay increases its rate of passage and intake in ruminants and probably horses, as indicated by a greater dry matter intake by horses fed pelleted alfalfa than when they are fed a coarse-chopped wafered alfalfa, and more of the wafered alfalfa than when fed unchopped long-stemmed alfalfa. In addition, it's been reported that most horses prefer chopped to long-stemmed grass hay. But the major advantage of chopping hay is so that it can be mixed with grain to slow the rate of grain consumption. However, horses are able to separate grain from chopped hay and eat only the preferred feed (usually the grain).

If preferred, or conditions are unsatisfactory for drying following cutting, harvested forage may be fed that day, or treated with acid or ensiled at a high moisture content (40 to 70%). Not allowing forage to dry minimizes feed and nutrient losses during harvesting and feeding and reduces the inhalation of dusts and molds, generally present in varying amounts in most dry hay. This assists in decreasing respiratory problems such as coughing and heaves. If green forage is not fed immediately following cutting, acid treatment, ensiling, or drying is necessary to prevent mold and bacterial growth resulting in its spoilage. If one of these three procedures is not done, fresh forage must be fed the day it is cut or it will spoil.

Fresh forage cut, chopped, and fed that day is called green chop or soilage. It must be harvested daily, and for the best feeding value the forage must be harvested at its optimum stage of growth or maturity. This limits its duration of use. Because of these limitations, green chop is not commonly fed to horses.

Hay Cubes (Wafers) and Pellets (Dehy)

Hay is usually fed in loose form, but it may be compressed into cubes, wafers, or pellets. Pellets containing primarily or entirely grains and supplements that are large enough (about thumb size or larger) to be fed on the ground, are also commonly referred to as cake or cubes, generally as range cake or range cubes. They are most often fed to cattle on pasture or on the range.

In cubing, hay is generally sun cured and either unground or only coarsely ground before it is compressed into about 1¼-inch squares that break apart every 2 to 3 inches (3 cm by 5 to 7 cm) (Fig. 4-5). In pelleting, hay is finely ground and often artificially dried or dehydrated (and thus the common name "dehy" pellets) before being compressed into pellets of approximately ¼ to ⅜ inch in

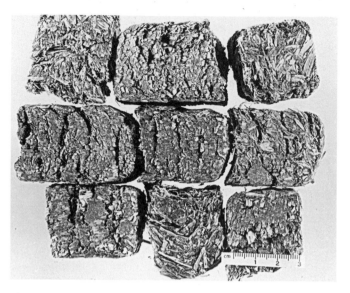

Fig. 4–5. Hay pressed into cubes. Cubes are 1 to 1¼ inches (3 cm) square and 1 to 3 inches (3 to 7 cm) long.

diameter by ½ inch long (0.6 to 1 by 1.3 cm) (Fig. 4-6). Cubing is done by farm equipment that moves across hay fields picking up windrows of hay, whereas pelleting is done in a pellet mill. In North America, dehy pellets are generally made from alfalfa and rarely a grass hay. Although heat is used in dehydrating and produced in pelleting hay, the amount of heat doesn't appear to greatly affect the nutritional value of most hay pellets. Excessive heating of forages lowers nutritional value by destroying vitamins and inducing formation of undigestible protein-carbohydrate

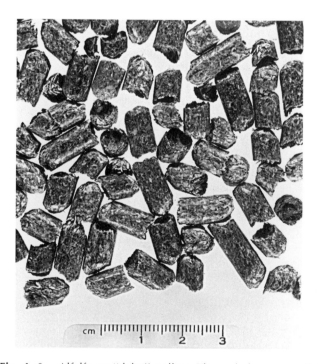

Fig. 4–6. Alfalfa or "dehy" pellets. These dark green pellets may be made from either sun cured or dehydrated alfalfa.

bonds. However, studies have shown no difference in nutrient digestibility by horses between loose, pelleted or cubed hay.

When pellets are made from good-quality alfalfa, they contain at least 17% crude protein as fed, and are often referred to as 17% dehy. When poorer-quality alfalfa is used, the pellets contain 15 to 17% crude protein as fed, and are referred to as 15% dehy. Generally, 15% dehy contains 26 to 28%, and 17% dehy 24 to 25%, crude fiber as fed.

Hay cubes offer the advantages of hay pellets with few of their disadvantages. The advantages of cubed and pelleted hay are the following:

1. Less wastage by the horse. With cattle, loss of baled hay stored inside and fed in racks was 9% in one study, as compared to a 4% loss when pelleted or cubed hay was fed. When loose hay is fed on the ground, losses during feeding may be 14 to 22% (Table 4-2). Losses similar to these might be expected for horses. Loss of leaves, particularly from legume hays, during harvesting, feeding, and when being eaten are lessened with cubes and pellets. Since leaves contain most of the nutrients in hay, decreasing their loss results in greater nutrient value being obtained from cubes and pellets than from long-stem hay.

2. Intestinal fill may be reduced when pellets are fed, so that as much as 20 to 30% more pelleted feed than loose forage can be consumed. This is of benefit if additional feed intake is needed. A decrease in intestinal fill also makes some horses look trimmer, with less of a "hay belly" appearance.

3. Less storage space. A ton of hay cubes occupies 60 to 70 cubic feet (1.8 or 2.2 cu m/metric ton), as compared with 200 to 330 cubic feet for each ton (6 to 10 cu m/metric ton) of baled hay and 450 to 600 cubic feet for each ton (14 to 19 cu m/metric ton) of loose hay (Appendix Table 8).

4. Reduced transportation costs.

5. Ease of transport for feeding away from home.

6. Minimal dust when eaten, if made properly. This is an important advantage for horses, in which the dust or fungal spores in loose hay cause chronic obstructive pulmonary disease or heaves and coughing.

7. Facilitated automation in both harvesting and feeding.

8. Reduced feces in horses eating pelleted hay. However, digestibility is the same. The lower amount of feces produced when pellets are fed is due to a lower fecal water content with no difference in fecal dry matter excreted.

It may take a few days for some horses to learn to eat hay cubes. However, once they do learn, they eat cubes and also pellets faster than loose hay. As a result of their more rapid rate of consumption, it is reported that some horses occasionally choke on pellets or cubes. Although this is an uncommon problem with hay cubes or pellets, their rate of consumption and, therefore, the risk of choking may be decreased in a number of ways as described later in this chapter (see end of section "Slowing Feed Consumption").

Wood and tail chewing may increase when cubes or pellets are the only forage fed. When wood chewing was measured, this observation was verified for pellets but not for cubes. In one study, nearly 4 times more wood chewing occurred when pellets were fed than when long-stem hay was fed. In contrast, there was no difference in the amount of wood consumed by mature mares when they were fed the same alfalfa hay loose twice daily, or when it was fed cubed either twice or three times daily. Thus, wood chewing did not increase when hay cubes were fed, nor decrease by feeding cubes more frequently. However, feeding pellets 6 times versus once daily did decrease wood chewing by about one-half. Other causes of and procedures for treating and preventing behavioral problems such as wood and tail chewing are described in Chapter 20.

Major disadvantages of hay cubes and pellets are that harvesting costs may be higher for cubing and pelleting than baling, and it is difficult to evaluate the quality of the hay in cubes and pellets without a laboratory analysis. In addition to containing as much or more protein, and crude fiber equal to or less than that given in Appendix Table 6 for a similar type of hay, good quality cubes and pellets are quite firm, not crumbly, and are free of mold, weeds, and foreign material. If pelleted feeds are too soft and crumbly, most horses don't like them, and they will break into fine material that is dusty, easily lost, and increases the risk of digestive problems. If they are well made, this is not a problem unless they get wet and then dry out. For this reason, pellets must be protected from the weather. If hay is cubed or pelleted when it is too dry, it will result in a soft crumbly cube or pellet; if it is too wet, mold growth and spoilage occur. The firmness and crumbling of feed pellets can be adjusted by adding varying amounts of binders and wet molasses. Too much wet molasses makes a soft pellet; too little results in a pellet that crumbles easily (7.5 to 10% generally results in a good pellet).

Horses' fecal water content is lower when pellets instead of long-stem hay are fed—in one study, 75.2% versus 81.5%. The effect on the horse of a lower fecal water content when pellets are fed isn't known. It theoretically may increase the risk of feed impaction in the intestinal tract, although there is no data indicating this. It has been reported that cattle fed only cubed or pelleted hay may develop a progressive indigestion and enteritis, but that feeding some loose hay (25% of the forage is the proportion recommended) will prevent this from occurring. Although this hasn't been reported or known to occur in horses, it is recommended that all horses, whether being fed hay cubes or pellets, receive at least ½ lb of long-stem hay or pasture forage/100 lbs body wt (½ kg/100 kg) daily. This may decrease the risk of gastrointestinal problems and decrease wood chewing from when pellets only are fed.

Hay Cuttings

Depending on conditions, from one to as many as eight cuttings of hay per year may be obtained in some areas. The first cutting of the season is generally high in nutri-

TABLE 4–3
Quality and Nutrient Content of Different Cuttings of Alfalfa Hay[a]

Cutting	No. of Samples	Visual Score[b]	Percent in Hay Dry Matter			
			Crude Protein (CP)	Acid Detergent Fiber (ADF)	TDN[c]	Lab Score[d]
1st	7	178 (157–186)	20.8 (17.9–23.4)	29.3 (23.6–33.6)	61.1 (58.9–64.8)	316 (271–388)
2nd	3	182 (172–188)	20.8 (18.8–22.0)	31.5 (30.3–32.8)	60.5 (60.0–61.4)	299 (287–313)
3rd	20	182 (172–189)	21.1 (18.4–23.9)	31.3 (25.6–35.2)	60.7 (58.0–64.8)	303 (252–388)
4th	7	183 (166–189)	21.1 (18.8–23.1)	31.2 (29.1–33.4)	60.8 (59.3–62.7)	304 (255–319)

[a] Top-quality hay entered in Western Washington Fair in 1992, Puyallup, WA (personal communication, Elmer N. Searls). Values given are the average (and the range).
[b] Based on: stage of cutting (40 pts), foreign matter (40), stem and leaf content (40), condition (40), color (30), bale shape and ties (10), for a total of 200 possible points as evaluated by a university agronomist. The higher the score, the better quality the hay.
[c] Total digestible nutrients (TDN) = $54.3208 + [(\%CP \times 0.7387) - (\%ADF \times 0.2915)]$.
[d] Lab score = $(\%CP + \%TDN - \%ADF) \times 6$.

tional value if harvested at the proper time and if it does not contain large numbers of weeds that have grown up since the last cutting the previous season. It is also least likely to contain blister beetles, which may occur in alfalfa cut after midsummer in some areas, and which are quite toxic to the horse as described in Chapter 19. However, first-cutting hay frequently contains more weeds, and in many areas, putting it up at the proper time without getting it rained on after cutting is more difficult than it is for later cuttings of hay. Plant growth is generally fastest during the hottest part of the growing season, if moisture is not a limiting factor. Fast growth results in more stem and fewer leaves, which decreases the plant's nutritional value. Later cuttings, when the temperature is cooler, generally have a higher leaf and nutrient content, the fewest weeds and, in many areas, the best opportunity of being harvested without being rained on after cutting, and, therefore, may have the highest feeding value. However, as shown in Table 4–3, there is no difference in either the appearance or nutrient content of different cuttings of alfalfa when only top-quality hay is evaluated. Thus, in selecting hay, the major consideration is not the type of hay or the cutting, but the quality of the hay, its availability, and its nutritional content in relation to its cost.

Hay Quality

Hay quality refers to the hay's nutritional value, its acceptability by the animal, and the type and amount of foreign material it contains. Good-quality hays are readily consumed in high amounts, are highly digestible, are high in available nutrients, and are low in foreign material. Characteristics of good-quality hay are that it is: (1) free of mold, dust, weeds, and other foreign material; (2) leafy, with fine stems; (3) soft and pliable to the touch; (4) of a pleasant, fragrant aroma; and (5) of a bright green, rather than a yellow or brown, color (least important criterion, although worth consideration). As a generality, the nicer that loose hay would be to sleep in, the better its quality. If it is nice and soft, lacks coarse stems, stalks, or weeds that would make it uncomfortable to sleep in, and has a nice, clean, fresh smell, with minimal dust or other particles, such as mold spores, that may be inhaled, it is probably good-quality hay.

The major factors that determine the quality of a hay are the stage of maturity when it's cut, its weathering and handling during harvesting, and the duration and conditions of its storage (Fig. 4–7). As the plant matures, its digestibility and energy and protein content decrease. Just prior to the time legumes flower (the bud or vegetative stage), and when grasses begin to show heads through the sheath (early head to boot stage), their leaf development has been completed and they should be harvested (Fig. 4–8). At this time, field grasses will begin to change from a deep green to a slight gray as the heads begin to appear. Legumes consist of about one-half leaves and one-half stems at the full bud stage. Allowing the plant to stand after first flowering and past the boot stage increases crude fiber and reduces crude protein about ¼% per day, and decreases digestible energy nearly ½% per day. As legumes mature from full bud to full bloom, and grasses mature from the boot stage to complete heading out, one-half of their protein and one-third of their energy content is lost. This is also true of pasture forage. These factors result in decreased total digestible nutrient intake and feeding value of that forage. Grass hay that has heads over ½ inch (1 cm) long and legume hay that is past full bloom are too mature to make a good feed.

The appearance of hay is the most commonly used and practical means of determining the presence of mold, dust, weeds, and other undesirable contaminants, and generally in estimating beta-carotene and vitamin E content based on color. However, appearance is a poor indication of the content of other nutrients in a hay. The only accurate and reliable means of determining the nutrient content of a hay is to have it analyzed. The crude protein content may vary as much as 2 to 3 times in grass hays that appear to be similar. In assessing forage quality, it should be analyzed, at least for moisture, protein, and crude fiber content as described in Chapter 6 (see section on "Nutrient Content of Feeds"). The crude protein content of forages directly correlates with that forage's digestible dry matter, NFE or nonfiber carbohydrate, and energy content, all of which directly correlate with the amount of that forage the horse will consume (i.e., the higher they are, the more the horse will consume, and, therefore, less is needed of the more expensive feed.

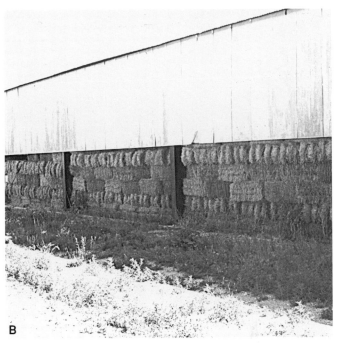

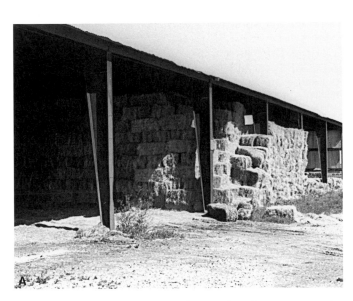

Fig. 4–7(A,B). Protect hay from the weather during storage. A 3-sided hay shed, as shown here, is adequate and relatively inexpensive. It will pay for itself within a few years in preventing weather-induced losses in the feeding value of the hay. If a hay shed or inside storage facilities are not available, waterproof canvas spread over the top and partially down the sides of the stack, and peaked so water will run off may be used. Plastic, instead of a waterproof canvas. is not recommended. Plastic will frequently puncture and allow water into the hay, but prevent its evaporation, resulting in more spoilage than would have occurred if the hay had been left uncovered.

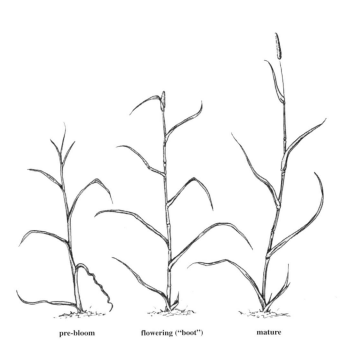

pre-bloom   flowering ("boot")   mature

Fig. 4–8. Growth stages of a typical grass, timothy. The grass should be harvested no later than the boot stage, which is when the head begins to show through the sheath (center figure). (Courtesy EQUUS, *32* (6), 1980.)

If a hay contains less protein or more fiber than the amounts given for that type of hay in Appendix Table 6, it is below-average-quality feed. It is important that this comparison be made on an equal moisture content basis, as described in Chapter 6. Average-quality forage contains 28 to 34% crude fiber and 0.9 to 1 Mcal digestible energy/lb (2.0 to 2.2 Mcal/kg) in its dry matter. A crude fiber content greater than 34 to 36% in dry matter indicates a poor-quality hay. If the moisture content of the feed is greater than 15% to 20% at baling or 15% when stored, excess heat is produced in the first few weeks of storage, which decreases protein digestibility, and it may become moldy during storage (Fig. 4–9). Moldy feed should not be fed. It may cause chronic obstructive pulmonary disease or heaves resulting in chronic coughing and decreased physical performance ability, and may contain mycotoxins, which can cause abortion and death (see Chapter 19). In addition, moldy feeds may be unpalatable and decrease growth rate.

The U.S. Department of Agriculture in 1946 set federal hay grades as U.S. Nos. 1, 2, and 3, and sample grade as an indication of the highest to the lowest hay quality. These grades, however, are based on an estimate of leafiness, color, and foreign material; they are not quantitative measurements of nutrient content. As a result, they are not a very accurate indication of hay quality and are not commonly used. A more accurate measure of feeding and market value of hay developed and proposed by the American Forage and Grasslands Council is shown in Table 4–4. Al-

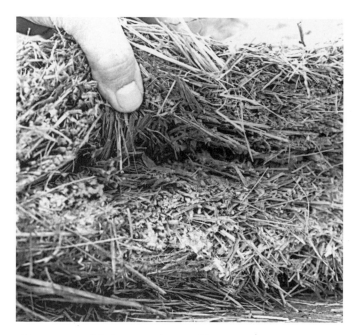

Fig. 4–9. Moldy hay. A white mold was present not only on the edges of this bale but throughout, and the hay was dusty. Moldy hay is unpalatable, contains fungal spores that cause heaves, coughing, and bleeders, and may contain mycotoxins. White dust in hay is usually fungal spores.

though this system is based on the hay's feeding value for ruminants, it would appear to be applicable to horses. As shown, a hay's feeding value is based on its crude protein (CP), acid detergent fiber (ADF), and neutral detergent fiber (NDF) contents. The NDF is the best indication of

TABLE 4–4
Market Hay Grades and Relative Feed Value of Hays

Grade	Description	Chemical Composition—% in DM			Relative Feed Value—%[a]
		CP	ADF	NDF	
Prime	Legume (prebloom)	>19	<30	<39	>132
1	Legume (early bloom) and 20% grass (vegetative)	17–19	31–35	40–46	118–132
2	Legume (midbloom) and 30% grass (early head)	14–16	36–40	47–53	101–117
3	Legume (full bloom) and 40% grass (headed)	11–13	40–42	53–60	88–100
4	Legume (full bloom) and 50% grass (headed)	8–10	43–45	61–65	75–87
5	Mostly grass (headed)	<8	>45	>65	<75

DM = dry matter; CP = crude protein; ADF = acid detergent fiber; NDF = neutral detergent fiber; > = greater than; and < = less than.
[a] Indicates the relationship between the feeding and economic values of different forages. For example: grade prime hay would be worth at least 1.76 times the cost of grade 5 hay (132 ÷ 75), and grade 1 hay 1.18 to 1.5 times the cost of grade 3 hay (118 ÷ 100 to 132 ÷ 88).

forage intake, and ADF the best indication of forage digestibility. Both intake and digestibility decrease with increasing NDF and ADF content of the forage, respectively, as shown by the following formulas.

Forage Digestible Dry Matter (% DDM) = 88.9 − (0.779 × % ADF)

Forage Dry Matter Intake (DMI) (as a % of body wt/day) = (120) ÷ (% NDF in forage dry matter)

Forage Relative Feeding Value (RFV) = (% DDM × % DMI) ÷ 1.29

The forage relative feeding value indicates the relationship between the feeding value and, therefore, economic value of different forages.

Although feeding good-quality hay is certainly preferred and recommended, if the only feed available is weathered, stemmy, weedy, or nutritionally deficient hay, lots of it should be fed. This allows the horse to sort through it and eat only the better portions. If lesser amounts are fed, the horse is forced to eat the poorer-quality portions of the feed, or consume inadequate feed to meet its needs. However, moldy or dusty hay should not be fed.

CEREAL GRAINS FOR HORSES

Grains are seeds from cereal plants that are members of the grass family Gramineae. In addition to the seeds, the entire plant can be grazed as described in the next chapter or harvested as a cereal grain hay or haylage, as discussed previously in this chapter. The primary use of cereal grain plants, however, is the utilization of their seeds for feed and the rest of the plant as chaff, stover, or straw for high-fiber, low-energy, and low-protein feeds for ruminants or idle mature horses, or the straw for bedding as discussed in Chapter 9. The seed is the nutrient store for the embryo or germ from which a new plant develops. It consists of a coat, starchy endosperm, and germ. In milling, the coat is removed as bran. Rice, oats, barley, husked sorghum and husked millet have a fused husk or hull; corn (maize), wheat, rye, and grain sorghum (milo) and millet do not. Hulls are high in fiber; grains with hulls are therefore much higher in fiber than those without hulls.

The density, nutrient content, and characteristics of the cereal grains most commonly available are given in Table 4–5. In contrast to forages, the nutrient contents of cereal grains vary little from the values given. These values, therefore, may be used in formulating diets for the horse. A laboratory analysis usually is not necessary. An exception to this is triticale, whose nutrient content is quite variable.

All cereal crops are annuals. Depending on the type and variety of grain, they may be either winter annuals (planted in the fall and grazed in the spring or harvested in the summer) or summer annuals (planted in the spring and harvested in late summer or early fall).

Wheat, corn, and rice each constitute about 25% of world grain production, barley 10%, and grain sorghum (milo), oats, millet, and rye 1 to 4%. How different grains are used varies from country to country. Corn, oats, grain sorghum, and barley constitute about 75%, 10%, 10%, and 4%, respectively, of the grains fed to livestock and poultry in the United States. However, production and feeding of corn is steadily increasing while that of oats is decreasing. Most wheat produced in the United States is consumed

TABLE 4–5
Cereal Grains: Density, Nutrient Content,[a] Relative Feeding Values, and Characteristics for Horses

Grains	Unground Density Lbs/qt (kg/L)	Digestible Energy[b] Mcal/qt (Mcal/L)	Mcal/lb (Mcal/kg)	Relative Feeding Value[b] (%) By wt.	By vol.	Decrease in Density if Ground (%)[c]	Crude Protein (%)	Crude Fiber (%)	Comments
Other Feeds for Comparison:									
Soybean meal	1.8 (0.85)	2.5 (2.7)	1.4 (3.1)				44	6	Most common protein supplement fed
Alfalfa, hay			0.9 (2.0)				17	26	Average to good quality
pellets	0.6 (0.3)	0.6 (0.6)	1.0 (2.2)				17	24	
Grass hay, good			0.9 (2.0)				9	27	
poor			0.7 (1.5)				5	33	
Cereal Grains:									
Oats (regular)	0.85 (0.4)	1.1 (1.1)	1.3 (2.8)	85	45	28	11–12	11	Most palatable and safest grain. Often most expensive & variable in quality.
Oats (heavy)	1.0 (0.5)	1.4 (1.5)	1.4 (3.1)	90	50	28	12.5	11	Also referred to as "race horse" or "jockey" oats
Oats (hull-less)	1.4 (0.7)	2.4 (2.5)	1.7 (3.8)	110	95		18	2.4	e.g., Pennula, Rhiannon, and Kynon varieties
Corn (maize)	1.7 (0.8)	2.6 (2.7)	1.5 (3.4)	100	100	14	8–10	2.2	Grain most prone to mold and most commonly overfed
Barley	1.5 (0.7)	2.3 (2.4)	1.5 (3.3)	95	85	25	12	5	Between oats and corn in safety but less palatable. Malting barley is higher in energy & lower in protein than regular.
Grain Sorghum (Milo)	1.7 (0.8)	2.5 (2.6)	1.45 (3.2)	95	95		11.5	2.6	Should be processed. Brown variety is high-tannin, less digestible & less palatable.
Wheat	1.9 (0.9)	2.9 (3.0)	1.55 (3.4)	100	110	14	11–14	1.5–3	Less palatable than oats and corn. Should be processed.
Rye	1.7 (0.8)	2.6 (2.7)	1.53 (3.4)	100	100	14	12	2.2	Feed processed with ⅓ maximum in grain mix. Ensure no ergot.
Rice, ground (rough)	1.2 (0.6)	1.85 (2.0)	1.55 (3.34)	100	75		7–9	7–9	
Millet	1.5 (0.7)	2.0 (2.1)	1.35 (3.0)				10–12	6–9	Should be processed. Used primarily as birdseed.
Emmer	1.1 (0.5)	1.2 (1.3)	1.1 (2.5)				11–12	9–10	Look like barley. Feeding values similar to oats.
Spelt	1.1 (0.5)	1.4 (1.5)	1.3 (3.0)				12	9–10	
Triticale	1.25 (0.6)	2.0 (2.1)	1.55 (3.45)				15	4	A hybrid of wheat and rye. Protein is high quality.

[a] All values given are for whole, unprocessed grain and are the amount of, or in, the grain as fed. All are 88 to 90% dry matter and contain the following: 1.5–4% fat (ether extract) except 5–6% in oats; 19–25% neutral detergent fiber (NDF) and 8–14% acid detergent fiber (ADF), except 10 to 16% NDF and 3.6% ADF in corn, wheat, and rye; 0.04–0.08% calcium, 0.27–0.37% phosphorus, 0.10–0.15% magnesium, 0.32–0.48% potassium, 0.01–0.06% sodium, 0.1–0.2% sulfur; in mg/kg (ppm), 4–8 copper, 0.04–0.11 iodine, 30–80 iron, 5–36 manganese, 0.1–0.4 selenium, 15–35 zinc, 0.06–0.14 cobalt, 4–7 thiamin, 1–3 riboflavin, 15–60 niacin, 5–30 pantothenate, 3–8 pyridoxine, 0.1–0.4 biotin, and 0.2–0.6 folacin; and in IU/kg, less than 1000 vitamin A and 5–15 vitamin E, except 30 in oats.

[b] For horses, these values for oats, corn, barley, and probably spelt and emmer are not affected by processing (rolling, cracking, crimping, flaking, pelleting, etc.), whereas for sorghum, wheat, rye, and probably millet and triticale they are increased 10 to 15% by processing.

[c] The weight or Mcal/qt or liter of ground (or rolled, flaked, or crimped) grain is the percentage given lower than the weight or Mcal/qt or liter as given above for whole grain. For example, as given above, ground regular oats density is 28% less than its unground density of 0.85 lbs/qt, which would be [0.85 × (1 − 0.28)], or 0.6 lbs/qt. Ground oats' energy content would also be 28% less than its unground energy content of 1.1 Mcal/qt, which would be [1.1 × (1 − 0.28)] or 0.8 Mcal/qt.

by people; in Europe, large amounts are considered the primary feed grain for livestock and poultry. In Mexico, many consider corn primarily a food for people, while grain sorghum is considered the primary feed grain for livestock and poultry. In most of the world much of the rice is consumed by people, and barley and rye are used in the brewing and distilling industries. All of the cereal grains, however, and their by products, are sometimes fed to horses and other animals.

Cereal grains have the following general characteristics. Compared to other horse feeds, cereal grains are:

1. Quite palatable for horses. Most horses prefer most cereal grains to other types and forms of forage and,

therefore, will eat all the grain available before they will eat forage.

2. Dense, with a high weight per unit of volume, which is 4 to 8 times that of baled hay and 10 to 15 times that of loose hay (Appendix Table 8).

3. Low in fiber and high in dietary energy. Cereal grains contain one-half to one-third the crude fiber and 50% more energy than average to good quality hay (Appendix Table 6).

4. Very low in calcium (below 0.1%) and most vitamins, including the vitamin A precursor beta-carotene (below 1000 IU/kg) and vitamins D, E, K, B_2, and B_{12} (Appendix Tables 2 and 3).

5. High in starch, which makes up 55 to 60% of grain dry matter, whereas starch is low in forages.

Some of the starch in grain is digested and absorbed as the simple sugar, glucose, whereas most other carbohydrates in horse feeds are converted by microorganisms to and absorbed as volatile fatty acids. As a result, the horse's blood-sugar (but not insulin) concentration increases more following consumption of grain than of hay. But there is no difference in the plasma concentration of either glucose or insulin in horses fed barley, corn, oats, or a sweet feed.

Starch digestibility by the horse is high (87 to nearly 100%) and similar in different feeds, but differs in where its digestion occurs. Starch not digested in the small intestine is converted by microbial organisms in the cecum to volatile fatty acids and lactic acid. A sufficiently rapid production of enough of these acids causes cecal acidosis. If cecal acidosis is severe, diarrhea, colic, and/or founder occur. The risk of this occurrence can be decreased by decreasing the amount of starch reaching the cecum. This can be done by each of the following procedures.

1. By feeding less grain.
2. By feeding, in order of preference, oats, grain sorghum (milo), corn, and last, barley. The amount of starch digested in the small intestine is highest from oats and lowest from barley (and thus the amount of starch reaching the cecum is lowest from oats and highest from barley).
3. By grinding and heat treatment (popping, micronizing, etc.) of grain, which increases the disintegration of the grain and its starch granule structure, but not by rolling or cracking, which do not do so sufficiently to have an effect on small intestinal starch digestion.
4. By not feeding forage for 1 hour or more before and for 3 hours or more after feeding grain. Forage, unprocessed or chopped, consumed with grain decreases the amount of the grain's starch digested in the small intestine.

Regardless of whether these procedures are used, the consumption of a sufficient amount of any cereal grain at one time will result in diarrhea, colic, founder, or death. Even if excessive amounts at one time aren't consumed, the consumption of excess amounts of grain results in excess dietary energy intake, which over time will result in obesity, frequently increased hyperactivity or nervousness, and may increase the risk of developmental orthopedic diseases in young horses (see Chapter 16). Because of these factors, grain or grain mixes should not make up over 50 to 70% of the total weight of the feed consumed by any horse, and need not be fed at all unless energy or nutrients in excess of that in the forages available are needed. A need for energy or other nutrients in excess of that in the forages available is the major reason nutritionally for feeding grains or grain-supplement mixes.

Grain Types

Any of the cereal grains given in Table 4–5 are nutritious, good feeds that may be fed to horses. Providing they are good quality and that excess amounts are not fed, none are harmful in any way. The major criteria that should be considered in determining which grain to feed are: (1) the quality of the grain, determined as described in the sections "Grain Quality" and "Grain Storage" later in this chapter, and (2) the characteristics of each grain most important for each feeding program and horses. When the amount of grain fed is not more than a few pounds (up to 6 or 7 lbs or 3 kg) daily, doesn't vary greatly from day to day, and the chances of feeding too much are minimal, the major criterion in determining which of similar-quality grains to feed is the relative feeding value of the grains with respect to their cost. Other than as a carrier to ensure that the desired amount of a supplement is consumed, the major reason nutritionally to feed grain is to provide dietary energy. Therefore, barring differences in quality, cost with respect to energy provided is the most rational factor to consider in determining which type of grain to feed.

The relative feeding values of equal-quality cereal grains for horses are given in Table 4–5. The usefulness of these values is as an indication of the relative amount that each grain is worth. For example:

1. If corn costs $8/100 lbs, heavy oats would be worth $8 times their relative feeding value with respect to corn, which as given in Table 4–5 is 90%. Heavy oats would therefore be worth $8 times 90%, or $7.20/100 lbs. If oats cost more than this, they aren't worth it nutritionally. Whether their other attributes, such as less chance of being overfed or harmful, is worth their additional cost must be considered for that feeding program.
2. If sorghum costs $10/cwt, regular oats would be worth $10 times their feeding value with respect to sorghum, which is regular oats' relative feeding value divided by sorghum's relative feeding value. As given in Table 4–5, this would be 0.85 ÷ 0.95, or 0.895. So, regular oats would be worth $10/cwt times 0.895, or $8.95/cwt.

The feed preference of most horses from the most to the least preferred is a mixed-grain sweetfeed, oats, cracked corn, whole corn, good-quality alfalfa hay, wheat, barley, rye, and soybean meal. However, there are large individual variations in feed preferences by horses, just as there are in people. Although some horses may, for exam-

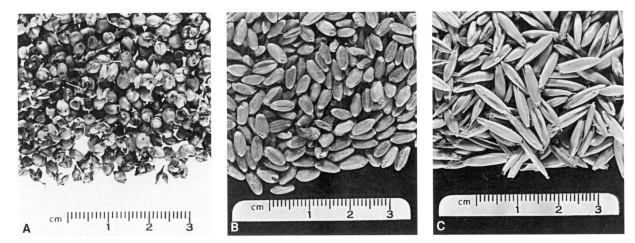

Fig. 4–10(A,B,C). Cereal grains. These are grain sorghum or milo (A), wheat (B), and oats (C). Oats are similar in appearance to barley.

ple, prefer rye to oats, just as some people may prefer liver to steak, for the majority the reverse is true. In addition, most horses prefer the type of feed to which they are accustomed. Thus, when the type of grain fed is changed, regardless of which type of grain is involved, initially most horses will show a preference for the one to which they are accustomed. This initial lack of preference for the newly introduced grain doesn't, therefore, indicate that it is unpalatable, even for that horse, but only that the horse is unaccustomed to it.

Oats

Oats (Avena sativa) are in many areas the most popular cereal grain fed to horses (Fig. 4-10) They are reported to make up 31% of all commercially prepared horse feed. Although they are fed to other livestock, they are less popular because of their lower energy density (Table 4-5), higher fiber content, greater variability in quality, and frequently higher cost. Oats are not as widely grown as many cereal grains and their production is decreasing because their yield per unit of ground is lower than it is for other cereal grains. Because oats require a low amount of water and a short season, and grow well in cool weather, their major production is in areas where other grains do less well, such as the northern plains states (Dakotas, Minnesota, Iowa, Wisconsin, Ohio, and Michigan). Their popularity as a food for horses is often due to habit, a lack of familiarity with feeding other cereal grains, and the fact that they are the safest and most palatable (in contrast to pigs) cereal grain for horses. Oats also have a relatively soft kernel that is easy for the horse to chew. Cooking and processing oats to crack the kernel aren't necessary or of much benefit, except possibly for very young horses or horses with poor teeth. This is a benefit not only because it alleviates the need for processing, but also because nutrient deterioration during storage is slower than in grains that are processed.

Oats are safer to feed to horses than other types of grains because they are higher in fiber, lower in digestible energy, lower in density, and less likely to have molds and myco-toxins (Table 4-5). Because they are several times higher in fiber (10 to 12% vs 2 to 5% in most other grains), they are less likely to cause founder or digestive problems. In addition, because on a volume basis they provide only about one-half as much digestible energy as other types of grain, and because grain is most commonly fed to horses by volume, the risk and the problems of excess grain intake are reduced when oats are fed. Problems with excess grain intake include not only founder and digestive problems, but also the possibility that the horse will become too spirited or high and too fat. In contrast to what is occasionally stated or believed by some, the consumption of excess oats will cause any or all of these problems. But more oats than any other type of grain (2 times greater volume) must be consumed to cause any of these problems.

The advantages provided by oats are often expensive and unnecessary if precautions are taken to ensure that the grain fed is of good quality and that excess amounts are not fed. Generally, oats are the most expensive type of grain, particularly when their cost is compared to their feeding value or energy content, which is how their cost should be compared since the major reason grain is fed is to provide dietary energy. Because of this, the production and use of oats in the livestock industry is declining while that of corn, particularly, is increasing.

Three major types of oats may be available: regular, heavy, and hull-less. Heavy oats are of better quality than regular oats. They contain less foreign material and weigh more per unit of volume (e.g., 36 vs 32 lbs/bu)—thus the name—heavy oats. The nutrient content of regular and heavy oats, however, is quite similar. Because heavy oats are preferred and fed by many racehorse people, they are often called "racehorse" or "jockey" oats. They do vary less in quality than regular oats, which tend to be the most variable of all cereal grains in quality. The lower variation in quality is generally the only benefit of the additional cost of heavy oats over regular oats.

In contrast to the small differences between regular and heavy oats, hull-less oats are higher in feeding value (Table 4-5). Most of the fiber in oats is in the hulls that cover the grain kernels. Hulls are over 30% crude fiber and make up 23 to 35% of the grain. This variation in hull content accounts for much of the variability in oats. The removal of the hulls decreases oats' fiber content similar to other grains that don't have hulls (corn, wheat, rye, and grain sorghum), and increases the concentration and digestibility of other nutrients in oats. Dehulled, naked, or clipped oats, or groats, of which there are several varieties, including Pennula, Rhiannon, and Kynon, are occasionally available. In ponies, the digestibility of Pennula hull-less oats as compared to heavy oats was: 84 vs 68% for energy, 86 vs 71% for dry matter, 86 vs 83% for crude protein, 55 vs 34% for neutral detergent fiber (NDF), 40 vs 30% for acid detergent fiber (ADF), and 62 vs 40% for hemicellulose, respectively. The hull-less oats as compared to heavy oats weighed 52 vs 36 lbs/bu (67 vs 46 kg/hl) and in their dry matter provided 3.8 vs 3.0 Mcal digestible energy (DE)/kg, 15.6 vs 10.6% digestible protein, 2.4 vs 12.9% cellulose, and 15.5 vs 34.2% NDF. Whether hull-less oats' higher energy and protein content is worth the cost can be determined from their relative feeding value given in Table 4–5 and as described previously. The lower fiber and higher energy and density of dehulled or hull-less oats, however, decrease their safety from excess consumption similar to that of other grains that don't have hulls (corn, wheat, grain sorghum, and rye).

Corn

Corn or maize (Zea mays) (Fig. 4–11) is the leading crop in the United States in terms of amount produced and value, and its production and use are increasing steadily. Of that produced, over 80% is fed to livestock and poultry, and it constitutes over 80% of all grains fed in the United States. It is commonly fed to horses, for whom it is a nutritious, palatable, and good feed, providing it is of good quality and not fed in excessive quantities. For most horses, it is only slightly less palatable than oats, and is more palatable than other cereal grains. Corn, however, is more prone to moldiness and lacks the safety margin against the effects of excess grain consumption that oats provide. Mold is most likely to occur in processed (cracked or flaked) corn. Moldy corn may contain mycotoxins, which cause the highly fatal moldy corn disease or less commonly aflatoxicosis as described in Chapter 19. Thus, moldy or even questionable corn should not be fed.

Corn, like other grains without hulls, is low in fiber and higher in both energy content and density than oats. It provides twice as much energy as an equal volume of oats (Table 4–5). Because of this, some feel corn has a tendency to cause obesity or to make a horse high spirited. If equal volumes of corn and regular oats are fed, this is true, since the horse is receiving twice as much energy from the corn. However, if equal amounts of energy, not equal volumes of grain, are fed, corn does not have any greater tendency to cause obesity or to make a horse too high spirited than other cereal grains. How spirited a horse acts is directly related to how good it feels and how much energy it has consumed compared to its needs.

Contrary to another popular belief, corn is not a "heating feed." It is sometimes fed during the winter and not during the summer because of this mistaken belief. Corn is a "hot feed" when hot implies high energy, but not when it implies high heat production. The heat produced in the utilization of corn is one-third less than that produced in the utilization of oats. Only 41% of the gross energy in corn is given off as heat, as compared with 66% of the gross energy in oats. This is because corn is lower in fiber, and the greatest amount of heat produced in feed utilization is from microbial fermentation of fiber; therefore, the lower a feed's fiber content, the less heat produced in its utilization. However, because corn has a high energy density and because energy needs are increased during cold weather, it is a good winter feed (see Chapter 10 for cold-weather care of horses).

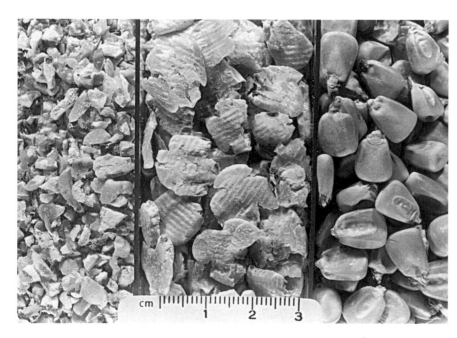

Fig. 4–11. Corn or maize—cracked, flaked or crimpled, and whole.

The risk of cecal acidosis, and as a result founder, diarrhea, and colic, is greater when corn than when oats is fed. This is because of corn's higher energy density, which increases the risk of excess intake, its lower fiber content, and because less starch from corn is digested and absorbed in the small intestine than from oats. As a result more starch enters the cecum after the horse eats corn than oats. More starch in the cecum results in a greater production of volatile fatty acids and lactic acid, and increased cecal acidity. At a high corn intake, a subclinical cecal acidosis occurred. However, no difference in founder, or in gastrointestinal disorders (including diarrhea and colic), occurred in horses in training that were fed corn as compared to those fed oats, with either grain making up 40% or 60% of the total diet.

Barley

Barley (Hordeum vulgare) has the distinction of being the most widely geographically cultivated cereal grain in the world, being suited for cool, dry climates. It can be grown in areas with too short a growing season for corn and can tolerate limited rainfall in the summer. Over one-half of that grown and used in the world is in Europe and the former Soviet Union. In the United States, of the barley grown, over 50% is fed to livestock, about 25% is used for alcohol production, and most of the remainder is exported.

Barley grain looks similar to, but is somewhat harder than, oats (Fig. 4-10). Because of this, many recommend that it should be crimped or rolled for horses, although this doesn't increase its feeding value for horses with normal teeth, and, therefore, processing barley is of questionable benefit. Like oats, most types of barley contain hulls. Because of the hulls, its fiber content is higher than the hull-less grains (corn, grain sorghum, wheat, rye, and dehulled or hull-less varieties of oats or barley). Barley might be best described as an in-between grain: in-between regular oats and corn in fiber and energy content, safety, and heat produced in its utilization. However, it is more similar to corn in density (Table 4-5) and even slightly less of its starch is digested in the small intestine. If it is of good quality, barley is a nutritious, palatable, and good cereal grain for horses, and may be fed as the only grain in the diet with no detrimental effects. However, for most horses, like wheat and rye, barley is less palatable than oats and corn and, therefore, is best and most commonly used in a grain mix with either or both oats and corn, and frequently molasses.

Sorghum (Milo)

Sorghum (S. vulgare) encompasses a wide range of varieties, including grain, grass, syrup, and broom corn sorghums. Grass sorghums include Johnson grass and Sudan grass used as pasture, hay, or haylage. Sorgo is the principle syrup sorghum and is used for the production of sugar and syrup, but can be used for hay. Broom corn sorghums produce stems and panicles suitable for use in brooms. Some green grain sorghum plants may be high in cyanide or prussic (hydrocyanic) acid and, therefore, shouldn't be grazed, as described in Chapter 18. However, many of the currently used sorghum species have been developed to have a low cyanogenic potential. Cyanide toxicosis is not a problem with feeding grain sorghum. Only grain sorghum is used as a cereal grain. In 1957, new, improved grain sorghum hybrids became available. Most were derived from milo-kafir crosses. Thus, this grain sorghum is often referred to as milo.

Grain sorghum is grown and used primarily in Asia and the United States, particularly in the central and southern plains states (Texas, Nebraska, Kansas, and Missouri). It is often considered to be a cereal grain suited to areas not conducive to corn due to inadequate or irregular rainfall, and where it is not too cold (mean temperature about 80°F [27°C]). Nearly all grain sorghum grown in the United States is fed to livestock, and it represents 6 to 8% of all grain fed. In a number of African and Asian countries it is primarily a food grain for people.

Grain sorghum, like wheat, has a small hard kernel (Fig. 4-10) that for efficient utilization must be steam flaked. Dry rolling is not adequate. Its feeding value varies with its tannin content. Tannins provide some degree of resistance to mold but decrease the grain's protein digestibility and palatability, giving it an astringent taste—enough so that birds won't eat it. High tannin content is present in brown-type grain sorghums (also called bird-resistant sorghums).

Under United States Grades and Standards there are four classes of grain sorghums. They are:

1. Yellow, although the seeds may be white, yellow or red. This is low- or no-tannin grain sorghum.
2. Brown, which is high in tannin. Its nutritional value may be lower than yellow grain sorghum.
3. Mixed, with more than 10% brown grain.
4. White, which has pure white kernels but is not presently available commercially.

It can be difficult to differentiate between yellow and brown varieties on a strictly visual basis.

Good quality, low tannin grain sorghum is a nutritious, good cereal grain for horses, and may be fed as the only grain in the horse's diet with no detrimental effects. However, because it is less palatable for most horses than are oats and corn, it is best and most commonly used in a grain mix with them and often molasses. For good utilization it should be preferably steam flaked. Its small hard kernels are hard for the horse to chew and efficiently digest. Like corn, it is high in energy density and low in fiber (Table 4-5) and, therefore, carries the same risk as corn in causing founder, colic, diarrhea, obesity, and too high a spirit if overfed. It is generally similar to oats and barley in protein content (Table 4-5) although it can vary from 8 to 14% depending on moisture adequacy during growth.

Wheat

Wheat (Triticum aestivum) is widely grown throughout the world. In the United States its production is second only to corn, with the greatest acreage being in the central plains and north central states. It is consumed primarily by people. Because of its high cost, it is not used extensively for animal feed, although at times it may be less expensive than other cereal grains. Most varieties of wheat grown for animal feeds are soft types. Even these types, however, have relatively small, hard kernels (Fig. 4-10), and, therefore, for efficient utilization by animals, including horses, they should be cracked, coarsely ground, or steam flaked. Fine grinding should be avoided because it increases wheat's dustiness and decreases its palatability.

Wheat is even higher in energy density than corn and provides about 2.5 times more energy than an equal volume of regular oats (Table 4-5). The energy and dry matter digestibilities of wheat are 4 to 5% higher than oats, whereas protein content and digestibility are the same (71 to 72%). As a hull-less grain it is also quite low in fiber. Thus, the risk of excessive grain and dietary energy intake and the problems associated with this—such as founder, diarrhea, colic, obesity, and being too spirited—are even greater with wheat than corn. In addition, wheat flour has a stickier consistency than other cereal grain flours, which is what makes it so valuable to the baking industry. Because of this and the fear that the stickiness will increase digestive problems, it is commonly recommended that wheat not make up more than one-half of the grain mix fed. However, no digestive disturbances occurred in eight horses fed a diet consisting of 40% grass hay and 60% ground pelleted wheat. These horses did as well with no differences noted as when they were fed oats instead of wheat. Thus, wheat is a good, nutritious feed that may be fed to horses as the only grain without detrimental effects. However, it should be processed to break the small hard kernels, and caution must be used to ensure that it isn't overfed. Because it is less palatable for most horses than oats and corn, it is best and most commonly used in a grain mix with them, often along with molasses.

Rye

Rye (Secale cereale) is not commonly grown or fed. It may be grown in poor sandy soils and in climates too cold for most other cereal grains. It is used primarily for pasture or hay but may be harvested and the grain fed. The grain is similar in energy, fiber, and feeding value to corn, but is higher in protein (Table 4-5). Like wheat and grain sorghum, rye kernels are small and hard and, therefore, for efficient utilization they should be cracked by some processing method. Rye may be fed to horses, but should be mixed with other grain as not over one-third of the grain mix because of poor palatability. Rye is the least palatable cereal grain for most animals. In addition, it should be inspected closely to ensure that it doesn't contain ergot, which is quite toxic to horses (see "Equine Ergotism" in Chapter 19).

Rice

Rice (Oryza sativa) is one of the most important grain crops in the world. It requires a warm, long growing season with an abundance of water. It is used as a food primarily for people and only to a limited extent for animals. It contains a thick fibrous hull, which constitutes about 20% of its total weight and gives it a fiber content only slightly lower than oats (8% vs 11%). The hull is removed for human consumption. Rice hulls, without the grain and unground are unsuitable for feeding horses because the sharp edges may cause irritation. However, rough or unpolished rice, which is the grain before removal of the hull and the form generally fed to animals, is a suitable feed for horses. Its energy content is similar to corn on a weight basis (3.4 Mcal/kg) but on a volume basis is lower (2.0 Mcal/L vs 2.7 for corn and 1.4 for oats) (Table 4-5). Its protein content is lowest of all cereal grains (Table 4-5).

Millet, Emmer, Spelt, and Triticale

Millet (Panicum milaceum and Sataria spp.) is most commonly used as birdseed. It has a small hard seed covered by a hull. It should be ground for use in feeding horses. It has a feeding value similar to oats but is slightly lower in fiber (Table 4-5).

Emmer and spelt, like wheat, are Triticum spp. (T. dicoccum, spelta and vulgare, respectively) but have hulls, look like barley, and have a feeding value similar to oats. In the United States, emmer is grown primarily in the Dakotas, spelt in the East.

Triticale is a hybrid of wheat and rye. It is high in high-quality proteins (usually 13 to 15% as fed) and in the essential amino acids lysine, threonine, and tryptophan, which are low in other cereal grains. However, it is lower yielding than wheat. Numerous studies have shown that it is a nutritious palatable feed for pigs, and probably also for horses.

Grain Processing

Grain, like harvested forages, may be dried, ensiled, or acid treated to prevent spoilage due to heating and molding during storage. High moisture ensiled and acid-treated feeds are discussed later in this chapter. Drying is most commonly accomplished by sun curing in the field. Artificial drying or dehydrating may be used but generally substantially increases the cost of the feed. Although drying to a moisture content of less than 20% is adequate for hay, less than 13% is necessary for grain because of grain's higher and more fermentable soluble carbohydrate content. A moisture content below 10% stops the development of most insects. However, as moisture level decreases, especially below 12%, breakage of grain kernels increases.

Dry grains may be processed cold or hot. Cold processing is generally hammermill or rollermill grinding, but also includes milling. Hot processing is most commonly steam flaking or crimping (Fig. 4-12), but may be popping, micronizing, extruding, or pelleting. Hot processing is more expensive. In one study, e.g., steam flaking cost $5/ton versus about $2/ton for grinding. It's reported that there is no advantage in cooking grains for horses that have good teeth and that steam treatment had no effect on the digestibility of ground corn for ruminants. However, protein digestion by the horse is 2 to 3% higher from both oats and milo when these grains are micronized than when they are crimped. In addition, it's reported that steam flaking milo improves its utilization by cattle, whereas cold rollermill grinding does not. Heating and grinding sufficiently to disintegrate grain and its starch granule structure increases the amount of its starch digested in the small

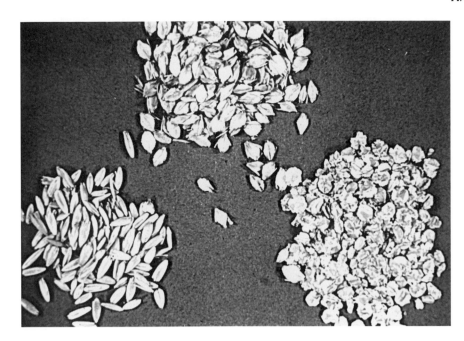

Fig. 4–12. Oats. From left to right, whole, rolled or crimped, and steam flaked. Rolling and steam flaking don't increase the feeding value of oats for most horses, but they do decrease the length of time oats should be stored.

intestine. In one study, small intestinal starch digestion of popped, ground, cracked, and whole corn was 90%, 46%, 30%, and 29%, respectively. Thus, small intestinal starch digestion was increased three-fold by popping and 50% by grinding, but it wasn't affected by cracking. Rolling oats or barley also does not increase the amount of their starch digested in the small intestine. Increasing the amount of starch digested in the small intestine decreases the amount of starch reaching the cecum, which decreases the grain's risk of causing diarrhea, colic, or founder if excessive amounts are consumed.

Although crushed grain for horses has been reported to result in a faster growth rate and generally has been thought to have a higher feeding value than whole grain, controlled studies have failed to confirm this. Neither rolling nor pelleting had any effect on dry matter or gross energy digestibility of either oats or barley by mature horses. Crimping also had no effect on dry matter, protein, or neutral detergent fiber digestibility of either oats or corn by ponies. There was no significant difference between whole unprocessed regular oats and chopped vacuum-cleaned oats, with or without the hulls, in the digestibility of dry matter, protein, fat, acid detergent fiber, neutral detergent fiber or gross energy by mature quarter horses.

Thus, it appears that cold or hot processing of the large kernel grains, oats, barley, and corn, does not improve their digestibility or feeding value for mature horses with good teeth, but grinding and heat treating corn and barley does decrease their risk of causing diarrhea, colic or founder in the horse. Processing in any manner is reported to be important in utilization of the small kernel grains such as rye, wheat, and milo by the horse, and has been reported to increase the grain's feeding value 10 to 15%. Thus, if processed milo, wheat, or rye can be purchased for not more than 15% above the cost of that grain whole, the processed feed is the best buy. If processing costs more than this, it isn't worth the added cost. The exception would be when large amounts (over 8 to 9 lbs or 4 kg/

day) of grain are fed, or when the grain is for foals or horses with poor teeth, such as some older horses that have trouble chewing feed properly. For these horses, all grains should be cracked, crimped, rolled, pelleted, or extruded and dental care provided as described in Chapter 9. Most horses, however, prefer processed to unprocessed grain, as has been shown for cracked versus whole corn.

Grain should not be finely ground. Utilization of fine ground grain generally is no better and may be worse than coarse ground grain. Fine grinding decreases palatability, increases dust and may increase the risk of gastric ulcers in horses as it does in pigs. Gastric ulcers commonly occur in both foals and young pigs, although their greatest incidence is in nursing foals who are generally consuming little grain. In addition, gastric acidity (an increase of which would increase gastric ulcers) is not affected by grinding or pelleting a grain mix.

Grain Quality

Cracking the cereal grain by any method decreases its stability during storage. Cereal grain with unbroken kernels, less than 13% moisture, and protected from insects and rodents may be stored for many years with little loss in feeding value. Cereal grains with broken kernels become oxidized during prolonged storage and develop a stale flavor that decreases their palatability. Mold and bacterial growth also occur more readily in grains containing broken kernels. The higher the temperature, humidity, and moisture content of the feed, the less time required for oxidation and for mold and bacterial growth to occur. The most important single factor is moisture. At 70% relative humidity or above, deterioration is almost certain to take place, even after only a few months and at temperatures as low as 41°F (5°C). If oxidation occurs, it causes vitamin and essential fatty acid deterioration. Once mold growth occurs, it generates metabolic water, enhancing further mold growth and water production; a vicious cycle occurs.

TABLE 4–6
Minimum Weight per Bushel in U.S. Grading Standards[a]

Grade	Barley	Corn, Rye, and Soybeans	Oats	Milo (Sorghum)	Wheat[b]	Wheat[c]
U.S. No. 1	47	56	36	57	58	60
U.S. No. 2	45	54	33	55	57	58
U.S. No. 3	43	52	30	53	55	56
U.S. No. 4	40	49	27	51	53	54
U.S. No. 5	36	46	—	—	50	51

[a] Amounts given are lbs/bu; to convert to kg/kl, multiple values given by 12.9, and to convert to lbs/qt., divide values by 32.
[b] Hard red spring or white club wheat.
[c] All other wheat.

Mold growth during storage causes heating, mustiness, caking, and decreased palatability and nutrient content, and eventually decay of stored feed. Some molds and bacteria may produce toxins that are quite harmful to the horse. Problems, and their treatment and prevention, that may occur as a result of feed contaminates such as these are described in Chapter 19. Antioxidants and antifungal agents or mold inhibitors, as discussed near the end of this chapter, may be added to grain to prolong the time before oxidation or mold growth occurs. It should be remembered that these feed additives merely help prevent oxidation and mold growth. They do not improve feed that is already rancid or moldy. The rate of deterioration of each nutrient in stored feeds is covered in the discussion of each specific nutrient in Chapters 1 and 3.

Insects such as grain weevils, beetles, and mites hasten grain deterioration. Like molds, they generate both heat and metabolic water. Rodents are harmful not only because they eat grain in amounts up to 10% of their body weight daily, but also because their excretions greatly decrease the feed's palatability and may contain infectious bacteria such as salmonella.

To prevent these problems, only good-quality grains should be purchased, and once acquired they should be stored properly to maintain their quality. Government grading standards are a good indication of grain quality. In the United States, the best-quality grain is graded U.S. No. 1, followed in order by Nos. 2, 3, 4, and, for some types of grain, 5. U.S. Sample grade is the poorest quality. The higher the weight per bushel and, for most, the lower the moisture content, foreign material, broken and damaged kernels, and discoloration, the lower the grading number and the better the quality of the grain (Table 4–6). A grade 2 grain is adequate for feeding most horses. A grade 1 or 3 may be considered if their cost as compared to grade 2 is appropriately low. However, the grain that is frequently available for feeding generally has not been graded. Therefore, you should obtain a guarantee from the seller that it is of good quality or may be returned, and you should evaluate it to ensure that it is of good quality before and while it is fed. In contrast to harvested forages, a physical evaluation of grain is usually adequate; a laboratory analysis is not necessary.

Grain should be evaluated and have the following characteristics indicating that it is of good quality:

1. Unless processed, there should be a minimal number of split, cracked, or damaged kernels (less than 5 to 10%) or discolored kernels (not over 1 or 2%). The color should be characteristic of that type of grain. Grain sorghum or milo should be white, yellow, or red with few or no brown kernels, which are high in tannin and low in feeding value and palatability.
2. Kernels should be well formed, plump, firm, and separated; i.e., there should be no clumps present.
3. There should be no areas or kernels that appear moist.
4. There should be a minimal amount of dust and fines, and the grain should be free of hulls, chaff, cobs, and foreign material such as noncereal-grain seeds, wood, stalks, dirt, etc.
5. The grain must be free of foreign material such as pieces of metal, plastic or paper, and ergot. Rye, in particular, should be closely examined for ergot, which is a brown-black, hard, banana-shaped mass from $\frac{1}{4}$ to $\frac{3}{4}$ inch long (0.6 to 2 cm) (see "Equine Ergotism" in Chapter 19).
6. The grain should be free of mold and oxidation as indicated by both appearance and odor. It should not smell moldy, stale, rancid, sour, or dusty. Corn particularly should be closely examined for any evidence of mold.
7. The grain should be free of insects and evidence of rodents (stools and urine). Weevils and beetles should not be seen. Watch the grain closely for several minutes, looking for the movement of grain particles as an indication of the presence of flour mites, which also give the grain a sour odor.

In summary, if the grain doesn't look, smell, and taste good enough for you to eat or feed to your family, don't feed it to your horses. Buy only good-quality grain and store it properly for as short a time as practical to ensure that it is of good quality when fed.

Grain Storage

Good storage facilities greatly reduce feed contamination and a loss of feed and feeding value during storage. A good storage facility should: (1) allow good ventilation of the feed; (2) maintain feed at a cool and uniform temperature and low humidity; (3) protect feed from direct sun-

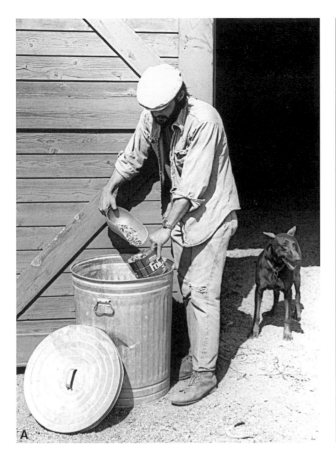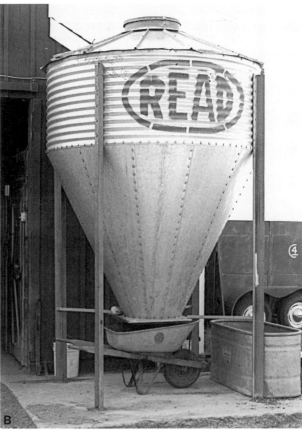

Fig. 4–13(A,B). Vermin- and moisture-proof grain bins should be used. Metal containers such as large garbage cans or wood bins, with tight lids, are excellent for limited feed storage. These should be kept in a feed room equipped with a latch so that a horse cannot get in. Mice and other vermin rapidly eat through sacks and plastic garbage cans. Hopper bottom bins are excellent for storing larger quantities of feed, and allow the purchase of grain in bulk. Purchasing grain in bulk may greatly decrease feed cost as compared with purchasing it in sacks. However, if the grain kernels are broken, as happens in processing, not more than several months' supply should be purchased at one time, to prevent grain from becoming stale and losing palatability and nutritional value prior to feeding.

light, moisture, rodents, birds, insects, mites, and especially from horses and other livestock; (4) be both clean and cleanable; and (5) be located in a location convenient for both filling and feeding. As storage temperature and humidity decrease, so also do problems, such as mold growth and insect and mite infestation. Control of moisture content of feeds is the single most important factor in prevention of spoilage during storage.

For the person with no more than a few horses, galvanized cans with tight-fitting lids work well to store grain (Fig. 4–13). Like all storage containers, they should be thoroughly cleaned prior to use. Rodents gain easy access to grain stored in sacks, plastic cans, and even wood containers. Grain in sacks may also become moist and moldy. For those with a number of horses, ventilated, galvanized metal, bulk storage bins work well (Fig. 4–13). Feed costs are reduced when bulk rather than sacked, grain or grain mixes are purchased. However, moisture condensation on the inner surface of metal feed bins and even cans with tight-fitting lids may occur and result in mold and even bacterial growth and insect proliferation, resulting in feed spoilage. This occurs particularly in feeds containing

greater than 12% moisture, or during warm humid days and cool nights. Painting the grain bin white or, preferably, keeping it completely shaded, and insulating and ventilating it at its highest point so warm damp air can escape, helps prevent condensation and maintain a cooler storage temperature. Mold or bacterial growth rarely occurs at feed moisture levels of 13% or below, and most insects need at least 11 to 12% moisture for prolific reproduction. Insect proliferation increases up to about 14 to 15% moisture, above which mold growth predominates. Troublesome insects include weevils as well as grain borers and moths, which develop inside grains and are therefore difficult to detect until they emerge from the grain kernels. Numerous types of beetles and grain mites also commonly infect stored grains.

HIGH-MOISTURE FEEDS FOR HORSES

Haylage, Silage, and High-Moisture Grains

Haylage and silage are green chop that, instead of being fed the day they are cut, are stored in a silo under anaerobic conditions. Cereal grains may also be harvested at a high-moisture content (22 to 40%) and ensiled. The silo may be an upright column, a trench in the ground, a bunker, a stack, or anything into which the high-moisture feed can be packed sufficiently tightly to prevent oxygen from getting to all but the exposed surface of the feed.

About any type of plant-source feed may be ensiled, including corn, sorghum, legumes, grasses, cereal grains, sunflowers, byproducts, and mixtures of different feeds. Those most commonly ensiled are alfalfa and corn (entire plant, grain, or ear). Ensiled plants containing grain, particularly corn and grain sorghum, are referred to as silage; ensiled legumes and grasses are referred to as haylage; ensiled grain is called high-moisture grain. With ensiling, a plant's maximum feed value is obtained by the animal because the plants can be harvested when they are at their greatest feeding value, and there is minimal loss of the feed and its nutrients during harvesting, storage, and feeding. Ensiling maintains the feeding value of protein, carbohydrate, carotene, and many vitamins better than any other practical method of animal feed preservation. However, since ensiled feed is not sun cured, it is low in vitamin D content.

Under anaerobic conditions, molds, yeast, and aerobic (with air or oxygen) bacteria die while anaerobic microorganisms present in the feed ferment its soluble carbohydrates, producing lactic and volatile fatty acids (e.g., the organic acids propionic, acetic, and butyric), just as occurs in the rumen and the horse's cecum and colon. As the acids are produced, the resulting acidification of the feed inhibits microbial growth, stopping fermentation and, in grain, killing the seed embryo. This process requires several weeks, after which, as long as anaerobic conditions are maintained, the feed is well preserved for many years. If too much air gets to the ensiled feed, as occurs if the feed doesn't contain the proper moisture content or isn't packed sufficiently, then when it is removed from the silo, yeast, mold, and bacteria grow and excess heat is produced, resulting in spoilage and heat damage.

A procedure for vacuum packing high-moisture forage in sealed heavy plastic, called "Horsehage" was developed in England and introduced to North America to assist in producing a good-quality haylage for horses. It results in a palatable haylage with a slightly improved digestibility of all nutrients except neutral detergent fiber. However, if the plastic is perforated allowing entry of air, some spoilage will occur in the bags. When used, every bale should be closely inspected and, if the plastic bag has been punctured, or if the fluid in the haylage isn't sufficiently acidic (has a pH above 4.5) the feed in that bag should not be fed.

Good silage, haylage, or high-moisture ensiled grain have a clean, pleasant acid odor. (Poor or spoiled feed has a foul or objectionable odor.) They have a pleasing, not bitter or sharp taste, and a pH of 3.5 to 5.0. There is no visible mold, and they are not mushy or slimy. They are uniform in moisture and color. Generally, good-quality silage or haylage is green or brownish. Tobacco-brown, dark brown, caramelized or charred-appearing and -smelling ensiled feed indicates that excessive heat occurred during fermentation; a black color indicates it is rotten.

Poor silage, haylage, or high-moisture ensiled grain

should not be fed. At best, they are poorly palatable, with decreased feeding value. At worst, they contain mold or bacterial toxins that if consumed may result in harmful effects, such as botulism, and death, as described in Chapter 19. Good silage, haylage, and high-moisture grain, however, although not commonly fed to horses, are excellent feeds for them. They are highly nutritious and palatable, although some horses are reluctant to eat ensiled feed until they become accustomed to it. It is commonly recommended that ensiled feed dry matter not constitute over one-half of forage fed to horses. Since ensiled feeds are high in moisture, containing only 25 to 60%—generally 25 to 35%—dry matter, whereas hay and grain are about 90% dry matter, it takes about 3 lbs (0.90 ÷ 0.30 = 3) of ensiled feed to replace 1 lb of dried feed.

Acid-Treated Feeds

Instead of preserving hay or grain by drying or ensiling them under anaerobic conditions, which allow microorganisms to ferment some of their soluble carbohydrates to organic acids, they can be preserved by spraying them with organic acids as they are harvested. Generally, a 0.5 to 2% mixture of primarily or entirely propionic acid is used. The acids used are not corrosive or harmful to the animal. They are normal products of microbial fermentation of ingested feeds in the horse's cecum and colon. They are absorbed and used for energy or glucose production. Several times more of these acids are produced in the horse's intestinal tract than would be ingested in a properly acid-treated feed. In contrast, lactic acid and bacterial cultures have been touted as hay preservatives but have been found to be ineffective.

If properly done, acid-treating hay or grain allows them to be stored without spoilage or molding at 20 to 40% moisture content. However, if not treated uniformly or with the proper amount of effective preservatives, spoilage and mold growth will occur. When purchasing hay treated with preservatives, it should be checked for mold and dustiness. A hay moisture content above 20% decreases leaf and nutrient losses during harvesting and feeding, and decreases the hay's dustiness. This is particularly beneficial for horses with chronic respiratory problems that are exacerbated by dry or dusty feed. However, beta-carotene and vitamin E deterioration occur more rapidly in acid-treated than in dry hay, and since there is less sun-curing, its vitamin D content is lower. Reduced vitamin levels in acid-treated hay, however, are not generally a problem or a reason to not feed it.

Acid-treated hay is readily consumed by most horses. In one study, mature horses ate three times more alfalfa hay dry matter when it was dry than when it was acid-treated. However, when not given a choice, there was no difference between the same hay acid-treated or dry in the amount of dry matter consumed or weight gained by yearling Quarter Horses, even during the first week of feeding. In another study, hay treated with buffered propionic acid (Early Bale, Agri-Concepts or Hay Pro II, American Farm Products) was neither consistently selected nor refused when mature horses were given their choice of one of the acid-treated hays or an untreated similar quality hay. All three hays were consumed in similar amounts and at a similar rate, both when first fed and after 35 days of having received only an acid-treated hay or an untreated hay. All 8 horses in the study readily consumed the acid-treated hay, and when only it was fed, they either gained or maintained their weight.

VITAMIN-MINERAL SUPPLEMENTS FOR HORSES

Vitamin-mineral supplements, like protein supplements or any nutritional supplement, are added to the diet to increase the diet's concentration and, therefore, the animal's intake of the nutrient(s) that are high in that supplement. Grains are an energy supplement to a high-forage diet; conversely, forage and many byproduct feeds are fiber supplements to a high-grain diet. The most concentrated energy supplements are fats and oils, as described later in this chapter.

The most common supplements for horses are protein, vitamin, and mineral supplements, and hair coat conditioners. An extensive list of sources of most additives or microingredient for animal diets is published annually. In addition, many companies produce and market one or more supplements high in several nutrients. These are sold under that company's trade name. Those intended to provide additional protein, as well as vitamins and minerals, are usually pelleted. Some may also contain various additives and make numerous claims as to their alleged, but rarely documented, benefit over that of similar amounts of the same nutrients provided individually. Skepticism is warranted for supplements for which unsubstantiated claims arc made, such as testimonials and studies with no controls, i.e., no unsupplemented animals fed the same feeds without the supplement as a comparison. Supplements such as these generally are an expensive means of obtaining nutrients. What the horseman gets for the additional cost is the benefit of the manufacturer's knowledge of nutrient amounts and for combining them in the proper amounts so as to provide an easy method of getting them to the horse.

Regardless of how good a supplement is or its cost, it is of no benefit and, therefore, no value unless the nutrients it provides are actually needed. If they aren't needed, not only is the supplement of no value, it may result in nutrient excesses that are detrimental. Even if some of the nutrients a supplement provides are needed or are of benefit, others may not be. For example, many supplements with added minerals contain calcium and selenium, both of which are needed by many classcs of horses consuming a grass forage. However, if the forage being consumed is a legume grown in high-selenium soils, additional amounts of calcium and selenium may be harmful. In one study of 50 horses fed one or more vitamin-mineral supplements because of the owner's belief in the benefit of doing so, but without any evaluation of its need, although supplementation did decrease the number of diets deficient in one or more nutrients from 28% down to 4%, it increased incidence of a significant excess of one or more nutrients 10-fold. Thus, supplements should not be given unless it is known that at least some of its nutrients are needed, and that it does not provide a harmful excess of any other

nutrient. The amounts of each nutrient needed by, and harmful to, horses are given in Appendix Tables 1, 2, and 3. How to combine various feeds and how to feed to provide the optimum amount of each nutrient are described in Chapter 6 and the feeding programs given in Chapters 10 to 15.

Many commercial supplements are high in unsaturated fatty acids, which are intended to give the horse a glossier, shinier hair coat or bloom and hasten shedding in the spring. As spring approaches, this generally occurs with or without the supplement and, therefore, if the supplement was given it misleads people into believing that it occurred because of the supplement. See the section on "Skin and Hair-Coat Care" in Chapter 9 for ways to give the horse a glossier hair coat and hasten shedding in the spring. Some supplements, particularly vitamin-mineral and protein supplements, are needed and are therefore quite beneficial in some situations. Fat or oil supplements are also often of benefit for horses with increased energy needs.

As shown in Appendix Tables 2 and 3, and as described in Chapters 2 and 3, cereal grains and forages may sometimes not contain enough vitamins and/or minerals to provide the amounts recommended or optimum. Inadequate intake of any one of these nutrients is harmful. To prevent these harmful effects and provide the additional vitamins and/or minerals needed when intake is inadequate, vitamin and/or mineral supplements must be fed.

Vitamin and mineral supplements are present in many commercial feed mixes available for the horse, and there are multitudes of vitamin-mineral supplements sold for the horse. Since excesses of many vitamins and minerals are just as harmful as deficiencies, they should not be given unless you know that they do contain nutrients that are or may be needed, and that they do not provide any ingredient or nutrient in an amount that may be harmful.

The vitamins that may be needed in various circumstances and a vitamin supplement that will satisfy these needs are given in Chapter 3. Other vitamin supplements may be compared to this information in evaluating their content and possible benefit or harm.

Many commercially prepared mineral mixes or supplements contain inadequate amounts of necessary specific minerals, such as calcium and phosphorus; and they frequently contain a multitude of other ingredients. Some of these ingredients, although needed by the horse, are already provided in optimum or excess quantities in the feeds already being consumed; others may be of no known benefit to the horse. The supplemental minerals that may be needed by the horse and the amount of each mineral in these supplements are given in Appendix Table 7. These are the same mineral supplements that commercial companies mix together in various amounts, often with additional ingredients, to make their mineral mixes and for which they generally charge substantially more than the cost of the mineral supplements given in Appendix Table 7. The higher cost for the commercially mixed and marketed mineral supplement is often accompanied by claims of greater availability of minerals as well as general supcriority and benefits. The validity of these claims is doubtful unless they are supported by controlled studies preferably performed by someone not paid by, supported by, and with no monetary interest in the product evaluated, which is often difficult to determine because these interests are rarely indicated.

The availability or absorption of the minerals from the supplements given in Appendix Table 7 is equal to or greater than the availability used in determining the amount of that mineral needed by or of benefit to the horse. In addition, although there are some exceptions, there is minimal difference in the availability of their minerals between most of these supplements and others. Thus, in most cases, mineral availability does not need to be considered in determining which mineral supplement to use. For example, 65 to 75% of the calcium and 55 to 60% of the phosphorus needed by the horse are available from bone meal, dical, calcitic limestone, calcium carbonate, and monophos. Calcium availability is also similar from calcium carbonate, calcium sulfate (gypsum), ground oyster shells, and marble dust. Dolmitic limestone is an exception in that its calcium is only 51 to 78% as available as that which comes from calcium carbonate. Other exceptions are chelated, proteinated or complexed minerals, often referred to as organic minerals, in which the mineral may be either more or less available than the same mineral not in this form.

Organic minerals are metallic or inorganic ions combined with an organic molecule to form cyclic structures. Minerals of nutritional concern most often bound to inorganic substances are iron, cobalt, copper, and zinc. The organic molecules to which they are most frequently bound are amino acids, inorganic or organic acids, ketones, acetone, dihydroxy compounds, disulfides, or, the one most often used for chelation is ethylenediamine tetraacetic acid (EDTA). Naturally occurring chelated mineral compounds include chlorophyll (chelated magnesium), phytate (chelated phosphorus), vitamin B_{12} (chelated cobalt), and hemoglobin and cytochromes (chelated iron). Chelation shields the mineral from external influences and thereby affects intestinal absorption of these minerals. It also affects interference that other minerals may have on the absorption of the chelated minerals. For example, unabsorbed calcium may bind zinc, decreasing its absorption. However, chelated zinc is protected from binding by calcium. If the compound to which the mineral is chelated is more readily absorbed than the mineral, chelation will increase the amount of that mineral absorbed. This is beneficial if the animal needs more of that mineral. If more is not needed, it may be harmful. However, if the compound to which the mineral is chelated is less readily absorbed than the mineral itself, chelation will reduce the absorption of that mineral; phytate is an example of this.

Chelated or organic minerals are occasionally promoted primarily by commercial companies marketing them as being superior to nonchelated or inorganic minerals. This may or may not be true, depending on: (1) the mineral and the compound to which it is chelated, (2) the animal's need for that mineral, and (3) other minerals in the diet. Having a mineral bound to an organic compound or chelated is beneficial if all three of the following criteria are met: (1) if chelation increases that mineral's absorption, (2) if more of that mineral is needed by the animal, and

(3) if there are excesses of other minerals or other substances in that diet that interfere with that mineral's absorption. If any of these three factors is not true, chelation is of no benefit and may be harmful. Even when all of these factors are true, the use of a chelated or organic mineral is rarely necessary. Instead, an additional amount of the mineral needed can be added to the diet in a nonchelated form, generally at a much lower cost. The higher cost of chelated minerals is usually much greater than the increase in their mineral availability. For example, if chelation doubles a mineral's availability but it costs much more than twice as much as the nonchelated mineral, economically there is little reason to use it.

PROTEIN SUPPLEMENTS FOR HORSES

Cereal grains and many forages do not contain enough protein to meet the requirements of the lactating mare or the growing horse, and some mature grass forages don't contain enough protein to meet other horses' requirements. Inadequate protein intake is quite harmful, as described in the section on "Protein Deficiency" in Chapter 1. To prevent these harmful effects and provide the additional protein needed when the protein content of the diet is inadequate, a protein supplement must be fed.

Protein supplements are feeds sufficiently higher in protein than other feeds so that when added to the diet they increase the diet's protein concentration. Since most other horse feeds contain less than 20% crude protein, a feed containing more protein than this when added to the diet would increase the protein concentration of the diet. As a result, a protein feed containing more than 20% crude protein is generally classified as a protein supplement. There are a number of different types of protein supplements. These different types are usually classified according to their origin as: (1) plant, (2) animal, (3) single cell, and (4) nonprotein nitrogen. As discussed in the section on "Nonprotein Nitrogen (Urea) for Horses" in Chapter 1, non-protein nitrogen is of little benefit or harm for horses. Any of the first three types of protein supplements are useful. In most areas, plant proteins are the most commonly used protein supplements for horses and other livestock. The major plant protein supplements used are the oilseed meals, although grain protein supplements are also commonly used.

By themselves, most plant protein supplements are not particularly palatable for most horses. For example, the one most commonly fed in the United States—soybean meal—is slightly less palatable for most horses than wheat, barley, and rye, and considerably less palatable than oats and corn. Because of this, it is best to feed the protein supplements well mixed with cereal grains. When included in a loose mixture, wet molasses is beneficial and commonly used both to increase the feed's palatability and to prevent the protein supplement from sifting out.

Oilseeds and Oilseed Meals

A number of high-oil-containing seeds are grown primarily for vegetable oils for human consumption, paint, and other industrial uses. These oilseeds include soybeans, cottonseeds, peanuts, flax or linseed, safflower seeds, sesame seeds, sunflower seeds, rapeseeds (canola), and coconut or copra. These seeds, usually cooked, may be used as a food for people and animals. However, most commonly their oil is extracted by a solvent, hydraulic, or expeller process. Currently, solvent extraction is the only method commonly used for most oilseeds. It leaves 1 to 1.5% oil in the remaining meal of most oilseeds, whereas 4 to 5% is left by the hydraulic and screw presses used in the other two processes, which mechanically squeeze the oil out of the meal. Following crushing, cooking, and solvent extraction, the remaining protein-rich meal is dried, which completely volatilizes the solvent (generally hexane).

Oilseed meals contain 35 to 50% crude protein (Table 4–7). Because they are used as a protein supplement, they are generally referred to according to their protein content. For example, 44% soybean meal indicates that it contains 44% crude protein as fed. Soybean meal is by far the most widely used of all protein supplements for animal feeds, constituting two-thirds of the total amount of protein supplements used in the United States in 1984. This total has increased gradually to three-fourths by 1992. All animal by-products constituted about 10%, all grain by-products and cottonseed meal 5% each, sunflower and canola meals 1.6% each, and linseed and peanut meals 0.5% each of the protein supplements used in the United States in 1992. Each of these protein supplements may be used effectively for horses and, at times and in some areas, some may be more economical than others.

Soybeans

The major feed derived from soybeans (Glycine max) is soybean meal, which is a by-product of oil extraction from soybeans. It contains about 53% crude protein in its dry matter. However, ground soybean hulls, which are high in fiber and low in protein, may be included with it to produce the protein content of usually 41, 44 or 48% as fed. Soybean meal contains the highest-quality protein and the highest amount of lysine of any of the plant-source protein supplements (Table 4–7). Because of this and the inadequacy of other horse feeds in supplying adequate lysine for growth (Table 1–5), soybean meal is the preferred plant-source protein supplement for the growing horse. It is the most common protein supplement fed to horses; soybeans are much less commonly fed.

Raw soybean seeds contain substances that decrease both the growth rate and feed efficiency of young pigs, poultry, rats, very young ruminants and probably other species. The major growth inhibitor in soybeans is a trypsin inhibitor. It inhibits the protein-digestive enzymes trypsin and chymotrypsin, which are secreted into the small intestine by the pancreas, and therefore decreases their digestion of protein. Soybean trypsin inhibitor also inhibits cholecystokinin-pancreozymin (CCK-PZ) release, which results in greater pancreatic enzyme secretion and enlargement. Ingestion of the trypsin inhibitor present in raw soybeans may also cause cartilage defects during growth, as the incidence of slipped tendon increases with increasing amounts in the chick's diet. However, it and other harmful substances (e.g., urease, goitrogens, and hemagglutinin) in raw soybeans are destroyed by heating in the prepara-

tion of soybean meal and in the roasting or extruding of soybeans. In addition, these substances don't appear to affect older animals. Raw soybeans high in antitrypsin activity don't affect: (1) the growth of pigs over 16 weeks of age, (2) lactation, reproductive efficiency, or feed intake of breeding swine, (3) mature poultry, or (4) cattle. There is no difference in the digestibility by cows of the protein, fat, or crude fiber present in raw versus roasted soybeans. Cows have been fed up to 13.2 lbs (6 kg)/day of either raw or extruded soybeans with no detrimental effects and only a minor decrease in milk fat as compared to when soybean meal was fed.

The effect of feeding raw soybeans to horses is unknown. The information described above would suggest that whole soybeans, raw or heat processed, may be fed without harm to mature horses, but unless heat processed, may not be safe to feed to growing horses. As shown in Table 4–7, whole soybeans are high in digestible energy and protein. They have the same caloric content as corn and, therefore, like corn, care must be taken to ensure that they aren't overfed. If overfed, they would not be expected to be as likely to cause colic or founder as a cereal grain since they contain less than one-third as much starch and 2 times more crude fiber than corn.

Cottonseeds

Cottonseed meal is a by-product of oil extraction from cottonseeds (Gossypium spp.), which themselves are a by-product of the cotton industry. By screening out the hulls, which are low in protein and high in fiber, the processor is able to make a cottonseed meal of the protein content wanted, usually 36, 41, 44, or 48% as fed. Cottonseed meal is reported to be more palatable for most horses than soybean meal, but is lower in protein quality and lysine (Table 4–7). Although this doesn't matter for mature horses, if it is used as the protein supplement for the growing horse, there will be inadequate lysine in the diet, resulting in a slower growth rate unless more protein than needed is fed (Table 1–5).

The major concern in feeding either cottonseeds or cottonseed meal is toxicosis due to their gossypol content. Gossypol toxicosis is rarely reported in horses, as they—like mature, but not immature ruminants—are fairly resistant to it. However, gossypol toxicosis does occur even in mature ruminants and, therefore, quite likely in horses: the younger the horse, the greater its susceptibility. Although cottonseed meal has been fed as the only protein supplement to horses ranging from 3 to 9 months of age with no noticeable detrimental effect when sufficient lysine was added to the diet, feeding cottonseed products to horses is not recommended, unless it is known that doing so does not exceed safe gossypol levels as described in Chapter 19. Excess gossypol intake may result in infertility, slow growth, and sudden death without other clinical or premonitory signs.

Unprocessed or whole cottonseeds are less commonly fed than cottonseed meal because they are generally more expensive and less available, and their free gossypol content and therefore toxicity are greater. In addition, there is a lint on cottonseeds' surface which tends to make the

TABLE 4–7
Protein Supplements: Nutrient Content and Characteristics for Horses[a]

Protein Supplement	Crude Protein (%)	% Lysine in Feed	% Lysine in Protein[b]	Mcal DE/ lb (kg)	Crude Fiber (%)	Fat (%)	Ca (%)	P (%)	Comments
Nonprotein Supplement Feeds for Comparison:									
Oats, regular	13	0.44	3.3	1.45 (3.2)	12	5	0.1	0.35	
Grass hay, good	8–12	0.4–0.5	3.8	1.00 (2.2)	30	3	0.5	0.3	
poor	5–7	0.3–0.4	3.8	0.75 (1.65)	36	3	0.3	0.15	Similar to straw
Alfalfa pellets "dehy" (17%)	19	0.9	4.9	1.07 (2.36)	24–28	2.5–3.5	1–2	0.2–0.3	Often used as a protein supplement
Oilseed Meals:									Many are available at protein levels different from that given
Canola meal (double low rapeseed)	35–44	2.3–2.5	5.9	1.4 (3.1)	10–13	3–4	0.5–0.8	1–1.4	Rapeseed meal that is not low in glucosinolates may cause goiter
Coconut meal (copra meal)	23	0.6	2.5	1.5 (3.3)[c]	15	5	0.2	0.65	
Cottonseed meal (41%)	45	1.8	4.1	1.4 (3.0)	13	1.7	0.18	1.2	Not recommended unless known not to exceed safe gossypol level (see Ch. 19)
Linseed (flax) meal (37%)	40	1.3	3.3	1.4 (3.0)	9	1.6	0.4	0.9	May soften stools but doesn't increase hair-coat glossiness.
Peanut meal (47%)	53	1.7–2.3	3.2–5.1	1.5 (3.25)	8.5	1.5	0.2–0.3	0.65	
Safflower seed meal (42%)	49	1.4	3.1	1.55 (3.4)[c]	9	1.9	0.3	1.8	
Soybean meal (44%)	50	3.2	6.5	1.6 (3.5)	7	1.6	0.4	0.7	Best plant-source protein supplement for growing horse. Most commonly used supplement.
Sunflower seed meal, dehulled (44%)	50	1.8	3.7	1.25 (2.8)	12	3	0.45	1.0	Too high an amount in grain mix may decrease palatability
Oilseeds:									
Canola or rapeseeds	20	1–2	5.9	1.95 (4.3)[c]	6	38	0.38	0.75	May cause goiter unless cooked or low in glucosinolates
Cottonseeds	24	1.0	4.1	1.95 (4.3)[c]	18–20	24	0.15	0.7	Not recommended unless known not to exceed safe gossypol levels
Flax seeds (linseeds)	22.8	0.9	4.1	1.6 (3.6)	6.5	38	0.25	0.6	May cause cyanide toxicosis unless cooked
Safflower seeds	19.5	0.6	3.3	1.8 (3.9)[c]	31	19	0.25	0.75	
Soybeans	33–43	2.3–3.1	6–7	1.6 (3.5)	4–6	18–19	0.2–0.3	0.6–0.8	Raw all right for mature horse but should be heat processed for young horse
Sunflower seeds with hull	18	2.3	4.2	1.65 (3.6)[c]	31	28	0.18	0.56	
Grain Protein Supplements:									
Brewer's grains	25–28	0.95	3.5	1.2 (2.7)	15.6	7.4	0.33	0.55	
Distiller's grains	29–34	0.75–0.9	2.2–3.0	1.2 (2.6)	12–13	7–16	0.10–0.15	0.3–0.6	Palatable for horses, particularly at higher levels (20%)
Distiller's solubles	22–30	1.0	3.3	1.4 (3.1)	5–6	9–12	0.3–0.4	1.3–1.4	Palatable for horses
Gluten meal, corn	47	0.9	2.0	1.4 (3.0)	5	2.4	0.16	0.5	Gluten feed contains some bran and germ, and about 2 times more fiber, 50% as much protein, and 10% less energy than gluten meal.
Gluten meal, wheat	56	1.7	3.0	1.5 (3.2)	6.7	4.9	0.2	0.6	
Pulse Proteins:									
Beans and peas	21–26[d]	1.3–1.8[d]	5–8[d]	1.6 (3.6)	5–7[d]	1.5–1.8[d]	0.1–0.2	0.4–0.6	Field (horse, broad) beans, field peas, chickpeas, & cowpeas safe uncooked. Most others are not.

(continued)

TABLE 4–7
Protein Supplements: Nutrient Content and Characteristics for Horses[a]–(Continued)

Protein Supplement	Crude Protein (%)	% Lysine in Feed	% Lysine in Protein[b]	Mcal DE/ lb (kg)	Crude Fiber (%)	Fat (%)	Ca (%)	P (%)	Comments
Animal-Source Proteins:									
Fish meal, menhaden	60–70	4.4–5.7	7.6	1.4 (3.1)	0.9	10–14	5.6	3.2	Major fish meal fed in U.S. May have low palatability.
Fish meal, white	60–70	4.0–5.0	7.5	1.5 (3.3)	0.8	2–8	8	3.9	Major fish meal fed in U.K. Preferred over menhaden.
Milk, cow's, skimmed	35.6	2.7	7.6	1.8 (4.0)	0.2	1	1.36	1.1	Excellent for young horse. Their high lactose content may cause diarrhea if enough is fed to mature horse.
Milk, cow's, whole	27	2.0	7.4	2.55 (5.6)	0.2	27.6	0.95	0.76	
Casein, dry	93	7.7	8.5	1.8 (4.0)	0.2	0.7	0.6	0.9	Excellent supplement for hypophagic horse
Poultry manure, no litter, dry	25–28[e]			1.0 (2.3)[c]	10–16	1.5–3	6–9	2–3	Content differs if it contains litter. A safe feed but may slow growth.
Single-Cell Proteins:									
Yeast, brewer's	47–51	3.3	6.9	1.5 (3.3)	3–7	1.1	0.15	1.5	Used primarily as a B-vitamin supplement. See Appendix Table 3.
Yeast, torula	52.5	4.1	7.8	1.5 (3.3)	2–3	2.3	0.65	1.8	

[a] All values given are in the feed dry matter.
[b] Greater than 5 to 6% is needed in most diets when the amount of protein supplement used is not in excess of that needed to meet the young horse's protein requirements. A lower value may decrease growth rate and feed efficiency as shown in Table 1–5. For the mature horse, the amount of lysine in the diet and, therefore, this value doesn't matter.
[c] Value given is for ruminants. Value for horses is probably about 15% lower for oilseeds and 20 to 30% lower for the other feeds.
[d] Field (horse or broad) beans contain 8.5% crude fiber, 35.6% protein, and 3.7% lysine (10.6% of its protein); chickpeas contain 3.4% lysine (15.7% of its protein) and 4.8% fat.
[e] The amount given is that provided for horses. About 20% of the nitrogen in poultry manure is not in protein. If all of its nitrogen were converted to protein, it would add an additional 7% protein to the amount given here. However, in contrast to ruminants little nonprotein nitrogen is used by the horse (as discussed in Chapter 1). Thus, the amount of protein poultry manure provides ruminants should be multiplied by 0.80 to get the amount it provides horses.

seeds stick together. This makes them more difficult to feed, particularly if a mechanized feeding system is being used.

Linseed (Flaxseed) Meal

Flax (Linum usitatissimum) in most areas is grown for the oil extracted from its seeds, leaving the by-product linseed meal. It has been a preferred horse feed by some because it was thought to give the horse a glossy hair coat—i.e., a "bloom" or "finish"—and to soften the stools without causing loose stools and thus treat or prevent constipation and impactions. Mechanically processed linseed meal contains more oil than solvent processed (over 4% versus under 2%). The higher oil content of mechanically processed linseed meal when fed may give horses not receiving green forage or an oil or fat supplement a glossier hair coat. However, most linseed meal currently available is solvent processed, which doesn't have any advantage over the other oilseed meals in giving the horse a glossier hair coat. Things that may be done to give the horse a glossier hair coat are described in Chapter 9 (see section on "Skin and Hair-Coat Care").

Linseed meal may, however, have a laxative effect because it is high in the soluble fiber mucilage (3 to 10%). Following its ingestion, some mucilage remains in the stools, which may soften the stools and, by binding water,

increase their water content without making them appear loose or watery. Because of its water-absorptive properties, some have recommended that flaxseed or linseed products not be fed dry because they may cause problems due to excessive swelling as they absorb water in the gastrointestinal tract. However, this does not appear to occur, at least, not when fed in the amount that would be needed as a protein supplement. In addition, wetting linseed products before feeding may increase their cyanide or prussic (hydrocyanic) acid content.

Flaxseeds and flax plants contain cyanogenetic glycosides and enzymes that allow these glycosides to release cyanide. Intact plants and seeds don't normally contain cyanide because these glycosides and enzymes are separate from each other. Damage to the plant or seed, such as that due to drought, frost, wilting, or processing, allows them to come together, resulting in the release of cyanide. Cyanide is readily absorbed from the gastrointestinal tract. It prevents oxygen release from the blood, which in sufficient quantity results in sudden death. However, glycosidase enzymes are destroyed in the stomach and intestinal tract so that no cyanide is released from ingested cyanogenetic glycosides. Glycosidase enzymes are also destroyed by heat, although that used in processing linseed meal may not be sufficient to completely inactivate its glycosidase enzyme activity. However, cyanide is fairly volatile, so much of what may form is lost from the processed feed. As a result of these factors, cyanide toxicosis is not known to occur in horses as a result of feeding linseed meal. Other causes of cyanide toxicosis, as well as its effects, treatment, and prevention, are given in Chapter 19.

Linseed meal is a palatable and adequate protein supplement for mature horses. Its protein, calcium, and phosphorus are all quite digestible (66%, 59%, and 54%, respectively, in weanling horses). However, linseed meal, like most plant-protein supplements, except soybean and canola meals, is low in lysine (Table 4-7). As a result, it will reduce growth and feed efficiency when used as the protein supplement for young horses unless the diet contains adequate lysine from other sources, or unless linseed meal is fed in sufficient excess of protein needs to provide adequate lysine (0.7%), which is rarely economical. The growth rate, feed efficiency and health of weanlings fed diets containing 15% linseed meal with added lysine were similar to those fed a milk-product-containing diet similar in nutrient content.

Peanut Meal

Peanut (Arachis hypogaea) meal is a by-product of peanut oil production. It is similar in nutrient content, including inadequate lysine for young horses, to cottonseed and linseed meals (Table 4-7). It is reported to be a palatable and good protein supplement, but to become rancid when stored too long (more than several months), especially in warm moist climates. However, currently this would be less likely to occur because the peanut meal generally now available is much lower in fat (1.5% versus 4 to 8%). Care must be taken to ensure that it doesn't contain the mold-produced aflatoxins that may be high in some peanut meal, as described in Chapter 19.

Sunflower Seed Meal

Sunflower (Helianthus annus) seed meal, a by-product of oil extraction, is used as a protein supplement in animal feeds in many areas of the world, particularly where it is an indigenous crop and, therefore, less expensive than other protein supplements. Sunflower meal varies from 23 to 59% protein and 8 to 32% crude fiber depending primarily on whether the seeds are dehulled before processing. Although high in sulfur-containing amino acids, it, like other oilseed meals excluding soybean and canola meals, when used as the protein supplement for the young horse, results in a diet with inadequate lysine (Table 4-7). Sunflower seed meal is a safe feed for horses, but at too high a concentration in a grain mix, it may decrease its palatability.

Rapeseed (Canola)

Rapeseed (Brassica napus and B. campestris) has become an important oilseed crop in various temperature-zone countries (e.g., Canada, northern Europe, and Asia) where most other oilseed crops do not thrive. Rapeseed (canola) meal contains more calcium, phosphorus, magnesium, manganese, selenium, and sulfur-containing amino acids, and only slightly less lysine, than soybean meal

(Table 4-7). But it does contain enough lysine to meet the growing horse's lysine requirements when the amount needed to just meet the horse's protein requirements is used. Its protein is 81 to 83% digestible by several species of animals as compared to 85 to 90% for soybean meal. It is quite high (14.5%) in pectin and low in mono- and disaccharides, and contains no starch.

Rapeseeds, and their extracted oil and meal, all contain both glucosinolates and erucic acid. Rapeseed and other oils from cruciferous plants differ from most vegetable oils in containing a significant amount of long-chain fatty acids with 20 and 22 carbon atoms (eicosenoic and erucic acids). Both erucic acid and gluconsinolates are toxic and unpalatable. However, varieties of rapeseed (Tower, Duo, Candle, Regent, and others) have been developed that contain low amounts of both compounds. The name canola was adopted in 1979 in Canada for these "double low" varieties of rapeseed. Since then and until recently, the production of other types of rapeseed has nearly ceased in Canada. High-erucic-acid rapeseed (HEAR) oil has been found to have unique lubricating properties and to be quite useful as a raw material for the manufacture of special plastics. Because of this, varieties of rapeseed high in erucic acid, and as a result also high in glucosinolates, have been developed and are being produced. Thus, rapeseed products both low (canola) and high (HEAR) in both erucic acid and glucosinolates are available.

Glucosinolates may vary tenfold in rapeseed meal from different varieties or cultivars of rapeseeds. Glucosinolates, per se, are nontoxic until hydrolyzed. Although some bacteria in the gastrointestinal tract may cause some hydrolysis of ingested glucosinolates, most hydrolysis is due to the enzyme myrosinase in the diet. Myrosinase is in the rapeseed but is separated from the seed's glycosinolates so hydrolysis doesn't occur unless the seed is damaged. In processing, although the seed is damaged, much of the myrosinase is destroyed by cooking. However, all varieties of rapeseed meal contain some harmful substances, with these substances being the lowest in canola meal and highest in HEAR meals. Harmful substances in rapeseed meals include not only those released from hydrolyzed glucosinolates and erucic acid but also sinapine, which has a bitter taste.

Upon hydrolysis of glucosinolates, free (aglucones) goitrogenic compounds evolve. These substances cause goiters. Although not secreted into the milk, they result in a low milk-iodine concentration; as a result, young receiving milk from animals consuming them may develop goiter that can be treated or prevented by increasing their iodine intake. Although a sufficient amount of either whole canola seeds or high-glucosinolate-rapeseed meal in the diet will cause goiter, there is no evidence that canola meal is goitrogenic at least to cattle and swine.

In addition to goitrogenic and unpalatable substances, rapeseed products may decrease growth rate and feed efficiency. To prevent this, the amount of rapeseed product that may be fed, at least to young pigs, is limited. However, canola meal may be used as the only protein supplement in swine finishing and reproduction diets, and for all cattle diets, without any undesirable effects. Canola meal and low glucosinolate varieties of rapeseed meal are also suitable as the only protein supplements in the horse's diet. They are equal to soybean meal as protein supplements for the horse. This was demonstrated in two studies in which there was no difference between either weanling or yearling horses fed diets containing 15% of either canola meal or soybean meal. All of these horses remained in excellent condition and health throughout the studies, and none showed any signs of any abnormalities.

Based on growth rate, feed efficiency, serum lysine concentrations, nutrient digestibility, and feed acceptance as indicated by free-choice feed intake, canola meal and low-glucosinolate rapeseed meal appear to be excellent protein supplements for the horse, are adequate as the only protein supplement for growing horses, and are equal to soybean meal as a protein supplement for horses.

Grain Protein Supplements

There are three major grain protein supplements used in feeding horses: gluten, dried brewer's grains, and dried distiller's grains with or without dried solubles. Unfortunately, considerable quantities of grains are used in the brewing of beer and the distilling of liquor; brewer's and distiller's grains, and yeast, are the resulting by-products. More of these, or similar by-products, may become available in the future from gasohol production. The characteristics of these products vary somewhat with the grain used, the area in which it is grown, and the procedures and processes used. What is described here is for the products most commonly available in the United States and Canada.

Brewer's Grains and Yeast

In the production of beer, barley usually (although other grains may be used) is soaked in warm water and allowed to sprout. The germinated kernels form malt, which is mixed with other grains (usually corn or rice) and hops (used as a flavoring agent) to form mash. The malt sprouts, which are separated from the kernels, are dried as a by-product feed. The mash is crushed and heated and its starch enzymatically converted to sugar. The sugar and other soluble materials (called wort) are removed and boiled with hops. Then yeast is added to convert its sugar to alcohol. The yeast that grows during the fermentation procedure is harvested as brewer's yeast. Mash solids are dried, producing brewer's grains.

Malt sprouts (or cums) contain 12 to 13% oil, 14% crude fiber, and, based on their nitrogen content, 24 to 25% crude protein. However, about one-half of their "crude protein" is from nonprotein nitrogen and, therefore, not usable protein for the horse. Malt sprouts are reported to be a good horse feed but rather dusty and having a bitter flavor. Brewer's, distiller's, and torula yeasts, although low in sulfur-containing amino acids, do provide adequate amounts for the horse and are similar in protein and lysine content to soybean meal (Table 4-7). However, they are generally too expensive to use as a protein supplement and instead are used primarily as B-vitamin supplements, usually in amounts of a few ounces (50 to 100 g) daily. As shown in Appendix Table 3, dried brewer's yeast is many times higher in all of the B-vitamins, except B_{12}, than other horse feeds.

Dried brewer's grains may be referred to by the name of the brewer, as in Coor's pellets. They are slightly lower in energy and higher in fiber than oats, but are 2 times higher in protein (Table 4-7). They are a nutritious and palatable feed for horses. Because of their high fiber and protein content, they are often used in complete pelleted feeds for horses. However, they contain only about one-half as much protein as most oilseed meals, and like most plant-source protein supplements, except soybean and canola meals, contain inadequate lysine for the growing horse unless more than needed to meet their protein requirement is used (Table 4-7).

Distiller's Grains

Following grain fermentation to produce alcohol, and distillation to remove it, what remains (called whole or wet stillage or slop) is separated into wet grains (solid portion) and thin stillage (liquid portion). These are dried to produce distiller's dried grains and solubles, respectively. They may be sold for use separately or combined to produce distiller's dried grains with solubles (DDG/S). Distiller's grains and solubles are similar in nutrient content except that crude fiber is lower (4 to 6% versus 12 to 13%) and phosphorus is higher (1.3% versus 0.4%) in dried solubles (Table 4-7).

Distiller's grains are similar nutritionally to brewer's grains. The yeast that grows during fermentation is harvested as distiller's yeast. It, like brewer's yeast, is used primarily as a B-vitamin supplement, being several times higher in all of the B-vitamins, except B_{12}, than other horse feeds.

Distiller's grains are similar in energy and crude fiber to oats, but are about 2.5 times higher in protein (Table 4-7). However, like brewer's grains, they contain only about one-half as much protein as most oilseed meals and inadequate lysine for growing horses (Table 4-7). For mature horses they are a good and palatable protein supplement, increasing the palatability of diets containing 20%, with lower amounts having no effect on diet palatability. However, different results may be obtained with different or poorer-quality distiller's grains.

Gluten

Gluten meal is the viscous, nitrogenous material remaining when the flour of wheat, corn, or other cereal grains is washed to remove starch. It is similar in nutrient content to most oilseed meals and is low in lysine (Table 4-7). Sometimes some of the cereal bran and germ are included with gluten meal, producing gluten feed. Gluten feed contains about twice as much fiber, one-half as much protein, and 10% less digestible energy than gluten meal. Both gluten feed and gluten meal may be fed to horses and are high in B-vitamins, but are reported to be relatively unpalatable for nonruminants.

Beans and Peas (Pulse Proteins)

Beans and peas, which are seeds of leguminous plants and are called pulses, are used primarily for human consumption, but some can be fed to horses when economically feasible. Most are similar in nutrient content to cereal grains except that they contain 2 to 3 times more protein, and their protein is much higher in lysine (Table 4-7). However, even the leguminous seeds used for human food contain antinutritional and potentially toxic substances. These include protease (trypsin) inhibitors, goitrogens, cyanogenic compounds, antivitamin factors, mineral-binding factors, hemagglutinins (lectins), and lathyrogens. Fortunately, cooking, particularly in water or steam, destroys or greatly decreases the toxicity of all these harmful substances so that many types of beans and peas may be safely fed to horses and other animals, or eaten by people.

Protease inhibitors decrease protein digestion. Lectins may decrease nutrient absorption by damaging the intestinal villi and causing diarrhea. Antivitamin and mineral-binding effects of leguminous seeds used for feed are minimal. The hypothyroidism and enlarged thyroid gland caused by their goitrogens are counteracted by increased dietary iodine. Their cyanogenic compounds decrease oxygen utilization by inhibiting cytochrome oxidase as discussed in Chapter 19.

Lathyrogens cause a neurologic disorder in animals and people referred to as lathyrism, which is characterized in most species by a spastic paraparesis. Lathyrism occurs when primarily the seeds of various Lathyrus and Vica spp. (primarily L. sativus or chickling vetch or pea, L. cicera or flat-podded vetch, and L. clymenum or Spanish vetchling) make up the majority of the total diet for more than a several-month period. The condition occurs primarily in epidemics in young men in India. Those affected develop stiffness of leg muscles, gradually progressing to partial paralysis and total loss of control of the legs with increased extensor muscle tone. Two experimentally induced disorders affecting bone collagen and elastin metabolism similar to that occurring as a result of a copper deficiency (see Chapter 2) have also been induced in various laboratory animal species. No reports of any of these conditions in horses are known. However, it has been reported, but without any supportive data or cases presented, that horses are particularly susceptible to lathyrogens, causing degenerative changes in the nerves and muscles of the larynx which may result in a sudden and transient laryngeal paralysis causing near suffocation brought on by exercise, and that severe hepatic and splenic inflammation may also occur.

Indian or grass peas or chickling vetch or peas (Lathyrus sativus), sweet peas (L. odoratus), wild winter peas (L. hirsutus), singletary peas (L. pusillus) and everlasting peas (L. sylvestris) after long periods of consumption by horses are reported to cause lathyrism. Although the whole plant contains the toxin, the seeds appear to be the most toxic source. Steeping and boiling, or roasting seeds at 300°F (150°C) for 20 minutes, removes or destroys up to 80 to 85% of the toxin.

Field (horse or broad) beans (Vicia faba), chick peas (Cicer arietinum), cowpeas (Vigna sinensis), field peas (Pisum satium and P. aruense) and tick beans are reported to be safe and palatable for horses, even without cooking. Most other beans and peas are not. Uncooked kidney (navy, pinto, haricot, or yelloweye) beans (Phaseolus vulgaris) contain antiproteases, lectins, antivitamin-E factors;

are unpalatable; and cause colic. Two hours of wet heat at 93°C (200°F) or greater are reported to be necessary before they can be safely fed. Lima beans (Phaeolus lunatus) contain antiproteases and lectins and are particularly high in cyanogenic compounds, all of which are detoxified to a large extent by wet heat.

Animal-Source Protein Supplements

Numerous protein supplements of animal origin are often available for feeding animals. Most are derived from milk or milk products and inedible or surplus tissues from meat-packing or rendering plants as well as from fish, poultry, eggs, and the by-products of their processing. Few are fed to horses because of their cost, poor palatability, and problems with spoilage and with bacterial contamination and growth. Milk products, and less commonly fish meal, may be used in some creep feeds and milk replacers for foals. However, even these feeds often will contain plant- instead of animal-protein supplements. For example, Calf Manna (Carnaton-Albers) contains soybean meal and not milk products. The major advantage of these animal-protein feeds is that they contain high-quality protein high in lysine. However, soybean and canola meals are nearly as high in lysine and provide adequate lysine for growth (Table 4-7), generally at a much lower cost and without the other disadvantages of most of the animal-source protein supplements.

Dried Milk Products

Dehydrated skimmed milk is the most commonly used animal-source protein supplement fed to horses. Other milk products also are sometimes available or are added to horse feeds, primarily milk replacers and creep feeds. These include dried whole milk, dried whey, cheese rind, and dried buttermilk. Milk proteins, such as casein and lactalbumin, although excellent feeds containing 75 to 90% protein, are rarely fed because of their cost. Dried whole milk is also usually too expensive and, therefore, not used. Whey, which is what remains after milk proteins have been removed following drying, still contains 17 to 18% protein, but is primarily lactose. Cheese rind or meal consists of cheese trimmings containing 50 to 60% protein, 1 to 1.4% calcium and 0.6 to 8% phosphorus, and provides about 1.8 Mcal/lb (4 Mcal/kg). Buttermilk and skimmed milk have about the same composition and feeding value as cheese by-products.

All of these milk products, in addition to containing high-quality protein high in lysine, are high in, with a good balance of, minerals. They are also highly palatable and digestible, unless excess heat, which decreases protein digestibility, is used in their production. Those in which most of their fat has been removed are quite low in the fat-soluble vitamins A, D, E, and K. In addition, all (except casein and lactalbumin) are high in lactose. Lactose, if consumed in sufficient quantity, causes diarrhea in mature horses because of their lack of the lactase enzyme necessary for lactose digestion and subsequent absorption. This is not a problem in younger horses, who have adequate lactase; horses over 3 years of age, however, have little lactase.

Fish Meals

Fish meals consist of ground whole fish or parts thereof, which are cooked and dried. All are high in a high-quality protein, high in lysine, and high in minerals and B-vitamins, including B_{12} which is not present in plant feeds except from bacterial contamination. But they are low in the fat-soluble vitamins A, D, E, and K, as these vitamins are removed with their oils. The lower the fish meals' fat content, the better it is considered as a feed. Although antioxidants currently added to most fish meals prevent its fat from becoming rancid under most conditions for 6 to 12 months, even nonrancid fish fat may impart an unpalatable flavor to the feed. The greater the fat content, the less that can be fed without decreasing feed consumption. For this reason, low-oil (under 5%) high-protein fish meal, such as white fish meal made from fish used for human consumption, such as cod and haddock, is preferred.

While white fish meal is the major fish meal produced in the United Kingdom, it constitutes only a small fraction of United States' production. Over 90% of the fish meal produced in the United States is made from menhaden herring, a high-oil-content fish. As a result, menhaden fish meal is higher in oil (Table 4-7) and generally considered a less desirable feed for horses and other herbivores than white fish meal. It's reported that 5 or 10% white fish meal in a creep feed or milk replacer is quite satisfactory for foals and should be a good safe feed.

Fish meal in cattle and sheep diets has been found in a number of studies to increase their growth rate and feed efficiency, with 90% of the benefit occurring with only 2% fish meal in the diet. Therefore, there is little added benefit from higher amounts in the diet and more may be detrimental. Whether similar results apply to the horse is unknown.

Dried Poultry Manure

Although not a very appealing sounding feed, dried poultry manure (DPM) has been shown to be a safe and acceptable feed for horses, cattle, and sheep. It is occasionally added to commercial feed mixes and is available in some areas as a protein supplement. In drying, it is heated sufficiently to kill bacteria so that it does not transmit infectious diseases. The heating may decrease its protein digestibility. About 20% of the nitrogen in DPM is from nonprotein-nitrogen-containing substances. Since (as discussed in Chapter 1) nonprotein nitrogen provides little protein to horses, DPM provides about 20% less crude protein than that determined from its total nitrogen content. For example, a DPM containing 35% crude protein determined from its nitrogen content would actually provide only 28% (35% × 0.80) crude protein to the horse. Up to 10% DPM can be used successfully in weanling and yearling horses' diets.

Dried poultry manure is low in dietary energy and high in minerals, (Table 4-7) both of which, as well as its protein content, are decreased if it contains litter. Litter may also increase its fiber content as much as twofold.

Single-Cell Proteins

Single-cell proteins (SCP) are derived from single-cell organisms such as yeasts, bacteria, and algae. These organisms may be grown on a multitude of different media, such as many types of industrial wastes. They are potentially, but not currently, a source of large amounts of protein. It has been calculated that a single-cell fermenter covering less than 4 square miles (10.4 sq km, about 25 acres, or 10 hectares) could produce enough protein to supply total world needs, and that an equal weight of single-cell organisms produces 100,000 times more protein than beef cattle and 1250 times more than soybeans. However, numerous problems with SCP are yet to be solved. These include poor palatability and digestibility, toxins produced by or from the growth media, poor protein quality, high nucleic acid content (particularly in that produced by bacteria), and economics. Work is being done to solve these problems.

SCP from yeast and algae, but not bacteria, are quite low in sulfur-containing amino acids. However, this is easily and inexpensively overcome by adding methionine hydroxy analog. Neither their low amount of sulfur-containing amino acids or their high nucleic acid content are likely to be a problem for horses. Currently there is a limited amount of SCP available from brewer's yeast and torula yeast, which result from the fermentation of wood residue and other cellulose sources. However, they are generally too expensive to use as a major protein supplement. Instead, currently they are most often used primarily as B-vitamin supplements, usually in amounts of only a few ounces (50 to 100 g) daily. They contain many times more of these vitamins, except B_{12}, than other horse feeds (Appendix Table 3). Their nutrient content is given in Table 4-7. Live yeast cultures, instead of killed dried yeast products, are occasionally fed to try to increase the efficiency of feed utilization. These are discussed later in this chapter in the section on "Digestion Enhancers."

A SCP that is available commercially is produced by the algae Spirulina. It is present in some equine supplements and is occasionally touted as being quite beneficial. It is high in protein, many trace minerals, and carotenoids. Its benefit or harm for the horse has not been demonstrated. Rats and chicks accumulate more hepatic beta-carotene and vitamin A when this SCP is fed than when synthetic beta-carotene is fed. However, at levels as low as 2.7% spirulina in the diet, plasma vitamin A (retinol) and plasma, liver and heart alpha-tocopherol (vitamin E) concentrations are reduced. This would increase the susceptibility of the liver and heart to lipid peroxidative damage. It appeared to inhibit vitamin A release from the liver. Levels of greater than 10% spirulina in a rat's diet reduce food intake and digestibility and slow growth rate.

FAT AND OIL SUPPLEMENTS FOR HORSES

Fats or oils may be added to the horse's diet: (1) to decrease dust; (2) to lubricate and thus lessen wear on feed preparation and mixing equipment; (3) as a binder for pelleting or to assist in preventing fine material, such as added vitamins, minerals or protein supplements, from sifting out; (4) to try to give the horse a glossier hair coat; and (5) to increase energy density of the diet. The purpose of increasing diet energy density is to increase energy intake and/or decrease the amount of feed needed to provide energy needs in order to increase athletic performance, milk production, reproductive efficiency, and growth rate and/or to maintain or increase body weight during hot humid weather and when energy needs are high. Fats or oils may be added to commercially prepared horse feeds for all five of these purposes, with the last two being the reason most horseowners add them to the horse's diet. Fat supplementation appears to be of benefit for all of these purposes, except perhaps in giving the horse a glossier hair coat (see section on "Skin and Hair-Coat Care" in Chapter 9).

The high amount of energy needed by horses during growth, lactation, training, or use generally necessitates an increase in their diet's energy density so that a sufficient amount of dietary energy can and will be eaten to meet their needs and, thus, allow the young horse to grow rapidly and the mature horse to maintain optimum body weight, condition, and reproductive or athletic performance. The increase in the energy density of the diet is generally accomplished by increasing the proportion of grain in the diet up to a maximum of 40 to 60% of the weight of the diet. More grain than this decreases forage intake too greatly, increasing the risk of founder, colic, diarrhea, and exertional myopathy. A decrease in forage intake also decreases the amount of water, electrolytes, and energy-providing nutrients present in the intestinal tract, which are quite beneficial for endurance type physical performance. A low-forage diet also increases the risk of boredom and stable vices in horses not on pasture. Fat supplementation can alleviate these detrimental effects of excess grain and inadequate forage intake, yet accomplish the needed and beneficial increase in the diet's energy density.

Supplemental fats are well used by the horse. Utilization does not vary between different sources, but tends to be lower for animal fats than for plant or vegetable oils. Added fat or oil generally increases the diet's total energy digestibility and increases or has little effect on the utilization of other nutrients. Fat supplementation also has no effect on the horse's blood parameters except for increasing plasma cholesterol concentration. This effect is not detrimental in horses as it is in people.

Adding fat to the horse's diet increases the amount of dietary energy available, even without an increase in dietary energy intake, by decreasing the amount of dietary energy used for heat production. This not only decreases the animal's body heat load, but also leaves more energy available for other body functions. This decreases the amount of dietary energy and thus feed intake required for the same amount of activity. The amount of feed the horse must consume is decreased further when fat is added to its diet because the added fat increases the diet's energy density.

As shown in Table 4-8 plant or vegetable oils provide about 3 times more digestible energy than an equal weight of cereal grain, and 3.5 to 6 times more than an equal volume of cereal grain. As a result, 1 cup (8 oz or 237 ml) of vegetable oil will replace or provide the same amount of digestible energy as 1.5 qts (or L) of oats, and 1 qt (or L) of other cereal grains. In one study, adding 5 or 10% fat to the total diet increased its metabolizable energy density

TABLE 4–8
Fats' and Oils' Density and Energy Content Compared to Grains'

	Density		Digestible Energy as Fed		
	lbs/qt	kg/L	Mcal/lb (kg)	Mcal/qt (L)	Mcal/cup[a]
Oil, vegetable	1.92	0.92	4.08 (8.98)	7.8 (8.3)	1.95
Fat, animal	1.80	0.86	3.61 (7.94)	6.5 (6.8)	1.62
Corn, cracked	1.50	0.72	1.54 (3.40)	2.3 (2.4)	0.57
Oats, regular whole	1.0	0.48	1.30 (2.88)	1.3 (1.4)	0.33

[a] 8 oz or 237 ml/cup

8.5 and 17%, respectively, which decreased the amount of grain mix needed for weight maintenance 21 and 25%, respectively. The decrease in feed intake needed when fat is added to the diet may be quite beneficial for horses whose energy needs are increased for growth, lactation, and work, and during hot/humid weather as described in the chapters on feeding during each of these situations (Chapters 15, 13, 11 and 10, respectively).

A number of different sources of fat or oil may be used. Although different fats and oils vary primarily in their degree of saturation (number of double bonds) and, therefore, their melting points, all are readily utilized by the horse to provide the same amount of energy. However, there may be a difference in other ingredients they contain and in their palatability. In products commonly available for feeding, animal fats tend not to be as pure as vegetable oils, which is the reason for their slightly lower energy density (Table 4-8), and may not be as palatable for horses. Of 10 different types and mixtures of fats and oils evaluated in one study, horses seemed to prefer corn oil. In another study, corn oil was found to be more palatable for horses than soy oil, and lecithin decreased the palatability of both oils. Most other vegetable oils, except coconut oil (often referred to as copra oil), also appear to be acceptable to most horses. Fats and oils generally cost 2 to 5 times more per unit of weight than cereal grains, but since they provide about 3 times more available energy, they may not be much more expensive on a digestible energy basis. To compare costs on an energy basis, divide the cost of each feed per unit of weight by the amount of energy the same weight of that feed provides (as explained in Chapter 7).

Plant or vegetable oils and feed-grade animal fats generally can be obtained most inexpensively from feed ingredient suppliers. Information on how to contact those in your areas usually can be obtained from manufacturers of feed, milk replacers, and either large or small animal feeds. In addition to price and availability, important selection criteria that should be provided by the supplier are: moisture less than 1.5%, insoluble impurities less than 0.5%, unsaponifiables less than 0.1% for animal fats and less than 2% for hydrolyzed fats, and, most important, free of oxidative rancidity as indicated by a peroxide value of less than 20 mEq/kg. To help prevent rancidity, the fat or oil should contain the maximum allowable amount of antioxidants.

Although common horse feeds contain only 3 to 6% fat, horses can utilize up to 20% added fat to the total diet and

30% in the grain mix without adverse effects. Higher levels may decrease feed palatability and cause loose stools. In addition, lower amounts appear to be optimum for increasing muscle glycogen content. Muscle glycogen content increased with increasing fat up to 10 to 12% of the total diet, but did not increase further or began to decrease with 15 and 20% fat added to the total diet. One pint of oil per 5 lbs of grain (200 g or 217 ml/kg) results in 20% added fat in the grain. If one-half of the total diet by weight is grain, adding this amount of fat to the grain will result in 10% added fat in the diet. If one-half of the diet is not grain, the amount of fat added to the grain should be adjusted accordingly so that the total diet doesn't contain over 10 to 12% added fat. For example, if the grain mix constitutes $\frac{1}{3}$ and forage $\frac{2}{3}$ of the weight of feed eaten, to add 10% fat to the diet add 30% to the grain mix (10% ÷ $\frac{1}{3}$, i.e. the percent fat wanted in the total diet divided by the proportion of grain in the diet equals the percent fat needed in the grain). The oil may be added and mixed with the grain at each feeding or beforehand. About 3 gallons added to 100 lbs (24 L added to 100 kg) of grain results in 20% added fat in the grain. Don't mix more than what is needed for over 1 to 2 weeks, particularly during warm weather. Store the fat in a cool dark place to reduce the likelihood of rancidity. Fats or oils with off-odors should not be fed. If the peroxide value of a fat or oil, which can be measured by most laboratories, is above 20 mEq/kg, that fat or oil should not be fed.

Remember, when supplemental fat is fed, less feed is needed to provide the same amount of energy. Five pounds (2.3 kg) of a 10% added-fat grain provides the same amount of energy as 6 lbs (2.7 kg) of the grain alone, and 7 lbs (3.2 kg) of a 20% added-fat grain provides the same amount of energy as 10 lbs (4.5 kg) of grain alone. Ensure that the horse eats at least 1 to 1.5 lbs of forage/100 lbs (1 to 1.5 kg/100 kg) body weight. If this amount of forage is not being consumed, decrease the amount of grain fed, with or without oil, until this amount of forage is consumed. Monitor the horse's body weight and condition, and adjust the amount of feed accordingly to maintain them at the horse's optimum.

GRAIN MIXES AND COMPLETE FEEDS FOR HORSES

Grain or concentrate mixes are cereal grains with supplements added to increase the mix's content of specific nutrients. A complete feed is a grain mix that is high in fiber generally because it contains a forage or high-fiber by-product feed such as hulls. To hold the mixture together, complete feeds are usually pelleted or extruded, which is discussed later in this chapter. A grain mix is needed only if the horses being fed have nutrient requirements greater than those which can be obtained from forage and cereal grain alone. If this is not the case, a grain mix is not needed, of no benefit, and an unnecessary expense, since grain mixes generally cost more than cereal grains alone. Most forages, with or without cereal grain and with no supplements given, provide an adequate amount of all nutrients needed except during growth and, for brood mares, during the last 3 months of pregnancy and during lactation. During these periods, a grain mix may be needed to provide

a higher concentration of the nutrients which may be inadequate in the forage being consumed with respect to the horse's requirement.

There are three types of grain mixes for horses: home, custom, and commercial. For home mixes, the amount of whatever feeds or supplements are wanted is added to the grain as it is fed. Custom mixes are those prepared by a feed mill according to specifications they are given. Both a home and a custom mix require a formula that gives the amount of each ingredient they should contain. How to determine this formula and obtain or prepare home and custom feed mixes are described in Chapter 6.

For most people in most situations, the most practical grain mixes are the ones that are commercially formulated and made. These may be made and marketed by international, national, or regional companies, or by a local feed mill. Those produced by local or regional businesses may be formulated specifically for that area, based on the nutrient content of the forages in, and any nutrient peculiarities unique to, that specific area. Thus, if properly formulated and prepared, they may be quite good. Larger companies may have the advantage of, but do not necessarily have, better research and development of their products and their formulations, preparation, and quality assurance.

The grain mix selected should meet the needs of the horses fed. Most companies indicate the class of horse for which each of their feeds is intended. However, one should make sure that the grain mix selected contains the amount of the nutrients needed for the type of forage fed so that the two (that is, the total diet) meet or exceed the nutrient requirements for each class of horse being fed. The information given in Table 4-9 can be used as a rough guide in doing this. Table 4-10 gives examples of grain mixes that contain these amounts of nutrients. These tables indicate the advantage of feeding all or some legume hay to growing horses and brood mares late in pregnancy and during lactation. When a legume is fed, the grain mix doesn't need to contain as much protein supplement, which is usually one of the most expensive ingredients in a grain mix. However, a less expensive or better-quality grass hay may make feeding a more expensive grain mix preferable and economical (see Chapter 7 for a description of how to minimize feeding costs).

Some information on the nutrient content of a grain mix is on the feed tag. The feed tag should give the minimum crude protein and crude fat, and maximum crude fiber, concentrations. Some companies also give the amount of calcium, phosphorus, and occasionally other nutrients. If the information needed is not on the feed tag, the dealer or the company may be able to provide it. If not, consider using a different feed or having the feed analyzed for the nutrients of concern. If the feed will be fed to young horses, the list of ingredients on the feed tag should indicate that it contains as its only protein supplement those ingredients whose protein contains greater than 5% lysine (Table 4-7), such as soybean, canola, fish or meat meals, or milk products. Ingredients are listed in order of decreasing preponderance in the feed either as individual ingredients or in collective terms. Collective terms commonly used for livestock feeds are: grain products (which include any

TABLE 4-9
Minimum Nutrient Contents Needed in Grain Mix[a]

		Type of Forage Fed		
Class of Horses	Nutrient	Legume Hay	Mixed Hay or Growing Grass	Grass Hay
Nursing foal	Crude protein[b]	16	16	16
	Calcium	0.9	0.9	0.9
	Phosphorus	0.6	0.6	0.6
Weanlings	Crude protein[b]	14	16	18
	Calcium	0.6	0.9	0.9
	Phosphorus	0.6	0.6	0.6
Yearlings, 2-yr-olds & Broodmares in last 3 mo. of pregnancy and lactation	Crude protein	10	14	16
	Calcium	0.3[c]	0.3[c]	0.7
	Phosphorus	0.5	0.5	0.5
Other mature horses[d]	Crude protein	8	8	10
	Calcium	0[c]	0[c]	0.3
	Phosphorus	0.3	0.3	0.3

[a] Amounts given are the percent of each nutrient needed in the grain mix as fed when average- or better-quality forages are fed. Higher amounts aren't harmful but may unnecessarily increase feeding costs. In addition to the nutrients shown, it is also recommended that the grain mix contain zinc and copper in ppm (mg/kg) of 60 and 50 for nursing foals, 60 and 25 for weanlings, and 40 and 25 for yearlings. The grain mix for all except other mature horses should also contain 1365 IU of vitamin A/lb (3000/kg) and 45 IU of vitamin E/lb (100/kg) unless green growing forage, which will provide adequate amounts of both, is being consumed. Grain mixes that contain these nutrient levels are available commercially or may be formulated and prepared as described in Chapter 6; examples are given in Table 4-10.

[b] Protein supplement in the grain mix should be one whose protein contains greater than 5% lysine (Table 4-7).

[c] Most grain mixes contain more than 0.4% calcium, which isn't harmful when adequate phosphorus is provided and is needed if a legume forage doesn't constitute at least one-half of the weight of the total diet consumed.

[d] A cereal grain alone is adequate for mature horses, except during late gestation and lactation. A grain mix isn't needed, unless more than 4 to 5 lbs (2 kgs)/day are being fed to the horse receiving grass hay, in which case a grain mix is needed since cereal grains alone contain inadequate calcium (0.04 to 0.1%).

cereal grain or combination of cereal grains), processed grain by-products (includes brewer's and distiller's grains, corn gluten, bran, and wheat middlings), plant or animal protein products, forage products (any forage or forage meal), and roughage products (that are high fiber nonforage ingredients, such as cereal grain hulls, straw, corn cobs, corn stover, beet pulp and fruit pomaces). When a collective term is used, individual ingredients within that group cannot be listed on the label. The use of collective terms usually indicates that the feed is a least-cost formulation and ingredients in it are varied according to their cost and availability. The individual ingredients listing permits a better evaluation of the feed and is preferred when quality and consistency of ingredients is deemed more important than the feed's possibly higher cost, and when it is preferred that the feed not contain specific ingredients.

If the feed is intended for species other than horses, ensure that it doesn't contain additives harmful to horses,

such as the ionophore antibiotics, monensin (rumensin) or salinomycin (see Chapter 19 for a discussion of these substances), or lincomycin. Lincomycin is an antibiotic added to swine diets to increase their growth rate and feed efficiently. In horses it causes severe fatal colitis and diarrhea.

Commercial grain mixes may be loose, pelleted, or extruded. Loose mixtures generally contain molasses. Because of this, and molasses' sweet taste, they are often referred to as sweet feeds. The previous factors discussed are what is important in selecting a grain mix not whether it contains things such as molasses, or is loose, pelleted, or extruded.

Pelleted and Extruded Grain Mixes and Complete Feeds

Pelleted and extruded feeds, often referred to in Europe or the United Kingdom as compounded nuts, are produced by forcing a ground compacted feed through die openings. With pelleted feeds, this occurs under low pressure; with extruded feeds, it occurs under high pressure. When the feed comes out of the die, the sudden release of high, but not low, pressure causes the feed to expand. Thus, both are extruded feed pellets, with what are referred to as pelleted feeds being compacted and what are referred to as extruded feeds being expanded. Pelleting, therefore, refers to a low-pressure—no-expansion process, and extrusion refers to a high-pressure—expansion process. As a result of this difference, extruded feeds are about one-half as dense as both pelleted feeds and loose feeds made with the same ingredients.

In both pelleting and extruding, the feed may be cooked by friction-produced heat, with or without injected steam, and by temperatures ranging from 140 to 230°F (60 to 110°C) for pelleted feeds, and up to 100°F (38°C) higher for extruded feeds, depending on the degree of expansion wanted. Heating and other processes involved decrease vitamin content. At fairly high processing temperatures and conditioning times, from 5 to 40% of the activity of the different vitamins needed by the horse are lost (Table 3-4). However, vitamins in excess of that lost may be added to the feed prior to processing so that the processed feed contains the desired vitamin content.

If too much heat is used in feed processing, protein digestibility will be decreased. Cooking gelatinizes the starch and generally increases its digestibility for dogs, cats, pigs, and poultry, but doesn't appear to for horses or ruminants. No difference in feed utilization, feed intake, or its effects on body condition, growth rate, feed efficiency, or eating or digestive behavior have been noted in horses fed complete feeds that were unprocessed, pelleted, or extruded.

In contrast to a complete feed, the digestibility of a grain mix may be increased by extruding. In one study, growth rate was faster and feed efficiency better in weanlings fed an extruded grain mix than in those fed the same grain mix pelleted. The difference, however, decreased with time on the diets. Rate of digesta passage may be faster when a complete feed is pelleted than when it is unprocessed, whereas there was no difference in the rate of digesta pas-

TABLE 4–10
Grain-Mix Examples[a]

Crude Protein	Ca	P	Any Cereal Grains	Soybean Meal	Wet Molasses[b]	Dicalcium Phosphate	Calcium Carbonate
18	1.0	1.0	73	18	5	4[c]	0
16	1.0	1.0	78	13	5	4[c]	0
14	0.6	0.6	86	7	5	1.5	0.5
10	0.3	0.5	93.75	0	5	1.25	0
10	0.4	0.3	94	0	5	0	1

[a] All values given are the percent wanted in the grain mix. In addition to the ingredients given, it is recommended for growing, reproducing, athletic performance, show, nervous, or hyperactive horses and those not eating well, that 0.3% of a vitamin supplement similar to that given in Table 3–5 be added to their grain mix, and for growing horses that 0.01% (100 ppm) copper sulfate (containing 25% copper) and 0.015% (150 ppm) zinc sulfate (containing 36% zinc) or an equivalent amount of other copper- and zinc-containing minerals be added to their grain mix. Adding a maximum of 20% fat or oil may also be beneficial for growth, lactation, athletic performance, or for the horse not maintaining optimum weight during hot/humid weather. If a grain mix is prepared, it is recommended that it be analyzed to see that it contains close to the nutrient contents given. If instead of having the grain mix prepared at a feed mill, the individual ingredients are fed, the amount of grain, soybean meal, and mineral needed can be determined from the following: 1% is 0.01 lbs, 0.16 oz or 1 tsp/lb (or 10 g/kg). Thus, for example, if a grain mix containing 13% soybean meal (SBM) and 4% dicalcium phosphate (dical) is wanted, and 5 lbs of grain mix/feeding is being fed, (13% SBM) × (0.01 lbs/1%) × (5 lbs grain mix) or 0.65 lbs of soybean meal, (4% dical) × (0.16 oz/1%) × (5 lbs grain mix) or 3.2 oz of dicalcium phosphate and (5 lbs grain mix) − (0.65 lbs SBM) − (3.2 oz dical ÷ 16 oz/lb) or 4.15 lbs of grain should be mixed together and fed. If the grain doesn't contain molasses, it may be necessary to wet the mixture to keep the soybean meal and mineral from sifting out.
[b] The amount of wet molasses can be varied from 0 to 15% (replacing cereal grain accordingly) as necessary to prevent the soybean meal and minerals from sifting out. More than 10 to 15% wet molasses may cause the mix to clump. In hot, humid weather, grain mixes containing greater than 5% wet molasses may become moldy.
[c] The 4% dicalcium phosphate in these grain mixes may be replaced with 2.5% calcium carbonate or limestone, and 1.5% of any calcium-free 20 to 24% phosphorus-containing mineral (Appendix Table 7). If this is done, the resulting grain mixes will contain 0.6% instead of 1.0% phosphorus, and the cost of the grain mix may be reduced.

sage when a grain mix was unprocessed, pelleted, or extruded.

Pellet size doesn't appear to be particularly critical. Most are about ¼ inch in diameter by ⅓ to ¾ inch long (6 to 8 by 8 to 20 mm, or about the size of a pencil). Those intended for young foals are often slightly smaller (4 to 5 by 5 to 12 mm), whereas those intended for feeding on pasture ground are larger or about thumb size (1 inch in diameter by 1 to 2 inches long, or 2.5 by 2.5 to 5 cm). The larger pellets, often referred to as range cubes or range cake, are generally intended for feeding cattle on pasture range and may be used for this same purpose for horses, providing they don't contain any additives harmful to horses (e.g., rumensin, as discussed in Chapter 19). Smaller pellets tend to be eaten more slowly, which is an advantage. Pellet hardness doesn't appear to affect acceptability, although most horses dislike pellets that crumble too easily, and those that are excessively hard have been reported to occasionally be consumed rapidly or bolted without adequate mastication, which increases the risk of choke.

Any of the four major types of horse feeds (grain mixes, complete feeds, hays, or supplements) may be pelleted or extruded. Pelleted supplements are generally high in protein (24% or greater, which will be given on the feed tag), with many having added vitamins and minerals. The hay pellets most commonly available in North America are dehydrated alfalfa, referred to as "dehy" pellets (Fig. 4–6).

For a complete feed, a grain mix and hay, or other high-fiber source, are ground, mixed together (generally with a binder such as molasses), and are usually pelleted or extruded to hold the mixture together. As the name "complete feed" implies, it is intended to be fed as the complete diet for the horse without any additional grain, supplements, pasture, or hay. However, when fed without addi-

tional forage, as discussed previously for hay pellets (dehy), wood and tail chewing, eating feces, and gastrointestinal problems such as diarrhea and colic may increase. To assist in preventing these, when a complete pelleted or extruded feed of any type is fed, feed at least ½ lb of long-stem hay/100 lbs of body weight (½ kg/100 kg) daily, or some pasture forage. A complete pelleted feed is eaten by most horses with good teeth at the rate of an amount equal to 1 to 1.3% of their body weight per hour and, therefore, most horses can meet their needs with two 1-hr feeding periods daily. With nothing else to do the remaining 24 hours, and particularly without companionship, boredom and as a result bad habits such as wood chewing may occur, as described in Chapter 20, in which ways to prevent these behavioral problems are described.

Any type of grain, supplement, and, in a complete feed, hay may be used in grain mixes and complete feeds. Complete feeds, depending on their intended use, may or may not contain protein, vitamin, or mineral supplements. They may contain anywhere from 10 to 70% grain. Those highest in grain are generally intended for young horses and, therefore, also contain supplements sufficient to provide all the nutrients in the amounts that the manufacturer thinks are needed. Those lowest in grain are intended for the mature idle horse and may contain no supplements, but only hay or a high-fiber feed such as hulls, straw, etc., and 10 to 25% grain. The more grain a feed contains, the more dietary energy it provides and the lower its fiber content, as shown in Table 4–11. This information is helpful in determining the type and energy content of a commercial feed since crude fiber, not energy, is given on the feed tag. A grain mix with no hay or high-fiber feed included will have a crude fiber content of 12% or less, whereas one that is entirely hay will have a crude fiber

TABLE 4–11
Digestible Energy (DE)–Crude Fiber Relationship in Horse Feeds[a]

Crude Fiber (%)	≤ 4	6	10	12	19	24	28	30	34–38
Mcal DE /lb[b]	1.6–1.7	1.5–1.6	1.3–1.4	1.2–1.3	1.1	1.0	0.9	0.7–0.8	0.65–0.7
/kg[b]	3.5–3.7	3.3–3.5	2.9–3.1	2.6–2.9	2.4	2.2	2.0	1.5–1.75	1.4–1.5
Grain (% in feed)	100%	100%	100%	100% if oats[c]	25–65%	0–40%	0–25%	0–15%	0[d]

[a] All values given are the amount in the feeds as fed.
[b] These values will be higher if the feed contains more fat than that present in grain and forages (2 to 6%), e.g., 1.8 Mcal/lb (4 Mcal/kg) in a commercial grain mix containing not more than 4% crude fiber and at least 14% fat (Athlete, Ralston Purina Co.).
[c] Unless the feed contains a lower-fiber grain and some high-fiber feeds such as hay, hulls, straw, or stover.
[d] Unless the feed contains a high-fiber forage or by-product feeds such as straw or hulls.

content of greater than 24%, unless some grain is added to offset a high-fiber-containing ingredient.

Pelleted and extruded feeds have several advantages and disadvantages compared to unprocessed feeds. Most of these are the same as given previously in this chapter for pelleted hay. One additional advantage of a pelleted or extruded grain mix, and particularly a complete feed, is that all vitamins, minerals, protein supplements, and anything else wanted in the diet can be added and will not sift out, so the horse is assured of getting them, and of getting them in the proper amount, providing the proper amount has been added.

A complete pelleted or extruded feed, particularly one containing added fat or oil, may be quite beneficial for hard-keeping horses, especially those with poor teeth, such as some older horses. Often, thin horses of this type that have been receiving hay or pasture forage and grain will put on weight and do much better when switched to a good pelleted or extruded feed. These feeds may also decrease the incidence of colic that can occur in the older horse with poor teeth that doesn't adequately chew its feed, particularly forages. A complete feed as high in grain and digestible energy as needed for horses of this type to maintain their optimum body weight and condition should be fed. If additional energy intake is necessary to gain or maintain body weight and condition, a cereal grain that has been processed, supplemental fat or oil, or a high (over 8%) fat-containing grain mix should be fed.

Some have feared that pelleted or extruded feeds in the stomach may absorb water and swell sufficiently to cause gastric distension, colic, and even fatal gastric rupture. This, however, doesn't occur. In addition, some have thought that if finely ground feeds, such as may be present in pelleted feeds, are ingested fast enough, gastric digestion and fermentation may result in sufficient gas production to cause gastric distension, colic, and enterotoxemia. However, studies have shown that this does not occur and that there is no difference in the rate of fermentation between a pelleted or an unprocessed sweet feed grain mix.

A rapid rate of consumption of pellets has also been thought to increase the risk of choke. Choke is more likely to occur if the pellets are very hard, as they may be swallowed without being completely pulverized by sufficient chewing. The rate of consumption, and thus the risk of digestive problems and choke, is lessened by feeding an extruded, rather than a pelleted or a loose grain mix.

In one study there was no difference in the rate of consumption between unprocessed and pelleted grain mixes by either horses or ponies, but was 22 to 32% slower for the same grain mix when extruded. Intake of the extruded feed was even slower until the horses became accustomed to it. Feeding pellets, containing either grain or forage, causes the quickest filling of the horse's stomach. The incidence of digestive disturbances, including gastric rupture, has been reported to decrease when young horses were changed from a pelleted to an extruded feed. A complete pelleted feed may also increase digestive problems such as gastric ulcers. A complete pelleted feed was found to cause a higher and more prolonged increase in the serum gastrin concentration than the same amount of a sweet feed, with or without hay available. Increased gastrin increases gastric acid secretion, which increases the risk of gastric and/or duodenal ulcers.

Slowing Feed Consumption

The rate at which feed is consumed, and thus the risk of digestive disturbances and choke, has been reported to be decreased by the following methods: (1) spread grain thinly over a large surface, (2) put several bars or compartments in the feed box, (3) put several large smooth stones in the feed box, (4) feed small amounts often, which may be accomplished with automatic feeders (e.g., On Time Feeders, Specialty Fabrication, Wichita, KS, 1-800-664-8463), (5) feed nervous horses first because some horses become excited when others are being fed and as a result eat faster, and (6) mix chaff or chopped hay with the grain. Although these methods appear logical, there are few studies in which their effects or their benefit have been quantified. It has been found that mixing equal parts of chopped timothy hay with grain decreases the rate of consumption of the grain alone. The rate of feed consumption also decreases with meal duration probably due to satiety. There is no correlation between dominance rank in a group of horses and the rate of grain consumption.

BY-PRODUCT FEEDS FOR HORSES
Bran

Bran is the outer layer of the grain kernel, or the endosperm, which is removed in milling wheat, corn, rice, and other cereal grains. Wheat bran is most commonly fed in North America; rice bran is commonly fed in other areas. Unextracted rice bran is relatively high in unsaturated fat. This fat becomes rancid with prolonged storage, particularly in the presence of moisture and heat. Rancidity destroys essential fatty acids and some vitamins, and decreases the feed's palatability. Much of the fat in rice bran may be removed, decreasing its fat content from about 15% to 1 to 2% and greatly increasing its storage stability. Wheat bran may be sold as giant, broad, or fine bran according to flake size, or most commonly as the entire fraction or "straight-run bran."

The nutrient content of brans are changed by inclusion of either kernels or hulls. Without either kernels or hulls, wheat bran and extracted rice bran are similar in nutrient content (digestible energy, crude fiber, fat, and calcium) to oats, but contain slightly more protein and 3 to 4 times more phosphorus (Table 4–12). However, bran is a fluffy, low-density feed (Fig. 4–14). Wheat bran's density (0.5 lbs/qt or 0.24 kg/L) is one-half that of regular oats and close to one-fourth that of corn and wheat, so for the same volume it provides one-half as much digestible energy as regular oats and about one-fourth as much as corn and wheat (in Mcal/qt or L, bran 0.7, oats 1.4, corn 2.6, and wheat 2.9) (Appendix Table 8). Rice bran is a little more dense than wheat bran with 0.7 to 0.8 lb/qt (0.34 to 0.4 kg/L) providing 1 Mcal DE/qt or L. Wheat and rice brans are relatively high in folate, niacin, thiamin, and riboflavin as compared to other feeds, although they are much lower than brewer's yeast in all of the B-vitamins. Rice bran frequently contains as much as 6% silica. Although this is not known to be harmful to horses, it may contribute to silicate urinary calculi formation in dogs and ruminants.

The high phosphorus content of bran is harmful if not balanced with adequate calcium. About 90% of the phosphorus in brans is in the form of phylate, which decreases calcium absorption. As a result, if excess bran is fed without the minimum amount of calcium consumed being close to the amount of phosphorus consumed, it will cause a calcium deficiency or "bran disease" as discussed in Chapter 2. When their high phosphorus content is balanced with calcium, wheat bran and rice bran are safe feeds for the horse. In addition, they are quite palatable, but they are generally expensive for the nutrients they provide.

Bran frequently is fed to the horse, not to provide specific nutrients, but instead as a laxative and as an aid in preventing colic. However, it has been shown that bran does not have a laxative effect, i.e., it does not increase fecal water content and therefore soften the stools. There is no evidence based on controlled studies either supporting or refuting the belief that feeding bran can treat or prevent colic, whether it is fed dry or as a mash. It is often fed as a hot bran mash. However, steeping bran in warm 122°F (50°C) water even for 1 hour does not affect its digestibility. Giving hot bran mashes may make a person feel good because they believe they are doing something that is good or nice for the horse, but this probably does little for the horse in the way of either benefit or harm.

Straw and Stover

Straw, the plant residue left after removal of the seeds, may be from cereal grains, lentils, peas, beans, clover, various grasses, corn, or grain sorghum. That from corn and grain sorghum without the ears or grain is referred to as stover, or stalks if they are left standing in the field, and fodder if the corn or grain hasn't been harvested and the ears or grain remain. Corn and sorghum stover or fodder may be cut and fed, or left standing in the field for the stalks to be grazed.

Both corn and sorghum stover and fodder have been used extensively as part of the forage for wintering idle horses, often by turning the horses into the field. The horses will eat any ears or grain that are there, as well as much of the rest of the plant. There is, however, some danger of moldy corn causing moldy corn disease under certain conditions (as discussed in Chapter 19). In one study, mature idle horses were adequately maintained on pelleted corn fodder (PCF) containing 6.2% crude protein at an intake equal to 1.8% of their body weight by feeding 1 lb (0.5 kg) of soybean meal daily to provide the additional protein needed. Pony mares fed a diet consisting of 33% PCF, 33% sunflower hulls, 13% corn, 13% dehydrated alfalfa, and 7% soybean meal gained 15% more than those fed the same diet with the PCF replaced by brome-grass hay. The PCF was readily consumed and resulted in well-formed stools.

Straw is used for horses primarily as bedding (as discussed in Chapter 9), but properly supplemented can make up a majority of their diet. Oat straw is generally considered the best feed among the cereal-grain straws, with barley second and wheat third. Oat straw is often softer than that of wheat and rye, is more readily eaten, and does not have the awns that are present in barley straw and some varieties of wheat straw.

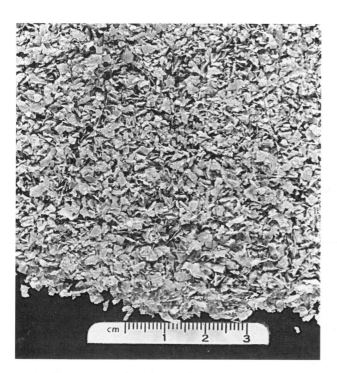

Fig. 4–14. Wheat bran, often called just bran.

TABLE 4–12
By-Product Feeds: Nutrient Contents and Characteristics for Horses

Feed	Mcal DE/ lb (/kg) DM	% in Feed Dry Matter[a]					Comments
		Crude Protein	Fat	Crude Fiber	Calcium	Phosphorus	
Non By-product Feeds and Horses' Maintenance Requirements for Comparison:							
Maintenance Need		8	1–1.5	<36	0.25	0.18	16.4 Mcal/d ± 3/100 kg body wt above or below 500 kg
Grass Hay, Good	1.0 (2.2)	8–12	3	30	0.5	0.3	
Poor	0.75 (1.65)	5–7	3	36	0.3	0.1	Similar to straw and stover
Oats, Regular	1.45 (3.2)	13	5	12	0.09	0.35	
By-Product Feeds							
Bran, wheat	1.5 (3.3)	16–17	4.3	10–12	0.14	1.27 ⎱	Not laxative. Help preventing
Bran, rice	1.3 (2.9)	14	1.6 or 15[e]	13	0.1	1.5–1.7 ⎰	colic doubtful. When fed, ensure Ca ≥ P in total diet.
Bran, corn	1.5 (3.3)	9	5.5	10.7	0.04	0.22	Unavailable in most areas
Straw, grains	0.7 (1.6)	3–4.5	2	40–42	0.15–0.3	0.05–0.1	Feed with adequate legume or grain mix
Corn, ears	1.5 (3.3)	9	3.7	9.5	0.07	0.27	With grain and no husks
Corn, fodder	0.9 (2.0)	7–8	1–2.5	26–32	0.5	0.25	Total plant ⎱ May cut and feed
Corn, stover	0.8 (1.7)	4–7	1.3	35–38	0.5–0.6	0.1	No ears ⎰ or graze in field. Feed with adequate legume or grain.
Corn, cobs	0.6 (1.4)	3	0.7	35	0.12	0.04	Not adequate for horses
Hulls, oats	0.6 (1.3)	4–6	1.5	33–36	0.15	0.1 ⎱	Ground hulls should be
Hulls, cottonseed	0.6 (1.3)	4	2	47	0.15	0.09	pelleted or mixed with
Hulls, soybean	0.8 (1.8)	11–13	1–2	36–45	0.4–0.7	0.15	molasses to decrease
Hulls, rice	0.24 (0.5)	3	1	43	0.1	0.07 ⎰	dustiness. They can replace hay in diet for mature idle
Hulls, peanuts	0.45 (1.0)	7–8	1–2	59–63	0.26	0.07	horse and help decrease
Hulls, sunflower	0.9 (2.0)	4–6	3–4	43–51	0.38	0.13	obesity and boredom. Diet should include at least 8 lbs (3.6 kg) of legumes or a 16% protein grain mix.
Hulls, almond	1.1 (2.4)	4–6	2–3	11–12	0.23	0.11	Well-accepted and safe feed.
Molasses	1.6 (3.5)	2–6[b]	0.2–0.9	0–0.5[c]	0.9–2[d]	0.1–0.3[d]	Increases palatability, decreases dust, and is a binder
Beet pulp, sugar	1.2 (2.6)	9–10	0.6	20	0.7	0.1 ⎱	May replace some hay or
Fruit or citrus pomace	1.3 (2.8)	8.5[f]	2–4	10–16	0.7–2[f]	0.18 ⎰	grain in horse's diet. Devoid of vitamins A & D. Pomace values are for apple, orange, lemon and grapefruit.
Potatoes, Irish	1.6 (3.6)	9.5	0.4	2.5	0.04	0.24	Can feed up to 20 lb (9kg)/day but sprouts are toxic
Lawn clippings	1.0 (2.2)	15–17	3.5–5.5	25	0.5	0.3–0.5	Best pelleted or green. Impaction risk for greedy eater. Dusty if dry.

[a] All the by-product feeds given, except lawn clippings, are devoid of vitamin A or its precursor, beta-carotene. All contain 8 to 12% moisture, except corn ears 14%, corn fodder 19%, fresh law clippings 65 to 70%, wet molasses or syrups 22 to 33%, dry or dehydrated molasses 5 to 6%, and fresh potatoes 77%.
[b] Much of the nitrogen in molasses is nonprotein, which is of little benefit or harm to horses. Molasses contains 2 to 6% true crude protein.
[c] Dehydrated sugar cane molasses contains 5 to 10% crude fiber.
[d] Beet molasses contains 0.15% calcium and 0.03% phosphorus.
[e] Available with or without fat extracted. High-fat rice bran often becomes rancid during storage.
[f] Dry apply pulp or pomace contains only about 5% protein and 0.1 to 0.15% calcium.

Straw and stover are only slightly lower in protein and higher in fiber than fully mature grass hay or pasture (Table 4–12); they are similar in digestible energy and mineral content. This doesn't indicate straw's or stover's nutritional quality or adequacy; instead, it indicates a lack in mature grasses. Straw and stover are very low in vitamin A and provide about one-half as much phosphorus and protein as the mature nonreproducing horse needs. However, these deficiencies can be corrected by feeding, along with all the straw or stover the horse (weighing 900 to 1100 lbs, or 400 to 500 kg) will eat, 1.5 to 2 lbs (0.7 to 0.9 kg) of soybean meal or 5 to 6 lbs (2.5 kg) of either a good legume hay or a 16% protein grain mix similar to that indicated for yearlings and brood mares receiving grass hay (Tables 4-9 and 4-10).

Straw is poorly digested even by ruminants because of its fibers' resistance to fermentation by intestinal microorganisms. Numerous chemicals have been used to treat straw and other high-fiber feeds to try to increase their digestibility. Ammonia treatment increased dry-matter digestibility of oat straw from 32% to 48%, and wheat straw from 36.4% to 46.5% by horses. The digestible-energy content of cereal straws is increased by 23 to 31% for horses by either sodium hydroxide or ammonia treatment. Generally no difference in the acceptability of the treated straws has been observed, although in one study sodium-hydroxide-treated straw was not as well accepted as ammonia-treated straw. Microbial treatments using molds or fungi have also been studied, but currently there is little data as to their effects.

Hulls

Hulls, or the outer covering of grains or other seeds, are high-fiber, low-energy feeds that may be used to replace all or some of the hay or forage in the horse's diet. There are two major reasons to consider them for feeding horses: (1) they are available at a lower cost than hay, or (2) they help limit dietary-energy intake while still allowing enough to be consumed to satisfy the horse's appetite and thus help prevent obesity, boredom, or stable vices. Either one of these factors would be a reason to consider the use of hulls in a feeding program; if neither is the case, there is little reason to feed them. In addition, even if they are inexpensive, because of their low energy content, the amount that can be fed to horses requiring increased dietary energy, such as during growth, late pregnancy, and lactation, and for the exercising or working horse, is quite limited. However, hulls may be quite beneficial and make up a majority of the diet for the mature idle horse.

Hulls from most cereal grains and seeds may be safely fed to horses. Most are about 50% lower in digestible energy, protein, and phosphorus, and 50% higher in crude fiber, than grass hay (Table 4-12), although their nutrient content will vary somewhat with the amount of kernels, linters, or other plant parts included. They are devoid of vitamin A or carotene. Because of their low-energy, high-fiber content, most horses may be fed all the hulls they will eat without excess energy intake occurring. In addition to all the hulls they will eat, the mature idle horse's diet should include by weight one-third either alfalfa or a 16% protein grain mix (Table 4-9) to provide the additional protein, calcium, and phosphorus needed. For the average-size light-breed horse (weighing about 1100 lbs, or 500 kg) this would be 8 to 10 lbs (3.5 to 4.5 kg) of either alfalfa or grain mix daily. Hulls may also be fed with about 3 lbs (1.5 kg) of a 30 to 40% all-natural protein supplement, providing that adequate phosphorus and vitamin A are provided.

Hulls are frequently ground and are quite dusty. As a result, they may produce respiratory problems if fed without pelleting or blending with wet molasses or some moist feed. Many types of hulls are available in a pelleted form. Oat hulls may have 30% oat dust added to them, which decreases their crude-fiber content from 33 to 36%, to 27%

or less and are referred to as oatfeed. Most hulls have a low density, which in lbs/qt (kg/L) is for: cottonseed hulls ground 0.37 (0.18) and pelleted 1.2 (0.56), soybean hulls ground 0.9 (0.4), and rice hulls ground 0.67 (0.32). Rice hulls unground are reported to be unsuitable for feeding horses because they have sharp edges which may cause irritation.

Soybean Hulls

These are the seedcoats of the soybean seeds; they are not the pod. The pod is left in the field by the combine; the soybean hull is removed from the soybean later in its processing. The soybean hull is toasted and ground, then blended back with soybean meal to decrease its protein content to 41 or 44% as fed. If high protein, or 48 to 49%, soybean meal is wanted, the soybean hulls are not blended back with the soybean meal but instead are sold, often as soy mill run or feed. Although soybean hulls are high in fiber, they are low in lignin (3.9%) and, therefore, are more digestible than most other types of hulls. This is reflected in their higher digestible-energy content (Table 4-12). They are reported to be very palatable, at least for beef cattle, and currently in the United States cost an average of 31% less than corn ($50 to $70/ton or $55 to $77/metric ton). They are also a viable alternative to cereal grains as an energy supplement for ruminants on a high-forage diet. However, they are less digestible for horses and, as a result, are an alternative to feeding horses forage, not grain.

In one study, 4-month-old weanling ponies were allowed free access to diets in which soybean hulls (SBH) were 0%, 50% or 75% of the diet, replacing alfalfa. Those fed either of the two SBH, but not the alfalfa, diets had loose, poorly formed, high-moisture feces and gained over a 48-day period, 2.5% less than those fed the diet not containing any SBH. Their slower growth rate was probably due primarily to a lower amount of the SBH diets being consumed. The weanlings consumed 12.9% and 25.6% less feed, and pregnant pony mares consumed 24.5% and 37.6% less, when SBH replaced 50% and 75% alfalfa in the diet, respectively. The mares fed the 50% SBH diet gained 0.9 versus 1.6 lb/day gain by those fed the 50% alfalfa diet; and those fed the 75% SBH diet gained 0.7 versus 1.0 lb/day gain by those fed the 75% alfalfa diet. Thus, SBH, like most hulls, cannot replace the hay in diets for horses with increased energy needs. However, the reduced feed intake on the SBH diets may be beneficial for the mature idle horse.

Sunflower Hulls

Without any seeds or meal, sunflower hulls are higher in both crude fiber and digestible energy than other types of hulls (Table 4-12). Six pregnant pony mares fed for 84 days an amount equal to 1.6% of their body weight of a complete pelleted diet containing one-third sunflower hulls ate the diet well, had normal well-formed stools, and increased their body weight by 2.4%. Yearling ponies fed amounts daily expressed as a percentage of their body weight (0.17% soybean meal, 0.57% corn, and 0.73% grass hay) which when the hay was reduced to 0.5% and to 0.34% were allowed free access to sunflower hulls consumed 1.0 and 1.34% of the hulls, respectively. All six yearlings on each diet ate the hulls readily and exhibited no depraved appetite or abnormal stools. Their total feed intake daily as a percent of their body weight, and their resulting body weight changes during the 188 days they were fed the:

No sunflower hull diet were 2.0% intake and 2.5% gain,

44% sunflower hull diet were 2.2% intake and 0.1% loss,

55% sunflower hull diet were 2.4% intake and 0.7% loss.

Thus, sunflower hulls, like other hulls, cannot replace the hay in growing horses' diets. But sunflower hulls are palatable, and they provide bulk and appetite satiation without causing any abnormalities or providing very much dietary energy, all of which are of benefit for the idle mature horse.

Almond Hulls

Almond hulls, which are similar to the fleshy part of a peach, are obtained by drying the portion of the almond fruit that surrounds the hard shell. They contain about one-third to one-quarter as much crude fiber as other types of hulls and are higher in digestible energy (Table 4-12). They are similar in digestible energy, calcium, and phosphorus, but generally lower in protein than, good-quality grass hay, although top-quality Nonpareil almond hulls may contain over 9% crude protein.

Almond hulls are commonly fed to cattle in some areas and have been shown to be a safe palatable feed for other ruminants, swine, and horses. In one study in mature geldings, a pelleted feed containing alfalfa hay and nearly 50% almond hulls was well accepted and more digestible than one containing 30% alfalfa and 70% oat hay. During the 56-day study, the horses' body weights increased 3% as a result of being fed about 50% more than needed to meet their dietary energy needs. There were no signs of any adverse reactions, such as lip sores, colic, or impactions, thus not supporting the speculation that tanins in almond hulls may cause lip sores in horses.

Molasses

There are several different types of molasses: cane, beet, refiner's, citrus, wood (hemicellulose), and starch (corn, sorghum, or hydrol). All are thick, viscous, black syrups. Cane, or blackstrap, molasses and beet molasses are the ones most commonly fed to horses. They are available in both liquid (22 to 33% moisture) and dehydrated (5 to 6% moisture) forms. Except for beet molasses, they are high in calcium because of substances used in processing. They are low in protein and vitamins A, D, B₁, and B₂, but are high in the B vitamins pantothenate and niacin. They are similar in energy content to oats (Table 4-12). However, in contrast to oats, most of their energy is from sugar rather than starch. About one-half of their dry matter is sugar, which gives them a sweet taste that most horses like. Beet molasses tends to have an unpleasant fishy aroma, whereas cane molasses has a very pleasant smell; most horses like both. Wood molasses is reported to be less palatable, at least for cattle, and citrus molasses to have a very acrid taste which doesn't affect the palatability for cattle but

does for pigs. All, particularly beet molasses, are reported to have a laxative effect. It has been reported that the reducing sugars in molasses may destroy lysine in feed—possibly 0.5% of the lysine per day. At this rate, more than one-third and one-half of the lysine content of the feed would be lost within 3 and 5 months, respectively. Because of this, it may be safest not to use, or to use minimal amounts of, molasses in the growing horse's diet, or to ensure that the feed is quite fresh and adequate in lysine.

Liquid molasses is added to grain mixes (1) to increase palatability, (2) to reduce dustiness, and (3) as a binder for pelleting, or to keep vitamin, mineral, or protein supplements and other ingredients from sifting out of a loose grain mix. More than 10 to 15% liquid molasses in a grain mix makes the feed sticky and difficult to handle. In hot humid weather, liquid molasses should be limited to 5% of a stored loose-grain mix; otherwise mold may develop. When used as a binder for pelleting, 7.5 to 10% may be used. Too much liquid molasses makes the pellets too soft and chewy; with too little, the pellet may be crumbly.

Either dehydrated or liquid molasses may be mixed with loose mineral mixes or protein supplements to encourage and increase their free-choice consumption, whereas salt (sodium chloride) may be added to limit their intake.

Condensed Molasses Solubles

New technology has enhanced the process of sugar extraction from sugar beets (Beta vulgaris) resulting in less molasses and large quantities of condensed molasses solubles from beets (CMSB). CMSB is less viscous and tends to be higher in sodium, potassium, iron, and pH than feed grade molasses. It appears to be an acceptable and safe ingredient for horse feeds at least at levels up to 1.6% of the diet for short periods, and there is no reason to think it would be harmful, although higher levels do appear to be less palatable than molasses.

Sugar Beet Pulp

After sugar extraction from beets the remaining pulp must be fed wet if used at once, or it can be ensiled or dried for storage. Dried beet pulp is generally the only form available. It is a good feed for horses that has been commonly fed for many years but frequently isn't available. In one study, replacing barley with 30% dried sugar beet pulp in the total diet did not significantly affect feed intake, plasma insulin or glucose concentrations or organic matter, neutral detergent fiber, or feed digestibility. In another study, when 0%, 15%, 30%, or 45% dry beet pulp by weight was mixed with alfalfa pellets, all four mature horses studied readily ate all of the diets fed in an amount equal to 0.9% of their body weight twice daily. They gained an average of 31 lbs (14 kg) during the 8-week study. A few of the horses occasionally tried to sort through the mixture of dried beet pulp pellets and alfalfa pellets to eat the alfalfa first, indicating its greater palatability. There were no signs of choke or any adverse effects from any of the diets, nor was there any change in the water content of their feces. Thus, in contrast to what has been recommended, it does not appear that dried beet pulp needs to be soaked in water before it is fed.

Dried beet pulp may be fed alone or blended with other

feeds, such as molasses, to increase its energy content. It may be used to replace either or both grain and hay in the horse's diet. Its digestible energy and fiber content are in between, and its protein content similar to, those of grain and good quality grass hay (Table 4–12). It is relatively high in calcium but very low in phosphorus and B-vitamins, and contains no carotene or vitamin D.

Fruit or Citrus Pulp

Fruit or citrus pulp remains following juice extraction and is available primarily from apples, oranges, and grapefruits. It may be ensiled or most commonly dried for feeding. Pomace is often used to denote dried fruit pulp. In drying citrus pulp, limestone (calcium carbonate) is generally used to bind pectin, in which it is high. As a result, dry citrus pulp is high in calcium. Fruit pomace's digestible-energy and fiber contents are in between, and its protein content similar to, those of grain and grass hay (Table 4–12). Fruit or citrus pulps are all quite low in phosphorus and vitamin A precursor. Citrus pulps are best fed incorporated into a pelleted feed as a replacement for either grain or hay. Their palatability varies with the way they are processed. In one study, diets containing 15% dried citrus pulp were readily accepted by horses, whereas higher levels were unpalatable.

Fresh Fruits and Vegetables

Most fresh fruits and vegetables are quite palatable to horses and are most often fed as a treat, rather than as a significant part of their diet. These include apples, pears, oranges, grapefruits, carrots, beets, etc. Fruits with pits, such as peaches, apricots, cherries, prunes, and plums, should not be fed unless the pit is removed, as horses may choke on them. Horses, as well as other livestock, may also choke on any of the fruits or vegetables if they are frozen and, therefore, the horse should not be allowed access to them when they are frozen. Although fresh fruits and vegetables contain 75 to 90% water, on a dry-matter basis they are comparable in digestible energy to grain.

Potatoes

Cull Irish potatoes (Solanum tuberosum) are sometimes fed to livestock. Although they need to be cooked to be safely fed to swine and poultry, this isn't necessary for other species. They are similar in nutrient content to corn (Table 4–12), but are reported to not be very palatable, and in large quantities they cause loose, watery stools. Choke is a risk but is said to be minimized by feeding at ground level. It is reported that horses and mules may be fed up to 20 lbs (9 kg)/head/day of Irish potatoes, fresh, raw, or cooked. Although 20 lbs may seem like a lot of potatoes, because of their high moisture content (77%), this would be equivalent to only 4 to 5 lbs (about 2 kg) of grain. Green, rotting, or sprouted potatoes should not be fed as they contain toxic solanine alkaloids, which as described in Chapter 18, cause colic, diarrhea, and if large amounts are ingested, cardiac arrest and death.

Lawn Grass Clippings

Fresh lawn clippings are a highly nutritious forage for horses (Table 4–12). Although occasionally dehydrated, pelleted, and sold by large grass sod companies, their availability is most commonly from periodic mowing of the horse owner's own lawn. Often the desire to feed them is as much to simply get rid of them as it is to nourish the horse, although both are laudable goals. Providing the lawn hasn't been sprayed or treated with chemicals, clippings less than a few hours old may be safely fed and are readily eaten by most horses. However, they dry out quickly and then tend to be quite dusty because they are so fine. In addition, horses that are greedy eaters may ingest large mouthfuls and fail to properly chew them because of their fineness. These poorly masticated clippings may result in impaction and colic. To help prevent this, ensure that the horse is not overly hungry when clippings are fed, i.e., has been just recently fed other feeds or is on good pasture.

FEED ADDITIVES FOR HORSES

Feed additives, in contrast to supplements, are not added to a feed to provide nutrients. They are added to be of benefit to the animal in other ways, such as increasing the feed's stability, palatability, or utilization, or improving the animal's response to the feed by, for example, increasing their growth rate, milk production, physical performance or bone strength. Occasionally, as a secondary benefit, an additive will provide a nutrient, such as the energy provided by organic acids used to preserve high-moisture feeds. Numerous additives are used in commercially available feeds for livestock, including horses.

In most countries, feed-additive producers are required to demonstrate safety of any proposed additive before it can be used. In the United States this includes: (1) acute toxicity of a single lethal dose, (2) short-term (3-month) studies showing the effects of different levels, and (3) long-term (2-year or more) studies to show effects of lifetime consumption. However, these studies are required and, therefore, safety at the levels recommended insured, only for the species of animals for which they are recommended. Some additives, such as ionophore antibiotics (see Chapter 19), are toxic to horses.

Zeolite

Zeolite is a bioavailable silicon containing compound available from several companies for adding to livestock feeds. Silicone enhances bone calcification and is high in connective tissue. Sodium zeolite A has been used for some years as a feed additive for poultry to improve egg quality. In poultry it also decreases the incidence of tibial dyschondroplasia and delays the loss of strength in unused wings. Feeding clinoptilolite, a naturally occurring zeolite, was found to increase feed efficiency of chickens and pigs by as much as 25%, and it has been suggested that it decreases diarrhea in young pigs.

Feeding 2% sodium zeolite A in weanlings' diets has been shown to increase the animals' plasma silicon concentration and radiographically measured bone density, and therefore may be beneficial in decreasing exertion induced bone injuries in young horses. This benefit was supported by a study in which Quarter Horses fed either 1.9 or 2.8% sodium zeolite A in their diets since 6 months of age when placed in race training at 18 months of age had faster racing times and covered more distance before injury than those with 0 or 0.9% sodium zeolite A in their diets (50, 72, 90 and 83 km before injury in those receiving 0, 0.9, 1.9 or 2.8% sodium zeolite A in their diet, respectively). In addition, there was a direct correlation between plasma silicon concentration and the distance traveled before injury occurred. Maximum benefit appeared to occur with 1.9% sodium zeolite A in the diet. It is doubtful that feeding zeolite resulted in any horse being able to run faster, but instead that it decreased injury in the faster horses, who are more prone to injury because of the greater stress the faster speed causes. Because of this horses receiving zeolite remained in the study decreasing their groups average race time, whereas faster horses not receiving zeolite were injured and removed from the study resulting in that group now consisting of only slower horses. Average racing times were 0.2, 0.4 and 0.5 sec slower at 274, 320 and 360 meters, respectively, in those receiving 0 or 0.9% zeolite than for those receiving 1.9 or 2.8% sodium zeolite A in their diets.

There was no difference with respect to the amount of zeolite in the diet and any of the horses' physiologic parameters either before or after training workouts or races. Thus, feeding 2% sodium zeolite A in the horse's diet during growth appears to be a safe and effective means of decreasing the risk of exertional induced injury when training and racing begins at a young age.

Flavoring Agents

Flavoring agents are occasionally added to commercial horse feeds, supplements, or medications intended for ingestion to increase their palatability and, therefore, acceptance. They are generally a marketing gimmick designed to appeal to the purchaser rather than the consumer of the product. Except for the sick horse and for unpalatable supplements or oral medications, what they are purported to do—i.e., increase feed acceptance and therefore increase either or both the rate of consumption or the amount consumed—is often more likely to be detrimental than beneficial. Overeating is a much more common problem than is inadequate intake, particularly of the grain mixes or supplements to which flavors are most commonly added. Nor is a rapid feed intake generally of benefit. Rapid feed intake has long been assumed to increase the risk of colic, choke, and with a high amount consumed, gastric rupture. However, many of the flavoring agents used have either no effect or decrease the rate of feed intake and, therefore, probably decrease rather than increase the palatability of the feed to which they are added.

In one study, when used at the manufacturer's recommended levels, peppermint flavor had no effect, and apple, caramel, and anise flavors increased the time required for horses to eat 4.4 lbs (2 kg) of a corn, oats, and barley mix sweet feed from 17.2 minutes to 25, 27, and 54 minutes, respectively. In another study, there was no difference in palatability for mature horses as measured by rate of consumption between molasses-containing an apple-flavored and orange-flavored feeds, whereas feeds flavored with peppermint, carrot, or wheat syrups were significantly less palatable. In amounts of 500 or 2500 g/ton, apple was preferred at the higher amount, orange and peppermint at the lower amount, and there was no preference difference for amount of carrot- or wheat-syrup flavors. Salivary flow was greatest on the molasses-containing feed, and its composition wasn't affected by feed flavoring agent.

Generalizations about the influence of flavoring agents on feed palatability cannot be made since the affect varies with the amount and type of flavor used, as well as the type, quality, and palatability of the feed, supplement, or oral medication to which it is added. If a flavoring agent does increase the palatability of the substance in which it is present and, therefore, increases both the rate at which it is eaten and the amount eaten, you should decide whether this is in fact beneficial or harmful.

Digestion Enhancers

A wide variety of substances are used to enhance feed digestion or utilization. Those substances applicable for horses include chelators, enzymes, probiotics, and production-stimulating drugs. Buffers or neutralizers are also used to enhance ruminants' feed utilization, whereas for horses they are used primarily to try to prevent azoturia or "tying-up" syndrome and to enhance athletic performance (as discussed in Chapter 11). Chelating agents are used in some mineral supplements to increase the availability of certain minerals and were discussed previously in this chapter in the section on "Vitamin-Mineral Supplements." Production-stimulating drugs are primarily antibiotics and, in swine, arsenicals; they are discussed in the following section on "Antibiotic Feed Additives." Enzymes used to enhance feed utilization for horses are primarily those present in and with, or produced by and separate from, live microbial or probiotic cultures. Digestive enzymes derived from animal and plant tissues are also available. Commercially available enzymes used as feed additives contain a variety of enzymes and are available in liquid, powder, and pill forms. They may be expected to be of benefit in enhancing feed utilization only if they are active or viable. Most are destroyed by feed processing and, following their ingestion, by gastric acidity.

A feed additive derived from the aloe vera plant has been found to have no effect on digestibility by horses being fed 10 lbs (4.5 kg) of a grain mix and Bermuda grass.

Probiotics (Yeast-Cultures)

Probiotics are used to provide digestive enzymes and to try to establish a desirable balance of gastrointestinal organisms. The most common probiotic products intended for horses are live bacterial cultures of lactobacillus (L. acidophilus), streptococcus (S. faecium), and bacillus (B. subtilis), and live yeast cultures, such as Saccharomyces cerevisia and Aspergillus oryza. Yeast culture products tend to be about 50% protein, 40% carbohydrate, 2% fat, and 8% minerals, but vary depending on the amount of media on which they were grown that is included with the product. The protein they contain includes enzymes such as proteases and amylases, which are also excreted by the live organisms. These enzymes may be the reason for the increase in fiber digestibility found in some studies when live yeast cultures, but not dead yeast cultures such as brewer's yeast, are added to the feed. The heat produced in pelleting and extruding kills most live probiotic culture organisms and the activities of their and other enzymes. Bacillus is the only one of the probiotic cultures listed above that can withstand the effects of pelleting with minimal loss of viability. Only probiotic products and enzymes guaranteed viable, with confirmation of that guarantee, should be expected to be of benefit for reasons other than the nutrients they provide, whose supply, because of the small amounts used, is insignificant and therefore presents a very expensive way to provide these nutrients.

Probiotic use for livestock has developed primarily over the last 40 years, ever since recognition of the benefits and use of low-level antibiotics in the diet. However, in contrast to antibiotics, which have been routinely found to increase growth rate and feed efficiency, the horse and livestock industries have been extremely skeptical of probiotics, placing them in the same category as snake oil and fufu powder. Probiotic promoters often refer to their product with names like "unidentified growth factors" or nutrilites, which are nutrients needed by microorganisms. A combination of variable field and experimental results, marketing of worthless products, and exaggerated unproven claims has hindered the acceptance of probiotics of all types. While there is still considerable bias against probiotics, the general feeling about their efficacy is gradually changing as quality products and demonstrated support of their efficacy become available. Although much skepticism is still warranted, it appears that some probiotics may be of some benefit to some animals under some conditions. However, which products under which conditions are of benefit, is in many instances yet to be clarified.

It appears that at least for the live yeast culture most studied (Saccharomyces cerevisiae, Diamond V Mills, Cedar Rapids, IA), it may be of some benefit for growing horses when added as 1 to 2% of their total diet, at least when they are receiving marginal diets. It may also be of benefit at one-half this amount for horses in training. In any amount, however, it does not improve diet utilization by mature horses.

Antibiotic Feed Additives

Numerous antibiotics or substances that inhibit or kill bacteria are used in low amounts in livestock feeds to increase growth rate and feed efficiency, and to decrease disease. Rarely are they included in feeds intended for horses, although they appear to have the same effect as for other species: they increase by 3 to 12% both growth rate and feed efficiency (i.e., reduce the amount of feed needed per unit of weight gain). In one study, eight Quarter Horse weanlings initially weighing 450 lbs (207 kg) fed a pelleted grain mix with chlortetracycline (to provide 27.5 mg/kg of total diet) for 112 days gained 11.5% more weight, 23% more height, 2.3% more heart girth, and 9.4% more cannon bone length, and feed efficiency was

7.4% better than controls fed identically but without chlortetracycline. No adverse health effects nor structural defects were observed in any of the weanlings fed chlortetracycline. However, several antibiotics used in diets for other species are toxic for horses. These include monensin (rumensin) and salinomycin used in cattle feeds, and lincomycin used in pig feeds. As discussed in Chapter 19, monensin and salinomycin cause signs similar to azoturia or "tying-up," and lincomycin causes a severe fatal colon inflammation and diarrhea.

Mold Inhibitors

Molds in feeds may cause one or more of several detrimental effects including: (1) a decrease in the nutrient value of the feed, (2) decreasing feed palatability and, therefore, acceptability, (3) respiratory problems or allergies from inhalation of spores, and (4) toxicosis from ingestion of mycotoxins, which are discussed in Chapter 19. Preventing these effects requires the prevention or minimization of the four primary conditions that promote mold growth: (1) a moisture level at any spot or location in the feed that exceeds 13% (or for ground oats or wheat, 12%) (2) temperatures in the feed during storage above 55°F (13°C), (3) damaged and broken grain, and (4) insect infestation. Grain storage to prevent these mold-promoting conditions were discussed previously in this chapter. If any of these factors are present or may occur (e.g., the humidity goes above 70% or the grain kernels are broken, such as in processing), or mold or any problems due to mold have occurred previously, having mold inhibitors thoroughly mixed with the feed may help prevent mold growth in the feed. Decreasing storage duration by buying smaller quantities of feed more often is also helpful and may be necessary. Much of the horse feed available commercially contains mold inhibitors.

Mold inhibitors, or antifungal agents, stop mold growth but do not kill molds or mold spores or destroy mycotoxins present. Most destroy seed germinability so treated grains can be used only as feed and not as seed grain. Propionic acid is the major mold inhibitor used, being the only active ingredient in 8 or 11 commercial products listed in one report. It is generally effective and added to grains at concentrations of 0.3 to 1.0%. Salts of propionic or other organic acids (such as calcium and sodium propionate, formate, acetate, and butyrate) are less effective. Butyrate also has an objectionable odor. These acids are corrosive to storage facilities but not to the animals eating them. Fungal resistance to them develops. While they decrease the vitamin E content of grain, they may slightly increase the grain's utilization, probably by increasing its digestibility. However, they are less effective in dry substrates. Their effectiveness is also decreased by buffering minerals, such as limestone, in the feed. Sorbic acid is an effective mold inhibitor but has some of the same disadvantages, and cost may preclude its use. A mixture of organic volatile acids may offer advantages over a single acid. These acids are not harmful to animals or people and, in fact, are produced in the gastrointestinal tracts of horses, ruminants, and other herbivores, and are absorbed and serve as an important source of dietary energy.

Enzyme antioxidants are effective as mold inhibitors without the corrosive effect of organic acids on storage facilities, but are not widely used. Formaldehyde is a marginally effective mold inhibitor, but it destroys enzymes, precipitates protein decreasing digestibility, is an irritant, and is highly toxic, as is pimaricin, which is not universally approved and is costly. Ammonia, copper sulfate, urea, chlorine, certain antibiotics, and various chemicals have been tested as mold inhibitors. Most have shown good mold inhibition activity but for numerous reasons have not been widely used.

Antioxidants

Oxidation is a degradative process by which oxygen reacts with various nutrients, particularly fats. The compounds resulting from oxidation (mainly peroxides) give feed an off-flavor or rancid taste and smell. This can occur in any feed, but occurs particularly in those high in unsaturated fatty acids. Although nearly all common horse feeds, except oilseeds, are low in fat, the fat present is relatively unsaturated and, therefore, quite susceptible to oxidation. Oxidation not only decreases the feed's palatability and, therefore acceptance, it also destroys vitamins. To prevent this, antioxidants may be mixed with the grain mix; they are present in many commercially available grain mixes as well as in fats or oils added to feeds.

The most commonly used antioxidant is ethoxyquin, followed by BHT (butylated hydroxytoluene). Both are quite safe, causing no harm to the animal, and have been used for many years. Vitamin E can also serve as an antioxidant both in the feed as well as in the body (as discussed in (Chapter 2). However, synthetic sources of vitamins E and A, although more stable than natural vitamins E and A, have little antioxidant activity in the feed. Antioxidants, such as ethoxyquin and BHT, although effective in the feed, do not prevent oxidation-induced damage in the body and, therefore, do not reduce dietary requirements for vitamin E.

Bioflavonoids

Citrus bioflavonoids such as hesperidin, have been called vitamin P to denote its effect on capillary permeability. However they do not have vitamin effects. They have been used and thought to be of benefit in various stress situations and conditions (nutritional, physical, environmental, and disease) in people, probably by enhancing the maintenance of capillary integrity. They have been used in horses during growth and training, and for the prevention and treatment of exercise-induced pulmonary hemorrhage (bleeders) and founder. However, they have been shown to be of no demonstrable benefit for either condition, or during growth or training.

In one study, exercise-induced pulmonary hemorrhage recurred in 84.4% of 45 horses given 28 g/day of hesperidin-citrus bioflavonoid in their feed for 90 days, as compared to 80% recurrence in 40 horses not given the bioflavonoid. There was no difference in any of several growth parameters, bone growth plates, numerous blood parameters, plasma enzyme activities, or microscopic appearance of capillary wall structure of skin or subcutaneous tissues of 12 Thoroughbred colts or fillies between those given a hesperidin complex and lemon bioflavonoid (44 to 58 mg/kg body wt/d) from weaning throughout a 342-day growth phase and a 153-day training phase, and those treated and fed the same but not given the bioflavonoid. In this study there were minimal health problems so that the bioflavonoids' effect on health problems could not be evaluated.

PASTURE FOR HORSES

Horse Pasture Purpose and Benefit	103	Planting Pastures	107
Horse Grazing Behavior	103	Forage Species to Plant	107
Grazing Management	104	Overseeding	110
Rotational Grazing	105	When to Plant	110
Pasture Fertilization	106	Soil Preparation for Planting	110
Weed Control	107	Planting	111
		Post-Planting Care	111

HORSE PASTURE PURPOSE AND BENEFIT

The most natural and, from the horse's point of view, preferred way to live is to have companionship and adequate pasture forage and space to run, buck, play, and bask in the sun or shade. The horse's preference is well demonstrated by its joy and exuberance upon being turned out on pasture following stall or paddock confinement. What person amongst us can observe this and not himself feel that joy and that freedom from confinement?

Pastures have a twofold purpose for the horse: to provide feed and to provide space for exercise. To provide a good space for exercise, pasture should be sufficiently dry and free of obstacles, holes, trash, and particularly wire and other items that might cause injury. Fences should be smooth wire, board, pipe, etc., with no barbed wire, as described in Chapter 9. Ideally, there should be ready access to salt, clean water, day-long shade, shelter from adverse weather, and adequate nutritious forage free of harmful plants. Adequate shelter does not necessarily mean man-made. Trees, brush, boulders, and the lay of the land, such as depressions or slopes, may be adequate and at times preferred by most horses. Companionship and pasture providing these amenities is all that's really needed, or quite likely desired, by the horse, barring injury, illness, and predators. Ah, but to have our needs and wants so simply met!

If properly managed, even a small pasture can greatly decrease feeding costs, stable cleaning, and other management chores, and quite likely greatly increase the horse's enjoyment of life. However, if not properly managed, pasture may not provide any of these benefits. Overgrazing and improper or inadequate irrigation, fertilization, weed control, and insect control may decrease, even to nothing, the amount of feed a pasture provides. In contrast, even relatively small pastures, properly managed, can provide all or a substantial amount of the feed and nutrients needed by the horse. The amount of the major nutrients of concern for the horse provided by various types of pasture forage are given in Appendix Table 6. Most pastures contain several different types of forage. For example, the average central Kentucky horse pasture is reported to contain about 50% bluegrass, 30% tall fescue, and 20% orchard grass, and to have the nutrient content given in Table 5-1. As also shown, forage nutrient content is highest during spring and fall growth.

The more immature the plant, the more nutritious and palatable but the smaller it is and, therefore, the less feed it provides. Digestible energy and protein content of grasses decreases by $\frac{1}{3}$ to over $\frac{1}{2}$ from midvegetative stage (2 to 4 weeks of growth and $\frac{2}{3}$ mature height) to seed-forming maturity (12 weeks of growth). These decreases are well demonstrated by the results of the study shown in Table 5-2. Although both types of forage in the study were high in nutritional value in the spring, by winter they were quite low. The concentration of some minerals also decreases with plant maturity. From 2 weeks to about 8 weeks of maturity, the concentrations of potassium, phosphorus, magnesium, manganese, and iron decrease by about one-half, whereas there is little change in calcium, zinc, or sodium. Phosphorus, copper, and protein concentrations in pasture forage decrease from spring to summer then increase with regrowth that fall (Table 5-3). Thus, if forage is grazed or cut late in maturity, its available dietary energy, protein, and palatability are low; if harvested too early, the amount of feed or forage obtained is low. A good balance between these factors and, thus, the best time to graze or cut pasture forage for hay is just prior to flowering (bud stage) or emergence of the heads. For alfalfa, this is generally when the plant is about 8 inches (20 cm) tall. Many pastures begin to change from an emerald green color to a darker green to a slightly gray color at the best time for harvesting, then with increasing maturity to full-bloom color, if it contains blooming species, then to yellowish brown. Proper pasture and grazing management are necessary if the horse is to obtain the maximum total amount of nutrients and, therefore, benefit from the pasture year after year.

HORSE GRAZING BEHAVIOR

Knowledge of the horse's grazing behavior may be helpful in managing grazing to maximize the nutrients obtained from pasture forages, and to maximize pasture benefit for the horse's physical and psychologic well-being. The amount of time horses devote to grazing and other activities varies considerably with changes in their environment. The time devoted to grazing decreases with severe weather (hot or cold), increased pasture forage availability, being alone, and flies, and is less in young horses. Variation in individuals commonly occurs. Mature horses, domestic and feral, on pasture with ample forage and no other feed

TABLE 5–1
Nutrient Content of Mixed Central Kentucky Pasture Forage[a]

Nutrient	Spring	Summer	Fall	Winter
Digestible Energy—Mcal/lb	1.17	1.10	1.27	1.11
Crude Protein—%	14.7	13.1	16.6	13.8
Calcium—%	0.37	0.40	0.43	0.47
Phosphorus—%	0.27	0.28	0.33	0.27
Magnesium—%	0.17	0.22	0.26	0.20
Zinc—mg/kg	28	20	31	28
Copper—mg/kg	15	10	17	20

[a] All values are the average in the forage dry matter from 11 pastures consisting of about 50% bluegrass, 30% tall fescue and 20% orchardgrass. Seasonal variation was the same in all three grasses but different in degree: variation in energy, and protein content, being greatest in orchard grass and least in fescue.

TABLE 5–2
Forage Maturity Effect on its Digestibility and Digestible Protein Content for the Horse

| Season | Tall Fescue (Ky31) | | Orchardgrass/Clover | |
	DM Dig.[a]	Dig. Prot.[b]	DM Dig.[a]	Dig. Prot.[b]
Spring	60	18	60	14
Fall	35	13	38	10
Winter	28	6	18	7

[a] % dry matter digestibility by the horse.
[b] % digestible protein in the forage dry matter.

during mild weather are reported to spend from 40 to 60% of a 24-hr period, and 60 to 80% of daylight hours, grazing, with the most continuous grazing, periods being early morning, late afternoon and evening, and the middle of the night. The normal pattern is to graze continuously for several hours, and to rest for longer or shorter periods, depending on weather conditions and distance that must be traveled to obtain water and sufficient forage. Grazing time is inversely proportional to the quality and amount of pasture forage, e.g., high quality and high amounts result in low grazing time. Horses also spend 9% of their time walking (more on poor pasture or if alone, presumably in search of companionship), and 5 to 10% of their time, primarily during the period 3 to 4 hours before dawn, lying down, with 25 to 30% of this on their side. Individually stalled horses with free access to hay spend a similar amount of their time eating: 73% of daylight hours when they could see other horses and 60% when they couldn't. When individually confined to a pen, mature horses spend 57% of the time eating hay, and 10% lying down. Even on the foal's first day of life, it spends 6 to 9% of its time grazing, with this increasing to 23% by 1 to 8 weeks of age, to 40 to 50% by 21 weeks, and as yearlings to the same as adults.

Horses are selective grazers. They do not simply eat from plants that are in the greatest abundance. They base their selection on palatability as well as availability. Until preferred forages are depleted, horses will eat only a few of many species available. Stage of growth, also determines seasonal difference in preference, the younger more immature plants being preferred. These preferences result in spotty grazing and incomplete utilization of pasture forage, which can be minimized with proper pasture grazing management.

GRAZING MANAGEMENT

The horse will eat, trample, or damage forage that is equivalent to at least 1000 lbs (454 kg) of hay per month. Forage production of pasture in most areas occurs during a 5- to 7-month period. During this period, one acre (0.4 ha) of good, improved pasture receiving the optimum amount of moisture (irrigation or precipitation) may yield the equivalent of 5 to 7 tons (11 to 16 MT/ha) of nutritious, high-quality forage. Thus, one acre (0.4 ha) of these types of pasture would support two mature light-breed horses during this period. In contrast, 30 to 60 acres (12 to 24 ha) of dry range pasture, typical of that in the Rocky Mountain-

TABLE 5–3
Plant Maturity Effect on Pasture Forage Nutrient Content[a]

	Spring	Summer	Fall
Crude Protein—%	21.8 (19–26)	11.5 (10–13)	18.9 (17–23)
Lysine—%[b]			
in feed	0.8–1.1	0.35–0.8	0.7–1.1
in protein	3.7–5.1	2.4–4.2	3.2–4.4
Calcium—%	0.39 (0.24–0.51)	0.36 (0.29–0.46)	0.40 (0.34–0.51)
Phosphorus—%	0.33 (0.28–0.43)[b]	0.22 (0.18–0.27)[b]	0.32 (0.25–0.47)[b]
Copper—mg/kg	6.7 (5.9–7.8)	5.1 (4.5–5.4)	6.9 (5.9–8.0)
Zinc—mg/kg	21.7 (19.1–23.2)	21.2 (14.8–26.9)	15.6 (12.6–18.1)
Manganese—mg/kg	170 (110–208)	207 (150–254)	175 (132–200)
Iron—mg/kg	139 (103–187)	187 (100–473)	266 (228–363)

[a] % or mg/kg (ppm) in dry matter of mixed legume and grass pasture forage in Buenos Aires province, Argentina. Values are means (ranges) from 8 pastures.
[b] 0.09 to 0.18% phosphorus and similar calcium levels were reported in pasture forage consisting primarily of grasses from three other areas of Buenos Aires Province. In one of these pastures during the summer, oxalate in forage increased from 0.4 to 0.66% and calcium:oxalate ratio decreased from 0.8:1 to 0.44:1. As described in Chapter 2, a ratio of less than 0.5:1 may cause calcium deficiency-induced bone problems, particularly in growing horses.

Great Plains area of the United States, may be needed to support a single horse for one year.

For maximum pasture forage production, horses should not be on the pasture during or shortly after precipitation or irrigation. Adequate time should be allowed for drying of pastures to minimize trampling, plant injury, and soil compaction. Irrigation should be at intervals that do not permit plants to be stressed. Ideally, the soil should not become dried out below the top two inches (5 cm). The approximate amount of total annual water (from precipitation or irrigation) needed for optimum pasture forage growth is 24 to 36 inches (60 to 90 cm).

On pastures of bluestem, smooth brome, crested wheat grass or legumes such as alfalfa or clover, or on native pastures in the Rocky Mountain-Great Plains area of the United States, only 50 to 60% of the forage should be removed by grazing. Grazing in excess of this is harmful to the plants and slows regrowth, so that over several years the average yearly yield is lowered. In contrast, Kentucky bluegrass, digit, bahia, and orchard and Bermuda grasses, which are the most common pasture grasses in many areas of the southern United States, do best when grazed intensively and cropped closely. These grasses should be grazed at early flowering or before, at which time their feeding value is greatest. At this time, they may provide up to 1.2 megacalories of digestible energy (Mcal DE/lb (2.6/kg) and over 20% crude protein in their dry matter, as compared to 1.45 Mcal DE/lb (3.2/kg) and 10 to 13% crude protein in oats. This illustrates why young horses grow rapidly and mature horses may become overweight on lush, green growing pasture forage, which is almost like allowing them to eat all the oats they want 24 hours a day, along with some additional protein and fiber.

Once the pasture forage is eaten down to the proper level, all grazing animals should be removed, and if the pasture is to be irrigated, it should be done at once. Overgrazing should be prevented. The short-term gain from the small amount of additional forage obtained by overgrazing is more than offset by the long-term loss of decreased forage growth. As a result, an increased amount of generally more expensive feed must be fed. Overgrazing is a good example of being "penny wise and dollar foolish." Overgrazing slows or prevents forage regrowth, which allows weeds to invade the pasture and replace desirable plants. To prevent this, the pasture forage preferred by the horse should not be grazed to less than 2 inches (5 cm) in height. However, to obtain the greatest forage production and thus benefit from pasture, it is better: (1) to remove all grazing animals from the pasture when the preferred forage is eaten down to the amount recommended, except in the late fall as the plant's dormant season nears, when 4 to 6 inches (10 to 15 cm) of plant height should remain; and (2) not to put them back on the pasture until shortly before plant growth but not seed production is nearing completion, as described in the previous section. To prevent overgrazing, horses must be removed from the pasture. Feeding additional feed and leaving them on the pasture won't prevent overgrazing. Even if they are fed grain and have ready access to good hay, they will continue to graze, particularly the more succulent young grass, so short that regrowth can't occur or is slowed.

The length of time horses may be maintained on a pasture without overgrazing it can be extended by shutting them off the pasture, having hay available for at least 4 hours or more before they are put back on the pasture, and leaving them on the pasture for only a few hours daily (or less, the longer you want to extend the number of days the pasture can be grazed). Although the horse continually on pasture will graze 14 to 16 hours per 24-hour period, if there are adequate quantities of good-quality pasture forage readily accessible, they can consume a sufficient quantity to meet their dietary energy needs for maintenance in 4 to 5 hours daily.

When horses are on a pasture providing an adequate amount of average quality forage for only a few hours a day, they will eat about one-third lb/100 lb body/wt/hr ($\frac{1}{3}$ kg/100 kg/hr). This is reduced to about one-tenth lb/100 lb body wt/hr (0.1 kg/100 kg/hr) when they are on pasture 24 hours a day. However, the rate of consumption varies directly with pasture-forage quality, digestibility, and palatability.

The key to obtaining the greatest feeding value from pasture is (1) not overgrazing it, and (2) utilizing its forages while they are in the young growing stages of development. As forages mature, their palatability and utilizable nutrient content decrease rapidly (Tables 5-2 and 5-3). As a result of the mature plants' reduced palatability, horses won't eat them, and instead will overgraze the more palatable plants which are trying to grow. The result is increased weeds in the overgrazed areas, and in the undergrazed areas wasted forage and increased feces. The increased manure contributes to uneven grazing because most mature horses avoid grazing fecally contaminated areas. The plants in these areas grow rapidly due to the added fertility from the manure, producing lush but rapidly maturing forage that, because of both the increased manure and plant maturity, remains ungrazed. To correct patchy grazing once it occurs, spray or mow the weeds, then mow the overmature forage close to the ground, and, finally, scatter the manure with a wire or chain drag or harrow. The way to decrease it from occurring is to not allow any portion of the pasture to be overgrazed and to either harvest the pasture forage or use rotational grazing.

Rotational Grazing

If there is adequate pasture available, the greatest benefit from it for grazing can be obtained by dividing it into two to four similar-size pastures and using rotational grazing (Fig. 5-1). Rotational grazing provides the best opportunity to obtain maximum forage yield. Ideally, each pasture should be just large enough so that the animals to be put on it will consume all the forage produced on it in 10 to 14 days during plant growing seasons. If the stocking rate is not high enough to totally utilize the pasture, spot grazing will occur and mowing may be necessary to rid the pasture of the tall mature grasses that the horses did not graze. Following the 10- to 14-day grazing period, the pasture should have about a month's rest for new forage growth to occur before the horses are rotated back onto it.

As shown in Table 5-4, in one study, more than twice

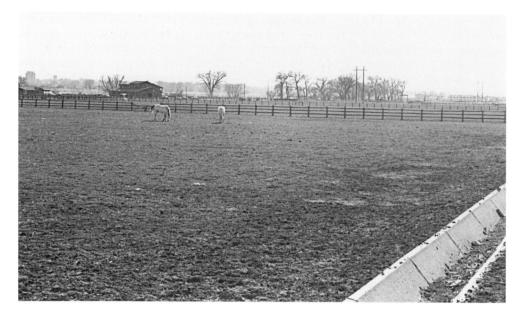

Fig. 5–1. Dividing an acreage into several pastures so that rotational grazing of each pasture may be used provides the best opportunity to obtain maximum forage production. (Courtesy of Moondrift Farm, Fort Collins, CO)

as much forage was obtained from the same amount of initially similar pasture by rotational grazing. The greater amount of forage obtained was due to the forage growth that occurred when the pasture wasn't being grazed, and because spot grazing didn't occur in the rotationally grazed pastures but did in the continually grazed pasture.

Although pasture can usually be divided easily using an electric wire, if several pastures are not available and, therefore, rotational grazing isn't possible, patchy grazing may be minimized using intermittent grazing. Put the horses on the pasture as its forage approaches maturity, or earlier, if necessary, so that all pasture forage will be eaten to the proper level within 10 to 14 days. At that time, the horses should be removed from the pasture until its forage is ready for the next grazing period.

Grazing cattle or sheep with horses will also decrease patchy grazing. Although horses and cattle show a large overlap in choice of forage, horses tend to graze only particular areas in the pasture while cattle and sheep graze more at random. Other types of livestock will also graze around manure piles left by horses while most horses tend to avoid these areas. In contrast to cattle, there is little

overlap between horses and deer in choice of forages and browse; thus, their presence on the same pasture doesn't decrease the feed available for the other species. Instead, a combination of livestock keeps pastures grazed more uniformly and helps maintain the pasture's forage in the high-quality growth stage. The combination not only makes more efficient use of the pastures, but also offers additional income from the pasture. Cattle, sheep, and horses may all graze the pasture at the same time, or the cattle or sheep may follow the horses on the pasture. Cattle also are able to utilize a greater amount of dietary energy, but less protein, from grass, but not alfalfa, than are horses. However, their protein requirement is lower than horses (6 versus 8%, except during lactation and growth). The more mature the forage, the greater the difference between horses' and cattles' digestibility of it. Thus, cattle may get by on more mature, lower protein forage than can horses.

PASTURE FERTILIZATION

Forage production and quality of established pastures can usually be greatly increased by proper fertilization. Proper fertilization requires applying the proper amount of the proper fertilizer at the proper time. To determine the optimum amount of the proper fertilizer to use requires a laboratory analysis of the predominant type of soil in the pasture. A soil analysis should be obtained every 3 to 5 years. At least twenty 1- to 2-inch (2- to 5-cm) diameter core samples of the top 4 inches (10 cm) of soil, excluding plants and surface litter, should be thoroughly mixed together. All tools used should be clean and free of rust, and the samples should be collected in a plastic or stainless steel container. Three to four handfuls of the mixture of soil samples from a single pasture or area should be thoroughly air dried and sent for analysis and fertilizer recommendations. These recommendations are best when they are based upon a recent soil analysis and the type of forage and its intended use. In the United States, the county or

TABLE 5–4
Rotational versus Continual Grazing Effects on Yearling Horses and Forage Production

Grazing Method[a]	Gain in lbs (kg)/day	Days of Grazing[b]	Total lbs (kg) Forage Dry Matter Eaten[c]
Continuous	0.5 (0.23)	25	2618 (1190)
Rotational	1.3 (0.6)	37	5350 (2431)

[a] Eight yearlings continuously grazed one 5.2-acre (2.1-ha) alfalfa pasture. Another eight rotationally grazed the same size pasture which initially was divided into six equal-size pieces.
[b] Until overgrazing first became apparent.
[c] Calculated from the amount of early-bloom alfalfa hay dry matter needed to provide the amount of digestible energy required for the growth obtained.

TABLE 5–5
Nitrogen Fertilization Effect on Bermudagrass Production, Protein Content, and Economic Value

Nitrogen Applied (lbs/acre)	Forage Produced (lbs/acre)	Forage Protein (% in Dry Matter)	Protein Produced (lbs/acre)	Additional Production from Fertilization				Fertilizer Cost ($/acre)[c]	Fertilization Value ($/acre)[d]
				Forage		Protein			
				tons/acre	Value[a] ($/acre)	lbs/acre	Value[b] ($/acre)		
0	2,100	4.5	95	0	0	0	0	0	0
50	4,312	5.7	245	1.11	55.50	150	36.75	13.33	78.92
100	7,448	6.9	515	2.67	133.50	420	102.86	26.67	209.69
200	10,834	8.0	867	4.37	218.50	772	189.06	53.33	354.23
400	16,339	10.7	1746	7.12	497.41	1,651	404.33	106.67	795.07
0–400 increase	7.8 times	2.4 times	18.5 times						

[a] If grass hay is worth $50/ton. For example, the value of additional forage produced by applying 50 lbs of nitrogen/acre is [(4312 lbs − 2100 lbs) ÷ 2000 lbs/ton] × $50/ton = $55.50.

[b] If soybean meal containing 49% protein in its dry matter costs $240/ton. Its protein would cost ($240 ÷ 0.49) ÷ 2,000 lbs/ton = $0.245/lb of protein. The value of additional protein produced by applying 50 lbs nitrogen/acre would be (245 lbs − 95 lbs) × $0.245/lb of protein = $36.75/acre.

[c] If 45% nitrogen fertilizer costs $12/100 lbs, its nitrogen would cost $12.00 ÷ 0.45 = $26.67/100 lbs of nitrogen.

[d] Additional forage value/acre + additional protein value/acre − fertilizer cost/acre. This doesn't take into account the cost of putting the fertilizer on the pasture.

local Extension Service is a good place to obtain this information, as well as recommendations on the best times of year to fertilize. Nearby universities and fertilizer companies and distributors may also be helpful in providing the needed services and information.

Nitrogen fertilization may be all that is needed on grass pastures in some areas; in other areas, phosphorus, lime (calcium oxide), potash (potassium carbonate), magnesium, sulfur, and minor elements such as copper, manganese, zinc, and boron application may be beneficial. Legume and grass-legume pastures containing more than 40% legumes generally do not need nitrogen fertilization, but many need minerals such as phosphorus, potash, and lime. Nitrogen fertilization of grass-legume pastures may be detrimental in that it may stimulate grass growth that crowds out the legumes. In contrast, it is especially important to maintain adequate levels of lime, phosphorus, and potash on legumes. As the levels of these nutrients decrease, legumes usually die out before the grasses.

One application of fertilizer yearly, generally 1 to 3 months before the beginning of the growing season, may be adequate. In other areas, fertilization near midsummer and/or in the fall may be beneficial.

Proper nitrogen fertilization of grass pasture will not only increase the amount of forage produced but also its protein content. As shown in Table 5–5, nitrogen fertilization of a Bermuda grass pasture increased the amount of forage produced nearly 8 times and its protein content 2.4 times; as a result, the amount of protein produced increased 18.5 times. The economic value of this increased forage and protein production can be substantial. For example, at the current cost of fertilizer, grass hay, and protein (soybean meal) in my area, the increased production from applying 400 lbs of nitrogen/acre would be worth almost $800/acre above the cost of the fertilizer (Table 5–5); that's a pretty good return on a $107/acre investment for fertilizer and good wages for applying it. Different results will be obtained on different pastures and with differ-

ent costs, but these results dramatically illustrate the benefit that can be derived from proper fertilization.

WEED CONTROL

The most important factors for minimizing pasture weeds are not overgrazing and proper fertilization. Overgrazing decreases or prevents growth of desirable plants, allowing undesirable plants, such as weeds, to flourish. Additional weed control measures include mowing or application of a herbicide. Either, if needed, should be done early in the spring before perennial weeds bud and before annual weeds seed. Mowing or herbicide application at this time gives much better weed control and will keep pastures from becoming reinfested longer.

PLANTING PASTURES

Types of forage best to plant, their productive capacities, and procedures for pasture establishment, improvement, and care differ widely based on the intended use of the pasture and in different areas based on things such as climate, soil type, drainage, plant diseases and pests, etc. Because of this, it is recommended that individuals familiar with this information for that specific area be contacted for recommendations best for that area. In the United States, the County Extension Service or state university are generally good and the most accessible places to obtain these recommendations. The following information is given as general advice and examples of factors that should be considered. These generalities may not be correct or optimum for your specific area and situation.

Forage Species to Plant

Pasture forage may be one or, often preferably, a combination of five different types of plants: warm- or cool-season perennial or annual grasses, or legumes. Annuals must be planted yearly; this isn't necessary or beneficial for perennials or legumes. Also, the productive season of annuals is limited. However, annuals are generally higher in nutrients than perennials, with the cool-season annuals generally being the highest.

Warm-season perennials (such as Bermuda grass, bahia grass, kleingrass, and digitgrasses such as pangola) produce their major growth during the summer and don't do well in areas having cold winters. In contrast, cool-season perennials (such as fescue, orchard grass, reed canary grass, brome, bluestem, and wheat grasses) are more adapted to cold winters, with their major growth occurring in the spring and fall and little or no growth during the summer. Both types generally respond well to proper fertilization.

Warm-season annuals (such as sorghums, Sudan grass, and Johnson grasses) generally are of limited value for horse pastures. Cool-season annuals (such as the cereal grains, however, can provide a high amount of high-nutritional-value feed for the horse for a short spring grazing period without decreasing their yield when harvested for grain and straw that summer.

In winter wheat (Triticum aestivum) growing areas, livestock, including horses, are commonly grazed on the young plants during early spring (February and March in central U.S.). This may be done without decreasing the amount of wheat obtained when it is harvested. One to two additional months of grazing can be obtained if the wheat isn't to be harvested. During this period, winter wheat pasture can provide 200 to 400 lbs/acre (225 to 450 kg/ha) of forage dry matter, depending on growing conditions. The forage obtained is higher in digestible energy and protein content than alfalfa, and is generally adequate in mineral content for all horses 18 months of age or older (Appendix Tables 1 and 6). Additional calcium particularly is needed for younger horses on winter wheat pasture during early spring.

Legumes (such as alfalfa, clovers, vetch, and birdsfoot trefoil) have a symbiotic relationship with bacteria that enables them to utilize atmospheric and soil nitrogen for production of plant protein. The bacteria are usually contained in root nodules. Thus, legumes, particularly their leaves, are much higher in protein, and also in calcium, than grasses. Under optimal growing conditions, legumes yield more protein, dietary energy, calcium, and most vitamins than do grasses. Grasses, however, can tolerate humid weather, cold weather, and poor soil conditions better than legumes, and can persist and maintain production with less management.

Legumes may be the sole pasture forage for horses, because they don't cause bloat in horses as some have a tendency to do in ruminants. The greatest benefit of legumes is derived when they are incorporated in with a pasture grass. Generally, only one, or at the most two, species of grass should be planted, since grazing will usually eliminate all but one. A legume should be seeded with the grass or overseeded into established pastures. Legumes provide additional nitrogen for the grass that is growing with them and, therefore, increase grass growth. In addition, legumes improve the physical condition of shallow clay soils, resulting in further improvement of grass growth on this type of soil. Legumes will grow during periods in which warm-

season perennial pasture grasses grow little or not at all; therefore, they prolong seasonal forage production from the pasture. The higher protein, calcium, and vitamin A precursor content of legumes, compared to grasses, also increases the nutritional value of the pasture forage for the horse. Legumes, such as alfalfa and red clover, are also more palatable for most horses than are equal-quality grasses. For these reasons, seeding legumes with grasses, or into established grass pastures, is generally beneficial. However, tall grasses tend to crowd out some legumes, such as clovers. If the amount of legume is thinning, keep the pasture grazed, or cut to reduce grass competition, and give the legume an opportunity to thicken. A balance of 40 to 60% of each (grasses and legumes) is ideal.

Alfalfa (Medicago sativa) is a deep-rooted legume that does best on well-drained soils with a pH of 6.5 or higher. Most varieties currently available do not do well in the southern United States because of a high susceptibility to insects, diseases, and hot humid conditions. **Birdsfoot trefoil** (Lotus corniculatus)—a yellow-flowered, stemmed, warm-season perennial legume—can tolerate more acidic soils that are less well drained than can alfalfa. However, alfalfa greatly outproduces it when conditions are good for alfalfa.

Many different types of clovers may be used as a legume forage for horses. **Alsike clover** (Trifolium hybridum) grows best in a cool moist climate and on heavy silt or clay soil. However, it is poorly palatable to horses and may cause photosensitization if grazed exclusively (see Chapter 18). **Crimson clover** (Trifolium incarnatum) is a cool-season annual legume that will grow under a wide range of soil conditions. It is widely used for winter grazing in southern United States. **Red clover** (Trifloium pratense) is a thick-stemmed legume that can be highly productive. It is one of the most widely grown of all clovers but has a low resistance to disease and pests and, as a result, a short life of often only a few years. In addition, a mold called black patch (Rhizoctonia leguminicola) may grow on red clover and produce the alkaloid slaframine, which causes excessive salivation by livestock consuming affected pasture or hay (see Chapter 18). Yellow- and white-flowered **sweet clovers** (Melilotus officinalis and M. alba) are rapid-growing legumes widely grown in areas such as southern Canada. They are quite drought and cold resistant and need only a short growing season. However, particularly when overmature, they have large coarse stems and, except for low-coumarin varieties, are high in coumarin. Coumarin is not harmful unless it is converted by a mold to dicoumarol, which inhibits vitamin K thus decreasing blood coagulation (see Vitamin K, Deficiency, Chapter 3). **White clovers** (Trifolium repens) grow best during cool moist seasons on well-drained soil. White clovers of the low- and intermediate-growing varieties (common or dutch clovers) are often present in pasture and lawns. The white clover most commonly used for livestock forage is **Ladino clover.** It can be highly nutritious but has a shallow root system and, therefore, cannot tolerate long dry spells. Ladino clover pasture is one of the most likely pasture forages to cause bloat in cattle but does not have this effect on horses.

Lespedeza and **crown vetch** are two additional perennial legumes that can be used for pasture forage. Lespedeza

(L. striata) was once widely grown as a hay crop in southern United States, but has decreased in popularity because usually only one cutting per season is obtained, it is low yielding, and it often has a high weed content. Crown vetch (Coronilla varia) is frequently used as a ground cover for soil conservation. It can be used as a pasture forage, but grazing reduces its persistence.

The grasses that are most productive on irrigated pastures, or pastures that receive adequate moisture throughout the growing season, are usually orchardgrass, followed by tall fescue, bromegrass, and intermediate or pubescent wheatgrass. Differences in productive capacity, however, exist in different areas and with different soil types.

The pasture grasses that generally produce the most forage and provide the best nourishment to the horse in different geographic regions of the United States are as follows:

Florida, south Georgia, and the Gulf coast—pangola or other digit grasses, bahia varieties, and coastal Bermuda grass.
Middle Atlantic—coastal Bermuda grass (southern area), orchard grass, bluegrass, tall fescue, and white, red, and ladino clovers.
Northeast—redtop, orchard grass, reed canary grass, Kentucky bluegrass, and timothy.
Midwest—smooth brome grass, buffalo grass, bluestem, grama, and tall fescue.
Southwest—coastal Bermuda grass and rye grass. Klein grass does well in much of the southwestern states but is not recommended because of its poor palatability for horses. Its hay or pasture also occasionally cause hepatotoxicosis, especially that from rapid early growth during hot humid weather.
Northwest—fescue, bent grass, bluestem, grama, and crested wheat grass.
Far West—orchard grass, coastal Bermuda grass, love grass, Rhodes grass, and rescue grass.

Tall fescue (Festuca arundinacea) has good tolerance to hot weather and drought, as well as wet, saline, and alkali, but not sandy, soils, and will withstand considerable trampling and heavy grazing. Although it is nutritious and horses will graze it if other grasses or legumes are not available, it is less palatable than most. Because of this, its presence in pasture with these forages will result in patchy grazing and wasted forage. Horses will greatly overgraze other more palatable plants before they will eat the fescue. In addition, particularly in warm humid climates, tall fescue may become infested by the endophyte, Acremonium coenophialum, which causes fescue toxicosis in pregnant and lactating mares and slows growth (see Chapter 19). Because of this, mares during late pregnancy or lactation, and horses less than 1 year of age should not be grazed on fescue pasture unless it is known to be endophyte free. However, other horses and mares, except at these two times, may safely graze fescue pastures. Cattle, but not horses, grazing endophyte-infected tall fescue may develop a lameness and dry gangrene of the legs called "fescue foot" or "summer syndrome," which is characterized by a rough hair coat, reduced growth or milk production, rapid breathing, and fever.

Orchard grass (Dactylis glomerata) grazed early produces excellent-quality forage but will not tolerate drought, wet or alkali soils, or as much trampling as fescue. Although it is more palatable than fescue, it is less palatable than most wheat grasses, timothy, and smooth brome. It is one of the earliest maturing of the common grasses and tolerates shade well. If full-season precipitation is less than 20 inches (50 cm), or irrigation water is not available, smooth brome grass, intermediate wheat grass, or pubescent wheat grass may be best.

Smooth **brome grass** (Bromus inermis) is excellent for pastures receiving more than 18 inches (45 cm) of rainfall. It will grow in soils with a higher moisture content than wheat grasses and requires a lower moisture content than fescue will tolerate. It is usually more winter hardy and more productive than fescue, reed canary grass, or orchard grass, and does particularly well when seeded with alfalfa. If mixed with alfalfa, and if several cuttings are made each growing season, however, the amount of brome grass may decrease.

Any of four **wheat grasses** (Agropyron spp.)—crested, pubescent, western, or intermediate (listed in order of most to lowest water needs)—are often quite good and recommended for seeding pastures that receive only 10 to 18 inches (25 to 45 cm) of water annually.

Bermuda grasses, in contrast to fescue, are well adapted to sandy soils but not to wet soils. Like fescue, Bermuda grasses tolerate trampling and overgrazing better than most other grasses. Coastal Bermuda grass (Cynodon dactylon) is higher yielding than the common variety and than bluegrass, wheat grasses, or timothy. It is one of the most extensively produced hay-crop forages in much of the southern United States. Its advantages are that it is high yielding, often providing three or more cuttings per year, and it maintains its stand indefinitely when properly fertilized. However, it can suffer from winterkill and loses much of its nutritional value when overmature. Because of this, it serves best as a hay crop or for rotational grazing. Bermuda grass may cause staggers or tremors in cattle and sheep, but not in horses (see section on "Grass Staggers" in Chapter 19).

Digit grasses (Digitaria spp.) such as pangola, slenderstem, and transvola), **Bahia grasses** (Paspalpum notatum), and to a lesser extent Bermuda grasses, are sensitive to frost and make little growth during cold weather. Very low temperatures may kill digit grasses and bahia grasses. Digit grasses are also quite sensitive to trace-mineral deficiencies, particularly copper. Bahia grasses will withstand prolonged periods of drought and overgrazing, but are not as productive as coastal Bermuda grass. The nutritional value of these three grasses, like all grasses, decreases as they reach maturity. This is particularly true for bahia grasses which, following maturity, become extremely fibrous and will not be eaten by horses. All make good hay. However, the digitgrasses, like alfalfa, and particularly sweet clover, dry quite slowly after cutting. In contrast, Bermuda grasses dry rapidly. Slow drying limits both digitgrass's and alfalfa's use for hay production in areas of high humidity or frequent rainfall.

Kentucky bluegrass (Poa pratensis), followed by timothy, are the most palatable pasture grasses for horses, whereas kleingrass is poorly palatable for horses. Although bluegrass makes excellent pasture for the horse, is winter hardy and tolerates close grazing or mowing, it does not produce as much forages as other grasses. It has low mid-summer growth and does not grow well in areas with less than 20 inches (50 cm) of annual precipitation or where there is not adequate moisture for growth during the summer. It is a long-lived perennial that forms a dense sod.

Timothy (Phleum pratense) and **reed canary grass** (Phalaris arundinacea) are quite winter hardy but don't do well in regions with high summer temperatures. For this reason they are generally grown in more northern states, and timothy in those with good rainfall as it does not withstand drought. In contrast, reed canary grass is one of the most drought-resistant grasses. Reed canary grass also grows well on wet soils. Because of this, reed canary grass is often used along waterways, ditch banks, and other areas with wet soil. It is a vigorous, tall-growing, coarse perennial. However, its palatability is low, particularly late in the growing season, because of a high alkaloid content. Some of these alkaloids (hordenine), as described in the section on "Grass Staggers" in Chapter 19, can cause disqualification of horses in athletic events in some states if detected in the urine. Reed canary grass following rapid growth conditions (sunny following wet weather) has been associated with two clinical syndromes in sheep and cattle, but not in horses. These are: (1) peracute collapse with cardiac arrhythmias and respiratory distress followed by death or recovery, and (2) Phalaris or reed canary grass staggers, which as described in Chapter 19, is characterized by generalized muscular tremors that progress to incoordination, stiffness, recumbency, and tetanic convulsions. These effects may occur as long as 5 months after sheep and cattle are removed from the pasture or hay. The administration of cobalt after exposure to the toxins, but before the onset of clinical signs, has been reported to prevent development of toxicosis. Toxicosis due to reed canary grass hasn't been reported in horses.

Rye grass (Lolium spp.) is one of the most widely used of all pasture grasses. It is an important cool-season grass worldwide. Both perennial and annual ryegrass are used. Ryegrass is finer-stemmed than most forage grasses and when grazed or cut early in maturity is high in nutritional value. Perennial ryegrass (L. perenne) may cause grass staggers in horses, and both it and annual ryegrass (L. rigidum) may cause grass staggers in cattle and sheep as described in Chapter 19.

Sorghum, Sudan grass, Johnson grass, Sudex and other sorghum grass pastures, haylage or silage, but not properly cured and stored hay, may cause cyanide (prussic or hydrocyanic acid) toxicosis resulting in cystitis, incoordination or, less commonly, sudden death as discussed in Chapter 18. They may cause cystitis in horses, but not ruminants, regardless of their stage of maturity or growing conditions. These types of pastures, therefore, should not be grazed by horses.

Millet (Pennisetum spp.) is a fast-growing, warm-season annual grass that produces lots of growth. It is especially useful as a supplemental forage during drought periods. However, German or foxtail millet has been reported to be unsafe and to cause excess urination in horses, although no reports that actually document this have been found.

Pearl millet (P. glaucum) appears to be a good pasture forage that is widely used in some areas for horses, with no problems reported. Grazing can begin when the pearl millet is 10 to 12 inches (25–30 cm) tall. It should not be allowed to exceed 24 to 36 inches (60–90 cm), or grazed closer than 4 inches (10 cm). Unless cut quite early in maturity, pearl millet is a coarse, poor-quality hay. As with all warm-season annual grasses, millet is killed by frost and must be reseeded each year, preferably in late spring, at about 20 lbs/acre (20 kg/ha) and a soil pH of 6.0 to 6.2 with a medium to high level of soil potassium and phosphorus. Prior to seeding, generally 50 to 60 lbs/acre (50 to 60 kg/ha) of nitrogen should be applied along with whatever potassium and phosphorus is needed. A second application of the same amount of nitrogen following the first grazing or cutting will encourage a second growth if adequate moisture is available.

Overseeding

Overseeding grass pastures with legumes (e.g., 0.5 to 1 lb of ladino clover and 4 to 5 lbs of red clover/acre or kg/ha) is one way to increase pasture forage production and quality. Successful overseeding of established pastures can usually be obtained by the following procedures:

1. Remove top growth or warm-season grass by heavy grazing or mowing just prior to seeding or cool weather in the fall.
2. Disk the area sufficiently to loosen top soil in order to get seed coverage. This will also retard growth of the warm-season grasses and allow the new seed to become established. Bermuda grass sods can be disked more heavily than bunch-grass types such as Klein grass or buffalo grass.
3. Apply fertilizer, based on the results of a soil test (for procedures see previous section on "Pasture Fertilization").
4. Seed legumes or cool-season annuals, such as ryegrass, or small-cereal grains such as wheat, oats, rye, or barley. Ryegrass and legumes can be broadcast over the surface. Small grains should be drilled in. In either case, some type of drag or harrow should be dragged across the area after seeding so that good seed coverage is obtained.
5. Withhold grazing until the newly seeded forage is well established.

When to Plant

Irrigated pastures and those receiving adequate precipitation throughout the growing season may be seeded from early spring through fall; however, in areas that have cold winters the ideal time is spring. Late fall seedings may not become sufficiently established to survive a cold dry winter. Early fall plantings, however, are recommended in some areas for cool-season grasses.

Soil Preparation for Planting

Before planting a pasture, a soil sample should be taken (for procedure see previous sections on "Pasture Fertilization"). If the soil is deficient in phosphorus or other minerals, an adequate supply of these minerals should be applied and, ideally, plowed under prior to planting. In addition, up to 50 pounds per acre (up to 50 kg/ha), of phosphorus (P$_2$O$_5$), nitrogen, and possibly other minerals (the amount of all are based on the soil test) should be applied just below the seed during planting. If the soil does not have the proper pH, or calcium or magnesium content, lime administration may be needed for best results. A soil test is also valuable in determining the species of grasses best suited to that soil.

For planting dryland pasture, a sorghum grain (milo) stubble, prepared the year prior to planting, makes a good seedbed and is recommended. Nurse crops or small-cereal grain stubble are not as good.

Planting

If legumes are going to be planted, the seed should be inoculated with nitrogen-fixing bacteria. An inoculum specific for the species of legume being planted must be used. The amount of bacterial inoculant needed varies from none to several times the amount recommended by the manufacturer. Individuals knowledgeable of the local situation should be consulted as to the amount recommended in that area.

In some areas, seed or soil inoculation may be unnecessary as the bacteria are already present in the soil. The directions for inoculation given by the inoculant producer should be closely followed. Inoculant and inoculated seed should never be exposed to direct sunlight or allowed to become heated or completely dry before planting. Seed should be planted within a few hours after inoculation; if not, the seed should be considered untreated.

The amount of seed to plant should be based on the amount of pure-live seed. The fraction of pure-live seed can be determined by multiplying "purity" by "germination." The amount of bulk seed to use can then be determined by dividing the amount of pure-live seed recommended by this fraction. The amount of pure-live seed to use should be obtained from those familiar with the area where it is to be planted, e.g., personnel from the County Extension Service or nearby university.

If legumes, such as alfalfa or clover, are being planted with a grass (which is generally recommended), the total amount of legumes should not exceed 25% of the seed mix. For example, if 3 lbs/acre of orchard grass, and 8 lbs/acre of alfalfa were the recommended amounts to use in your area, the seed mix should contain 0.75 × 3, or 2.25 lbs/acre (kg/ha), of orchard grass and 0.25 × 8, or 2 lbs/acre (kg/ha), of alfalfa.

Planting depth should be ¾ to 1 inch (2 to 2.5 cm) in sandy soils and ¼ to ½ inch (0.6 to 0.2 cm) for small seeds in ideally textured soils.

Post-Planting Care

New plantings need water frequently to keep the seed moist and the emerged seedlings developing. Weed control is also important to prevent shading of the newly developing plants and to decrease competition for moisture. This may require frequent spraying or mowing. Spraying or mowing before perennial weeds bud and before annual weeds seed will give much better control and keep pastures from becoming reinfested longer.

After reseeding, the pasture should not be grazed during its first growing season after planting and not until it is 6 inches (15 cm) tall during the second season. During the first 2 to 3 years after planting, it is best not to graze it for 1 year to allow the plants to go to seed.

Chapter 6

DIET EVALUATION, FORMULATION, AND PREPARATION FOR HORSES

Why Diet Evaluation and Formulation are Needed 112
Feed Selection by the Horse 112
Information Needed for Diet Evaluation and Formulation . . . 113
Nutrients Needed in the Horse's Diet 113
Nutrient Content of Feeds 114
Methods of Expressing Feed Nutrient Content 117
Amount of Feed Needed by the Horse 118
Obtaining a Horse's Weight 118
Determining Total Amount of Feed Needed by the Horse . 120

Example 1—Idle Mature Horse 120
Example 2—Working Horse 122
Diet Evaluation and Formulation Procedures 122
Example 1—Weanlings on Pasture 123
Example 2—Weanlings Fed Alfalfa (Lucerne) Hay 128
Example 3—Lactating Mares on Growing Grass Pasture . 133
Example 4—Lactating Mares Fed Grass Hay 134
Preparation of Grain Mixes 136

This chapter describes: (1) why it is necessary and beneficial to know how to evaluate and formulate the horse's diet, (2) how to obtain the information needed to evaluate or formulate the diet, (3) how this information is used to evaluate or formulate the diet, and (4) how to use this information to prepare a diet that meets the horse's nutritional needs. How to do this most economically, so as to minimize feeding costs without sacrificing optimum nutrition, is described in Chapter 7.

WHY DIET EVALUATION AND FORMULATION ARE NEEDED

Feeding a correctly formulated and prepared diet is the only way to ensure that the horse receives the proper amount of the nutrients needed. However, diet formulation is not necessary if it is known that the feeds being consumed meet, but do not greatly exceed, the horse's requirements for all nutrients. This is the case if average- or better-quality commonly used horse feeds are fed without nutrient supplements, except during growth and for brood mares during the last 3 months of pregnancy and during lactation. For other horses being fed average- or better-quality common feeds, it is only necessary to ensure that the proper amounts of these feeds are fed as described later in this chapter in the section on "Determining Total Amount of Feed Needed by the Horse."

Even determining the amount of feed needed isn't necessary if it is ensured that ample quantities of feed are available for the horse to consume enough to maintain optimum body weight and condition. However, feeding costs can be minimized, and problems from excess dietary energy intake can be prevented, by restricting the amount fed to that just sufficient to meet the horse's needs. However, during growth, pregnancy, and lactation, or when poorer- or questionable-quality or uncommonly used feeds are being fed, feeding diets formulated to meet the horse's needs is necessary. In contrast to popular belief by some, the horse will not select and consume most nutrients, or feeds high in those nutrients, according to its needs for those nutrients.

Feed Selection by the Horse

Some mistakenly believe that animals, including the horse, have "nutritional wisdom," i.e., have an innate wisdom, appetite, or craving for the nutrients needed. This

misconception is prompted by those selling products based on this belief, such as cafeteria-style vitamin and mineral products, i.e., individual vitamin and/or mineral supplements in multicompartment feeders. Horses, like other animals, choose to either consume or reject feeds containing certain nutrients for one of three reasons:

1. A true appetite, in which, if available, a sufficient amount of that nutrient or feeds high in that nutrient are sought out and consumed to meet the animal's needs for that nutrient.
2. A learned appetite, in which the animal learns that a given food or nutrient results in feelings of well-being or sickness. However, the horse won't reject a food that causes illness if the food is too palatable, and if the illness does not occur within 30 minutes after the food is eaten, the horse will not associate the food with the feeling of illness. Palatability and a feeling of illness soon after eating are how horses learn to avoid some poisonous plants but not others.
3. A taste preference, with no relation to nutritional need or learned appetite, but instead due to feed characteristics affecting palatability.

The only nutrients for which animals are known to have a true appetite are water, sodium (such as in sodium chloride, or common salt), and those required to meet the animal's energy needs. All animals tested select a diet with a salt concentration of 0.5 to 1% in preference to diets deficient in sodium chloride or those with excessive levels (15 to 20%). Animals that are depleted of sodium actually seek sources of the mineral.

Taste, odor, texture, feed to which the animal is unaccustomed, and environmental influences (such as fear of other horses' getting their feed or of the activity of being fed) all influence the immediate control of feeding activity, i.e., what is eaten. Because of these factors, although horses will consume enough water, sodium, and dietary energy to meet their needs, they will generally consume more of all three than needed. For water and sodium this isn't known to be harmful for horses, but for dietary energy it may be. The rate at which the horse's relatively small stomach for its size empties is a major factor limiting the amount of feed eaten at one time.

A sudden intake of a large excess of a palatable feed, such as grain, results in colic, diarrhea, and founder. The intake of even a small excess of dietary energy from any feed may make the horse too high or spirited and over a prolonged period will result in obesity and its effects (as described in the section on "Dietary Energy Excess" in Chapter 1). In addition, it takes horses many days to adjust their intake to changes in the energy content of their diet. Horses tend to stabilize their body weight at levels well above those considered optimum by most people. This may reflect their adaptation to diets low in energy and high seasonal variability in feed available and its nutritional value. In their natural environment, horses' ability to accumulate fat in the spring and fall enhances their chances of survival through hot dry summers and cold winters. Of course, with people feeding them, accumulated fat often isn't lost during periods of lower pasture forage quality or availability. Moderately cold temperatures increase feeding activity whereas extremely cold, wet, windy, or hot weather decreases feeding activity.

With the exception of sodium, all other minerals and also substances high in vitamins or protein, if available, are consumed or are not consumed according to taste preference. Horses have large individual variations in taste preference, as do people and other animals. For example, some horses and people don't like a sweet taste whereas most do.

Many diseases, nutritional as well as non-nutritional, cause a change in taste preference. For example, horses, as well as cattle, normally prefer grain but may reject grain in favor of hay or even straw bedding when they are sick. When a change in taste preference and, as a result, the feed consumed occurs due to a nutritional deficiency, it is sometimes cited as evidence that the animal knows that it is deficient in that nutrient and is trying to obtain it, i.e., as evidence that the animal has a true appetite for that nutrient. However, numerous examples may be given that indicate this is not true, and instead that there is a change in taste preference with no innate knowledge of what nutrient is deficient.

Animals deficient in phosphorus may chew bones, which are high in phosphorus. However, they may also eat dirt and chew on wood and rocks, which are poor sources of phosphorus. Horses on a calcium-deficient diet will not consume more calcium than those on an adequate calcium diet. Conversely, when ponies fed a phosphorus-deficient diet were offered free access to various mineral salts, including phosphorus, they preferred and consumed more calcium than phosphorus. Calcium ingestion would worsen their deficiency because the additional calcium would decrease phosphorus absorption. Foals on a protein-deficient diet reduce rather than increase their intake of the diet, as would be necessary to consume the additional protein needed to meet their protein needs. Numerous studies such as these with different nutrients have shown similar results. Thus, horses do not consume protein, vitamins, or minerals (with the exception of sodium) according to their needs, and when they are allowed to freely consume nutrients or feeds high in them, there is much individual variation in the amounts consumed. The amount consumed is completely unrelated to dietary needs.

Average consumption of individually offered vitamin and/or mineral supplements by a group of animals may in some cases, by chance only, result in nearly proper levels of intake of some of the vitamins and/or minerals offered. However, intake by the individual animal will vary from too little to excessive. Free-choice, or cafeteria-style, feeding of vitamin, mineral, or protein supplements should never be relied upon to meet the animal's requirements. The only way to ensure that each animal receives its needed vitamins, minerals, and protein is to have the proper amount present in the animal's water or energy-providing feeds. In most instances and for most nutrients, having them present in, or consumed from, the water is not possible; therefore, the nutrients needed must be present in the animal's energy-providing feeds.

Occasionally, vitamins, minerals, or protein supplements, and drugs are added to salt. Although animals have a true appetite for sodium, sodium chloride, or salt, intake is erratic and depends upon the sodium and water content of feeds, so the consumption of substances when added to salt may be quite variable, as described in the section on "Sodium Chloride Salt" in Chapter 2.

INFORMATION NEEDED FOR DIET EVALUATION AND FORMULATION

To formulate or evaluate a diet, three things must be known. These are:

1. The amount of each nutrient needed by or harmful to the animal, i.e., the animal's nutrient requirements and tolerance to excessive or inadequate amounts.
2. The nutrient content of the feeds being consumed or available for feeding.
3. The amount of each feed being consumed or needed to provide the amount of nutrients needed.

How this information is obtained is described in the following three sections of this chapter. Following this is a description of how this information is used to formulate and evaluate the horse's diet, and to prepare a diet based on this formulation that will meet the horse's nutritional needs.

Nutrients Needed in the Horse's Diet

All horses need in their diet the proper amount of energy and protein (as given in Appendix Table 1), 15 different minerals (as given in Appendix Table 2), plus chlorine, 14 vitamins (as given in Appendix Table 3), plus beta carotene, fiber, fat, linoleic acid, and at least four amino acids (lysine, methionine, tryptophane, and threonine). Fortunately, it isn't necessary to formulate or evaluate the horse's diet for each of these 40 different nutrients.

Most nutrients needed are known to be provided in adequate, but not excessive, amounts in common diets for the horse and, therefore, need not be evaluated, unless the specific situations that may result in an excess or deficiency described for each nutrient in Chapters 1, 2 and 3 are present. If one of these situations is present, procedures for formulating or evaluating the diet for any nutrient are identical to that for all other nutrients. With the exception of these uncommon situations, the only nutrients which may be inadequate or excessive in the horse's diet and, therefore, for which the diet generally needs to be formulated or evaluated are: (1) adequate amounts of feed to supply sufficient dietary energy, (2) protein, (3) calcium, (4) phosphorus, (5) in some geographical areas selenium, and for growing horses, (6) zinc and (7) copper. In addition, unless growing forage is being consumed it may be worthwhile to evaluate the vitamin A and E content of the growing horse's and performance horse's diets or to add sufficient amounts of vitamins A and E to their diets to meet their needs. Additional amounts of these vitamins may be beneficial in enhancing rapid growth and resistance to infectious diseases, and in preventing or minimizing exertion-induced muscle damage, although rarely are additional amounts of vitamins A or E necessary to prevent a deficiency. However, for any nutrient or supplement high in specific nutrients that the horse is receiving, the amount of these nutrients being received should be determined to ensure that the amount is not harmful.

Nutrient requirements can be expressed as either the concentration needed in the total diet or the amount needed daily. The concentrations of the major nutrients of concern needed in the horse's total diet are given in Appendix Table 1. The concentrations in the diet of all the minerals and vitamins needed by the horse, as well as the maximum or upper safe concentrations recommended, as compared to the mineral and vitamin concentrations present in horse feeds, are given in Appendix Tables 2 and 3, respectively. The amounts of the major nutrients of concern needed daily by horses weighing 200 to 900 kg (440 to 1980 lbs) are given in Appendix Tables 4-200 to 4-900.

Nutrient Content of Feeds

The contents of the major nutrients of concern in horse feeds (digestible energy, protein, fiber, calcium, and phosphorus) are given in Appendix Table 6 and the compositions of mineral supplements are given in Appendix Table 7. The nutrient contents of mixed grass horse pastures during different seasons of the year are given in Tables 5-1, 5-2, and 5-3. The nutrient content of cereal grains, and of protein and mineral supplements, varies little from the values given; as a result, an analysis of their nutrient content generally isn't necessary. In contrast, the nutrient content of forages (hay, pasture, or silage) may be quite different with differing stages of maturity when cut or grazed, with different cuttings, and with that obtained from different fields and in different years from the same field. Therefore, the values given in Appendix Table 6 for forages should be considered only approximations. Even similar-appearing hay can vary widely in nutrient content. For example, 30 top-quality and similar-appearing alfalfa hays varied from 17 to 25% crude protein, 24 to 38% acid detergent fiber, and 1.1 to 1.35 Mcal digestible energy (DE)/lb of dry matter, while poorer-quality alfalfa may contain less than 15% crude protein, over 40% acid detergent fiber, and less than 0.9 Mcal/lb of dry matter. Thus, alfalfa hay may vary from less than 15% to 25% protein, and 24% to over 40% acid detergent fiber, and provide from less than 0.9 to over 1.35 Mcal/DE/lb. It may also vary from

less than 1 to over 2% calcium and less than 0.10 to near 0.5% phosphorus in its dry matter. In addition, the amount of minerals other than calcium and phosphorus, and of vitamins, in all horse feeds is quite variable. Because of this, only the ranges of the amount of these nutrients present in different types of horse feeds are given (Appendix Tables 2 and 3).

The most accurate way to determine the nutrient content of a feed is to have it analyzed. Local extension services, universities, feed mills, or feed stores can usually provide the information on where to have feeds analyzed. For an analysis to be of benefit, the sample analyzed must be representative of the feed being consumed or considered. Obtaining more leaves and fewer stems than is representative of a forage will result in values higher for all nutrients, and lower in fiber, than are valid. The reverse will occur if more stems and fewer leaves are taken. For example, core samples, grab samples high in leaves, and grab samples with few leaves all from the same square bales of alfalfa hay contained 30, 23, and 40% acid detergent fiber, and 16.4, 20.8, and 11.6% protein, respectively. Even a sample taken from a ground entire flake of the hay, as compared to the core samples, contained 34 versus 30% acid detergent fiber and 14.5 versus 16.4% protein.

Thus, the most important step in determining the nutrient content of a feed is proper sampling. The best method of sampling bales or stacks of hay, haylage, or silage is to use a special hay probe or coring tool that can be used to bore into the feed and remove a core sample (Fig. 6-1). Sample square bales of hay diagonally across the long axis of the bale rather than straight through the center. The feed analysis laboratory, extension service, feed mill, or feed store may have a hay sampling probe available. If one is not available, grab instead of core samples may be taken. A core or grab sample from inside the bale or stack should be taken ideally from 20 small bales from different parts of the field or stack, or for large bales, stacks, or silos obtain samples from 20 different sites. To obtain a meaningful pasture forage sample, unless there is only one species of forage, take samples of only the species that the horse selects when grazing. This may require watching horses grazing that pasture to determine which sites are grazed and forages consumed. A sample should be taken from preferably 10 or more sites. At each grazed site sampled, all forage within about a 1-ft (0.3-m) square, except forage known to be avoided by the horse, should be clipped to 1 inch (2 cm) from the ground. For grain, 2- to 4-oz (50- to 100-g) samples should be taken from at least 20 sites and from a variety of depths in binned or bulk feeds. For grain in sacks, samples should be taken from at least two sites from 10 bags. For grain mixes, ensure that samples are obtained from both the top and bottom to avoid bias due to settling of fines. All samples of each feed obtained should be cut up or ground if long stemmed, and combined and mixed together thoroughly. Then about a 1-lb (0.5-kg) sample of each feed should be placed in an air-tight plastic bag to prevent moisture evaporation, and used for analysis (Fig. 6-2).

Feeds should be analyzed for a minimum of moisture, fiber (crude or preferably acid detergent fiber), crude protein, calcium, and phosphorus contents and calculated di-

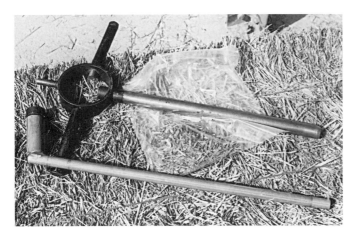

Fig. 6–1. Hay probe used for taking a sample for nutrient analysis. At the top of the figure is the probe, which is sharp at one end to cut into the hay and which has handles at the other end to twist the probe into the hay. Below it is a solid rod used to push the core of hay out of the probe. In the center is a plastic bag containing the hay sample and at left is a cap that is inserted over the sharpened end of the probe when it is not in use.

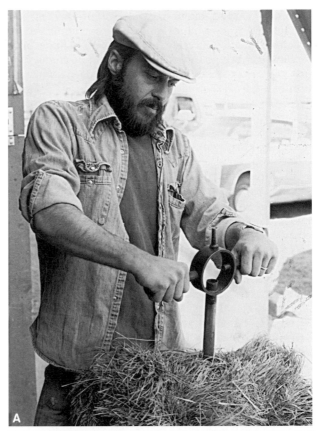

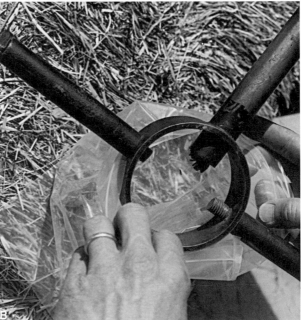

Fig. 6–2(A, B). Taking a hay sample for nutrient analysis using a hay probe. After the probe is bored into the hay (A), the core of hay it contains is removed. Several cores of hay should be taken, put into a plastic bag (B), sealed, and sent to a feed analysis laboratory. Local agricultural extension agents or veterinarians usually know the location of the nearest laboratory. The minimum analysis required to formulate a feeding program for the horse is for crude protein, calcium, and phosphorus. Analysis for moisture, and either crude fiber, TDN, or energy, may also be necessary to assess the quality of the hay.

gestible energy contents for horses. Protein, calcium, and phosphorus contents of the feeds used are needed to formulate or evaluate the diet for these nutrients. Moisture content must be known so that the feed's nutrient content can be put on an equal-moisture basis with other feeds in the diet and with the animals' nutrient requirements. This is necessary to properly evaluate, formulate, or prepare a diet so that the proper amount of nutrients may be fed. Moisture and fiber content are also an indication of feed quality. If the moisture content of hay is greater than 15%, and of grain or a protein supplement is greater than 12 to 13%, the feed may mold or heat sufficiently to decrease protein digestibility and destroy vitamins during storage. If the moisture content of hay is less than 6 to 8%, leaf crumbling and loss, and as a result, nutrient losses, are greater when it is fed.

As the fiber content of a feed increases, its digestible energy, as well as its protein and dry matter digestibility, decrease. Because of this, a relatively good estimate of a feed's digestible energy content may be obtained by using the digestible energy value given in Appendix Table 6 for a similar type of feed with a similar fiber content, or by using the information shown in Table 4–11, which gives the relationship between the crude fiber and digestible energy contents of horse feeds. Values obtained in this manner may be more accurate for the horse than are the values calculated for ruminants, which are what are used by many feed analysis laboratories. However, if utilization values for horses are used by the laboratory in calculating the feed's energy content, that value should be used. The digestible energy content of the feeds used is needed to formulate and evaluate the diet, and to estimate the correct amount to feed. However, there is little correlation between the concentration of one nutrient and that of another nutrient in hay. Thus, inferences about the concentration of nutrient(s) based on the concentration of other nutrient(s) in a hay can be misleading. For example, a hay with a low fiber and high protein concentration may have a calcium or phosphorus content lower, or higher, than average for that type of hay. Thus, formulations and evaluations whenever possible should be based on actual analysis, rather than on averages obtained from feed tables. Analysis values outside of the normal range for that feed, as given in Appendix Table 6, should be evaluated closely, as errors in analysis do occur. If there is any question about a value, a re-analysis, preferably a new sample, should be obtained.

For vitamins and trace minerals of concern in the horse's diet, it is generally less expensive and more practical to add them to the grain mix in a sufficient amount, or to use a grain mix that by itself contains a sufficient amount, to meet the horse's requirements than it is to analyze the feeds for each of these nutrients and determine and add the exact amount needed to the diet. If the feeds being fed don't already contain a sufficient amount of these nutrients to meet the horse's requirements, that added is quite beneficial; if they do, although the additional amount added is of no benefit, it isn't harmful. If the feeds contain a harmful excess, the amount added sufficient by itself to meet the horse's requirements contributes little to the excess. This is because the horse's requirement for these vitamins and minerals is a small percentage of the amount that is harmful; e.g., 2 to 5% for selenium, 1 to 3% for copper, 1 to 12% for zinc, and 10 to 20% for vitamin A. However, to determine if an excess, or a deficiency, of any nutrient is present—i.e., to evaluate the diet for any nutrient—all feeds consumed should be analyzed for that nutrient. In addition, you should determine the amount of that nutrient being received from sources other than the feeds that are being evaluated—e.g., the water, or nutrients being given orally or injected.

Feeds are analyzed by many different methods. The most common method used historically is the proximate or Weende analysis. As shown in Figure 6-3, the proximate analysis of a feed determines its content of moisture, crude fat or ether extract, total minerals or ash, crude fiber and nitrogen, and from it crude protein (which is sufficiently accurate only if all nitrogen in the feed is from protein). By subtracting the percentage of each of these from 100, the percent nonfiber or soluble carbohydrate in the feed, which is often referred to as the nitrogen free extract or NFE, is determined. From the values obtained, the digestible energy, the total digestible nutrient (TDN), content of the feed is frequently calculated. This calculation, however, may be based on values for ruminants, which for forages results in an erroneously high digestible energy content, and for grains and protein supplements an erroneously low value for horses. A major problem with the proximate analysis is that specific minerals or types of fiber aren't determined. The type of fiber may be obtained by the detergent or Van Soest analysis. The higher a feed's fiber content, the greater the benefit of this analysis in obtaining that feed's digestible energy content. Thus, obtaining a feed's acid or neutral detergent fiber content is of most benefit for forages and of little benefit for grain or protein supplements.

Near infrared reflectance spectroscopy (NIRS) is a newer method of feed analysis. It is based on predictive equations. The nutrients in the feed are not measured directly. Because of this, its accuracy is questionable for feeds outside the standard or normal range for that laboratory and, therefore, its results should not be relied on for

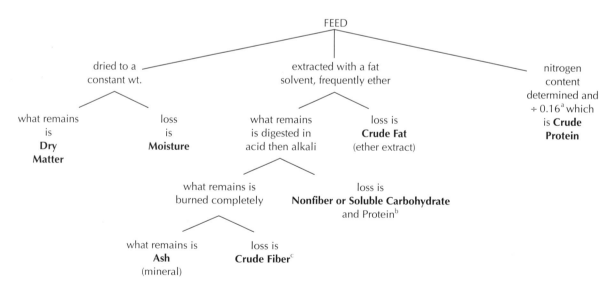

Fig. 6–3. Proximate Analysis of Feeds
[a] Proteins contain 16 ± 2% nitrogen. Crude protein = nitrogen × 6.25, or nitrogen ÷ 0.16. Protein determined by this method will be erroneously high if the food contains nonprotein nitrogen such as urea or ammonia.
[b] It also consists of variable amounts of both soluble and nonsoluble fibers. It is frequently called nitrogen-free extract, or NFE, since it is the extract of acid and alkali digestion less the amount of protein determined from its nitrogen content. It is determined as the difference between 100% and the amount of everything else in the feed, i.e., 100% − % moisture − % crude protein − % crude fat − % crude fiber − % ash. Any errors in these analyses will also appear in the NFE value.
[c] Which is insoluble fibers, primarily cellulose and hemicellulose, not lost by acid and alkali digestion.

analysis of exotic or nontraditional feeds. It is also reported to be unreliable for evaluating grain mix and protein supplements. Its advantages are that it is fast, relatively inexpensive, and usually reports results for acid and neutral detergent fiber, TDN or digestible energy, crude protein, calcium, phosphorus, magnesium, and potassium. However, like other analysis procedures, energy values are frequently those valid for ruminants and not horses.

Methods of Expressing Feed Nutrient Content

Some laboratories report the nutrient content of a feed as the amount present in the feed dry matter; others report it as the amount present in the feed as fed, or as the laboratory received it. If it isn't stated, it will generally be the amount present in the feed as fed. The amount given on the feed tag of commercially available feeds or supplements is the amount present in the feed as fed. The only way that a feed or diet can be accurately formulated, evaluated, or compared to other feeds or the animal's requirements is if all are expressed on an identical moisture, or most accurately on an available calorie, basis. Concentrations on an available-calorie basis can be obtained by dividing the concentration in a feed by that feed's available calories. For example: A feed provides 2 Mcal of digestible energy/kg and contains 1% calcium, i.e., 1 g of calcium/100 g of feed or 10 g of calcium/1000 g or/kg of feed. The feed would therefore contain the following:

$$\frac{10 \text{ g of Ca/kg of feed}}{2 \text{ Mcal DE/kg of feed}} = \frac{10 \text{ g Ca}}{2 \text{ Mcal DE}} = \frac{5 \text{ g Ca}}{\text{Mcal DE}}$$

However, the available calories provided by a feed or diet frequently aren't known; therefore, most commonly the nutrient content of feeds, and animals' requirements, are expressed on or converted to an equal-moisture basis. The best way to ensure that all are on an equal-moisture basis is to determine the amount of all nutrients in the feed or diet dry matter, i.e., the concentration of each nutrient that would be in the feed or diet if it did not contain any water or moisture.

Although for formulating and evaluating the diet it is necessary to have the amount of nutrients in all feeds and needed by the animal expressed on an equal-moisture basis, in preparing and feeding a diet the amount of all feeds must be on an as-fed basis. For example, you don't feed 9 lbs of hay dry matter, you feed 10 lbs of hay, which in this example happens to contain 1 lb of, or 10%, moisture.

Thus, it is necessary to be able to convert back and forth from a dry matter to an as-fed basis. There are two rules that must be remembered to do this. These are:

1. Always use the dry-matter fraction; never the moisture fraction. Since a feed or diet consists of two parts—dry matter and moisture—the dry matter fraction is 1 minus the moisture fraction. For example, a feed containing 12% moisture contains a dry-matter fraction of 1 − 0.12 = 0.88, or 88% dry matter.
2. Stop and think: should the value wanted be larger or smaller than the value being converted, then either multiply or divide the value being converted by the

dry-matter fraction, whichever is necessary, so that the answer obtained is larger or smaller, whichever you know the answer should be. For example:

a. Since the weight of a feed as fed contains some water, it will always be larger than that amount of feed dry matter, so you would either multiply or divide the weight of feed being converted by that feed's dry-matter fraction so that your answer is either smaller or larger than the value being converted, whichever you know the answer must be. For example: 18 lbs of feed dry matter, which as fed contains 10% moisture and therefore a dry-matter fraction of 1 − 0.10 or 0.90. The pounds of this feed as fed—i.e., containing 10% moisture—would have to be greater than the 18 lbs of the feed without any moisture. Therefore, you would divide the

$$\frac{18 \text{ lbs of feed dry matter by}}{\text{the feed's dry matter fraction of } 0.90}$$

$$= \begin{array}{l} \text{to get 20 lbs of feed as} \\ \text{fed, which is correct.} \end{array}$$

If instead you multiplied the

18 lbs of feed dry matter by
the feed's dry-matter fraction of 0.90,
you would get
16.2 lbs of feed as fed, which is wrong.

You know this cannot be correct since the feed with some water in it cannot weigh less than it did without that water in it.

Conversely, for 20 lbs of feed as fed, which contains 10% moisture, if the moisture isn't there, what's left (i.e., the amount of dry matter) must be less than 20 lbs. Therefore, you would multiply the

20 lbs of feed as fed by
the feed's dry-matter fraction of 0.90 to get
18 lbs of the feed dry matter, which is correct.

If instead you divided the

$$\frac{20 \text{ lbs of feed as fed by}}{\text{the feed's dry matter fraction of } 0.90}$$

$$= \begin{array}{l} \text{you would get 22.2 lbs of} \\ \text{feed as fed, which is wrong.} \end{array}$$

You know this cannot be correct since the feed without any water cannot weigh more than it did when it contained some water.

b. The concentration of a nutrient in a feed as fed is always smaller than it is in the feed's dry matter because when the feed is diluted by including with it some water, it will decrease the concentration of everything else in the feed. So you would either multiply or divide the nutrient concentration in the feed by that feed's dry-matter fraction so that the answer is either smaller or larger than the nutrient concentration being converted, whichever you know the answer should be.

For example: 20% protein in a grass's dry matter, which as fed contains 75% moisture and, therefore, a dry-matter fraction of 1 − 0.75, or 0.25. The percent protein in the grass as fed, i.e., containing or diluted with 75% moisture, would have to be less than the 20% in its dry matter. Therefore, you would multiply the

20% protein in the grass's dry matter by
the grass's dry-matter fraction of 0.25 to get
5% protein in the grass as fed, which is correct.

If instead you divided the

$$\frac{\text{20\% protein in the grass dry matter by}}{\text{the grass's dry matter fraction of 0.25}}$$

= you would get 80% protein in the grass as fed, which is wrong.

You know this cannot be correct since the concentration diluted by including some water with the feed cannot be greater than the concentration that exists when the feed doesn't contain any water diluting the concentration of everything else in the feed.

Conversely, 5% protein and 75% moisture in a grass as fed. If the moisture is removed, it will increase the concentration of the protein in what is left, i.e., in the grass's dry matter. Therefore, you would divide the

$$\frac{\text{5\% protein in the grass as fed by}}{\text{the grass's dry matter fraction of 0.25}}$$

= to get 20% protein in the grass's dry matter, which is correct.

If instead you multiplied the

5% protein in the grass as fed by
the grass's dry matter fraction of 0.25, you would get 1.25% protein in the grass's dry matter, which is wrong.

You know this cannot be correct since the grass without water cannot have nutrient concentrations lower than they were when the grass contained water, or when everything in it was diluted by its water content.

Amount of Feed Needed by the Horse

The amount of feed needed depends on the horse's energy needs and the energy content of the feeds consumed. The energy contents of horse feeds are given in Appendix Table 6. The horse's energy needs depend on numerous factors, including its body weight, function (e.g., growth rate or stage of pregnancy or lactation), physical activity, and environment, and varies between individuals as discussed in the section on "Energy Needs" in Chapter 1. The average energy needs for the horse, based on its weight, function, and physical activity, can be obtained from Appendix Tables 4 and 5. To obtain this information, the weight of the horse must be known or determined.

Obtaining a Horse's Weight

Obtaining the horse's body weight is useful for many purposes, including:

1. Determining the amount of feed needed.
2. Determining the adequacy of the feeding program so, if needed, feeding practices can be changed accordingly.
3. As an early indication of health problems.
4. As an aid in training and competing optimally.
5. To assist in maximizing breeding efficiency.
6. To determine the proper amount of drugs or other substances to give.

Overfeeding or underfeeding, resulting in a gradual weight change, generally isn't apparent until changes are severe. Inadequate or excessive growth rate also may not be readily apparent. Inadequate feed intake resulting in weight loss is one of the first indications of many illnesses. Horses, like other athletes, have an optional performance weight. Racehorses' optimal racing weight has been reported to be within a 16-lb (7.3-kg) range; much less than can be detected from the horse's appearance. Reproductive efficiency is also greatest within a certain body-weight range. Thus, there are many reasons for obtaining and monitoring the horse's weight. The best way to do this is by using a walk-on scale. However, the horse's weight can vary greatly with degree of hydration and gastrointestinal fill. Up to a 5% decrease in body weight due to dehydration cannot be detected visually, and the horse's body weight may vary from 5 to 10% depending on the time since feeding and feed type. To alleviate errors in the body weight obtained, and to correct for changes in body weight due to variations in the degree of hydration and gastrointestinal fill, the horse should be weighed at a consistent time prior to feeding, watering, and physical activity, such as training or competing. If a scale isn't available, a fairly accurate estimate of the horse's weight can be obtained from accurate body measurements.

A girth measurement alone is fairly accurate, but accuracy can be improved by also measuring the horse's length and by using the following formulas.

Lb body wt = [Heart girth (in)^2 × length (in)] ÷ 330

Kg body wt = [Heart girth (cm)^2 × length (cm)] ÷ 11,880

A fairly accurate estimate of the horse's body weight can be calculated from this equation or from the nomogram derived from it and shown in Figure 6-4.

For light horse breed foals 1 to 6 weeks of age, a more accurate weight may be obtained from the following formulas.

Lb body wt = (Heart girth in inches − 25.1) ÷ 0.07

Kg body wt = (Heart girth in cm − 63.7) ÷ 0.38

The actual weight of light horse breed foals at 1, 2, 3 and 4 weeks of age was found to be within 5% of that calculated from this formula. However, to obtain this accu-

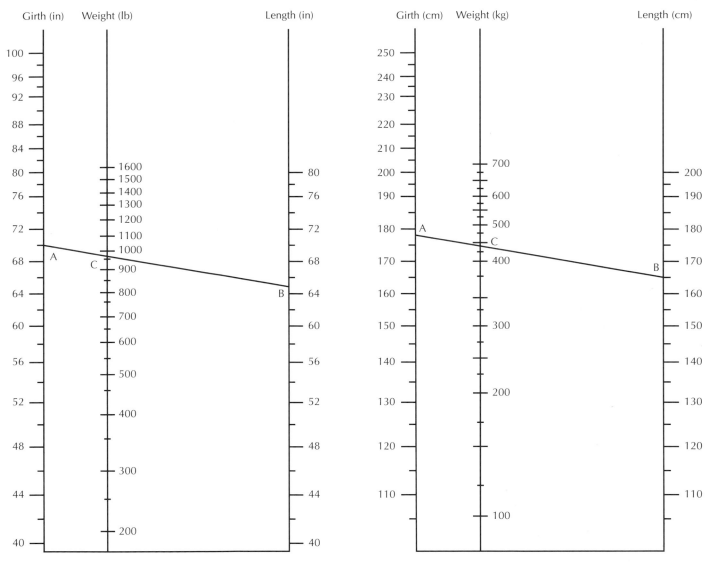

Girth (in)   Weight (lb)   Length (in)   Girth (cm)   Weight (kg)   Length (cm)

Fig. 6–4. Nomograms for estimating a horse's weight from girth and length measurements. Girth is measured just behind the withers and elbows following respiratory expiration, and length is measured from the anterior point of the shoulders to the posterior point of the buttocks (tuber ischii) (illustrated in Fig. 6–5). Example: A horse's girth is measured as 178 cm (70 in), which is plotted on the girth scale above as point A, and length is measured as 165 cm (65 in), which is plotted on the length scale as point B. Where a straight line drawn from point A to point B crosses the weight scale, indicated above as point C, is the horse's weight, which in this example is 440 kg (968 lb).

racy for foals at birth and at 12 weeks of age 17%, or ⅙, must be added to the weight obtained using this formula.

Heart girth should be measured just behind the withers and elbows (where the cinch goes) following respiratory expiration; body length should be measured from the anterior point of the shoulder to the posterior point of the buttocks (tuber ischii) (Fig. 6–5). For accuracy in measuring length, two people are needed—one to hold each end of the tape.

A slightly less accurate but still good estimate of the horse's weight can be obtained from the girth measurement alone and the information given in Table 6–1, or by using a horse-weight tape (Fig. 6–6). A horse-weight tape is used to measure the heart girth and is marked in pounds or kilograms of body weight corresponding to the girth

measurement for the average horse. However, a heart girth measurement without the correction indicated in Table 6–1 is not accurate for pregnant mares. A heart girth measurement is also not sufficiently accurate to detect small changes in weight that influence physical performance, but it is quite adequate for estimating the amount of feed needed, and is much more accurate than a body-weight estimate based on visual examination.

Many horse people believe they can estimate fairly closely the horse's weight just by looking at the horse. Perhaps some can, but most cannot, as shown by the following study. Seventy-seven farm managers and 62 veterinarians with an average of 17 and 21 years of professional experience with horses, respectively, from visual examination estimated the weight of five horses of varying size.

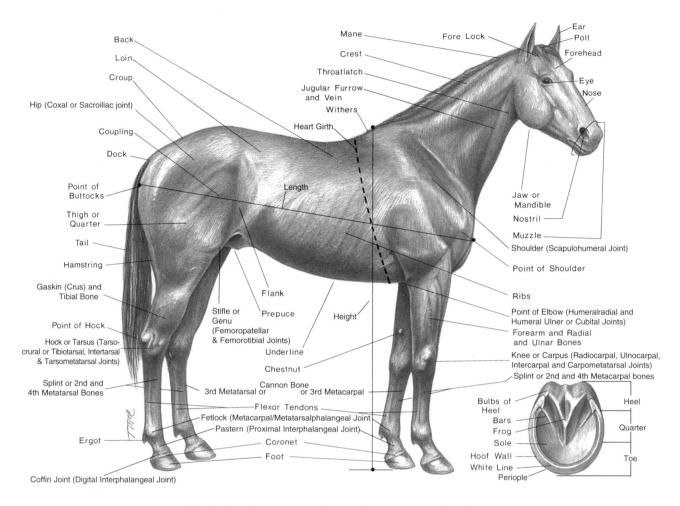

Fig. 6–5. Major external anatomic structures of the horse.

Of the 695 estimates, 12.5% were over the horses' actual weight by an average of 92 lbs (42 kg)/horse, and 87.5% were under by an average of 186 lbs (85 kg)/horse. Nearly 60% underestimated all five horses. There was no correlation between accuracy and years of professional experience with horses.

Determining Total Amount of Feed Needed by the Horse

The amount of feed needed can be calculated, as shown in the following examples, by dividing the horse's dietary energy needs by the energy provided by the feed(s) consumed. When done correctly, the amount obtained will be quite accurate for the average horse, or group of horses, under similar conditions and fed feeds similar to that used in the calculation. However, the feed needed by the individual horse may be more or less than the amount determined because of (1) variations among horses in their dietary energy needs, (2) variations in the amount of feed consumed and the amount wasted or lost, (3) differences in environmental conditions, and (4) differences in the energy content of the feeds consumed. Always feed the

amount needed to maintain the horse at optimum body weight and condition. To ensure that this is done, monitor each horse's weight periodically and change the feeding program as needed.

Example 1: Idle Mature Horse. Determine the amount of feed needed by a 900-lb (409 kg) idle mature horse. This value can be obtained by interpolating between the amounts needed by the 400- and 500-kg horse, as given in Appendix Tables 4 as 13.4 and 16.4 Mcal/day, respectively. The 409-kg horse therefore would need the following amount:

$$13.4 + (16.4 - 13.4) \times (409 - 500/500 - 400)$$
$$= 13.4 + (3) \times (0.09)$$
$$= 13.4 + 0.27 = 13.67 \text{ Mcal/day}$$

To determine the amount of feed needed to provide this amount of energy, divide the amount of energy needed by the energy that the feed provides. Thus, if early-bloom alfalfa hay, which provides 1.1 Mcal/lb of dry matter (DM) (as given in Appendix Table 6), were the only feed con-

TABLE 6–1
Estimating a Horse's Weight from Girth Measurement*

Girth Length (inches)	Weight (lbs)	Girth Length (cm)	Weight (kgs)**
32	100	80	45
40	200	90	70
45	275	100	90
50	375	110	120
55	500	120	150
60	650	130	185
62	720	140	230
64	790	150	285
66	860	160	345
68	930	170	410
70	1000	180	475
72	1070	190	545
74	1140	200	615
76	1210		
78	1290		
80	1370		

* Girth is measured just behind the withers and elbows (as shown in Figures 6–5 and 6–6).
** For pregnant mares, multiply the value obtained by 1.02, 1.06, 1.11, and 1.17 for their weight at 8, 9, 10, and 11 months of pregnancy, respectively.

sumed, this horse would need to consume the following amount of it.

(13.67 Mcal DE/day needed) ÷ (1.1 Mcal/lb DM)

= 12.4 lbs of hay dry matter/day needed

However, dry matter isn't being fed. Hay is being fed, and, as given in Appendix Table 6 or from its analysis, it contains 90% dry matter. Therefore, to obtain 12.4 lbs of dry matter, the horse would need to consume the following amount of hay:

(12.4 lbs hay DM/day) ÷ (0.90 DM fraction)

= 13.8 lbs of hay as fed/day needed

Generally, an additional 10 to 15% of hay must be fed to allow for that wasted and lost. Thus, in this example the following amount should be fed:

(13.8 lbs of hay/day needed) × (1.15 loss factor)

= about 16 lbs of hay/day

If small square bales weighing 60 to 65 lbs each are being fed, about ⅛ of a bale/horse each morning and night would provide the amount of hay needed.

If 2 lbs of regular oats were fed daily, they would provide the following:

(2 lbs) × (0.90 DM fraction from Appendix Table 6)

= 1.8 lbs of DM

(1.8 lbs DM) × (1.45 Mcal/lb DM from Appendix Table 6)

= 2.6 Mcal/day

Feeding 2 lbs of oats/day would reduce the amount of hay needed by 3 lbs/day, as determined below.

(2.6 Mcal/day from oats) ÷ (1.1 Mcal/lb of hay DM)

= 2.36 lbs hay DM/day

(2.36 lbs of hay DM/day) ÷ (0.90 DM fraction)

= 2.6 lbs of hay/day

2.6 lbs of hay/day × 1.15 loss factor = 3.0 lbs of hay/day

Thus, if 2 lbs of oats/day were fed, you would also need to feed about 13 lbs of early-bloom alfalfa hay/day. This is instead of the 16 lbs/day that should be fed when no oats are fed.

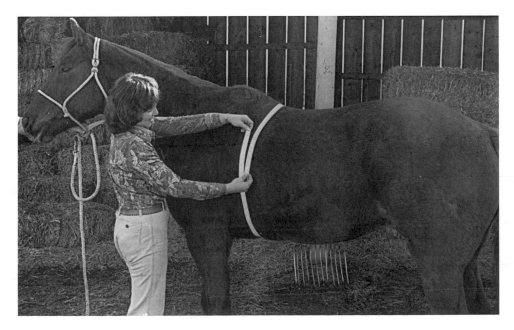

Fig. 6–6. Estimating the horse's weight from measurement of the girth. A weight tape marked in pounds of body weight (which for the average horse correlates well) is available from some feed stores and tack shops. A tape measure and the information given in Table 6–1 may be used instead.

Example 2: Working Horse. A 1400-lb (636-kg) horse ridden at a slow trot for 3 hours/day for 3 days/week needs:

1. For maintenance from Appendix Table 4 or the formula:
   DE = 1.4 + (0.03 × kg body wt). Thus
   1.4 + (0.03 × 636 kg) = 20.5 Mcal/day
2. For work (from Appendix Table 5) DE = 0.6 Mcal/hr/100 kg × 9 hrs/week × (636 kg of horse + 64 kg of tack and rider) = 37.8 Mcal/week or 5.4 Mcal/day.
3. Total = 20.5 + 5.4 = 25.9 Mcal/day needed.

If the physical activity in this example is equivalent to light work, two other ways to estimate total energy needs for this 636-kg horse would be:

1. DE = 1.25 × (maintenance needs of 20.5 Mcal/day from step #1 above) = 25.6 Mcal/day.
2. By interpolating between the values given for a 600- and for a 700-kg horse, as given in Appendix Tables 4–600 and 4–700, as shown below:

600-kg horse needs of 24.3 Mcal
+ (700-kg horse needs of 26.6 Mcal − 24.3 Mcal)
× [(636 − 600) ÷ (700 − 600)]
= 24.3 Mcal + [(2.3 Mcal)] × (0.36)]
= 24.3 + 0.83 = 25.1 Mcal/day

If good-quality (early-growth) grass hay providing 0.9 Mcal/lb of dry matter and containing 90.5% dry matter (such as given in Appendix Table 6) is being fed, the following amount would be needed:

(25.9 Mcal/day needed) ÷ (0.9 Mcal/lb DM)

= 28.8 lb DM/day needed

(28.8 lb DM/day) ÷ (0.905 DM fraction)

= 31.8 lbs hay/day needed

To receive 31.8 lbs of hay/day, the following amount should be fed:

(31.8 lbs hay/day) × 1.15 loss factor = 36.6 lbs hay/day

Finally, determine if the horse can consume the amount of hay needed. The amount of hay needed daily is equal to 2.6% of the horse's body weight (36.6 ÷ 1400 = 2.6%). As given in Appendix Table 1, the mature horse can consume a total amount of air-dry feed equal to 3% of its body weight daily. Since the amount needed (2.6%) is less than 3%, the horse could consume enough hay to meet its energy needs. If energy needs were sufficiently high, and/or the energy density of the hay was sufficiently low, so that the amount of feed needed daily was more than 3% of the horse's weight, a higher-energy-dense feed, such as grain, would need to be fed to provide sufficient energy to meet the horse's needs in a lower amount of feed.

Another feeding program, and one frequently preferred, is to feed a sufficient amount of hay to supply energy needs for maintenance, and enough grain to supply the additional energy needed for physical activity. Thus, the amount of hay fed would remain constant and the amount of grain fed would be gradually increased or decreased as needed. In this example, if this type of feeding program were used, and cracked corn was the grain fed to provide the energy needed for physical activity, the feeding program would be the following.

1. Hay needed for maintenance is:
   20.5 Mcal/day needed for maintenance (from first step, above) divided by 0.9 Mcal/lb hay DM (from Appendix Table 6) = 22.8 lbs hay dry matter and, therefore, (22.8 lbs hay DM) ÷ (0.905 DM fraction from Appendix Table 6) = 25.2 lbs hay/day needed.
   (25.2 lbs hay/day needed) × (1.15 loss factor) = 29 lbs hay/day to feed
2. The amount of corn, which provides 1.7 Mcal/lb of dry matter and contains 88% DM (from Appendix Table 6) needed for physical activity is:
   (5.4 Mcal/day from the second step, above) ÷ (1.7 Mcal/lb DM) = 3.2 lbs corn DM/day
   (3.2 lbs corn DM) ÷ (0.88 DM fraction) = 3.6 lbs corn/day
   (3.6 lbs corn/day) ÷ 1.6 lbs cracked corn/qt from Appendix Table 8 = 2¼ qts cracked corn/day
   Thus, the feeding program would be to feed either 35 to 40 lbs of hay/day, or 29 lbs of hay and 2¼ qts of cracked corn daily.

DIET EVALUATION AND FORMULATION PROCEDURES

The most important attributes needed to accomplish anything are first the desire to do it and second taking the initiative to start it. The most important thing needed to get started is knowing where to start and how to proceed. For diet evaluation or formulation, the place to start and the way to proceed is to begin with the nutrient needed in the greatest amount, then proceed to that needed in the next greatest amount, etc., until the diet has been evaluated or formulated for all nutrients of concern.

Although all nutrients are necessary for life, the amounts needed vary tremendously and in the following order of magnitude, from greatest to least:

1. *Water*—Even at rest in a comfortable environmental temperature, 2 to 3 times more water is needed than feed supplying all of the other nutrients; and nutrient needs for physical activity or a warmer environmental temperature increase more for water than for any other nutrient.
2. *Energy-providing nutrients*—From 80 to 90% of all food consumed by the horse is needed and is used for energy.
3. *Protein*—From 8 to 14.5% of food dry matter ingested by the horse is needed for protein functions other than as a source of energy, although for nursing foals it is as high as 25% early in life.
4. *Minerals*—Only 2 to 3% of the total diet is needed to provide all of the many minerals needed by the horse.
5. *Vitamins*—All vitamin needs are met with only 0.2 to 0.3% of the diet as vitamins.

If there is inadequate intake of more than one nutrient, the first and major effect will be as a result of the nutrient for which there is the greatest deficit. For example, if an animal is not eating or drinking, although a body deficit for all nutrients develops, the major deficit is water, since more of it is needed than any other nutrient. If the animal is drinking but not eating, dietary energy will be the major deficit. If water and either carbohydrates, fats, or both are provided in a sufficient quantity to meet the animal's needs, the greatest deficit will be protein, and so on for each nutrient.

Not only will the first and major effect of inadequate nutrient intake be as a result of the nutrient for which there is the greatest deficit, but the body will forsake other nutrient needs to try to correct or minimize the deficit which is greatest. For example, with inadequate water intake, animals will decrease their water needs by reducing feed intake. With inadequate feed intake, the body will use protein, both in the diet as well as that in the body, for energy, again forsaking protein needs to try to minimize the greater deficit for energy. Thus, you cannot meet an animal's needs for dietary energy unless you first meet its needs for water. Nor can you meet the animal's protein needs unless you first meet its energy needs, and so on for other nutrients. Because of this, the diet should always be evaluated, formulated, and corrected in the order of the nutrient needed in the greater amount first. First ensure that there is adequate water and feed to meet the horse's water and energy needs. Then ensure that the feed contains adequate protein, then minerals, and last vitamins. This should also be done within each class of nutrient. For example, for minerals, ensure that calcium and phosphorus needs are met before evaluating, and, if necessary, correcting, a zinc or copper deficiency. The amount of each nutrient needed in the horse's diet and, therefore, the order in which the diet should be evaluated or formulated are given in Appendix Tables 1, 2, and 3.

Don't become enamored with a currently in-vogue nutrient before ensuring that there is adequate intake of other nutrients that are needed in greater quantity. However, if it is known that in a particular situation a deficiency or excess of a certain nutrient doesn't occur, the diet does not need to be formulated or evaluated for that nutrient. In doing this, you have not forgotten or ignored that nutrient, you simply know that its intake is neither inadequate nor excessive. For example, even though over 100 times more sulfur than copper is needed in the horse's diet, because neither a sulfur deficiency nor excess has ever been reported or known to occur in the horse consuming natural feeds (whereas inadequate copper intake does occur), the diet should be evaluated or formulated for copper but not for sulfur.

The nutrients that may be inadequate or excessive in the horse's diet are the following, listed in the order of the amount needed in the diet and, therefore, the order in which the horse's diet should be formulated or evaluated and, if necessary, corrected: (1) water, (2) feed to supply sufficient energy, (3) protein, (4) calcium, (5) phosphorus, (6) common salt, or sodium chloride, (7) in some geographic areas, selenium, and, (8) zinc, copper, and vitamin A for growing horses, and (9) vitamin E for physical exertion. If adequate water, feed, and salt are available, this reduces the number of nutrients of concern in the mature horse's diet in most areas and circumstances to only three (protein, calcium, and phosphorus) with two additional nutrients (zinc and copper) of concern for growth. In addition, unless growing forage constitutes most of the horse's diet, additional vitamins A and E may be beneficial, although rarely are they necessary to prevent a deficiency. The horse may suffer from a variety of diseases or problems as a result of deficiencies or excesses of nutrients other than these in the situations described for each mineral and vitamin in Chapters 2 and 3. However, under normal conditions, using average- or better-quality feeds, it is generally not necessary to consider nutrients other than these in feeding programs for horses. The exception would be if feeds or supplements high in other nutrients are being given to the horse, in which case the amount of these nutrients that the horse is receiving should be determined to ensure that the amount being received is not harmful.

Thus, in evaluating or formulating the horse's diet, begin by ensuring that there is adequate feed intake to meet energy needs, then ensure that the feeds ingested meet the horse's requirements for: (1) protein, (2) calcium, (3) phosphorus, (4) for the growing horse, zinc and copper, (5) for the horse receiving only brown or yellow forage (hay or pasture), vitamin A, and (6) for the performance horse in use or training not receiving growing forage, vitamin E. Computer programs for evaluating and formulating horse's diets are available and can be quite helpful in rapidly obtaining the information needed. For example, one available from Purdue University calculates the horse's nutrient requirements when the horse's category, weight, and activity are entered. These requirements can be customized for a particular situation or horse, if desired. The program contains the average table values for the nutrient content of feeds, such as given in Appendix Table 6, but different feed nutrient contents can be used to reflect the actual feeds being fed if more accurate values for these are known. Based on this information, the program analyzes the diet for digestible energy, crude protein, calcium, phosphorus, magnesium, and potassium, and compares these values to the horse's requirements for these nutrients. The program calculates the amount of additional major minerals needed and formulates a grain mix that, with the forage being consumed, will meet the horse's requirements. However, to use this or any computer program successfully, you should know and understand what the program is doing. Frequently, it is necessary to evaluate and formulate diets for nutrients not included in the computer program being used. The following examples describe how to evaluate and formulate a diet.

Regardless of the nutrient for which a diet is being evaluated or formulated, the same procedures described in the examples given are used. The reader ought do the mathematics for each sample to become familiar with the procedure. Note that the same procedures are repeated for each nutrient and in each feeding situation or example.

Example 1—Weanlings on Pasture. A 6-month-old, 475-lb (216-kg) weanling is on average-quality mature grass pasture with ample forage for the weanling to eat all it wants. Based on its parents, it's anticipated that its mature weight will be 1100 lbs (500 kg). Formulate a grain mix that, when fed in the amount necessary to obtain a rapid growth rate, will, along with the pasture forage, meet the weanling's requirements for all nutrients of concern (energy, protein, calcium, phosphorus, zinc, copper, and vitamin A).

1. Obtain the nutrient content of the forage being consumed
   a. most accurately and preferably by having clippings of the pasture grasses being eaten analyzed for protein, calcium, phosphorus, and fiber, from which an estimate of the forage's energy content can be made, or
   b. from feed tables (e.g., Appendix Table 6) which indicate that mature grass pasture forage generally contains in its dry matter: 0.75 Mcal digestible energy/lb, 8% protein, 0.25% calcium, and 0.2% phosphorus.

2. Determine what percent of the diet should be a grain mix. Since in this example a rapid growth rate is wanted and a forage that is not high in energy or protein is being consumed, the maximum percentage of grain mix should be fed, which, as given in Appendix Table 1, is 70%. Therefore, the diet will consist of 70% grain mix and 30% forage. If a higher energy and protein forage, such as a good-quality alfalfa or alfalfa-grass mix forage, was being eaten, a diet consisting of no more than 50% grain mix would be quite adequate and preferred.

3. Determine the amount of each nutrient that the forage contributes to the total diet by multiplying the fraction of forage in the diet by the amount of each nutrient in the forage. For example, as shown below for protein, the forage contains 8% protein, but since the forage only makes up 30% (or the fraction 0.3) of the diet, it only contributes 0.3 times 8%, or 2.4%, protein to the diet.

		Nutrients in Feed Dry Matter (from step 1)								
	Fraction of Feed in Diet	DE (Mcal/lb) in		Protein (%) in		Calcium (%) in		Phosphorus (%) in		
Feed	(from step 2)	feed	diet	feed	diet	feed	diet	feed	diet	
Forage	0.3	× 0.75 =	0.225	× 8 =	2.4	× 0.25 =	0.075	× 0.20 =	0.06	

4. Obtain the amount of each nutrient needed by the horse. In this example, it indicates in Appendix Table 1 that the 6-month-old weanling's diet dry matter should contain 1.3 Mcal DE/lb, 14.5% protein, 0.7% calcium, and 0.4% phosphorus.

5. Determine the amount of each nutrient that the grain mix must contribute to the diet so that it, plus the nutrients provided by the forage, will provide a sufficient amount of each nutrient to meet the

horse's needs. As shown below, this is done by subtracting each nutrient provided by the forage (as obtained in step 3) from total needs for that nutrient (as obtained in step 4) to get the amount of each nutrient the grain mix must contribute to the diet. For example, as shown below for protein: 14.5% protein needed (from step 4) − 2.4% protein provided from forage (from step 3) = 12.1% protein needed from the grain mix.

	Fraction of Feed in Diet	DE (Mcal/lb) in		Protein (%) in		Calcium (%) in		Phosphorus (%) in	
Feed	(from step 2)	feed	diet	feed	diet	feed	diet	feed	diet
Forage (from step 3)	0.3	0.75	0.225 ↓	8	2.4 ↓	0.25	0.075 ↓	0.20	0.06 ↓
Grain mix	0.7		1.3–0.225 ↑		14.5–2.4 ↑		0.7–0.075 ↑		0.4–0.06 ↑
Total or needed (from step 4)			1.3		14.5		0.7		0.4

6. Determine the amount of each nutrient that must be in the grain mix so that it will provide the amount of nutrients that it must contribute to the diet. As shown below, this is done by dividing the amount of each nutrient that the grain mix needs to contribute by the fraction of grain mix in the diet. For example, the grain mix needs to contribute 14.5 − 2.4, or 12.1%, protein to the diet (from step 5), but since

the grain mix makes up only 70% (or the fraction 0.7) of the diet (from step 2), for it to contribute 12.1% protein to the diet it must contain 12.1% ÷ 0.70, or 17.3%, protein.

7. Thus, from step 6 we have determined that the grain mix should contain in its dry matter 1.075 ÷ 0.7 or 1.54 Mcal/lb, 12.1 ÷ 0.7 or 17.3% protein, 0.625 ÷ 0.7 or 0.893% calcium, and 0.34 ÷ 0.7 or 0.486%

	Fraction of Feed in Diet	DE (Mcal/lb) in		Protein (%) in		Calcium (%) in		Phosphorus (%) in	
Feed	(from step 2)	feed	diet	feed	diet	feed	diet	feed	diet
Forage (from step 3)	0.3	0.75	0.225	8	2.4	0.25	0.075	0.20	0.06
Grain mix	0.7	1.075 ÷ 0.7	1.075	12.1 ÷ 0.7	12.1	0.625 ÷ 0.7	0.625	0.34 ÷ 0.7	0.34
Total or needed (from step 4)			1.3		14.5		0.7		0.4

phosphorus. If the grain mix contained 10% moisture and, therefore, a dry matter fraction of 0.90 as fed, it would need to contain 1.54 × 0.90 or 1.4 Mcal/lb, 17.3% × 0.90 or 16% protein, 0.893% × 0.90 or 0.8% calcium, and 0.486 × 0.90 or 0.45% phosphorus. Thus, the grain mix should contain the following.

Nutrients Needed in Grain Mix

	DE (Mcal/lb)	Protein (%)	Calcium (%)	Phosphorus (%)
Dry Matter	1.54	17.3	0.893	0.486
As Fed	1.4	16	0.8	0.45

A grain mix containing these, or greater, amounts of each of these nutrients might be purchased and fed. If this were done, steps 8 and 9 that follow are unnecessary and you would skip to step 10.

8. The amount of ingredients to use in a custom or home-prepared grain mix containing these nutrient levels may be determined in the following manner. As always, begin with the nutrient needed in the greatest quantity first, then the next greatest quantity, etc. Thus, begin with energy, then protein, next calcium, and last phosphorus.

a. *Energy*—For the grain mix to provide 1.54 Mcal/lb of dry matter needed as determined in step 7, as indicated in Appendix Table 6, any combination of corn, barley, and wheat could be used, and 50 to 70% oats, but not more as oats provide only 1.45 Mcal/lb of dry matter.

b. *Protein*—From Appendix Table 6, we find that barley, corn, and wheat (soft) contain 13, 8 to 10, and 11 to 12% protein in their dry matter, respectively. A mixture of these cereal grains will, therefore, contain about 11% protein, and we want 17.3% in the grain-mix dry matter (as determined in step 7). Thus, a protein supplement must be added to the grain. Since the grain mix is for the growing horse, the protein supplement used should be high in lysine. The protein supplement generally most available in the United States and high in lysine is soybean meal (SBM), which contains 50% protein in its dry matter (Appendix Table 6). From 5 to 10% wet molasses, fat, or oil would be needed in a mixture of grain and SBM to keep the SBM from sifting out. Molasses contains 2 to 6% protein (Appendix Table 6). Therefore, a mixture of 92% grain plus 8% molasses would contain 11% × 0.92 = 10.1% protein from grain, plus about 4% × 0.08 = 0.3% protein from molasses, for a total of 10.1 + 0.3 or 10.4% protein.

Next we must determine the amount of SBM that needs to be added to increase the protein content of the grain mix from 10.4 to the 17.3% needed. One of the easiest ways to determine the proportional amount of two feeds needed to provide a certain nutrient concentration in their mixture is by using a procedure called Pearson square. This procedure is performed in the following manner. As shown below, the percent of the nutrient wanted in the mixture of the two feeds is placed in the center of the square, in this example, 17.3%. The percentage of that nutrient in the one feed or the diet (or in this case, in the grain mix) is placed at the upper left corner. In this case, it is 10.4%. The percent of that nutrient in the other feed or supplement is placed at the lower left corner. Here it is 50%. Next, the number in the middle is subtracted from the number at the lower left corner, and the result is placed at the upper right corner: in this case 50 − 17.3 = 32.7. Then the number at the upper left corner is subtracted from the number in the middle, and the answer is placed at the lower right corner: in this case 17.3 − 10.4 = 6.9. Add the two numbers at the right corners: in this case 32.7 + 6.9 = 39.6. Then divide the number at each right corner by this sum: in this case 32.7 ÷ 39.6 = 0.826 and 6.9 ÷ 39.6 = 0.174.

The values obtained (0.826 and 0.174) are the fractions of each of the feeds, whose nutrient contents were placed at the corresponding upper or lower corner, that are needed in the mixture of the two feeds so that the resulting mixture contains the amount of that nutrient placed in the center of the square: in this example, 0.826 parts grain mix and 0.174 parts of the protein supplement SBM. Thus, in order for the mixture of cereal grains and molasses, and SBM to contain 17.3% protein, there must be 82.6% grains and molasses, and 17.4% SBM in the mixture. However, since we may need to add some mineral supplements to the grain mix, which will dilute its protein content slightly, it is best to round the amount of SBM up from 17.4 to 18%. The resulting grain mix should contain the amount of protein shown below.

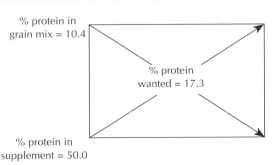

% protein in grain mix = 10.4

% protein wanted = 17.3

% protein in supplement = 50.0

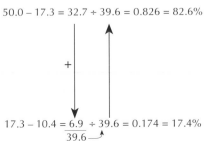

50.0 − 17.3 = 32.7 ÷ 39.6 = 0.826 = 82.6%

17.3 − 10.4 = 6.9 ÷ 39.6 = 0.174 = 17.4%
          ───
          39.6

Feed	Fraction in Grain Mix Dry Matter		Protein (%) in feed		in mix
Grain	0.74	×	11	=	8.14
SBM	0.18	×	50	=	9.00
Molasses	0.08	×	4	=	0.32
Total	1.00	×			17.46

c. *Calcium and Phosphorus*—From Appendix Table 6 we find that the feeds contain the amounts of calcium and phosphorus in their dry matter shown below; therefore, the grain mix contains the amount of calcium and phosphorus shown as compared to that wanted.

Feed	Fraction of Grain Mix Dry Matter		Calcium (%) in feed		in mix	Phosphorus (%) in feed		in mix
Grain	0.74	×	0.05	=	.037	0.35	=	0.259
SBM	0.18	×	0.40	=	.072	0.7	=	0.126
Molasses	0.08	×	1.0	=	.080	0.2	=	0.016
Total in grain mix	1.00	×			0.189			0.401
Wanted in DM (from step 7):					0.893			0.486

Since both additional calcium and phosphorus are needed, a mineral providing both could be used, such as bone meal, which contains 30 to 32% calcium and 12 to 14% phosphorus (Appendix Table 7). The amount needed could be determined using the Pearson square procedure as shown.

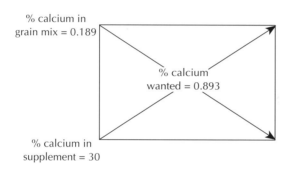

% calcium in grain mix = 0.189

% calcium wanted = 0.893

% calcium in supplement = 30

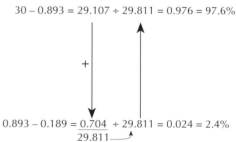

30 − 0.893 = 29.107 ÷ 29.811 = 0.976 = 97.6%

+

0.893 − 0.189 = 0.704 ÷ 29.811 = 0.024 = 2.4%
29.811

Thus, in order to increase the calcium content of the grain mix from 0.189% to 0.893%, we need to add 2.4% of the supplement bone meal. This would result in the following grain mix containing the nutrient levels shown.

Feed	Fraction in Grain Mix DM		DE (Mcal/lb) in feed		mix	Protein (%) in feed		mix	Calcium (%) in feed		mix	Phosphorus (%) in feed		mix
Grain	0.716	×	1.6	=	1.146	11	=	7.9	0.05	=	0.036	0.35	=	0.251
SBM	0.18	×	1.6	=	0.288	50	=	9.0	0.4	=	0.072	0.7	=	0.126
Molasses	0.08	×	1.6	=	0.128	4	=	0.3	1	=	0.080	0.2	=	0.016
Bone Meal	0.024	×	0	=	0	0	=	0	30	=	0.720	12	=	0.288
Total	1.000				1.56			17.2			0.908			0.681
Wanted in DM (from step 7)								17.3			0.893			0.486

9. Thus, the grain mix dry matter should consist of the fraction of each feed dry matter shown above. However, the feeds as fed, not feed dry matter, will be mixed and fed. Therefore, you must determine the fraction of each feed as fed that should be in the grain mix. This may be done as shown below. The percent of each feed as fed in the grain mix is the amount of each that must be used in making up the grain mix.

Dry Matter and Percent of Ingredients in Grain Mix As Fed

Feed	Fraction of Mix DM (from step 8)		Dry Matter (%) (from Appendix Tables 6 & 7) feed		mix				Percent of Mix As Fed
Grain	0.716	×	89	=	63.72	÷	0.88	=	72.4
SBM	0.18	×	89	=	16.02	÷	0.88	=	18.2
Molasses	0.08	×	74	=	5.92	÷	0.88	=	6.7
Bone Meal	0.024	×	99	=	2.38	÷	0.88	=	2.7
Total	1.000				88.00				100.0

10. Determine the amount of grain mix that should be fed. The total amount of air-dry feed (air-dry feed is that containing 90% dry matter) that a 6-month-old weanling will consume is an amount equal to 2.5 to 3.5% of its body weight daily (Appendix Table 1). The better the quality of the forage, the more of it that will be consumed. Since in this example the pasture forage quality is average, 3% total feed intake would be a good approximation. Thus, this weanling, which weighs 475 lbs, would consume a total of about 0.03 × 475 lbs or 14.2 lbs of air-dry feed daily, which would provide 14.2 × 0.90 dry-matter fraction or 12.8 lbs of dry matter/day.

Since 30% of this is to be forage and 70% grain mix (from step 2), you would feed 0.70 × 14.2 or about 10 lbs of grain mix/day, which would provide 0.70 × 12.8 or 9 lbs of grain mix DM/day. This would provide 9 × 1.56 Mcal/lb of dry matter (from step 8) or 14 Mcal/day. In addition, the weanling would be consuming about 0.3 × 12.8 or 3.8 lbs forage dry matter/day, which would provide 3.8 × 0.75 Mcal/lb of DM (from Appendix Table 6), or 2.9 Mcal/day, for a total of 14 + 2.9 or 16.9 Mcal/day. These calculations are shown more clearly in the following table.

Feed	Fraction of Feed in Diet (from step 2)		Total Lbs Diet DM/ day Eaten*		Lbs Feed DM/day Eaten		Mcal of DE per lb of feed DM		eaten /day
Forage	0.3	×	12.8	=	3.85	×	0.75	=	2.9
Grain	0.7	×	12.8	=	9.0	×	1.56	=	14.0
Total	1.0								16.9
Needed (from Appendix Table 4-500), for rapid growth,									17.2
for moderate growth									15.0

* (475 lb body wt) × (will eat 3% of body wt in air-dry feed/day, from Appendix Table 1) × (90% dry matter in air-dry feed) = 475 × 0.03 × 0.90 = 12.8 lbs diet dry matter/day eaten. Slightly more or less than this may actually be consumed depending primarily on forage palatability and digestibility.

Thus, feeding 10 lbs of grain mix/day plus pasture forage would provide about 16.9 Mcal/day, as compared to 17.2 Mcal/day needed for rapid growth and 15.0 Mcal/day needed for moderate growth.

11. The next step is to compare the nutrient content

of the total diet as formulated to the horse's needs as shown below.

Thus, as shown, the total diet just meets or exceeds the horse's requirement for each of these four major nutrients of concern.

Amount of Feed Dry Matter and Energy Consumed, and Nutrient Content of Diet Dry Matter versus That Needed

Feed	Lbs DM/day Fed or Eaten (from step 10)		Mcal of DE lbs of feed DM		eaten /day	Fraction of Feed in Diet		Protein (%) in feed		in diet	Calcium (%) in feed		in diet	Phosphorus (%) in feed		in diet
Forage	3.8	×	0.75	=	2.85	0.3	×	8	=	2.40	0.25	=	0.075	0.20	=	0.06
Grain	9	×	1.56	=	14.04	0.7	×	17.2	=	12.04	0.908	=	0.636	0.729	=	0.51
Total	12.8				16.89	1.0				14.44			0.71			0.57
Needed (Appendix Table 4-500)					17.2					14.5			0.70			0.40

12. Check the calcium phosphorus ratio (Ca:P) in the total diet to ensure that it is in the acceptable range of 1:1 to 3:1 for the growing horse, by dividing both the amount of calcium (0.71%) and the amount of phosphorus (0.57%) in the total diet by the amount of phosphorus (0.57%), as shown.

13. *Trace Minerals and Vitamins*—To ensure that the weanling receives adequate amounts of trace minerals and vitamins of concern for growth (copper, zinc, and vitamin A), the amount of each needed should be added to the grain mix. As given in Appendix Table 2, 25 and 60 mg of copper and zinc/

kg (ppm) of total diet dry matter, respectively, are recommended. The weanling in this example is consuming 12.8 lbs/day of diet dry matter (from step 10), which is 12.8 ÷ 2.2 lbs/kg, or 5.82 kg of feed dry matter/day. Therefore, the weanling should receive 25 × 5.82, or 145 mg, of copper/day and 60 × 5.82, or 349, mg of zinc/day. The weanling should also receive 10,000 IU of vitamin A/day (Appendix Table 4-500). Since 10 lbs of grain mix/day (from step 10) are being fed, the grain mix should contain 145 ÷ 10 = 14.5, and 349 ÷ 10 = 34.9, mg/lb of copper and zinc respectively, and 10,000 ÷ 10 = 1000 IU of vitamin A/lb. Thus, the grain mix should contain the following (from above and step 7).

Nutrient Content Needed in Grain Mix As Fed

DE (Mcal/lb)	Protein (%)	Calcium (%)	Phosphorus (%)	Zinc (mg/lb)	Copper (mg/lb)	Vitamin A (IU/lb)
1.4	16	0.8	0.45	34.9	14.5	1000

If zinc oxide, which contains 78% zinc, and copper sulfate, which contains 25.4% copper (Appendix Table 7), are used to provide the zinc and copper needed, the grain mix would need to contain 34.9 ÷ 0.78 = 45 mg of zinc oxide, and 14.5 ÷ 0.254 = 57 mg of copper sulfate/lb as fed. If the vitamin A supplement used contains 1,000,000 IU/lb, the grain mix should contain about 0.5g of it/lb of grain mix, as shown below (1 lb = 454 g from Appendix Table 9).

$$\frac{1,000,000}{lb\ of\ supp.} \times \frac{1\ lb}{454\ g} = \frac{2200\ IU/g}{of\ supplement}$$

$$\frac{1000\ IU\ wanted}{lb\ of\ grain} \times \frac{1\ g\ of\ supp.}{2200\ IU} \simeq \frac{0.5g\ of\ supp.}{lb.\ of\ grain}$$

14. Instead of having the grain mix prepared at a feed mill, or buying a grain mix containing the desired nutrient levels or greater, and then feeding 10 lbs of it daily (as determined in step 10), the ingredients could be mixed at each feeding. If this were done, the following amounts would be needed daily, as determined by multiplying the fraction of each ingredient in the grain mix (as determined in step 9), or for zinc, copper, and vitamin A, the amount of each needed/lb of grain mix (as determined in step 13), times the amount of grain mix fed daily as shown below.

Amount of Each Feed to Feed the 6-mo, 475-lb Weanling on Mature Grass Pasture for Rapid Growth

Feed	Fraction of Mix As Fed (from step 9)		of mix (from step 10)		of feed		Feed Wt/Unit Vol. (from Appendix Table 8)		Volume/ day to Feed
Grain	0.724	×	10	=	7.24	÷	(1.7 lbs/qt)	=	4.25 qts
SBM	0.182	×	10	=	1.82	÷	(1.8 lbs/qt)	=	1 qt
Molasses	0.067	×	10	=	0.67	÷	[(3.0 lbs/qt) ÷ (4 cups/qt)]	=	1 cup
Bone Meal	0.027	×	10	=	0.27	÷	(1 lb/16 oz)	=	4.3 oz wt

Supplement	Mg/lb of Mix As Fed (from step 13)		Lbs/d of Mix Fed		Wt to Feed Daily		Feed Weight/ Unit Volume (from Appendix Table 8)		Volume/day to Feed
Zinc oxide	45	×	10	=	450 mg	×	1 tsp/4000 mg	=	1/8 level tsp
Copper sulfate	57	×	10	=	570 mg	×	1 tsp/4000 mg	=	1/8 level tsp
Vit A supp. (10⁶ IU/lb)	500	×	10	=	5000 mg	×	1 tsp/5000 mg	=	1 level tsp

Example 2—Weanlings Fed Alfalfa (Lucerne) Hay. A 9-month-old weanling is being fed good-quality full-bloom alfalfa hay. Based on its parents, it's anticipated that the weanling's mature weight will be 1200 lbs (545 kg). Formulate a grain mix that, when fed in the amount necessary to obtain a rapid growth rate, will, along with the alfalfa, meet the weanling's requirements for all nutrients of concern (energy, protein, calcium, phosphorus, zinc, copper, and vitamin A).

1. Obtain the nutrient content of the alfalfa, preferably by laboratory analysis or alternatively from feed tables (e.g., Appendix Table 6).

2. Determine what percent of the diet should be grain mix. In Appendix Table 1, 70% is given for the 6-month-old weanling and 60% for the yearling as the maximum percent grain mix recommended. Since the weanling in this example is 9 months old and, therefore, for its feeding program from 9 to 12 months of age, 60% would be a good maximum to use. A lower percentage of course could be used

and may result in a slightly slower growth rate but no decrease in mature size.

3. Determine the amount of each nutrient the alfalfa contributes to the diet by multiplying the fraction of alfalfa in the diet by the amount of each nutrient in the alfalfa as shown below.

		Nutrients in Feed Dry Matter (from step 1)									
	Fraction of Feed in Diet	DE (Mcal/lb)			Protein (%) in			Calcium (%) in			Phosphorus (%) in
Feed	(from step 2)	feed		diet	feed		diet	feed		diet	feed		diet
Alfalfa	0.40	× 1.0	=	0.40	× 17	=	6.8	× 1.2	=	0.48	× 0.2	=	0.08

4. Obtain the amount of each nutrient needed by the horse. The 9-month-old weanling would need the amount midway between the needs given in Appendix Table 1 for a 6-month-old and a 12-month-old horse.

5. Determine the amount of each nutrient that the grain mix must contain so that it and the alfalfa will provide the amount of nutrients needed in the total diet. This is done as shown below. An explanation of these procedures is given in Example 1, steps 5 and 6.

		Nutrients Needed in Grain Mix Dry Matter									
	Fraction of Feed in Diet	DE (Mcal/lb) in			Protein (%) in			Calcium (%) in			Phosphorus (%) in
Feed	(from step 2)	feed		diet	feed		diet	feed		diet	feed		diet
Alfalfa	0.4	× 1.0	=	0.4	× 17	=	6.8	× 1.2	=	0.48	× 0.2	=	0.08
Grain mix	0.6	1.5[b]	=	0.9[a]	11.2[b]		6.7[a]	0.2[b]		0.12[a]	0.45[b]		0.27[a]
Needed (from step 4)				1.3			13.5			0.60			0.35

[a] Obtained by subtracting the amount provided by alfalfa from that needed, e.g., 13.5% protein needed − 6.8% provided by alfalfa = 6.7% needed from the grain mix.

[b] Obtained by dividing the amount needed from the grain mix by the fraction of grain mix in the diet, e.g., 6.7% protein needed from the grain mix ÷ 0.6 fraction of grain mix in the diet = 11.2% protein needed in the grain mix dry matter.

If the grain mix contains 10% moisture (and therefore a dry matter fraction of 0.90), it should contain the following:

Nutrient	Amount in DM (from above)	×	DM Fraction	=	Amount in Grain Mix as Fed
Mcal/lb	1.5	×	0.90	=	1.35 Mcal/lb
Protein	11.2%	×	0.90	=	10.1%
Calcium	0.20%	×	0.90	=	0.18%
Phosphorus	0.45%	×	0.90	=	0.405%

A commercial grain mix containing these amounts, or greater, of these nutrients could be purchased and fed, or a custom or home mix could be prepared as shown below.

6. Formulate a grain mix that contains the amount of nutrients needed.

a. *Energy*—Regular oats provide 1.45 Mcal/lb of dry matter whereas all others provide about 1.7 Mcal/lb (Appendix Table 6). The amount of oats that could be used and still result in a grain mix that provides at least 1.5 Mcal/lb could be determined using the Pierson square as shown below.

Thus, the grain-mix could contain up to a maximum of 80% oats.

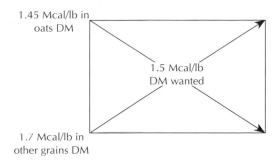

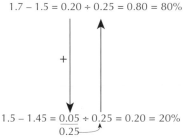

1.45 Mcal/lb in oats DM

1.5 Mcal/lb DM wanted

1.7 Mcal/lb in other grains DM

1.7 − 1.5 = 0.20 ÷ 0.25 = 0.80 = 80%

+

1.5 − 1.45 = 0.05 ÷ 0.25 = 0.20 = 20%

0.25

b. *Protein*—The amount of protein needed in the grain-mix dry matter (11.2%) is close to that present in most cereal grains; however, the amount of calcium and phosphorus needed is greater, and therefore a mineral and possibly protein supplement will be needed. To prevent these from sifting out, the grain mix should include 5 to 10% wet molasses, fat, or vegetable oil. A mixture of 95% grain containing 11% protein, and 5% wet molasses containing 4% protein, would contain 11% × 0.95, or 10.4%, protein plus 4% × 0.05, or 0.20%, protein for a total of 10.6% protein, as compared to 11.2% needed. There are two ways the additional protein needed could be provided. One is to add a protein supplement to the grain mix; the other is to feed less grain mix, therefore requiring the horse to consume more of the higher-protein feed: alfalfa. Feeding less grain mix would result in a small decrease in energy intake and, therefore, growth rate. If this were done, the percentage of grain mix and alfalfa to feed can be determined using the Pearson square as shown.

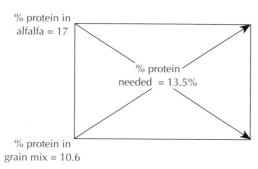

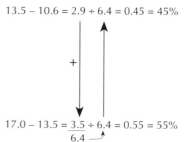

Thus, if the diet consisted of 55% grain mix, no protein supplement would be needed. This is recommended. However, if 60% grain mix were fed, the amount of soybean meal (SBM) containing 50% protein in its dry matter (Appendix Table 6), needed to increase the protein in the grain mix from 10.6% to 11.2%, can be determined using the Pearson square as shown.

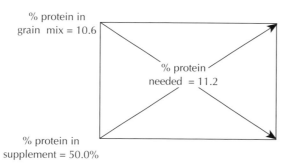

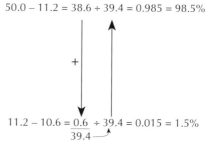

Thus, only about 2% soybean meal is needed in the grain mix.

c. *Calcium and Phosphorus*—As obtained from Appendix Table 6 the feeds contain the amount of calcium and phosphorus given below and, therefore, the grain mix contains the amount determined below as compared to that wanted. Dicalcium phosphate, which contains 21% cal-

Feed	Fraction of Grain Mix Dry Matter		Protein (%) in feed		Protein (%) in diet	Calcium (%) in feed		Calcium (%) in diet	Phosphorus (%) in feed		Phosphorus (%) in diet
Grain	0.93	×	11	=	10.2	0.05	=	0.046	0.35	=	0.326
Molasses	0.05	×	4	=	0.2	1.0	=	0.050	0.20	=	0.010
SBM	0.02	×	50	=	1.0	0.40	=	0.008	0.70	=	0.014
Total	1.00				11.4			0.104			0.35
Wanted in DM (from step 5)					11.2			0.20			0.45

cium and 18% phosphorus (Appendix Table 7) may be used to provide the additional amount of these minerals needed. The amount needed is determined using the Pearson square as shown on the following page. Because more phosphorus than calcium is needed, and the mineral supplement used is lower in phosphorus than in calcium, determine the amount of the mineral needed to provide sufficient phosphorus. This amount will also provide the amount of calcium needed.

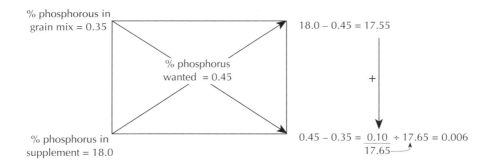

Thus, the grain mix should consist of the following:

Ingredient Amounts and Nutrient Content in Grain Mix Dry Matter

| Feed | Fraction in Mix DM | | Mcal/lb DM | | | | Protein (%) | | | | Calcium (%) | | | | Phosphorus (%) | | |
			in feed		in mix		in feed		in mix		in feed		in mix		in feed		in mix
Grain	0.924	×	1.6	=	1.48		11	=	10.2		0.05	=	0.04		0.35	=	0.323
Molasses	0.05	×	1.6	=	0.08		4	=	0.2		1	=	0.05		0.20	=	0.010
SBM	0.02	×	1.6	=	0.03		5	=	1.0		0.04	=	0.06		0.70	=	0.014
Dical	0.006	×	0	=	0		0	=	0		21	=	0.13		18	=	0.108
Total	1.000				1.59				11.4				0.30				0.455
Wanted in DM (from step 5)					1.54				11.2				0.20				0.45

7. The amount of each ingredients as fed needed in the grain mix is determined as shown below.

Dry Matter and Percent of Ingredients in Grain Mix As Fed

| Feed | Fraction in Mix (from step 6) | | Dry Matter (%) (from Appendix Table 6) | | | | Dry-Matter Fraction in Mix | | Percent of Mix As Fed to Use | |
			feed		mix					
Grain	0.924	×	89	=	82.2	+	0.883	=	93	use 92
Molasses	0.05	×	74	=	3.7	+	0.883	=	4.2	use 5
SBM	0.02	×	89	=	1.8	+	0.883	=	2	use 2
Dical	0.006	×	98	=	0.6	+	0.883	=	0.67	use 1
Total	1.000				88.3				100	100

8. The nutrient content of the grain mix as fed would be the following.

Nutrient Content in Grain Mix As Fed

| Dry Matter Fraction (from step 7) | | Mcal/lb | | | Protein (%) | | | Calcium (%) | | | Phosphorus (%) | | |
		DM		As fed	DM		As fed	DM		As fed	DM		As fed
0.883	×	1.59*	=	1.40	11.4*	=	10.0	0.30*	=	0.265	0.455*	=	0.40

* From step 6.

9. Determine the amount of grain mix that should be fed. The total amount of air-dry feed the 6- and 12-month-old horse will consume daily is an amount equal to 2.5 to 3.5%, and 2.0 to 3.0%, of their body weight, respectively (Appendix Table 1). Thus, for the 9-month-old weanling in this example, it would be 2.25 to 3.25%. The higher the forage quality, the more that will be consumed. Since in this example the forage being fed is of average quality, a good estimate of the total amount of air-dry feed con-

sumed daily would be an amount equal to 2.75% of body weight. The horse's weight should be obtained preferably by weighing or, if a scale is unavailable, by using the procedures described previously in this chapter in the section on "Obtaining a Horse's Weight." If the weanling weighs 675 lbs, it would consume about 0.0275 × 675 lbs, or about 18.56 lbs, of air-dry feed daily, which would provide 18.56 lbs × 0.90 dry-matter fraction, or 16.7 lbs of dry matter. Since 40% of this is to be alfalfa and

60% grain mix (from step 2), you would feed these amounts of each, and they would provide the amount of energy, shown below. The energy content of the grain mix was determined to be 1.59 Mcal/lb of dry matter from step 6, and of the full-bloom alfalfa hay to be 1.0 Mcal/lb (from Appendix Table 6).

Amount of Feed Dry Matter and Digestible Energy Consumed

Feed	Fraction of Feed in Diet (from step 2)	Lbs Diet DM/ day Eaten		Lbs Feed DM/day Eaten	Mcal of DE		
					/lb of feed DM		eaten/ day
Alfalfa	0.40	× 16.7	=	6.7	× 1.0	=	6.7
Grain mix	0.60	× 16.7	=	10.0	× 1.59	=	15.9
Total	1.00			16.7			22.6

Because the dry matter content of the grain mix is 88.3% (from step 7) you would feed daily 10.0 lbs of grain-mix dry matter ÷ 0.883 dry-matter fraction, or 11.3 lbs as fed.

10. Compare the nutrient content of the total diet to the horse's needs as shown below.

Thus, as shown, the total diet meets the horse's requirements for all of these nutrients.

Amount of Feed Dry Matter and Energy Consumed, and Nutrient Content in Diet Dry Matter versus That Needed

Feed	Lbs DM/day Fed or Eaten (from step 9)		Mcal of DE		Fraction of Feed in Diet		Protein (%)		Calcium (%)		Phosphorus (%)	
			lbs of feed DM	eaten /day			in feed	in diet	in feed	in diet	in feed	in diet
Alfalfa	6.7	×	1.0	=	6.7	0.4	×	17	=	6.8	1.2	=	0.48	0.2	=	0.08
Grain	10.0	×	1.59	=	15.9	0.6	×	11.4	=	6.8	0.30	=	0.18	0.455	=	0.27
Total	16.7				22.6					13.6			0.66			0.35
Needed (from step 4)										13.5			0.60			0.35

11. The calcium: phosphorus ratio is 0.66:0.35.

$$\frac{0.66}{0.35} : \frac{0.35}{0.35} = 1.9:1.$$

This is within the acceptable range for growth of 1:1 to 3:1.

12. *Trace Minerals and Vitamins*—To ensure that the horse receives the amount of trace minerals and vitamins of concern (zinc, copper, and vitamin A), the total amount needed may be added to the grain mix. The amount needed is 60 and 25 mg of zinc and copper, respectively, per kg diet dry matter (Appendix Table 2). In this example, 16.7 lbs DM (from step 9) ÷ 2.2 lbs/kg (from Appendix

Table 9), or 7.6 kg of feed dry matter/day, is being consumed and, therefore, as shown below, the weanling should receive daily 7.6 × 60, or 456, mg zinc and 7.6 × 25, or 190, mg copper. The 9-month-old weanling should also receive 13,250 IU of vitamin A/day (from interpolation between needs given in Appendix Tables 4–500 and 4–600, for the 6-month- and 12-month-old weanlings whose anticipated mature weights are 500 kg and 600 kg). Since 11.3 lbs of grain mix/day are being fed (from step 9), as shown below, each pound of grain mix would need to contain 40.2 and 16.7 mg of zinc and copper, respectively, and, if the vitamin A supplement contained 2200 IU/g, 1167 IU of vitamin A.

Nutrient	mg Needed/kg Diet DM (Appendix Table 2)		kg Diet DM/day		mg or IU/ day Needed		lbs Mix Fed/day		mg or IU /lb Mix
Zinc	60	×	7.6	=	456	÷	11.3	=	40.4
Copper	25	×	7.6	=	190	÷	11.3	=	16.8
Vit A (from Appendix Tables 4–500 & 4–600)					13,250	÷	11.3	=	1173

Thus, the grain mix would need to contain the following (from above and step 8).

Nutrient Content Needed in Grain Mix As Fed

| Mcal/lb | Protein (%) | Calcium (%) | Phosphorus (%) | Zinc (mg/lb) | Copper (mg/lb) | Vitamin A (IU/lb) |
| 1.40 | 10 | 0.265 | 0.40 | 40.4 | 16.8 | 1173 |

If zinc oxide, which contains 78% zinc, and copper sulfate, which contains 25.4% copper (Appendix Table 7) are used, the grain mix would need to contain 40.4 ÷ 0.78, or 52, mg of zinc oxide, and 16.8 ÷ 0.254, or 66, mg of copper sulfate/lb as fed. If the vitamin A supplement used contained 2200 IU/

g, the grain mix would need to contain 1173 IU ÷ 2200 IU/g, or 0.53 g of it.

13. The following amounts would be needed daily, as determined by multiplying the fraction of each ingredient in the grain mix, or, for zinc, copper, and vitamin A, the amount of each needed/lb of grain mix.

Amount of Each Feedstuff to Feed the 9-month-old, 675-lb, Weanling in Addition to All the Alfalfa Hay It Will Consume

Feed	Fraction of Mix As Fed (step 7)		Amount/day As Fed of mix (step 9)		of feed		Feed Wt/Unit Volume (from Appendix Table 8)		Volume/day to Feed
Grain	0.92	×	11.3 lb	=	10.4 lb	÷	(1.7 lbs/qt)	=	6 qts
Molasses	0.05	×	11.3 lb	=	0.57 lb	÷	[(3.0 lbs/qt) ÷ (4 cups/qt)]		
SBM	0.02	×	11.3 lb	=	0.23 lb	÷	(1.8 lbs/qt)	=	0.2 qts
Dical	0.01	×	11.3 lb	=	0.11 lb	×	(454 g/lb) × (1 tsp/4 g) × (1 tblsp/3 tsp)	=	4.3 tblsp

	mg/lb Grain Mix As Fed (from step 12)								heaping tsp
Zinc oxide	52	11.3	=	590 mg	×	1 tsp/4000 mg	=		$\frac{1}{8}$
Copper sulfate	66	11.3	=	749 mg	×	1 tsp/4000 mg	=		$\frac{1}{8}$
Vit A. Supp. (2200 IU/g)	530	11.3	=	6000 mg	×	1 tsp/5000 mg	=		1

14. The average daily grain (ADG) that this feeding program can be expected to result in for this weanling can be calculated from these formulas.

$$\text{Maintenance DE} = 1.4 + 0.03 \text{ (kg body wt)}$$

$$DE_g = \text{(maintenance DE)} + [4.81 + (1.17 \times \text{mo of age}) - (0.023 \times \text{mo of age squared})] \times \text{(ADG in kg/day)}$$

For the 9-month-old weanling weighing 675 lbs (306.8 kg) and being fed 22.6 Mcal/day (from step 10), the following would be calculated from these formulas.

$$22.6 = [1.4 + (0.03 \times 306.8)]$$
$$+ [4.81 + (1.17 \times 9) - (0.023 \times 9^2)] \times ADG$$
$$22.6 = [10.60] + [4.81 + 10.53 - 1.863] \times ADG$$
$$22.6 = [10.60] + [13.477] \times ADG$$
$$(22.6 - 10.60) \div 13.477 = ADG$$
$$0.89 = ADG$$

Thus, with this feeding program this horse should gain 0.89 kg/day, or about 2 lbs/day.

Example 3—Lactating Mares on Growing Grass Pasture. Develop a feeding program for 1000-lb (454-kg) mares during the first 3 months of lactation. Ample good-quality growing fescue-brome-mix grass pasture forage is available.

1. Obtain the content of the nutrients of concern (energy, protein, calcium, and phosphorus) in the pasture forage, preferably by laboratory analysis, or alternatively from feed tables (e.g., Appendix Table 6), and compare it to the mares' needs (Appendix Table 1).

	Percent in Dry Matter		
	Protein	Calcium	Phosphorus
Grass	18	0.5	0.4
Needed	13	0.50	0.35

Thus, the pasture forage alone will provide adequate protein, calcium, and phosphorus. Since it is green, it will also provide very ample amounts of the vitamin A precursor, beta-carotene, as well as other vitamins.

2. The 454-kg mares' energy needs can be obtained by interpolation between the values given in Appendix Table 4-400 and 4-500 for 400- and 500-kg mares, respectively, which are 22.9 and 28.3 Mcal/day. Thus, these mares would need the following:

$$22.9 + (28.3 - 22.9)(0.54)$$
$$= 22.9 + 2.92 = 25.8 \text{ Mcal/day}$$

3. During the first 3 months of lactation, mares will eat an amount of air-dry feed equal to 2.5 to 3.0% of their body weight daily (Appendix Table 1). The higher the quality of the forage, the more they will eat. Thus, these 1000-lb mares on green pasture will eat about 0.03 × 1000 lbs, or 30 lbs, of air-dry feed daily, which would be 30 lbs × 0.90 dry matter in air-dry feed = 27 lbs of forage dry matter.

4. From Appendix Table 6, we find that this pasture forage provides 0.95 to 1.15 Mcal/lb of dry matter. Thus, if these mares ate as much as they wanted, they would consume the following amounts of dietary energy:

$$(27 \text{ lbs DM/day}) \times (0.95 \text{ to } 1.15 \text{ Mcal/lb DM})$$
$$= 25.6 \text{ to } 31 \text{ Mcal/day}$$

This would meet or exceed the 25.8 Mcal/day needed (as determined in step 2).

5. The feeding program for these mares would be to allow them free-choice access to trace-mineralized salt, water, and the growing grass pasture forage. No other feeds would be needed.

Example 4—Lactating Mares Fed Grass Hay. Develop a feeding program for 1100-lb (500-kg) mares during the first 3 months of lactation. The forage available is grass hay analyzed to contain 33% crude fiber, 8% protein, 0.3% calcium, and 0.2% phosphorus in its dry matter.

1. Compare the nutrient content of the hay to that needed (Appendix Table 1). The energy content of the hay is obtained from Appendix Table 6 for a similar-type hay containing a fiber and protein content similar to the hay in question, in this example an average-quality late-growth grass hay.

	Mcal/lb of DM	Percent in Dry Matter		
		Protein	Calcium	Phosphorus
Hay	0.8	8	0.3	0.2
Need	1.2	13	0.5	0.35

Thus, a grain mix must be fed to provide the nutrients needed in excess of that provided by the hay.

2. Determine the percentage of the diet that must be a grain mix. This amount is based on that needed to meet the horse's dietary energy needs and can be determined using the Pearson square as shown.

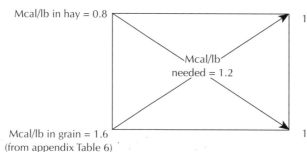

Mcal/lb in hay = 0.8

Mcal/lb needed = 1.2

Mcal/lb in grain = 1.6 (from appendix Table 6)

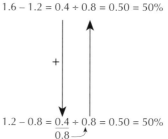

$1.6 - 1.2 = 0.4 \div 0.8 = 0.50 = 50\%$

$1.2 - 0.8 = 0.4 \div 0.8 = 0.50 = 50\%$

Thus, the diet should consist of 50% grain mix, providing 1.6 Mcal/lb of dry matter.

3. Determine the amount of each nutrient of concern (energy, protein, calcium, and phosphorus): contributed to the diet by the hay, and needed in the grain mix, as shown below:

			Nutrients Needed in Grain Mix Dry Matter													
Feed	Fraction of Feed in Diet (from step 2)		DE (Mcal/lb) in			Protein (%) in			Calcium (%) in			Phosphorus (%) in		
			feed		diet	feed		diet	feed		diet	feed		diet
Hay	0.50	×	0.8	=	0.4	8	=	4	0.3	=	0.15	0.2	=	0.10
Grain mix	0.50	×	1.6[b]	=	0.8[a]	18[b]	=	9[a]	0.7[b]	=	0.35[a]	0.5[b]	=	0.25[a]
Needed (from step 1)					1.2			13			0.5			0.35

[a] Obtained by subtracting the amount provided by the hay from that needed, e.g., 13% protein needed minus 4% provided by the hay = 9% needed from the grain mix.

[b] Obtained by dividing the amount needed from the grain mix by the fraction of the grain mix in the diet, e.g., 9% protein needed from the grain mix divided by 50% grain mix in the diet = 18% protein needed in the grain-mix dry matter.

4. Formulate a grain mix that contains the amount of nutrients needed.

a. *Energy*—Since regular oats provide 1.45, and other grains about 1.7, Mcal/lb of dry matter (Appendix Table 6) and 1.6 is needed, little regular oats, but any amount of other cereal grains, could be used.

b. *Protein*—Most cereal grains with 5 to 10% molasses will contain about 10%, and soybean meal (SBM) 50%, protein in their dry matter (Appendix Table 6). The amount of SBM needed to increase the protein content of the grain mix from 10% to 18% as determined below is 20%.

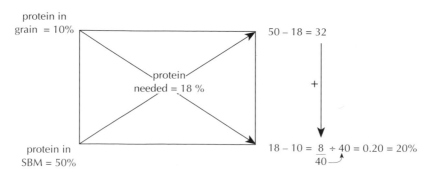

protein in grain = 10%

protein needed = 18 %

protein in SBM = 50%

$50 - 18 = 32$

$18 - 10 = 8 \div 40 = 0.20 = 20\%$

c. *Calcium and Phosphorus*—The feeds contain the amount of calcium and phosphorus shown below (Appendix Table 6); therefore, the grain mix contains the amount determined below as compared to the amount needed.

Feed	Fraction in Mix		Protein (%) in			Calcium (%) in			Phosphorus (%) in	
			feed	mix	feed		mix	feed		mix
Grain	0.72	×	11 =	7.9	0.05	=	0.036	0.35	=	0.252
SBM	0.20	×	50 =	10.0	0.40	=	0.080	0.70	=	0.140
Molasses	0.08	×	4 =	0.3	1	=	0.080	0.20	=	0.016
Total	1.00			18.2			0.196			0.408
Needed (from step 3)				18			0.7			0.5

If bone meal containing 30% calcium and 12% phosphorus (Appendix Table 7) is used to provide the additional amounts of these minerals needed, the amount of bone meal needed, as determined, is 0.017, or 1.7%.

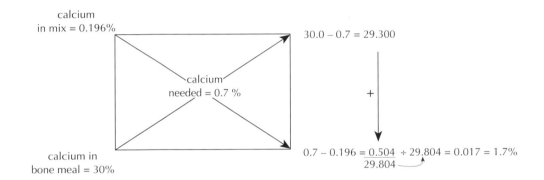

calcium in mix = 0.196%

calcium needed = 0.7 %

calcium in bone meal = 30%

30.0 – 0.7 = 29.300

+

0.7 – 0.196 = 0.504 ÷ 29.804 = 0.017 = 1.7%
29.804

5. Thus, the grain mix will consist of the following and have the nutrient content shown.

Ingredient Amounts and Nutrient Content in Grain Mix Dry Matter

Feed	Fraction in Mix DM		Mcal/lb of DM			Protein (%)			Calcium (%)			Phosphorus (%)		
			in feed	in mix		in feed	in mix		in feed	in mix		in feed		in mix
Grain	0.703	×	1.6 =	1.12		11 =	7.7		0.05 =	0.03		0.35 =		0.246
SBM	0.20	×	1.6 =	0.32		50 =	10.0		0.40 =	0.08		0.70 =		0.140
Molasses	0.08	×	1.6 =	0.13		4 =	0.3		1 =	0.08		0.2 =		0.016
Bone Meal	0.017	×	0 =	0		0 =	0		30 =	0.51		12 =		0.204
Total	1.000			1.58			18.0			0.70				0.606
Needed (from step 3)				1.6			18			0.7				0.5

6. The amount of each ingredient as fed in the grain mix is determined as shown below.

Dry Matter and Percent of Ingredients in Grain Mix As Fed

Feed	Fraction of Mix DM (from step 5)		Dry Matter (%) (from Appendix Table 6)			Dry Matter Fraction		Percent of Mix As Fed
			in feed		in mix			
Grain	0.703	×	89	=	62.57	÷	0.88 =	71.1 use 71
SBM	0.20	×	89	=	17.80	÷	0.88 =	20.2 use 20
Molasses	0.08	×	74	=	5.92	÷	0.88 =	6.7 use 7
Bone Meal	0.017	×	99	=	1.68	÷	0.88 =	1.9 use 2
Total	1.000				88.0			99.9 100

7. The nutrient content of the grain mix as fed would be the following.

DM Fraction (step 6)		Mcal/lb in		Protein (%) in		Calcium (%) in		Phosphorus (%) in	
		DM	As Fed	DM	As Fed	DM	As Fed	DM	As Fed
0.88	×	1.58* =	1.39	18* =	15.8	0.7* =	0.62	0.606* =	0.53

Nutrient Content in Grain Mix As Fed

* From step 5.

8. Determine the amount of grain mix that should be fed. There are at least two ways this may be done, as shown below.
   a. One way to determine the amount of grain mix that should be fed is by determining the amount of feed intake from energy needs as shown.

$$\text{Lbs Total Diet DM Intake} = \frac{\text{Mcal/day Needed (Appendix Table 4)}}{\left(\begin{array}{c}\text{Fraction of}\\\text{Mix in Diet}\end{array} \times \begin{array}{c}\text{Mcal/lb}\\\text{Mix DM}\end{array}\right) + \left(\begin{array}{c}\text{Fraction of}\\\text{Forage in Diet}\end{array} \times \begin{array}{c}\text{Mcal/lb}\\\text{Forage DM}\end{array}\right)}$$

Putting in the amounts applicable for this example would give the following:

$$\text{Lbs Total Diet DM Intake} = \frac{\begin{array}{c}28.3 \text{ Mcal/day Needed}\\ \text{(from Appendix Table 4–500)}\end{array}}{\left(\begin{array}{c}0.5 \text{ from}\\\text{step 2}\end{array} \times \begin{array}{c}1.58 \text{ from}\\\text{step 5}\end{array}\right) + \left(\begin{array}{c}0.5 \text{ from}\\\text{step 2}\end{array} \times \begin{array}{c}0.8 \text{ from}\\\text{step 1}\end{array}\right)}$$

$$= \frac{28.3}{1.19} = 23.8$$

Thus, 23.8 lbs of diet dry matter/day consisting of 50% grain mix providing 1.58 Mcal/lb of dry matter and 50% forage providing 0.80 Mcal/lb of dry matter will provide 28.3 Mcal/day. This meets the 1100-lb (500-kg) mare's dietary energy needs during the first 3 months of lactation. The amount of grain mix that should be fed then is the following.

23.8 lbs diet DM × 50% grain mix in the diet
= 11.9 lbs grain mix DM

11.9 lbs mix DM ÷ 0.88 DM fraction (from step 6)
= 13.5 lbs mix as fed

   b. The second way to determine the amount of grain mix that should be fed is by determining the amount of feed intake from expected consumption. During the first 3 months of lactation, mares will eat an amount of air-dry feed equal to 2.5 to 3.0% of their body wt/day (Appendix Table 1). The higher the quality of the forage, the more that will be eaten. In this example, a hay low in energy and protein, and high in fiber, is being fed; therefore, it is a poorer-quality forage. Since a poorer-quality forage is being consumed, total air-dry diet intake of an amount equal to 2.5% of her body weight would be expected. For this 1100-lb mare, feed intake expected would be:

Total diet intake = 0.025 × 1100 lbs
= 27.5 lbs of air-dry diet

27.5 lbs air-dry diet × 0.90 dry matter fraction
= 24.75 lbs diet dry matter

Versus that determined above from energy needs, which was = 23.8 lbs diet dry matter

9. The feeding program for these 1100-lb (500-kg) mares during their first 3 months of lactation would be:
   a. Feed 13.5 to 14 lbs/day of a grain mix (from step 8a), which, as determined in step 7, should contain at least 16% protein, 0.6% calcium, and 0.5% phosphorus.
   b. Feed all the grass hay they will clean up without wastage. This would be about 14 lbs plus 10 to 15% for wastage, or 15 to 16 lbs/day.
   c. Have trace-mineralized salt and water always available. An alternative would be to include 1% salt in the grain mix, which would provide 0.01 × 14 lbs × 16 oz/lb, or 2.24 oz, of salt/day.

PREPARATION OF GRAIN MIXES

There are two major types of prepared diets for the horse. One is a total diet, or a "complete feed," which consists of hay or other high-fiber ingredients, grain, and all needed supplements so that it meets all of the horse's nutritional needs except water and sometimes salt. A complete feed is intended to be the only feed consumed by the horse. The second type of prepared diet for horses is the concentrate, or grain mix, which in addition to grain generally contains various amounts of one or more supplements, but no hay or ingredient high in fiber (greater than 24, and generally not greater than 14%, crude fiber). Therefore, when grain mixes are fed, the horse must receive adequate forage, hay or pasture.

Commercially prepared grain mixes and complete feeds for horses are discussed in Chapter 4. Diet formulation, as described in this chapter, may be necessary to determine the nutrient content needed and, therefore, the proper commercially prepared feed to use. Diet formulation is necessary to obtain the formulas needed for the preparation of custom and home-prepared grain mixes or complete feeds.

For home-prepared grain mixes, amounts of desired supplements or ingredients are added to the grain as it is fed. This allows each horse to be fed the exact diet wanted. This is of benefit only if the horse has specific needs different from those of other horses being fed, or that are not met by custom or commercial grain mixes that are available. Home-prepared mixes may be necessary in treating specific conditions, such as sick horses or horses with known abnormalities. In feeding a home-prepared grain mix, if the loose grain to which dry supplements or ingredients are added does not contain a sufficient amount of something like wet molasses, fats, or oils, the dry ingredients will sift out and may not be eaten. If this occurs, it can be prevented or decreased by adding and mixing wet molasses, vegetable oil, or water with the grain before the dry ingredients are added. Wetted grain should be consumed within a few hours or spoilage may occur. However, adding substances to grain as it is fed frequently is not a very efficient, safe, or economical way to feed, and, therefore, it is better not to feed this way unless necessary. Mistakes are easily, and unfortunately not uncommonly, made, resulting in harmful deficiencies or excesses, or waste of the nutrients added. When practical and possible, it is better to have a custom mix made or to buy a commercially prepared mix.

Custom mixes are those prepared by a feed mill according to specifications they are given. These specifications may be for a specific formula, such as 80% of any cereal grain, 12.5% soybean meal, 5% wet molasses, and 2.5% dicalcium phosphate. Or the specification may be that the grain mix contain within a specified range a given amount of certain nutrients. For example, for weanlings you may want a grain mix that contains 18% or more crude protein, 12% or less crude fiber, 0.8 to 1.6% calcium, 0.6 to 1%

phosphorus, 0.3 to 0.6 ppm selenium, 50 to 100 ppm copper, 100 to 200 ppm zinc, 2000 to 5000 IU vitamin A/lb, and 100 to 200 IU vitamin E/lb. In addition, you may want it to contain certain feeds—such as soybean, canola, fish, or a milk-based meal—as the only protein supplement used to ensure that the grain mix contains adequate lysine. You may also want it to contain a certain amount of certain ingredients, such as 0.5% salt and 5% brewer's yeast, as sources of sodium, chloride, and B vitamins, respectively. In contrast, you may not want it to contain some feeds, such as cottonseed meal, unless the amount of gossypol in the cottonseed meal or grain mix containing it is below a certain level (as described in Chapter 19).

The advantage of a custom mix over a commercial mix is that it may be less expensive and that the amount of each nutrient needed can be included in the custom mix so that when it is fed with the specific forage being consumed, it will meet the requirements for the particular horses being fed. However, which nutrients and in what amounts they are needed in the grain mix must be known, as determined in the examples given previously in this chapter. In addition, a relatively large quantity generally must be purchased at one time (usually several tons), and errors and poor mixing of grain mixes unfortunately are not uncommon. For this reason, several samples from different parts of the mix should be analyzed to see that it contains the correct amount of nutrients. The feed mill should be informed before the grain mix is prepared that the mix will be analyzed and cannot be used if it is not what is wanted. This will necessitate working with the feed mill to ensure that the formula and ingredients used will provide what is wanted if the grain mix is correctly prepared. A custom mix is impractical and uneconomical for those not feeding a large number of horses. However, for those that are, and that have the capability of formulating or obtaining a custom mix, it may be less expensive and result in a better feeding program than buying a commercially prepared grain mix. Procedures for obtaining the formula needed for a home-prepared or a custom grain mix so that it, along with the forage being consumed, will meet the horse's requirements for all nutrients were described previously in this chapter.

Chapter 7

MINIMIZING HORSE FEEDING COSTS

Buying Feed Economically 139
Determining Least-Cost Feed 140
   Example 1—Hay Considering One Nutrient 140
   Example 2—Protein Supplement 140
   Example 3—Mineral Supplement 141

Example 4—Hay Considering Two Nutrients 141
Example 5—Grain Considering Two Nutrients 142
Example 6—When Grain is Less Expensive than Hay . . . 143
Minimizing Waste 144

The major factors helpful in minimizing feeding costs are:

1. To buy only feeds and supplements actually needed by or likely to benefit to the horse.
2. When available, to obtain maximum forage production and utilization of pasture, as described in Chapter 5.
3. To buy feeds economically.
4. To use feeds that provide the nutrients needed at the lowest cost.
5. To minimize feed losses with proper storage, as described in Chapter 4.
6. To minimize feed wastage by the horse.

These procedures can often greatly reduce feeding costs and do so without decreasing the nutritional quality of the diet or the horse's health, appearance, performance, or nutritional status.

Substantial savings can often be realized by not feeding unneeded vitamin/mineral supplements, blood builders, coat conditioners, snake oils, fu fu powders and the numerous other items often given to horses that are of no known or demonstrated benefit, are not needed, or are already provided in ample quantities in normal feeds. See Chapters 2 and 3 and the sections on "Vitamin-Mineral Supplements" and "Feed Additives" in Chapter 4 for when and what vitamins, minerals, and additives may be of benefit. Giving nutrients or additives that are not needed—i.e., that aren't deficient in the diet—is of no benefit and may be harmful. For example, a number of nutrients are needed for red blood cell production; when deficient, anemia and impaired performance occur. However, giving more of these nutrients than needed will not increase the number of red blood cells above normal or enhance performance; in contrast, this may be harmful. Examples of this type could be given for most nutrients—i.e., that a deficiency of that nutrient causes an impairment or problem, but that giving more of that nutrient than needed doesn't increase that factor above normal and, in contrast, causes harm. An excess of many nutrients is harmful, and many of the additives given to horses have resulted in detrimental effects, including death. The rule that should be followed is: If it's not known or there isn't good reason to believe that a nutrient is needed, or a substance hasn't been documented in controlled studies to be of benefit, don't give it.

Controlled studies are those in which a nutrient, substance, or treatment is given to one group of animals and not to another group of, as near as possible, identical animals, in identical environments and receiving identical diets and treatment, except for the specific item being tested or evaluated. Ideally, no one involved with conducting the study should know which group is, or is not, being given the substance or treatment being tested. This is called a blind study if those administering the diets or treatment don't know, and a double blind study if both they and those obtaining the effects being evaluated or measured don't know, until all effects have been obtained, i.e., the study has been completed except for analyzing the results. Blind studies are necessary to ensure against investigator bias, and greatly add to the credibility of the results obtained. Without such efforts, both intentional and unintentional bias is not only possible, but also probable, even by the most careful and honest investigators.

Testimonials are an extremely poor indication of need or benefit of a substance or treatment, no matter how valid their observations or results. If the observations or results were obtained without a control group, they may have occurred without the substance or treatment to which they are credited.

Not giving unneeded nutrients, supplements, and additives can not only be of benefit to the horse, it can also substantially reduce feeding costs.

A factor that may decrease the amount of feed needed and, therefore, feed costs, is to maximize feed utilization by dividing the amount needed into as many meals as practical. For example, in one study 10 ponies lost an average of 3% of their body weight in 2 weeks when fed once daily, whereas their body weight increased by 0.6% when fed the same amount of the same complete pelleted diet divided into six meals daily (see section on "Feeding Frequency" in Chapter 8). Feeding frequently, without increased time or labor costs, can be accomplished using mechanized timed feeders (such as, On Time Feeders, Specialty Fabrication, Wichita, KS, 1-800-664-8463).

When the procedures described in this chapter are followed, you will find that, at least in the United States, oats and commercially prepared grain mixes are generally the most expensive cereal grains to feed, and that corn is the least expensive, although in some areas and at some times other cereal grains or by-product feeds may be less expensive than corn. Any of the cereal grains may be fed to horses. Differences in their quality and cost as a source of dietary energy are generally the only factors that need to be considered in selecting which to feed. Other factors to consider are described in the sections on each type of feed in Chapter 4.

BUYING FEED ECONOMICALLY

A number of factors are often quite helpful or necessary in order to buy feeds economically. These include knowing feed prices, weights, and factors indicating quality, as well as knowing which feeds, when, and how much to buy. The first rule in buying anything at a fair price is knowing what a fair price is for what you're buying. Time should be taken to determine the current market price. This information may be obtained from other animal owners, feed mills, and feed suppliers. If a price is substantially higher or lower than prevailing prices, you should attempt to determine why. Is it because of the feed's quality? availability? something unique about it? or simply because it's being sold as a horse feed? Typically, a premium is charged for horse feeds, which may be of poorer quality than similar feeds sold to food animal producers. This is done because many people buying feeds for horses are not familiar with current prices and how to evaluate feed quality (see Chapter 4 for determining feed quality). Most things, including feeds, are sold for what the seller can get for them, which is not necessarily their worth. Thus, you should expect to buy at a fair price only if you know what a fair price is. Ignorance is not bliss; it's expensive.

Feeds should be purchased by weight. Even cereal grains may vary by more than 10 lbs/bu (1.3 kg/decaliter); hay varies much more than this. For example, similar-sized small square bales of hay may weigh 35 to 120 lbs (16 to 55 kg). Thus, on a per-bale price, for the same amount (weight) of hay, the lighter bales would cost over 3.4 times more than the heavier bales. If the weight of the hay being considered for purchase isn't to be weighed by the load, weigh a number of randomly selected bales to obtain their average weight (Fig. 7–1), and from this the number of bales/ton, and obtain a price per ton.

Buying at the proper time can make a great difference in both the price and quality of the feed obtained. The best price for hay and the best-quality hay can generally be obtained during and shortly following the growing season. Hay prices routinely increase, and quality and availability decrease, often by large amounts, during the winter or spring before the first cutting the following spring is available. Buying or contracting in the fall for enough hay to last until after the first cutting the following spring assures that the hay needed has been obtained at a fair price.

Generally, the greater the quantity purchased or contracted for at one time, the better the price. Buying hay by the ton rather than by the bale, and grain in bulk rather than sacked, usually results in substantial savings. Proper storage facilities are needed when larger feed purchases are made. Although the initial cost of these storage facilities may be quite expensive, the savings they permit will frequently more than offset this cost in a few years or less.

It is best not to buy more than a few months' grain supply at one time to prevent grain from becoming stale and losing palatability and nutritional value prior to feeding (see section on "Grain Storage" in Chapter 4). For hay, to

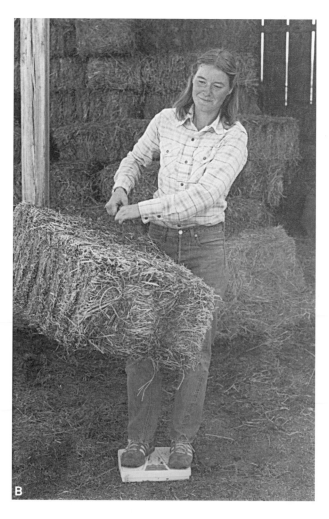

Fig. 7–1(A,B). Buy feed and provide it to the horse according to weight, not volume. To do this, weigh several of the bales of the hay being fed or that you are considering for purchase. The hay may be weighed by hanging it on the type of scale shown in A, or by standing on a bathroom or walk-on scale and subtracting the weight without the bale from the weight with the bale (B).

preserve the greatest nutritional value, it should be protected from the weather. If a hay shed or inside storage facilities are not available, waterproof canvas spread over the top and partially down the sides of the stack, and peaked so water will run off, may be used. Plastic will frequently puncture and allow water into the hay, but prevent its evaporation, resulting in more spoilage than would have occurred if the hay had been left uncovered (see section on "Hay Quality" in Chapter 4).

DETERMINING LEAST-COST FEED

Determining the least-cost feed is one of the most beneficial ways to decrease feeding costs. To determine the least-cost feedstuff, the costs of the major ingredient of concern in each feed should be compared. The major ingredient of concern is either the ingredient present in the greatest amount in that feedstuff, or the reason a particular feed is being fed. For a protein supplement, this would be protein. For a mineral mix, it might be either calcium or phosphorus. However, since the cost of phosphorus is routinely much greater than the cost of calcium, phosphorus is the major ingredient of economic concern in most calcium-phosphorus-containing mineral supplements. For all cereal grains, grain mixes and sweet feeds, fats, and oils, and generally for hay, haylage, or ensilage, the major ingredient of concern is energy, since as a source of energy is the major reason they need to be or are fed.

A nutrient in a feed that is not needed by the animal adds no value to the feed and, therefore, should not be taken into consideration. For example, if a horse needs 8% protein in its diet and a hay containing 8% or more protein is being fed, the protein content of the grain fed is of no concern—i.e., a grain mix containing 16% protein is of no greater benefit than one containing 8% protein. Thus, in this example the only nutrient that should be considered in the grain is its energy content.

To determine the cost of the major nutrient of concern in a feedstuff, divide the cost of the feed by the fraction of that nutrient in the feed, as shown in the following examples. It is important that comparisons be made among feeds equal in moisture content. To ensure that this is done, it is best to convert either the cost of the feed or the amount of nutrients in the feed to the amount present in the feed dry matter. How this is done and obtaining the amount of nutrients in the feed are described in the section on "Nutrient Content of Feeds" in Chapter 6.

Example 1—Determining the Least-Cost Hay Considering One Nutrient. Determine which of the following two hays is more economical to feed.

	Cost ($/ton)	Mcal/lb	Protein (%)	Ca (%)	P (%)
Alfalfa	120	1.1	17	1.2	0.25
Grass	110	0.9	8	0.4	0.25
Needed by the Horses Being Fed (Appendix Table 1)			8	0.25	0.2

Since both hays contain enough protein, calcium, and phosphorus to meet the horse's requirements, the differences in the amount of these nutrients in the two hays need not be taken into consideration. The only nutrient of concern economically in the hays is the energy they will provide, so we compare their cost on an energy basis as shown.

Alfalfa: $120/ton ÷ (1.1 Mcal/lb × 2000 lbs/ton)

$$= \$109.09/2000 \text{ Mcal}$$

Grass: $110/ton ÷ (0.9 Mcal/lb × 2000 lbs/ton)

$$= \$122.22/2000 \text{ Mcal}$$

Although the grass costs less per ton of hay, because of its lower energy content it costs more per calorie of digestible energy; therefore, the alfalfa is a better buy.

To further demonstrate this, calculate the cost of feeding both hays. In calculating which feed costs the least if the previous procedure is conducted, the procedure given below is not necessary but is done here to emphasize that the answer obtained using the previous procedure is correct and to demonstrate how to determine the feeding cost difference. The idle 1100-lb (500-kg) horse needs 16.4 Mcal DE/day (Appendix Table 4). The amount of each hay needed to provide this, and the associated cost, would be:

Alfalfa: 16.4 Mcal/horse/day ÷ 1.1 Mcal/lb alfalfa =

14.9 lbs alfalfa/horse/day

14.9 lbs alfalfa/horse/day × $120/ton alfalfa ÷

2000 lbs/ton = $0.89/horse/day

Grass: 16.4 Mcal/horse/day ÷ 0.90 Mcal/lb grass =

18.2 lbs grass/horse/day

18.2 lbs grass/horse/day × $110/ton grass ÷

2000 lbs/ton = $1.00/horse/day

Example 2—Determining the Least-Cost Protein Supplement. Determine which of the following protein supplements is the least expensive.

Protein Supplement	Cost ($/ton of Supp.)		Protein (%/100)		Cost (%/ton of Protein)
Range Cubes A	194	÷	0.39[a] − 0.13	=	746
Range Cubes B	174	÷	0.28	=	621
Dehy pellets	120	÷	0.17	=	705
Horse Supplement	246	÷	0.30	=	820

[a] With 13% protein equivalents from urea, which is subtracted from this value to obtain the amount of usable protein for the horse. Little urea, or other nonprotein nitrogen sources, is used by horses (see Chapter 1).

The reason these supplements will be used is as a source of protein. To find the one that provides protein most economically, determine the cost of protein from each by dividing the cost of the supplement by its usable protein content. For Range Cubes A, this would be 39 − 13, or 26% protein, not 39%, since the horse utilizes little nonprotein nitrogen such as urea. Thus, as shown above, Range Cubes B provide the least-expensive source of protein. If the supplement was to be used for mature horses, its source of protein doesn't matter, i.e., whether it contained soybean meal, cottonseed meal, or any other source of protein.

However, if the supplement was to be used for growing horses, you should ensure that the supplement's protein contains 5% or more of the essential amino acid lysine (Table 4-7 gives this information).

Example 3—Determining the Least-Cost Mineral Supplement. If the following mineral mixes are available, which is the least expensive?

Mineral Supplement	Cost ($/cwt) of Supplement		Ca	P		Cost ($/cwt) of Mineral
			(Fraction in Supplement)			
Monosodium phosphate (monophos)	16.25	÷	0	0.24	=	67.71 cwt of P
Dicalcium phosphate (dical)	13.00	÷	0.24	0.19	=	68.42 cwt of P
Limestone (calcium carbonate)	2.30	÷	0.35	0	=	6.57 cwt of Ca

As shown here, and as is routinely the case, phosphorus is much more expensive than calcium. Calcium is quite inexpensive. If in this example additional phosphorus, but not calcium, is needed in the diet, monophos would be the most economical supplement to use. The calcium provided by the dical is not needed and, therefore, is of no benefit. It also is of no harm unless it results in a calcium:phosphorus ratio in the total diet outside of the acceptable range (as given in Chapter 2). However, if both calcium and phosphorus are needed, the value of both must be considered. To do this, first determine the amount of monophos and limestone needed to provide the same amount of calcium and phosphorus as provided by the dical, which in the example as given in the table is 24 lbs Ca and 19 lbs P/100 lbs of dical.

1. It would take 24 lb Ca ÷ 0.35 lb Ca/lb limestone, or 68.6 lb of limestone, to provide 24 lbs of calcium.
2. It would take 19 lb P ÷ 0.24 lb P/lb monophos, or 79.2 lb of monophos, to provide 19 lbs of phosphorus.
3. Thus, a mixture of 68.6 lbs of limestone and 79.2 lbs of monophos would provide the same amount of calcium and phosphorus as 100 lbs of dical.

Next, determine the cost for the amount of each mineral mix needed to provide the same amount of calcium and phosphorus as 100 lbs of dical. The cost for the limestone plus monophos mixture is:

68.6 lb limestone × $2.30/100 lbs limestone = $1.58

plus

79.2 lbs of monophos × $16.25/100 lbs = $12.87 monophos

for a total cost of the mixture = $14.45
versus the cost of 100 lbs of dical, which is = $13.00

Thus, if both calcium and phosphorus were needed, in this example dical would be the most economical mineral supplement to use.

Example 4—Determining the Least-Cost Hay Considering Two Nutrients. Determine which of the following two types of hay is the least expensive for feeding weanlings.

	Mcal/lb	Protein (%)	Cost ($/ton)
Alfalfa	1.1	17	62
Grass	0.9	8	45

If only the cost of dietary energy is considered, the grass hay would be the least expensive?

Alfalfa: $62/2000 lbs ÷ 1.1 Mcal/lb = $56.36/2000 Mcal

Grass: $45/2000 lbs ÷ 0.9 Mcal/lb = $50.00/2000 Mcal

However, if the hays are being fed to horses who need more protein in their total diet (as shown in Appendix Table 1) than that present in the hay that is least expensive on an energy basis, then both the energy and the protein content of the hays must be considered. The cost of both protein and energy provided by a feed can be determined using the following formulas.

Formula A:

$$a = \frac{\left[\begin{array}{c}\text{(\% protein in} \\ \text{feed evaluated)}\end{array}\right] - \dfrac{\left[\begin{array}{c}\% \text{ protein} \\ \text{in grain}\end{array}\right] \times \left[\begin{array}{c}\text{Mcal/lb in} \\ \text{feed evaluated}\end{array}\right]}{\text{(Mcal/lb in grian)}}}{\left[\begin{array}{c}\% \text{ protein in} \\ \text{protein supp.}\end{array}\right] - \dfrac{\left[\begin{array}{c}\text{Mcal/lb in} \\ \text{protein supp.}\end{array}\right] \times \left[\begin{array}{c}\% \text{ protein} \\ \text{in grain}\end{array}\right]}{\text{(Mcal in grain)}}}$$

Formula B:

$$b = \frac{\left[\begin{array}{c}\text{Mcal/lb in} \\ \text{feed evaluated}\end{array}\right] - \left[\begin{array}{c}\text{(Mcal/lb in} \\ \text{protein supp.}\end{array}\right] \times (a)}{\text{(Mcal/lb in grain)}}$$

Formula C:

$$\left[\begin{array}{c}\text{Value of feed} \\ \text{evaluation with} \\ \text{respect to grain} \\ \text{\& protein suppl.}\end{array}\right] = \left[(b) \times \left[\begin{array}{c}\text{cost} \\ \text{of} \\ \text{grain}\end{array}\right]\right] + \left[(a) \times \left[\begin{array}{c}\text{cost of} \\ \text{protein} \\ \text{supp.}\end{array}\right]\right]$$

If the value of the feed being evaluated is greater than its purchase price, it is a good buy. In contrast, if its value is less than its cost, it is not a good buy with respect to the cereal grain and protein supplement with which it was compared. Although these formulas may look formidable, they are easy to use. Simply insert the values for the feeds and do the arithmetic involved, as shown below for this example.

In this example, let's say that the grain and protein supplements available are as follows:

Feed	Cost/ton ($)	Mcal/lb	Protein (%)
Oats	110	1.36	12
Corn	100	1.60	10
Soybean Meal	190	1.48	44
Cottonseed Meal	180	1.36	41

First, it is necessary to determine which of these grain and protein supplements to use. If the decision is based only on cost (for other considerations see the discussion of cereal grains and protein supplements in Chapter 4), corn and soybean meal would be used. Since in this example corn is higher in energy and lower in cost than any of the other concentrates, it is obviously the most economical source of energy, while soybean meal is the most economical source of protein, as shown below.

Feed	Cost/ton ($)	÷	Protein (%/100)	=	Cost/ton of Protein ($)
Oats	110	÷	0.12	=	917
Corn	100	÷	0.10	=	1000
Soybean meal	190	÷	0.44	=	432
Cottonseed meal	180	÷	0.41	=	439

Using corn and soybean meal as the grain and protein supplements, and inserting their values and the values of the feed being evaluated into formulas A, B, and C, both the value of the evaluated feeds with respect to corn and soybean meal, and which of the evaluated feeds is the best buy considering both energy and protein, can be determined, as shown.

Alfalfa Evaluated

Formula A:

$$a = \frac{(17) - \left[\frac{(10) \times (1.1)}{(1.6)}\right]}{(44) - \left[\frac{(1.48) \times (10)}{(1.6)}\right]} = \frac{17 - 6.875}{44 - 9.25} = 0.291367$$

Formula B:

$$b = \frac{(1.1) - [(1.48) \times (0.291367)]}{(1.6)} = 0.418$$

Formula C:

Value of alfalfa with respect to corn & SBM = [(0.418) × ($100/ton corn)] + [(0.291367) × ($190/ton SBM)] = $41.80 + $55.36 = $97.16/ton alfalfa

Value of alfalfa with respect to its cost
= (Value) ÷ (Cost) = $97.16 ÷ $62.00 = 1.57

Thus, the alfalfa is worth 1.57 times the cost of an equal amount of energy and protein provided by corn and soybean meal.

Grass Evaluated

Formula A:

$$a = \frac{(8) - \left[\frac{(10) \times (0.9)}{(1.6)}\right]}{(44) - \left[\frac{(1.48) \times (10)}{(1.6)}\right]} = \frac{2.375}{34.75} = 0.0683$$

Formula B:

$$b = \frac{(0.9) - [(1.48) \times (0.0683)]}{(1.6)} = 0.4993$$

Formula C:

Value of grass with respect to corn & SBM = [(0.4993) × ($100/ton corn)] + [(0.0683) × ($190/ton SBM)] = $49.93 + $12.99 = $62.92/ton grass

Value of grass with respect to its cost =
(Value) ÷ (Cost) = $62.92 ÷ $45.00 = 1.40

Thus, the grass is worth 1.40 times the cost of an equal amount of energy and protein provided by corn and soybean meal.

Alfalfa versus Grass Value. Since the value of alfalfa hay with respect to its cost is more than the value of the grass hay with respect to its cost (1.57 times versus 1.40 times), the alfalfa hay is a better buy than the grass hay. In addition, both are more economical than the least-expensive cereal grain and protein supplement and, therefore, to feed most economically you should feed as much hay and as little grain mix as possible.

Example 5—Determining the Least-Cost Grain Considering Two Nutrients. Determine which of the following two cereal grains is more economical to use in a grain mix for weanlings being fed grass hay.

Grain	Mcal/lb	Protein (%)	Cost ($/100 lbs)
Barley	1.5	12	5.20
Corn	1.6	10	5.30

If only the cost of energy is considered, corn, as shown below, is more economical.

Barley: $5.20 ÷ 1.5 = $3.47/100 Mcal

Corn: $5.30 ÷ 1.6 = $3.31/100 Mcal

In contrast, if only the cost of protein is considered, as shown below, barley is more economical.

Barley: $5.20 ÷ 0.12 = $43.33/cwt of protein

Corn: $5.30 ÷ 0.10 = $53.00/cwt of protein

If the hay and grain being fed contain less than the amount of protein needed in the diet (as shown in Appendix Table 1) a protein supplement must be fed to provide the additional protein needed. This is routinely the case for weanlings fed a grass hay, as in this example. Thus, in this example both the energy and the protein provided by the grains must be considered in comparing their relative values. This can be done by inserting the cost, energy, and protein content of the feeds into formulas A, B, and C given in Example 4. In this example, let's say that the soybean meal (SBM) as given in Example 4, is available and is the most economical source of protein. Therefore, it will be used to compare the cereal grains too. Either cereal grain may be used in the formulas as the feed being evaluated; the other may be used as the grain with which it is being compared. Let's use barley as the feed being evaluated.

Formula A:

$$a = \frac{\left[\begin{array}{c} \% \ protein \\ in \ barley \end{array} \right] - \left[\dfrac{\left[\begin{array}{c} \% \ protein \\ in \ corn \end{array} \right] \times \left[\begin{array}{c} (Mcal/lb) \\ in \ barley \end{array} \right]}{(Mcal/lb \ in \ corn)} \right]}{\left[\begin{array}{c} \% \ protein \\ in \ SBM \end{array} \right] - \left[\dfrac{\left[\begin{array}{c} (Mcal/lb) \\ in \ SBM \end{array} \right] \times \left[\begin{array}{c} \% \ protein \\ in \ corn \end{array} \right]}{(Mcal/lb \ in \ corn)} \right]}$$

Formula B:

$$b = \frac{(Mcal/lb \ in \ barley) - [(Mcal/lb \ in \ SBM) \times (a)]}{(Mcal/lb \ in \ corn)}$$

Formula A:

$$a = \frac{(12) - \left[\dfrac{(10) \times (1.5)}{(1.6)} \right]}{(44) - \left[\dfrac{(1.48) \times (10)}{(1.6)} \right]}$$

$$= \frac{12 - 9.375}{44 - 9.25} = \frac{2.625}{34.75} = 0.07554$$

Formula B:

$$b = \frac{(1.5) - [(1.48) \times (0.07554)]}{(1.6)} = 0.8676$$

Formula C:

$value of barley = [(0.8676) × ($5.30/cwt of corn)] + [(0.07555) × ($9.50/cwt of SBM)] = $5.32/cwt

Thus, in regard to both protein and energy, if soybean meal costs $190/ton and corn $5.30/100 lbs, barley is worth $5.32/100 lbs. Yet it costs only $5.20/100 lbs. Since barley is worth more than its cost, as compared with corn, it is more economical than corn. In contrast, if its value was found to be less than its cost with respect to the cereal grain with which it was being compared, then the other cereal grain would be more economical.

Example 6—Determining the Least-Cost Feed When Grain Is Less Expensive Than Hay. The following feeds are available. Design a least-cost feeding program for mature, nonreproducing horses.

Feed	Cost ($/cwt)	Energy (Mcal/lb)	Protein (%)	Ca (%)	P (%)
Corn	8.00	1.6	9	0.05	0.35
Hay	5.40	0.9	15	1.2	0.2
Horses Needs (Appendix Table 1)			8	0.25	0.2

Since both feeds meet or exceed the amount of protein needed, the least expensive to feed will be the one that provides the least expensive source of dietary energy. This is determined as shown below by dividing their cost by their energy content.

Corn: $8.00/100 lbs ÷ 1.6 Mcal/lb = $5.00/100 Mcal

Hay: $5.40/100 lbs ÷ 0.9 Mcal/lb = $6.00/100 Mcal

Since corn is the least expensive source of energy, the least-expensive feeding program would be one consisting of as much corn and as little hay as possible. However, some hay must be fed to prevent colic, founder, and behavioral problems, as described in Chapter 20. Although the amount of forage consumed daily may be as little as that equal to 0.5% of the horse's body weight, which may be less than one-third of total feed intake, it is safest if forage makes up at least one-half of the weight of the total diet, i.e., if the maximum grain mix in the diet by weight is 50%. Thus, in this example the least expensive, but still safe, feeding program would be a diet consisting of 50% corn and 50% hay. As shown below, this diet would provide an ample amount of nutrients to meet the horse's needs.

Feed	Fraction of Diet		Mcal/lb in feed		diet	Protein (%) in feed		diet	Calcium (%) in feed		diet	Phosphorus (%) in feed		diet
Corn	0.5	×	1.6	=	0.80	9	=	4.5	0.05	=	0.025	0.35	=	0.175
Hay	0.5	×	0.9	=	0.45	15	=	7.5	1.2	=	0.6	0.2	=	0.1
Total	1.0				1.25			12.0			0.625			0.275
Horses Need (from Appendix Table 1)					0.9			8			0.25			0.2

The amount of corn and hay to feed would depend on the horse's dietary energy needs, which can be calculated as described in the section on "Determining the Total Amount of Feed Needed" in Chapter 6. For the idle 1100-lb (500-kg) horse, 16.4 Mcal/day are needed (Appendix Table 4). The following amount of this diet (which as shown above provides 1.25 Mcal/lb) would be needed to provide this amount of dietary energy.

16.4 Mcal/day needed ÷ 1.25 Mcal/lb of diet

= 13.12 lbs of diet/day needed

The amount of corn to feed therefore would be one-half of 13.12, or about 6.5 lbs/day. As much hay as the horse will consume with minimum waste should be fed, which would be about 7.5 lbs/day (assuming 10 to 15% may be lost or wasted). If the corn is to be fed by volume, the amount to feed would be the following:

6.5 lbs/day ÷ 1.6 lbs cracked corn/qt

from Appendix Table 8 = 4 qts/day

MINIMIZING WASTE

Horses, given the opportunity, will waste a substantial amount of forage, both pasture and hay. Procedures for minimizing the waste of pasture forage from trampling and spotty grazing is described in Chapter 5. Horses are particularly wasteful of excess hay. Most horses will usually empty a feed bunk regardless of how much it contains or how much of the feed they need. Once the feed is on the ground, it may get wet and become contaminated with urine and feces; then horses won't eat it. Hay wastage can be reduced by using the following procedures.

1. Feed only as much as the horse will consume with little or no wastage, and as needed to meet its needs. The amount of hay fed may be decreased until the horse just maintains optimum body weight and condition.
2. Feed in feeders that have solid sides and bottoms. Feed bunks that are not solid allow the loss of leaves, which are the most nutritious part of forage. Feeding on the ground is likely to result in much greater waste.
3. Feed each horse separate from others if possible. When fed in groups, those at the top of the dominance or pecking order will overeat and waste feed, while those near the bottom of the pecking order may not receive enough feed unless a substantial excess is fed and, therefore, wasted.

Feed losses from storage conditions should also be minimized by following the procedures described in the section on feed storage in Chapter 4.

Section Two

FEEDING AND CARE OF HORSES

Chapter 8

GENERAL HORSE FEEDING PRACTICES

Water Feeding 147
Forage Feeding 147
   Forage Necessity 147
   Methods of Feeding Harvested Forages 148
Grain Feeding 149
   Grain Necessity 149

Methods of Feeding Grain 149
Feeding Frequency 150
Monitoring Horses' Nutritional and Health Status 151
Group Socialization, Communication, and Feeding 152
Changing Diets 154

WATER FEEDING

Before and during prolonged exercise, the horse should be allowed and encouraged to consume as much water as it will drink. However, following exercise, the horse should be cooled down before being allowed to drink as much as it wants. Consumption of a sufficient amount of water by the hot horse after physical exertion may cause colic and acute laminitis or founder. However, at all other times adequate quantities of good-quality palatable water should be readily available. Whether the horse drinks before or after feeding does not affect feed digestibility, but it does affect feed intake. Thirsty horses will reduce their feed intake, or not eat at all, if water isn't available before or during feeding.

FORAGE FEEDING

Forage Necessity

Water and forage are the two feeds required for life by all horses in all situations. Other feeds such as grain various supplements, and salt are not needed by many classes of horses and in many situations, or are optional—i.e., they may be beneficial but they are not required. Horses should be allowed all of both the water and forage that they will consume without waste. An exception is the overweight horse, in which forage intake should be restricted and no grain fed.

Forage is required in the horse's diet as a source of fiber. Usable or digestible fiber is necessary as a source of energy by microorganisms in the horse's cecum and large intestine, and, although not required, does provide a source of dietary energy for the horse. However, indigestible fiber, which is low in all nonforage feeds (except for some by-product feeds) is required for the maintenance of normal gastrointestinal pH, motility, and function. Indigestible fiber also helps prevent too rapid an intake of readily digested carbohydrates, which are high in cereal grains. Too rapid an intake of an excess amount of readily digested carbohydrates will cause diarrhea, colic, and acute laminitis or founder. Thus, an adequate amount of fiber, which can be provided only by feeding sufficient forage or some by-products such as hulls, are required by the horse for normal intestinal function and by microbial organisms, both of which are necessary for the horse's health and well-being.

Horses have been maintained in good health by feeding as little as 0.5 lbs of forage/100 lbs body weight daily (0.5 kgs/100 kg), with the remainder of their dietary energy needs provided by grain. This low amount of forage results in a diet consisting of 15 to 35% forage and 65 to 85% grain, and puts the horse at risk of the problems caused by inadequate fiber intake. If at any time, for any reason (such as not feeling well, weather or environmental change, etc.), the horse eats less feed, the reduction will generally be in the amount of forage and not the amount of grain eaten, resulting in an even lower fiber intake, which may be sufficient to cause diarrhea, colic, or acute laminitis. In addition, the high grain intake increases the risk of exertion myopathy (see Chapter 11) and, over time, obesity due to excess energy intake. For these reasons it is recommended that forage make up at least one-half of the total weight of feed dry matter consumed, or at least 1 lb of forage dry matter/100 lbs body weight daily (1 kg/ 100 kg) be consumed. If less forage than this is consumed, either as determined by actual measurement or by calculating the amount of forage that the horse needs to consume to provide its dietary energy needs above that provided by the amount of grain fed (for a description of how to determine this, see the section on "Determining the Total Amount of Feed Needed by the Horse," in Chapter 6), the amount of grain fed should be reduced.

Feeding inadequate forage to the horse not on pasture greatly increases the risk of not only diarrhea, colic, and founder, but also eating wood, feces, and, particularly in young horses, tail chewing and, less commonly, mane chewing. Increased wood chewing with decreased forage intake is known to occur for two reasons: (1) decreased eating time, resulting in increased boredom, and (2) increased gut acid. Wood chewing is detrimental for at least three reasons: (1) damage to facilities, (2) occasionally wood splinters in the oral cavity, and (3) intestinal obstruction, which if untreated may be fatal. Tail and mane chewing are not only cosmetic problems but may also cause intestinal obstruction. Although there are other causes of wood chewing, eating feces, and tail and/or mane chewing than boredom and inadequate forage in the diet (such as mineral and protein deficiencies, play, and mimicking other horses), these are the most common causes, and alleviating them is the most commonly successful means of stopping or preventing these behavioral problems.

Methods of Feeding Harvested Forages

Forage should be fed in a manner that minimizes: (1) forage losses, particularly of leaves, which are the component highest in nutritional value; (2) forage fecal contamination, which not only increases forage losses but increases intestinal parasitism; and (3) dust inhalation, during their consumption, which increases respiratory problems. To accomplish these objectives, harvested forages should be fed in a container or rack that catches leaves and loose forage, and that keeps as much forage as possible off the ground. There are numerous types of hay racks, feed troughs, or feed bunks that may be used, as shown in Figure 8-1.

Feed losses are considerably higher when the feed is consumed from the ground instead of from a feeder. Even when ground conditions are ideal (firm and dry), feeding hay on the ground can decrease growth rate and feed efficiency nearly 20% below that with the same amount of the same hay in a feeder. Feed losses are greater when hay is fed on the ground because of: (1) a greater loss of the hay, particularly leaves, and (2) greater fecal and urine contamination of the hay, resulting in feed the horses won't eat. If they do eat fecally contaminated hay, it increases the risk of intestinal parasite egg intake and, therefore, intestinal parasitism and all the detrimental effects this causes (as described in Chapter 9). Stalled horses defecate an average of once every 1.5 hrs and, even if adequate space is available, walk away from their feeding area before defecating less than one-half of the time. Thus, horses defecate and urinate frequently while eating, and the majority of the time do so in their feeding area, contaminating feed that is on the ground. However, even when hay is placed in a feed bunk, most horses will pull much of it out of the

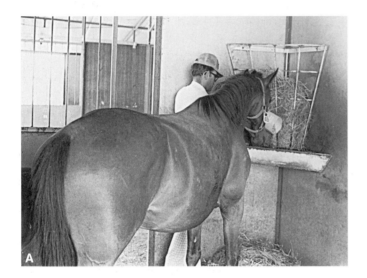

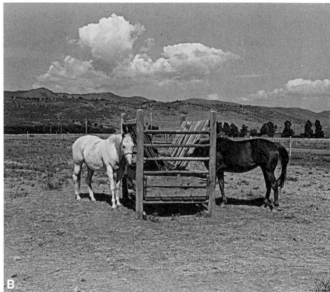

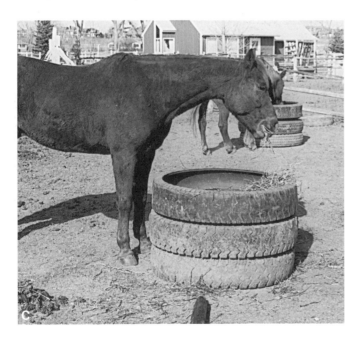

Fig. 8–1. Three types of feeders for horses for use in stables, paddocks, or pasture. Hay rack-type feeders (A and B) allow the horse to see while eating; catch leaves and loose hay, thereby minimizing their loss; minimize dust inhalation; and can be used for feeding grain as well as hay. Tire hay feeders (C) may be made by removing most of the sides of all except the bottom side of the bottom tire, on which a solid but not water-tight platform may be attached, and fastening the tires together. Hay losses may be greater for this type of feeder, and for feed troughs or bunks, than for hay rack-type feeders because many horses pull much of the hay out of them so they can see while eating it. Tire feeders and feed troughs would also be expected to result in greater dust inhalation.

bunk and eat it from the ground. This may occur because of their desire to see better what is going on around them while eating. This is an understandable desire: they can better avoid being hurt by other horses wanting their feed; it is also a residual antipredator behavior. When the hay is eaten from a feed bunk, the horse will lift its head frequently (in one study 25 times/hr) so they can be more aware of what is happening around them.

Hay consumption from a feed bunk or from a feeder placed above the horse's shoulder increases material getting into their eyes and dust inhalation while eating, which in turn increases the risk and occurrence of respiratory problems such as coughing, emphysema, heaves, exercise-induced pulmonary hemorrhage, and probably susceptibility to infectious respiratory diseases. For these and the reasons described above, it is recommended that all harvested forage be fed from hay racks designed to catch falling leaves and loose hay (Fig. 8-1 A and B), and that they not be higher than the horse's shoulder level.

GRAIN FEEDING

Grain Necessity

No grain or concentrates are needed by many horses all or the majority of the time. Grain or grain mixes are fed:

1. When necessary to provide the nutrients needed but not provided in adequate amounts by the forage consumed (most often this is during growth, lactation, and intense training or use).
2. When good-quality forages are poorly available or more expensive than grain (see Example 6, Chapter 7).
3. When desired for other reasons, such as a treat, training or behavior modification aid, to help get horses in or to catch them, etc.

Although horses may be gradually adapted to a diet consisting entirely of cereal grain, the greater the proportion of grain in the diet, the greater the risk of diarrhea, colic, acute laminitis or founder, exertion myopathy, hyperactivity, and obesity. For these reasons it is recommended that a grain or concentrate mix not make up over one-half of the total amount of feed of similar moisture content consumed, except for horses less than 1 year of age or those being used intensely for sprint-type activity in which up to 70% grain mix may be fed (Appendix Table 1). However, even for these horses, a maximum of 50% grain mix in the diet is safer. This would be a maximum of 0.7 lbs/100 lbs body wt (0.7 kg/100 kg) daily.

Methods of Feeding Grain

Grain and forages are generally fed at the same time. Because cereal grains are more palatable, most horses will eat all of the grain before eating any of the forage. Some believe that feeding grain after most of the forage has been consumed is beneficial because it will result in a slower rate of grain consumption. This doesn't appear to occur, however. The rate of grain consumption, as well as chewing behavior, also appears to be unaffected by the fiber content of the grain.

In addition, forage consumed with grain decreases the amount of the grain's starch digested in the small intestine and, therefore, increases the amount that reaches the cecum (Fig. 1-1). Excess starch in the cecum causes cecal acidosis, which if sufficiently severe results in diarrhea, colic or founder. The risk of this is decreased by not feeding forage for one hour or more before and for 3 or more hours after feeding grain. However, this risk can be better minimized in most feeding programs by feeding less grain. Not feeding forage and grain at the same time, increases feeding time and labor, and may not be practical in some situations. In addition, grain consumption before forage, as occurs when both are fed at the same time, results in a more intense mixing of ingesta and less variation in the concentration of substances in the horse's large intestine.

Grains, like harvested forages, should be fed in a feeder to decrease feed losses and dirt consumption, which, if sufficient over time, may result in sand-induced colic, and/or, intestinal impaction. Wooden, plastic, or rubber feeding pans may be used for nonstabled horses (Fig. 8-2) or feed bags may be used (Fig. 8-3A, B). To prevent injury, metal feed pans are not recommended. Lipped feeding pans, and troughs with rings mounted on top, will help prevent horses from rooting grain out on the ground if this is a problem with a particular horse. This is not a problem with most horses unless they are being overfed.

Many people feed by volume, i.e., by so many coffee cans, scoops, quarts or liters of grain, and by flakes of hay. There is no disadvantage in feeding by volume provided it is known what weight of feed that volume provides. The weight of feed per unit of volume, or density, varies widely, as shown in Appendix Table 8. For example, a 1 qt, 1 lb. or 1 liter (1-L) coffee can holds 0.5 lbs (0.25 kg) of bran, 0.85 to 1 lb (0.4 kg) of oats, and 1.9 lbs (0.9 kg) of wheat, which provide 0.75, 1.1, and 2.9 Mcal respectively, or nearly a fourfold difference in the amount of dietary energy provided by the same volume of feed. The small standard-size square bale may weigh anywhere from 35 to 120 lbs (16 to 55 kg), although it usually weighs 60 to 80 lbs (27 to 36 kg). A flake of it may weigh anywhere

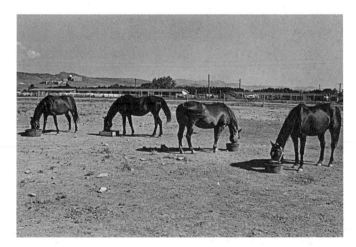

Fig. 8-2. Nonstabled horses may be fed grain in wooden, plastic, or rubber feeding pans. Metal pans are not recommended as they may cause injuries.

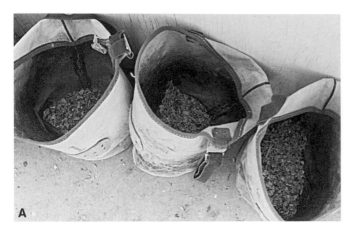
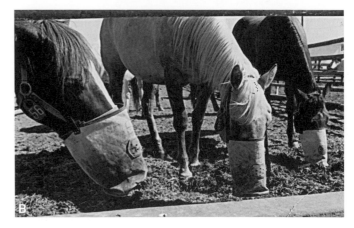

Fig. 8–3(A, B). Feed bags work well for feeding horses in a group. Each horse is assured of receiving the correct amount of the specific grain mix fed without any being wasted. Care should be taken to ensure that the feeding bags are removed as soon as the horse finishes eating the grain.

from a few to 15 lbs (1.5 to 7 kg). Thus, to determine the correct amount to feed, you should weigh the amount that the container you are using holds of the grain mix being fed, and the average size flake of the hay being fed (Fig. 8-4A, B).

FEEDING FREQUENCY

Horses have relatively small stomachs (Fig. 1-1) whose capacity constitutes only about 7 to 8% of that of their gastrointestinal tract, as compared to 60 to 70% for cattle.

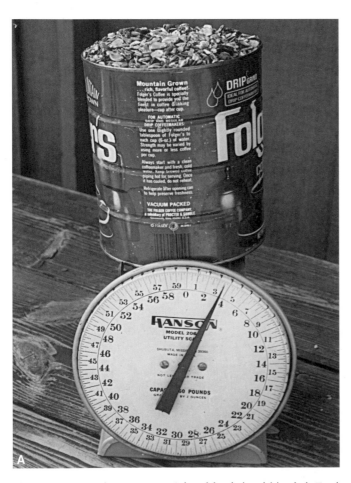
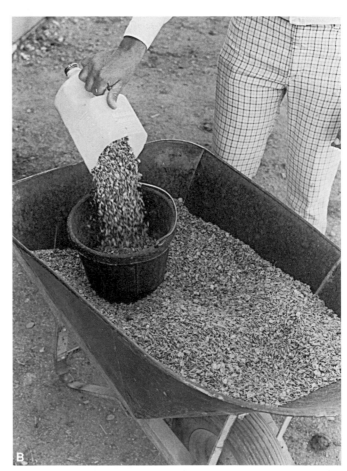

Fig. 8–4(A,B). The correct weight of feed should be fed. To do this, weigh the amount that the container being used to feed with holds of the grain mix being fed. Any type of container may be used, such as a coffee can (A) or an ice cream bucket. A grain scoop can also be made by cutting the bottom out of a plastic jug (B).

This limits the amount that can be eaten in a single meal. A small stomach is an advantage for enhancing wild horses' ability to flee from danger, and has no disadvantage for them since they are on pasture and able to eat small amounts continually. Horses on pasture spend 50 to 70% of their time, 24 hrs/day, grazing, during which small amounts of grass are ingested continually during the grazing periods. Regardless of the type of feed (hay, grain, or a complete pelleted feed), if it is available, most horses will eat hourly during the day and every 2 to 3 hours during the night. However, even when the feed is always available, the amount of time spent eating decreases from 50 to 70% when on pasture, to 30 to 70% when fed only hay, to 35 to 40% when fed a complete pelleted feed, and to 13 to 19% when fed a grain mix only. The decreased amount of time spent eating means more feed is consumed at one time. The amount consumed at one time is even greater when feed is not always available, as is the case and necessity for most horses not on pasture.

The greater the amount consumed at one time, the greater the stomachs distention, increase in gastrointestinal motility, and alteration it causes in the horse. However, horses can safely be fed even a high-grain diet as infrequently as twice daily when the total amount of feed is no more than the amount needed for maintenance, which would be up to 0.8 to 0.9 lb of grain/100 lbs body weight (0.8 to 0.9 kg/100 Kg) daily. However, for safety a maximum of one-half this amount of grain at a single feeding is recommended.

To prevent digestive dysfunctions (excessive gas production, colic, laminitis, and impaired fiber fermentation) grain intake in the horse fed 2 to 3 meals daily should be limited to about 0.5 lb of grain/100 lbs body weight (0.5 kg/100 kg) per feeding. When grain ingestion exceed these amounts, there is a dramatic increase in the amount of starch that escapes digestion and absorption from the small intestine, which greatly increases the risk of these problems.

Infrequent meal-induced changes in intestinal motility and blood flow increase the risk and occurrence of colic, a disease primarily of stabled or paddocked horses. This major disease of horses is uncommon in those on pasture. Since these changes, which increase the risk of colic, do not occur in response to small amounts consumed frequently, their occurrence and, therefore, the risk and occurrence of colic in horses not on pasture, can be decreased by: (1) having any forage, but preferably long-stem hay, available for the horse to eat to satiation and for as much of the time as possible; (2) feeding as frequently, at as regular, and at as even intervals as practical; and (3) feeding as little grain as necessary. Long-stem hay or pasture forage should be the basis for all feeding programs, and grain should be fed only if necessary and in as small amounts as possible. This doesn't mean that grain shouldn't be fed if desired or needed, but that forage should constitute the majority of the feed consumed. Two exceptions would be for the horse with poor teeth that may do better on a complete pelleted feed and/or more grain, and when good-quality forage is poorly available or considerably more expensive than grain (see Example 6 in Chapter 7).

In summary, it is recommended that all feeds be fed to all horses: (1) in equally divided amounts, (2) as near the same time each day and at as even intervals as practical, and (3) at least twice daily, but as many more times daily as practical. If the amount of grain fed is small (less than 0.25 lb/100 lbs bw daily) there may be little advantage in feeding it more than once daily. Feed working horses, lactating mares, and growing horses receiving large amounts of feed (an amount equal to more than 2.5% of their body weight daily) at least 3 times daily. It may be of benefit to feed grain to horses in intense training or use 4 to 5 hours prior to exercise, and not to feed them for at least one hour after strenuous exertion (see Chapter 11).

MONITORING HORSES' NUTRITIONAL AND HEALTH STATUS

Regardless of the types of horses or what or how they are fed, their nutritional and health status should be observed at least once and preferably twice daily. Each horse should be observed individually for injuries, attitude, and feeding behavior, including appetite, eagerness to eat, and rate and amount eaten or not eaten. A sore tongue or mouth, or bad teeth are common causes of decreased feed intake. Moldy or contaminated feed may cause a sudden decrease in feed intake. Any uneaten feed should be closely evaluated to determine if there is a problem with it, if too much was fed, if there is inadequate water, or if there is something wrong with the horse. Boredom may also be a cause of decreased feed intake, in which case exercise, a change in diet, or providing the companionship of another animal may be helpful. Decreased eagerness to eat, amount eaten, or attitude are frequently the first effects of, and, therefore, indications of, illness. The presence, source, and cause for any abnormal feces should also be determined. The horse showing any deviation from normal should be examined thoroughly. This includes taking a rectal temperature of any horse whose appetite, feed consumption, or attitude appear decreased. Rectal temperatures more than 1°F (0.5°C) outside the normal range of 99 to 101°F (37.3 to 38.3°C) should be evaluated further and treated accordingly.

To ensure that the proper amount of feed is being fed and consumed, the horse's body weight should be monitored at least every few months. The horse's weight can be obtained as described in that section in Chapter 6. If necessary, the amount fed should be altered accordingly. This is the best and only accurate way to ensure that the proper amount is being consumed, and that the horse is at the body condition desired for optimum physical performance, show performance, growth rate, reproduction, and comfort during both hot and cold seasons. Many horses are either overfed or underfed. Chronic gradual weight gain or loss may not be readily apparent to a person who observes the horse daily until the change becomes severe. Obtaining all horses' weights periodically prevents this from occurring.

Horses, like other athletes, have optimal performance weights. Weight loss may occur as a result of inadequate dietary energy for the work being performed, or from dehydration. In either case, weight records are helpful in detecting weight loss so that it can be corrected. It has been shown that horses have an optimal weight for physical performance and for maximum breeding efficiency. Most horses in most situations should be kept in moderate to moderately fleshy condition as described in Table 1–4.

Excess fat is usually a result of overfeeding rarely is it due to a hormonal problem. Factors that result in overfeeding include:

1. The satisfaction people get from feeding their horses. For many, feeding, not use, constitutes their major association with the horse.
2. Inadequate use and exercise, which are common for many horses.
3. Purposely overfeeding show horses and sale horses because fat may help hide blemishes, and fat horses traditionally place and sell higher than thin horses.
4. Erroneously assuming the mare needs more feed before the last 2 to 3 months of pregnancy and, therefore, overfeeding before this time.
5. The horse being high on the pecking or dominance order in a group and as a result getting too much of other horses' feed.

Conversely, some common causes of thin horses include:

1. Poor quality or inadequate amounts of forage available.
2. Dental problems as described in Chapter 9.
3. Excessive amounts of internal or external parasites, as described in Chapter 9.
4. High energy needs due to lactation or hard work.
5. Prolonged hot/humid weather which increases energy needs and decreases feed intake as described in Chapter 10.
6. Chronic disease that decreases intake or utilization of feed
7. The horse's being low in the pecking or dominance order in a group and as a result being chased away or, because of fear, staying away, from adequate feed.

GROUP SOCIALIZATION, COMMUNICATION, AND FEEDING

Horses are very sociable animals that desire and seek companionship; horses, people, or other animals. Two or more horses living together in the same pasture or paddock usually band together. Castration and life in a small pasture or stable don't eliminate the horse's desire and propensity to form specific associations with other horses. Horses frequently develop strong psychologic attachments for each other, which appears to be more for social need than security. They are selective in whom they pick as a preferred buddy if there are several horses available, but in the absence of another horse, they may develop affection for other animals, including a dog, goat, or person. They use sight, sound, and particularly smell to identify other horses, animals, and people. It is believed by some that horses can detect fear in people by smell, which makes them nervous. When a horse is separated from its friends, some become very restless, agitated, and even quite afraid. This strong desire and psychologic need for companionship question the welfare of horses left alone, and the lack of concern, care, or knowledge of those responsible.

However, it is difficult to train or sometimes even use a horse until it learns not to be too dependent on being with its friends. Some techniques to accomplish this include feeding it separately, using it more frequently, and removing it to a separate area in a well-fenced or safe area. Some horses replace social dependence with barn dependence, becoming "barn sour." A barn-sour horse resists being ridden away from the barn and may repeatedly turn back; persistently turning the horse all the way around and walking away from the barn is necessary. Once well away from the barn, most barn-sour horses will stop trying to return to it and gradually become less barn sour the more they are made to leave the barn.

Horses in a band develop a dominance hierarchy or "pecking order" which minimizes fighting that may result in injury. Forming a dominance hierarchy requires that each horse recognize every other horse and determine through initial aggressive (e.g., biting or kicking) and submissive acts (e.g., moving away) which of two horses is dominant and which is subordinate. The relationship is established among all horses in the band. Each horse in the band knows to which horses it is dominant and to which it is subordinate. Once this dominance hierarchy is formed, fighting is minimal. Conflicts are resolved by showing the teeth, laying back the ears, and moving toward or away from the other horses without any physical contact unless the subordinate horse can't get away fast enough. The size, age, and time in the group have been found to not be relevant in determining dominance rank in some groups, whereas all have been found to be factors in other groups, with size being important in higher ranks of dominance, particularly in domestic horses, and age being important in lower ranks of dominance, particularly in wild horses. The sex of the horse doesn't appear to be a relevant factor, at least in situations in which the individual's sex has little or no influence on its motivation to be dominant. Paradoxically, horses that are aggressive toward other horses and tend to be high in dominance hierarchy are usually not difficult for people to manage. They don't tend to be aggressive toward people. Procedures for preventing or correcting overaggression against people or other animals are described in Chapter 20.

Dominance hierarchies between horses are at times affected by special situations, generally those relating to the individual's motivation to win. For example, the mare not in estrus invariably wins over stallions' sexually aggressive actions towards her, whereas the stallion invariably wins in driving mares from his band away from a foreign stallion.

When a new horse is introduced to a group, its order in the dominance hierarchy will be established. This may result in physical injury, particularly when horses are shod or can't get away from one another. Injuries occur most often to the horse new to the group, but may also occur to those already in the group. To minimize injury, a physical barrier should be placed between strange horses when they are introduced. Ideally, horses should be put in adjacent paddocks so they can see, hear, and smell each other but cannot kick or strike each other and can easily move away from each other. The barrier between them should be one that poses minimal risk to the horses, such as a solid fence or a series of poles close enough and high enough so the horse can't get a foot through or over it. Horses are frequently injured when fighting across unsafe barriers such as those with wire, sharp edges, splinters, protrusions, or openings big enough to catch a horse's foot. Although the horses can bite across the fence, one horse can easily escape the other. The dominant-subordinate relationship can be established between them with minimal chance of injury. Later they can be placed in the same paddock or pasture. Some aggression may still occur, however, when they are placed together. Regardless of the procedures used prior to putting horses unfamiliar with each other together, avoid a crowded environment and one where a horse is unable to get away from a more aggressive horse without getting bitten or kicked. Crowding increases aggressiveness and decreases the subordinate horse's ability to escape; consequently, it may be kicked and bitten repeatedly.

Horses use many means to communicate their feelings and intentions. Knowing these can be quite helpful. Vocal sounds include and mean the following: (1) snort = warning, (2) neigh or whinny = distress, (3) nicker = greeting, (4) squeal = anger, (5) repeated throaty sounds by stallion with flared nostrils = mating, (6) rolling snort = pleasure, and (7) gentle nickering by mare to her foal = maternal care and affection.

The horse's ears are relaxed when the horse is relaxed and are usually positioned in the direction in which it is looking. Both ears pointing forward and relaxed indicates interest, whereas both forward and body tense suggests fear. A responsive horse may keep one ear cocked back for the rider's cues and one cocked forward to focus on what's ahead. A spoiled horse may do the same, however, with one eye and ear to catch a careless handler or rider unaware and the other to see where to run after it bucks, kicks, or shies. The horse can focus and look at separate objects with each eye, or focus both eyes on the same object, as we do for binocular vision. The height of the horse's head indicates whether it's focusing on near or far objects. A horse with a high head may be dangerous to ride because it's focusing on far objects and not watching its footing. It's also dangerous to approach a horse unexpectedly from the back, as they cannot see behind themselves without turning their head and they are easily startled from behind. As an old Yiddish proverb states—don't approach a horse from the back, a goat from the front or a fool from any side. Care should also be taken when the horse has both ears turned back and laid down on the head as this usually indicates anger, although during strenuous exertion it can indicate determination. A frightened horse will have its eyelids wide open and its nostrils flared, and may snort a warning or whinny a distress and tuck its tail between its legs. The tail held between the legs may also indicate that the horse is ready to kick, or that it is giving up in a fight. Constant switching that is not fly induced may indicate irritation—that something is annoying the horse—and can become a habit. A kink in the tail and a bowed back, which is indicated by increased space be-

tween the back of the saddle and the horse's back, indicates the horse is ready to buck. A kink in the tail or the tail held high also occurs during play, at which time, in addition to running, bucking, kicking, and squealing, the horse may trot or canter with stiff legs.

A horse's degree of dominance may be a factor to consider in riding with a group. Dominant horses tend to move to the front; passing by less dominant horses can result in kicking, biting, and shying. This can be a safety problem. Dominance order is also important in feeding and managing horses within a group. One should know and reinforce a group's dominance hierarchy by feeding the most dominant horse first, and then on down the line to the least dominant horse last. This assists in minimizing injuries to both horses and people, and helps keep order within the group. The rate of feed intake does not correlate with dominance rank; therefore, lower-ranking horses have the time and opportunity to eat if their feed is separated sufficiently from that of more dominant horses. Since most threats occur at distances of less than 50 ft (15 m), individual feeders should be separated by at least this distance (Fig. 8-2) and be well away from fences, especially corners. Feed bags may be used instead for feeding grain (Fig. 8-3). For feeding hay, small racks that accommodate only two to four horses (Fig. 8-1 C), with enough of them for all horses placed at least 50 ft (15 m) apart, are best. Alternatively, hay may be fed at scattered locations on the ground (Fig. 8-5).

However, feeding on the ground increases waste, feeding costs, parasitism, and dirt ingestion, the last of which increases the risk of sand colic, and intestinal impactions. It often works well to place individual feeders, hay racks, or hay in a large circle. Aggressive horses that eat rapidly and then run other horses away from their feed can be

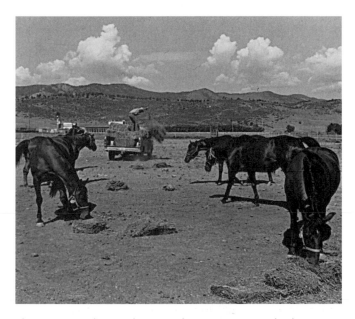

Fig. 8-5. Feeding on the ground increases waste, feeding costs, parasitism, and dirt ingestion, the last of which increases the risk of sand colic, and intestinal impactions.

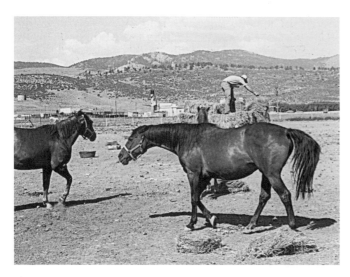

Fig. 8–6. Effect of dominance when horses are fed as a group. The mare on the right is driving the less-dominant mare away from the hay being fed. Less-dominant horses may be repeatedly driven from feed; after a time, they may make little effort to obtain their share, and become thin and in poor condition if adequate amounts of other feed are unavailable. To help minimize this, when group feeding is necessary, feed in a large circle and ensure that there is a feeder for each horse. It may be necessary to group horses according to dominance, or to feed very dominant or more commonly submissive horses away from the group.

managed by using one or two more feeders than there are horses, with proportionately less feed put in the aggressive horse's initial feeder.

If these group feeding procedures are not followed, aggressive horses will eat more than their share and need, and horses low in the dominance hierarchy may be continually driven away from feed (Fig. 8-6). Consequently, these horses may not receive an adequate amount of feed unless an excess of what is needed by the group is fed, which increases feeding losses and cost. Partitions between feeders and feed troughs frequently are not satisfactory alternatives. Dominant horses may be able to control too much space at the feed trough; subordinate horses may be hurt because of partitions obstructing and slowing their ability to get away from dominant horses.

In contrast to mature horses, immature horses generally can be group fed from a single feed trough if there is adequate space. Horses under 3 years old display a lot of play but little aggression toward one another even when vying for food. At least 2 ft (0.6 m) of trough per immature horse and 3 ft (0.9 m) for mature horses is recommended. The feed trough should have no splinters, sharp edges, points, or corners and should be narrow enough that all horses can reach feed on its far side.

CHANGING DIETS

The horse's diet (type of forage or grain, or the amount of either) should be changed gradually over several days or weeks. Increasing the amount of grain fed at a rate of no more than about 0.5 lb (0.2-0.3 kg) daily until the desired level is reached is a safe approach. Increasing the amount of grain fed too rapidly may cause colic or founder. It is also best to gradually decrease the amount of grain fed, particularly for horses on a high-grain diet, such as those returned home from strenuous performance training or competition. Their diet and amount of exercise should be reduced gradually over a 2-week period.

When given a day off, horses normally subject to strenuous daily exertion should have their grain decreased that day, be given some exercise, and preferably stay in an enclosure of sufficient size to allow them to run. On the first day of work or training following the day of rest, they should be warmed up slowly to prevent exertion myopathy (as discussed in Chapter 11).

When either the type of hay or grain is being changed, replace only about 25% of the current feed every other day so that it takes about 1 week before the new feed completely replaces the old. Many horses prefer the feed to which they are accustomed, so when the type of feed is changed, feed intake or eagerness to eat may be reduced unless the new feed is substantially more palatable than the old.

Horses being put on lush, green pasture should be given all of the hay to which they are accustomed before being turned out on the pasture. If possible, increase the time the horses are on the pasture by 1 hour each day. After the 4th to 5th day, they can be left on the pasture. The more lush and plentiful the pasture forage the more important these procedures.

Chapter 9

GENERAL HORSE CARE MANAGEMENT PRACTICES

Internal Parasite Problems	155
Large Strongyles	155
Small Strongyles	155
Ascarids	156
Bots	157
Pinworms	158
Stomachworms	158
Less Prevalent Equine Internal Parasites	158
Hairworms	158
Threadworms	158
Tapeworms	158
Lungworms	159
Onchocerca cervicales	159
Internal Parasite Control	159
Dewormer Drug Selection	159
Dewormer Administration Schedules	160
Interval Deworming Programs	161
Seasonal Deworming Programs	161
Continual Deworming Programs	161
Environmental Control of Internal Parasites	162
Monitoring Internal Parasite Control	162
Internal-Parasite Control Program	163
External Parasite Problems and Control	164

Infectious-Disease Problems and Vaccination Programs	165
Tetanus	168
Equine Encephalomyelitis (Sleeping Sickness)	169
Equine Influenza	171
Rhinopneumonitis (Equine Herpes Virus)	171
Equine Viral Arteritis	172
Strangles	173
Potomac Horse Fever (Equine Monocytic Ehrlichiosis)	174
Rabies	174
Anthrax	175
Equine Infectious Anemia (Swamp Fever)	175
Dental Problems and Care	175
Age Estimation by Horse's Teeth	177
Foot Care	178
Skin and Hair-Coat Care	179
Record Keeping	180
Housing for Horses	180
Open-Front Sheds	180
Stalls	181
Stable Ventilation	182
Bedding	184
Fencing for Horses	184
Supplemental Reading Recommendations	185

INTERNAL PARASITE PROBLEMS

One of the most important aspects in maintaining the health of the horse is the control of internal parasites. Parasite infestations are one of the most costly, insidious, and harmful disease problems of the horse. The most prevalent, harmful and, therefore, important internal parasites of the horse, listed in the order of the importance in controlling them, are: (1) large and small strongyles, (2) ascarids or roundworms, (3) bots, (4) pinworms, and (5) in foals also, threadworms. Stomachworms, tapeworms, and lungworms are not sufficiently common to warrant routine control procedures in most areas but may cause problems in specific groups or individuals.

Large Strongyles

Adult large strongyles, or blood worms, are 0.5 to 2 inches (1 to 5 cm) long (Fig. 9–1A). They live in the horse's large intestine. Their eggs are passed in the feces and hatch into what become infective larvae. Infective larvae crawl up pasture forage, where they are ingested by grazing horses (Fig. 9–1B). They affect all ages of horses. Following their ingestion by the horse, they penetrate the intestinal lining and migrate through the tissue, causing damage. There are three different species of large strongyles: Strongyles vulgaris, edentatus, and equinus. The most common species, S. vulgaris, migrates in the walls of arteries, particularly those supplying the intestinal tract. This may result in thickening of the arterial wall and decreased blood supply to the tissues supplied by that artery (Fig. 9–1C). This effect has been reported to be a predisposing cause of most cases of colic in the horse. Although there are numerous immediate causes of colic (including a rapid change in the type, quantity, or amount of feed ingested; stress; excessive cold water ingestion by a hot horse; lack of water; and ingestion of sufficient sand or dirt), in most cases these factors would not cause colic if the pre-existing strongyle-induced damage was not present. In one study, 61 to 93% of colic cases were prevented by a good strongyle control program. Migrating strongyle larvae may also damage arteries and decrease blood supply to the back legs, resulting in decreased endurance and strength of affected legs.

The second most prevalent large strongyle, S. edentatus, migrates in the veins to the liver. S. equinus, which is much less prevalent than the other two species, migrates through the abdominal cavity to the liver and pancreas. After 6 to 11 months, the immature adults of all three species of large strongyles develop and migrate back to the intestine, where they mature and lay their eggs which are passed in the feces. In addition to the damage caused by strongyle migration through body tissues, the strongyles suck blood. If sufficient, this causes anemia, weakness, poor condition, and may result in subcutaneous edema. Diarrhea may occur with heavy infestations.

Small Strongyles

Small strongyles (cyathostomes) (Fig. 9–1A), like large strongyles, affect horses of all ages, although younger horses are most susceptible. Over the past decade there has been a shift in small and large strongyle populations favoring an increase in small strongyles. Nearly all grazing horses are infected with small strongyles, and frequently they account for over 95% of fecal parasite eggs and infec-

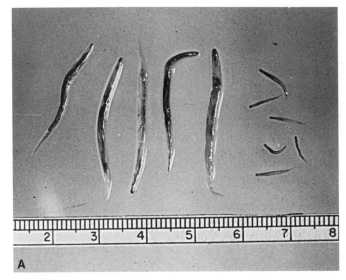

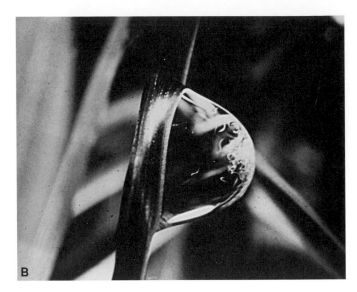

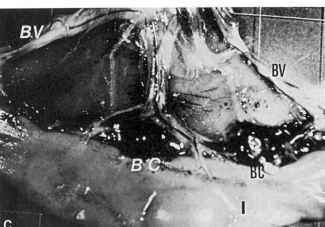

Fig. 9-1 (A,B,C). Adult large strongyles (blood worms) and small strongyles (cyathastomes) with a scale marked in centimeters (1 cm = 0.4 or about ⅜ of an inch) (A). Both live in the large intestine and cause damage which may result in colic, diarrhea, and poor condition. Their eggs are passed in the feces and hatch into what become infective larvae. Infective larvae crawl up pasture forage, shown in a drop of moisture on a blade of grass (B), where they are ingested. Large strongyle larvae migrate in the walls of arteries supplying the intestinal tract. This may cause damage and thrombi or blood clots (BC) in the blood vessels (BV) to the intestine (I), which passes across the width of the bottom of Figure C. This is a predisposing cause of most cases of colic in the horse.

tive larvae in pastures. In contrast to large strongyles, ingested small strongyle larvae don't migrate through body tissues. Because of this, they have in the past been thought to be less harmful than large strongyles. However, they may cause profound clinical disease. Following ingestion, infective larvae burrow into the large intestinal lining where they suck blood, ingest intestinal lining, and become encysted until they reach maturation. These effects may cause a profuse persistent or intermittent diarrhea, recurring low-grade colic, decreased appetite, slow growth or chronic weight loss, debilitation, listlessness, and can cause death. Encysted larvae emerge approximately 14 weeks after ingestion, usually in the winter and spring. When this occurs, it may result in a sudden onset of diarrhea with profuse cow-pie-consistency stools, mild colic, weight loss, delayed shedding of winter coats, recurring colic, pot belly, and subcutaneous edema, especially of the muzzle, legs, abdomen, and sheath.

Ascarids

Ascarids (Parascaris equorum) are large roundworms usually 6 to 12 inches (15 to 30 cm) in length (Fig. 9-2). They are a problem only in young horses. Horses exposed

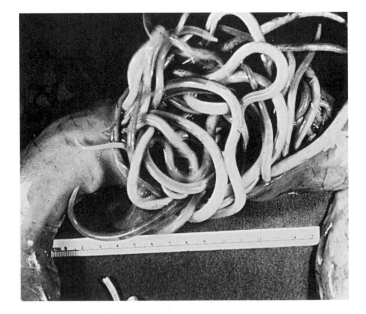

Fig. 9-2. Adult ascarids (Parascaris equorum) that became so numerous that they blocked and caused the rupture of the small intestine, resulting in the death of the horse.

to ascarids develop an immunity to them so that by 1 year of age they are no longer affected. Adult ascarids inhabit the small intestine, where they lay eggs which are passed in the feces. The eggs are very resistant to destruction in the environment. After their ingestion, they hatch in the small intestine, releasing larvae that penetrate the intestinal wall. The larvae migrate through the portal vein to the liver, and then to the lungs, where they are coughed up and reswallowed to become mature egg-laying adults in the small intestine, completing a 10- to 12-week life cycle. Their migration damages the liver and lungs, which may result in a lifetime reduction in the functional capacity of these organs. In addition, large numbers of ascarids in the intestine may cause intestinal impaction, colic, perforation, and death (Fig. 9–2). Large numbers migrating through the lungs may cause coughing, intermittent fever, and a nasal discharge, resulting in a condition sometimes referred to as a "summer cold." The lung damage they cause can permanently decrease the horse's future athletic performance. They may also cause alternating constipation and diarrhea; poor growth, condition, hair coat, and appetite; colic; and a pot-bellied appearance. Treatment is to give an avermectin, a broad-spectrum antibiotic, and nursing care during recovery.

Bots

Bot flies (Gastrophilus spp.) lay eggs on the horse's hair—primarily around the forelegs, shoulders, chest, neck, throat, jaws, and lips—during the summer and late fall (Fig. 9–3A, B). The bot flies are killed by the first hard

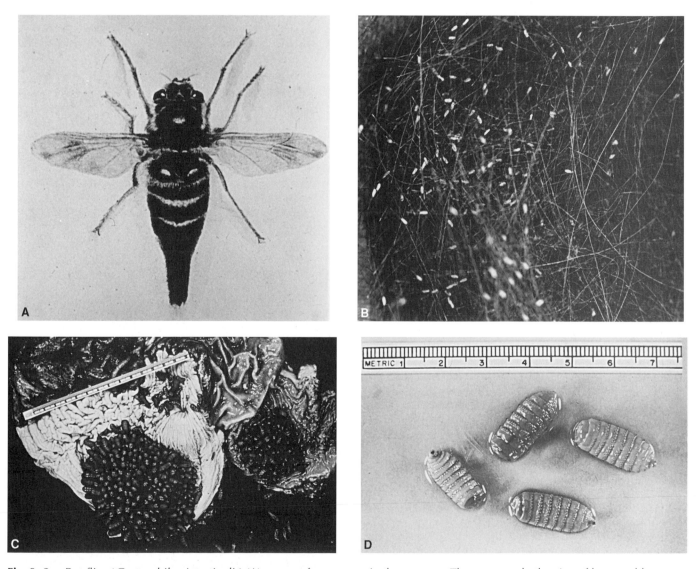

Fig. 9–3. Bot flies (*Gastrophilus intestinalis*) (A) emerge from pupae in the summer. They are nearly the size of bees and have no mouth, so they do not bite, as is commonly believed. During their 3- to 5-week life, they lay eggs or nits on the horse's hair (B) around the lips, jaws, neck, head, forelegs, and shoulders. This activity may cause horses to bunch, seek protection in dense shrubbery or in water, or run erratically. Larvae from these eggs migrate to the oral cavity and to the stomach, where they develop into adults over the following 9 to 10 months attached to the lining of the stomach (C). The following spring, they detach, are passed in the feces (D), and after 2 to 4 weeks, pupate to the bot fly (A), completing their 1-year-long life cycle.

freeze in the fall. After ingestion of the bot eggs, or migration of larvae into the mouth, larvae develop in the oral and pharyngeal tissue. Later they emerge and are swallowed or migrate to the stomach and upper small intestine where they attach (Fig. 9–3C). The following spring, after living for 9 to 10 months in the horse, they are fully grown and are about 0.8 to 1 inch (2 to 2.5 cm) long and reddish orange (Fig. 9–3D). These detach and are passed in the feces. Some, as they are passed, may reattach around the anus for a few days. Once excreted, they burrow into the manure or soil and, after 2 to 4 weeks, pupate to the bot fly, thus completing their 1-year-long life cycle. Without treatment, they are present in most horses.

The immature larvae may damage the oral and pharyngeal tissue. However, the greatest damage is to the stomach and duodenum, where they cause inflammation, which may result in colic, ulcers, or even perforations.

Pinworms

Adult pinworms (Oxyuris equi) occur primarily in the horse's colon and rectum. Their sticky yellow eggs are deposited around the anus, causing irritation. As a result, the horse may scratch its rump against walls and posts, wearing away the hair at the base of the tail and rump. This is thought to be the pinworm's only harmful effect. Similar symptoms occur as a result of tail mange mites (Chorioptes equi), the biting louse (Damalinia equi) and allergic dermatitis due to hypersensitivity to biting midges (Culicoides spp.). Diagnosis of oxyuriasis is made by clinical signs and by finding the eggs. Clear tape applied to the anal and perineal region will remove the eggs. The tape should be placed in mineral oil on a glass slide and examined for the characteristic eggs (Fig. 9–6C). Larvae hatched from pinworm eggs are ingested and pass to the colon, where they develop into the egg-laying adult. The life cycle takes about 5 months.

Stomachworms

Larvae of stomachworms or spirurids (Habronema and Draschia spp.) develop inside the maggots of the common horsefly or stablefly found in manure. These flies carry the larvae and deposit them around the horse's lips, nostrils and eyes as well as in wounds. Swallowed larvae develop into adults in the lining of the stomach, where they lay eggs which are passed in the feces. They are not commonly present in horses in the United States. In one study, they were present in only 3 to 13% of Thoroughbreds in Kentucky. Their presence in the stomach rarely causes problems, although a heavy infestation may cause stomach inflammation. Ivermectin administration is an effective treatment.

The major problem caused by stomachworms comes from larvae deposited around the eyes, causing persistent inflammation, or in skin wounds, causing skin sores sometimes referred to as "summer sores." The larvae cannot penetrate normal intact skin, but when deposited in the wound they migrate, extending the wound, and prevent healing. Yellow granular type lesions develop and can enlarge rapidly. Diagnosis is generally made from the history and appearance of the lesions, but if necessary can be confirmed by finding larvae in a skin biopsy.

Treatment of stomachworm larvae is to administer ivermectin twice 3 to 6 weeks apart. This kills the larvae and leads to a rapid resolution of lesions. Large or secondarily infected lesions may require additional therapy, including removing excess granulation tissue and applying antimicrobial ointment and corticosteroids to decrease inflammation. Prevention of reinfection requires fly control and immediate wound care. Lesions may be covered and fly repellents applied to the covering. Topical pastes containing organophosphates and anti-inflammatory agents may be used instead. For inflammation around the eyes caused by stomachworm larvae, application of antibacterial and corticosteroid ointments to the eye several times daily is usually an effective treatment.

Less Prevalent Equine Internal Parasites

Internal parasites not sufficiently prevalent to warrant routine control measures, although they may occur in sufficient number to cause problems in some specific areas or situations, include hairworms, tapeworms, threadworms, lungworms, and Onchocerca cervicalis.

Hairworms

Hairworms (Trichostrongylus axei) occur in the stomach of horses and other species. They usually occur only in horses grazed or housed with ruminants. Adults, which live deep in the stomach lining lay eggs which are passed in the feces. Infective larvae develop from these eggs and are ingested. Usually hairworms cause few problems. However, heavy infestations can cause poor condition and anemia. Treatment is to administer an avermectin.

Threadworms

Threadworm (Strongyloides westeri) adults can live both in the ground and in the small intestine. Infective larvae from their eggs can be excreted in the mare's milk. The larvae infect the foal by ingestion or by penetrating the foal's skin. In the infected foal, larvae migrate into the blood, which carries them to the lungs. They are coughed up, swallowed, and become adults in the small intestine. Because they stimulate a sufficient immune response, they rarely occur in other than nursing foals. Adult worms in the small intestine cause inflammation and, in sufficiently large numbers, can cause diarrhea and unthriftiness in 2- to 3-week-old foals. Treatment is to administer ivermectin or oxibendazole to the foal. Threadworm infestation is prevented by administering ivermectin to the mare the day of foaling and to the foal at 2 to 3 weeks of age.

Tapeworms

Tapeworms (Anoplocephala spp.) are flatworms present in the intestine of 10 to 67% of horses in North America. Although they have been associated with severe gastrointestinal disease and death, and utilize ingested nutrients, they usually do not cause clinical signs. However, they may cause chronic unthriftiness, intermittent colic, diarrhea, progressive emaciation, and anemia. Occasionally, heavy infestations may cause acute problems due to (1) clusters of the worms obstructing the intestine, or (2) cecal perforations resulting in colic and death. Pyrantel pamoate administered at 2 to 3 times the normal dose is effective for the treatment and prevention of tapeworms. Benefit is optimized by treating 2 weeks prior to and at the conclusion of the grazing season.

Lungworms

Lungworm (Dictyocaulus arnfieldi) infected horses generally but not always have been exposed to donkeys, or pastures used by donkeys, within the past several years. Donkeys serve as a reservoir whose infective larvae are passed in the feces. Infection in donkeys is generally relatively harmless to them. In horses, however, infection may cause airway inflammation and an accumulation of pus in the airways. Diagnosis is based on finding infective larvae in the feces or the parasite in the lungs. Affected horses should be separated from donkeys, removed from contaminated pastures, and administered ivermectin.

Onchocerca cervicales

O. cervicales is transmitted to horses by the bite of its intermediate host, the biting midge (Culicoides spp.), whose control is given in Tables 9–3 and 9–4. O. cervicales was found in the crest of the neck of 59% of Thoroughbreds in Kentucky, with the incidence being higher the older the horse. None were found in the ligaments or tendons of the legs. Although no clinical signs were present, some older horses had massive mineralization of caseous material around the parasite.

INTERNAL PARASITE CONTROL

To minimize parasite infestation and, therefore, reduce the likelihood of harm due to parasitic diseases, an internal-parasite control program must decrease the potential for the transmission of parasites between horses and their environment. To accomplish this objective requires the selection and utilization of effective dewormers along with sound management practices that enhance environmental control. Control programs should be developed based on climate, management practices, and economics for each specific farm. The program should be aimed at controlling (1) large and small strongyles for all horses, plus ascarids for yearlings and younger horses; (2) bots in all horses; and (3) other intestinal parasites that may be a problem in that farm, stable, or individual.

With a good internal-parasite control program, colic, anemia, diarrhea, poor growth or weight loss, reduced stamina, and reduced performance due to intestinal parasites are prevented. A good internal-parasite control program is particularly important for young horses. Young horses are generally more heavily infested than older horses, and horses affected early in life may have their entire future health and performance impaired.

There are four aspects of importance for the control of internal parasites in horses: (1) choice of dewormer (anthelmintic), (2) dewormer administration schedule, (3) nondewormer management practices, and (4) monitoring the results so the program can be modified as indicated.

Dewormer Drug Selection

A multitude of dewormers or anthelmintics and combinations of them are available in different forms for treating and preventing internal parasite infestation in horses. The many different dewormers currently available and recommended can be divided into five major chemically and pharmacologically similar classes: (1) avermectins, which currently include only ivermectin: and moxidectin, (2) organophosphates, (3) tetrahydropyrimidines, which currently include only pyrantel, (4) benzimidazoles and probenzimidazoles, and (5) piperazine, which is often used in combination with phenothiazine and benzimidazoles (Table 9–1). The spectrum of efficiency and resistance is similar for all the drugs in each of these five classes. Dewormers containing the same class of drug are called by different names by each manufacturer marketing them. Therefore, rely on the name of the active drug listed on the label and not on the marketer's name for the product.

A dewormer effective against the parasites you want to treat should be selected. The routine recommendation has been that a dewormer from a different class should be used on a rotational basis: i.e., a dewormer from a different class should be used than was used the previous time the horses on that farm were treated. It was believed that this procedure assisted in preventing the development of parasites resistant to the dewormers used. Recent studies in both horses and sheep, however, have demonstrated that alternating dewormer classes neither delays nor enhances the development of resistance to them. Consequently, as suggested, deworming treatment programs that alternate between dewormer classes, or that use the same dewormer for 1 year or as long as it is effective, appear to be equally acceptable procedures for the control of equine internal parasites.

Small strongyles resistant to piperazine, phenothiazine, and all of the benzimidazole drugs have been reported. No other parasites have been reported to have developed a resistance to any of the other dewormers. Once resistance to a drug develops, it may be 3 years or more before that drug will again be effective against those parasites on that farm. Benzimidazole-resistant small strongyles are susceptible to benzimidazole + piperazine combination products and ivermectin, pyrantel, and the organophosphate dichlorvos.

Deworming medications may be added to the feed, given by stomach tube, or put in the back of the horse's mouth as a drench or in a paste form with a syringe. One method of administration is no more or less effective than another if all of the correct amount of the medication reaches the animal's stomach within a fairly short period of time. Thus, dewormers added to the feed are effective only if all of the dewormer is consumed within a few hours or less.

Avermectins, one of the newest and most broad-spectrum class of parasite medications, have a wide margin of safety, including for pregnant and reproducing horses and for foals. They have a greater than 95% efficacy against parasites of the skin, respiratory tract, and blood, as well as the gastrointestinal tract. They are also effective against blood-sucking lice, flies, and mites as well as both the adult

TABLE 9–1
Deworming Drugs for Horses

Dewormer	Formulations Available[a]	Normal Dose (mg/kg)	Safety Index[b]	Efficacy[c] Large Strongyles	Small Strongyles	Bots	Ascarids	Pin Worms	Migrating Larvae
Avermectins[d]									
Moxidectin	P	0.4		+	+	+	+	+	+
Ivermectin	P,T	0.2	10	+	+	+	+	+	+
Organophosphates[e]									
Dichlorvos pellets	F	35	3	+[f]	+	+	+	+	+
Trichlorfon	P,T	40	1	0	0	+	+	+	0
Pyrantel pamoate	P,F,T	6.6	20	+[f]	+	0	+	−	+
Pyrantel tartrate	P,F	12.5[g]	>100	+	+	0	+	+	+
Benzimidazoles[h]									
Thiabendazole	P,F,T	44	13	+	±	0	−	+	2@10×[i]
Mebendazole	P,F,T	8.8	45	+[f]	−	0	+	+	0
Fenbendazole	P,F,T	5	200	+	±	0	1@2×[i]	1@2×[i]	5@2×[i]
Cambendazole[e]	P,F,T	20		+	±	0	+	+	0
Oxfendazole	P,F,T	10	10	+	±	0	+	+	1@2×[i]
Oxibendazole	P,T	10	60	+	±	0	+	+	0
Febantel	P,F,T	6	33	+	±	0	+	+	0
Piperazine	T	88	17	−	±	0	+	−	0
Phenothiazine	F,T	55		−	±	0	0	0	0
Carbon disulfide[e,j]	T	53	j	0	0	+	−	0	0

[a] For administration, P = orally as a paste, F = in the feed, and T = by stomach tube or as an oral drench.
[b] Safety Index = dose at which clinical signs of toxicosis first occur divided by the minimum therapeutic dose.
[c] + indicates 90 to 100% efficacy at the dosage given; − indicates 10 to 80% efficacy; 0 indicates less than 10% efficacy; ± indicates 90 to 100% efficacy unless a resistance has developed against that deworming drug. Benzimidazole-resistant small strongyles are susceptible to benzimidazole-piperazine combinations, ivermectin, pyrantel and dichlorvos.
[d] Also effective against blood-sucking lice, flies, and mites, and the adult and migrating larvae of most internal parasites of the horse, including ascarids, threadworms, stomach worms, cattle grubs (Hypoderma spp.), and others of the skin, respiratory tract, blood, and gastrointestinal tract. These drugs are not effective against cestodes (tapeworms), trematodes (flukes), Micronema deletrix, or eyeworms (Thelazia spp).
[e] Not recommended by most during pregnancy. Organophosphates are also not recommended for foals.
[f] May be less than 90% effective against the large strongyle (Strongylus edentatus).
[g] When fed continually, 2.64 mg/kg body wt daily is recommended.
[h] Not recommended during the first trimester of pregnancy.
[i] Effective when given daily for the number of days indicated at the number of times the normal dosage indicated, e.g., 2@10× indicates daily for 2 days at 10-times normal dose.
[j] Administer carbon disulfide by stomach tube only. It is quite toxic, irritating, and not recommended as there are now better alternatives for treating bots.

and migrating larvae of nearly all of the major parasites of the horse. In addition to its broad spectrum of activity, ivermectin suppresses fecal intestinal parasite egg excretion by the horse for 8 to 10 weeks following its administration, as compared to 4 to 5 weeks for all other nonavermectin dewormers currently available. As a result, it gives equal or better protection when administered one-half as often as other dewormers. However, avermectins are not effective against tapeworms (cestodes), trematodes (flukes), or eyeworms (Thelazia lacrymalis). Although avermectins don't cause the death or detachment of ticks, they do prevent their molting and egg production.

It has been suggested from field observation that degradation of feces from ivermectin-treated animals is slowed because its excretion in the feces may kill dung-degrading organisms. However, studies indicate this doesn't occur. No difference was found in the rate of decomposition of feces from horses treated bimonthly for 2 years with ivermectin and those either untreated or treated with other dewormers. There was no difference in the amount of fecal-fouled pasture where horses were treated only with ivermectin as compared to pasture used by horses on a rotational deworming program.

Although most deworming medications, except cambendazole and organophosphates, are safe for use throughout pregnancy, it is best not to give any medication not required for the life of the horse during the last few weeks of pregnancy. If any problems occur at foaling, any medication recently administered may be blamed. Cambendazole, carbon disulfides, and organophosphates should not be given to the mare during the first 3 months of pregnancy because of possible, but unproven, inducement of teratogenicity. Organophosphate dewormers are also not recommended for foals.

Dewormer Administration Schedules

Three different types of dewormer administration schedules or programs have been recommended and used: interval, seasonal, and continual. Interval programs, if done properly, are effective for all horses. Seasonal programs should be used only for mature horses not on a good interval program. Continual dewormer administration is a good alternative for individual horses where all horses on the premises are not on the same or on an effective internal parasite control program.

Interval Deworming Programs

In the mid-1960s, year-round bimonthly administration of dewormers for all horses was proposed and has been widely recommended and used since that time. Less frequent dewormer administration has been recommended and used by some for nonbreeding farms with lower concentrations of less valuable horses. Following these recommendations maintains adequate internal-parasite control at some farms and stables, whereas at some it hasn't provided satisfactory strongyle control or prevented environmental contamination with strongyle ova. At such farms and stables, satisfactory control was obtained by administering non-avermectin dewormers monthly or ivermectin every 2 months. This, as well as the effect of inadequate parasite control on colic incidence has been well demonstrated. In one study, a moderate incidence of colic was occurring even though a non-avermectin dewormer was being administered every 2 months. In horses given a non-avermectin dewormer monthly, and in those given ivermectin every 2 months, the incidence of colic decreased 61 to 93%, whereas there was no change in colic incidence in the other horses, who continued to be given a non-avermectin dewormer every 2 months.

Seasonal Deworming Programs

In addition to interval dewormer programs for horses of all ages, as described above, seasonal dewormer programs for mature horses have been developed to try to improve or maintain good internal-parasite control with less frequent administration of dewormers. The object of seasonal control programs is to administer dewormers at the right time to minimize fecal strongyle egg excretion and, therefore, pasture contamination, thus prolonging subsequent reinfestation of the horse. In cooler climates (e.g., the northern United States, the United Kingdom, and northern Europe), peak egg excretion occurs in the spring and summer. In warmer climates (e.g., the southern United States to Buenos Aires), pasture infectivity decreases during the hot summer months.

To prevent peak egg excretion in cooler climates, avermectin dewormers should be given just before grazing new spring pasture and again in the middle of the summer (e.g., in the northern hemisphere in May and again in July). Alternatively, a non-avermectin dewormer should be given twice, 1 month apart, beginning at each of the two times or monthly from spring through the middle of summer. In the fall following a freeze, a dewormer effective against bots should be given (e.g., an avermectin or an organophosphate).

In warmer climates, an avermectin dewormer should be given in late summer and early winter (e.g., in the southern United States, in August and October); instead, a non-avermectin dewormer should be given twice, 1 month apart, beginning at each of these two times, or monthly from late summer through early winter. Studies in Ohio and England found that this program resulted in a sixfold decrease in pasture infectivity, thus allowing the horse to graze in relative safety long after dewormers were administered.

Seasonal control programs should not be used for horses less than 1 year of age. Since adult and immature ascarids, as well as strongyle and bot control, are necessary in young horses, they should be given a dewormer every 2 months beginning at 6 to 8 weeks of age until 1 year of age. If the treatment interval is lengthened to even 10 weeks, there is a sharp increase in their fecal ascarid and strongyle egg excretion. To avoid treatment complications, the dewormer administered to young horses should not cause a sudden parasite kill, as occurs with organophosphates and piperazine. Slow-kill dewormers, such as ivermectin, pyrantel, or benzimidazoles, are less likely to cause complications. After foals are 1 year old, at which age they have developed an immunity to ascarids, they may be switched to a seasonal control program.

For bot control, the most important treatment is in the fall. In areas where it freezes, a dewormer effective against bots (e.g., avermectins or an organophosphate) should be given to all horses right after the first hard freeze, which will kill bot flies. It has been recommended that this fall bot treatment be delayed until 1 month after a hard freeze so that all ingested larvae will have reached the stomach. However, if a dewormer effective against migrating bot larvae is administered (e.g., avermectins or organophosphates), this 1-month wait isn't necessary or recommended. In addition to giving a dewormer effective against bots, anytime bot eggs or nits (Fig. 9–3B) are present, they should be removed from the hair or killed by topical application of insecticides such as 0.06% coumaphos, 0.12% malathion, or 0.03% lindane. Ideally, or if bots are considered a major problem on that farm, additional bot treatments should be given bimonthly beginning 1 month after bot eggs first occur on the horse's hair.

Continual Deworming Programs

A third intestinal parasite control program, besides interval and seasonal programs, is the continual feeding of low amounts of a deworming medication. However, many small strongyles developed a resistance against the dewormers used in this manner in the past, making them ineffective. One in which no parasite resistance has been demonstrated, and the only dewormer currently on the market recommended and found to be effective when fed continually, is pyrantel tartrate. It is available in alfalfa-flavored pellets (Strongid C, Pfizer). When fed continually at its recommended dosage, it is effective against both adult and larval stages of large and small strongyles, ascarids, and pinworms, and may prevent tapeworm infestation. Unlike dewormers used in interval or seasonal parasite-control programs, a continuously administered dewormer need not be given to all horses on the premises to maximize control in an individual. Thus, this is a beneficial alternative in boarding facilities where deworming is left up to individual owners rather than all horses being treated at the same time. Regardless of the control programs used by others at a facility, internal parasites, except bots, can be prevented in horses fed pyrantel tartrate daily. Before beginning this control program, a deworming dose of ivermectin should be administered. In addition, bot treatment as described previously for seasonal deworming programs is necessary since pyrantel tartrate is not effective against bots. One study suggested that feeding pyrantel tartrate daily decreased the risk of colic as compared to horses dewormed interchangeably with benzimidazoles and ivermectin an average of 5 times annually. Although in 1993 it cost about $15/month to feed the 1000-lb (454-kg) horse pyrantel tartrate daily, the company selling it claims, but without presenting supportive data, that pyrantel tartrate increases feed utilization and offsets its cost. Like all claims lacking valid supportive data, especially when a reason for a bias exists, skepticism is warranted.

Environmental Control of Internal Parasites

There are a number of management practices besides the administration of deworming medications that are beneficial in minimizing internal parasites in horses. One of the most important is to minimize ingestion of fecally contaminated feed and water. Almost all infected larvae are near a fecal mass. The concentration of infective larvae is 15 times higher in fecally contaminated areas of a pasture than in noncontaminated areas. Thus, decreasing fecal contamination of feed and water, and fecal proximity to grazing, is quite beneficial in minimizing the horse's ingestion of infective larvae. Procedures to do this include the following.

1. Minimize consumption of feed from the ground (as described in Chapter 8).
2. Remove manure from stables, paddocks, and small pastures regularly and frequently.
3. If manure is to be spread on horse pastures, let it compost for 1 year first so that all parasite eggs and larvae are killed by the heat of fermentation. If this is not done, spreading manure on horse pastures is not recommended. Instead, it can be spread on cropland or other ungrazed areas.
4. Don't overgraze pastures so horses are not forced to graze forage close to the ground and fecally contaminated areas. Most mature horses will not graze fecally contaminated areas of a pasture unless forced to do so because of inadequate feed. Young horses, particularly foals, are less discriminatory.
5. Harrow pastures to break up fecal masses and expose larvae to desiccation-induced death during hot dry weather. Harrowing should not be done in damp weather as it disperses infective larvae over a greater area without killing them.
6. Horses must be kept off a pasture for 4 to 12 months before all parasite larvae are dead. The damper and cooler the climate, the longer the time required. Survival and development of infective larvae increases with increased moisture, and parasite egg viability may be maintained over the winter even in cold climates.
7. Feces and, therefore, parasite eggs and larvae can be removed by sweeping pastures with a mechanized sweeper. Fecal removal by pasture sweeping twice weekly has been shown to control parasites as well as, and without, the administration of dewormers, and to increase grazing areas by 50%. With proper equipment, pasture sweeping takes about 4 hours/10 acres (1 hr/ha), but is effective only on relatively

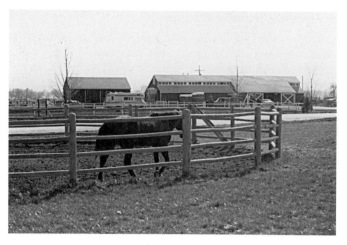

Fig. 9–4. On arrival to a new farm, all horses should be vaccinated (as described in Table 9–5), receive a non-benzimidazole dewormer, and be kept isolated for a minimum of the first 7 and preferably 14 days. Most infectious diseases are contagious for 7 to 14 days before the appearance of clinical signs of that disease, and viable strongyle eggs are excreted for up to 4 days after an effective dewormer is administered. If a horse is from a recent disease outbreak area, 30 days of isolation is recommended. The isolation pen should be well away from the stables and other horses.

flat even ground. Pasture sweeping and disposal of removed feces is impractical for some farms, but is an alternative that may be useful for others. When pasture sweeping is done, dewormer administration is unnecessary and should not be used except for bot control. Bot treatment is still necessary, as bots are transmitted by bot flies, not by the ingestion of fecally passed eggs or infective larvae.

8. All newly arriving horses or returning horses to the farm should be:
   a. Given a nonbenzimidazole dewormer (Table 9–1) and vaccinated.
   b. Isolated for a minimum of 7, and preferably, 14 days, or longer if signs of disease occur (Fig. 9–4). Four days after the administration of an effective dewormer, horses are no longer excreting viable strongyle eggs and, therefore, can be turned out on pasture without contaminating it. However, most infectious diseases are contagious for 7 to 14 days before the appearance of clinical signs of that disease and, therefore, a minimum 14-day quarantine is preferred.

Monitoring Internal Parasite Control

To monitor the efficiency of an internal-parasite control program, fecal samples can be examined for the presence and number of intestinal worm eggs or oocysts that they contain. This is done as described in Figures 9–5 and 9–6. It should be done at least twice yearly, once before and once 7 to 14 days after a dewormer is administered. Fecal samples should be checked from at least 10%, or 6, of the horses in each age and housing or pasture group. If the control program is effective, fecal egg counts on all sam-

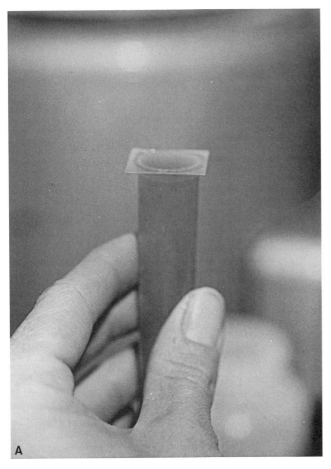
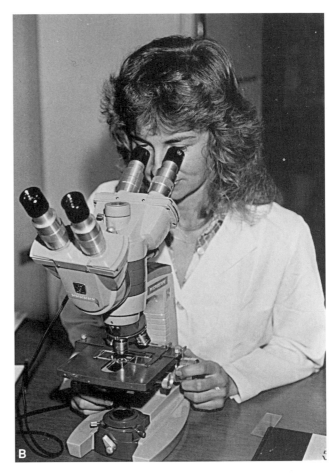

Fig. 9–5. Fecal flotation to determine the presence of intestinal parasites. A small amount of feces ($\frac{1}{2}$ to 1 tsp or 2 to 5 g) is mixed in a salt or sugar solution in a test tube. A microscope slide cover slip is placed on top of the tube, in contact with the solution (A). Oocytes, or eggs from intestinal worms, if present in the feces, float to the top of the solution and adhere to the cover slip. The cover slip is placed on a glass slide and viewed under a microscope (B). If the amount of feces used is determined, the number of eggs per gram can be determined as an indication of the adequacy of that farm's control program.

ples should be less than 50 eggs per gram (epg) or fewer than 10% of the fecal samples should contain parasite eggs. If this is not found, the control program should be modified accordingly. Over 80% of the post-treatment samples should be free of all parasite eggs, and there should be greater than a 90% reduction in pre-treatment to post-treatment egg counts. If this does not occur, it indicates ineffective treatment, either because the proper amount of deworming medication wasn't received by the horse or because the dewormer used was ineffective, which may occur because of the development of parasite resistance to that dewormer.

Internal-Parasite Control Program

The best internal-parasite control program for each farm or stable may be determined by the following procedures:

1. Give one avermectin treatment, or two non-avermectin treatments 1 month apart, to all horses on the same day beginning just before grazing spring pastures.
2. Obtain fecal egg counts monthly on all horses.

3. When egg counts in any of the horses exceeds 50 epg, re-treat all horses with the same dewormer and on the same day.
4. Treat all horses for bots after the first hard freeze in the fall and in problem areas 1 month after bot eggs first appear on the horse's hair.
5. After 1 to 2 years it should be possible to determine the timing and frequency that dewormer administration is needed for internal-parasite control on that farm or stable without the monthly fecal exams.
6. To ensure that the program is still satisfactory, once yearly obtain a fecal parasite egg count from 6 horses, or 10%, whichever is fewer, of each age group and each group of horses in the same pasture or stable, before and again 7 to 14 days after dewormer administration
7. Treat foaling mares with an avermectin dewormer the day of foaling, each time the foals are treated, and both the mare and foal before they join other mares and foals on pasture. This schedule minimizes the foal's exposure to internal parasites, including threadworms (S. westeri).

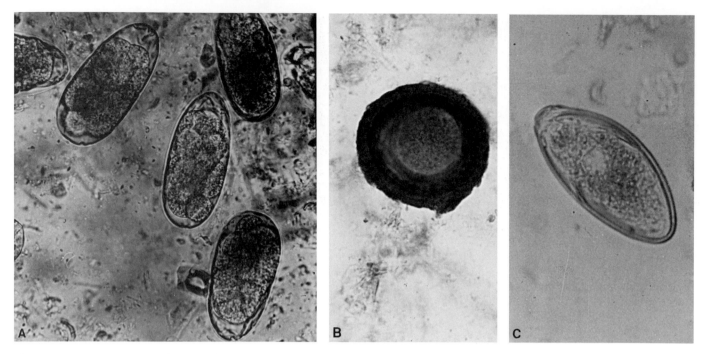

Fig. 9–6. Oocysts, or eggs of intestinal parasites, as viewed under the microscope at 100× magnification. Shown here are oocysts from strongyles (A), ascarids (B), and pinworms (C).

8. At 6 to 8 weeks of age, begin treating foals every 2 months until they are 1 year of age, at which time put them on the mature-horse internal-parasite control program. On large farms, averaging the age of all foals housed together to determine dates for deworming is easier and more efficient than deworming based on exact ages.

9. Keep weanlings and yearlings separate from mature horses.

10. All horses on the farm should be included on the same deworming program if possible. If this isn't possible, feed pyrantel tartrate continually as described previously for "Continual Deworming Programs."

11. Treat for other internal parasites if needed as described previously for that specific parasite.

EXTERNAL-PARASITE PROBLEMS AND CONTROL

In addition to internal parasites, there are numerous external parasites, or ectoparasites, that annoy farm horses and transmit numerous diseases. These diseases include encephalomyelitis (sleeping sickness), Rocky Mountain spotted fever, Colorado tick fever, tuleramia, Powassan encephalitis virus, anaplasmosis, piroplasmosis or babesiosis, equine infectious anemia or swamp fever, tick paralysis, and Lyme disease, whose incidence is increasing. Although less commonly affected by Lyme disease than dogs and people, horses can be affected, resulting in a reluctance to move and/or a transitory lameness with joint swelling sometimes apparent. Lyme disease is caused by a bacterium, spread by Ixodes ticks (e.g., deer or bear tick or western black-legged tick) when they are attached for 24 hours or longer. In addition to spreading these diseases,

a horse may develop a localized reaction or infection, or an allergy to ticks or other external parasites, which can result in hair loss or hives (Fig. 1–5). Most external parasites are a problem for horses only during warm weather. Lice, mites, and some ticks, in contrast, are a problem primarily during the winter or early spring. This is because their life cycles occur entirely on the animal, whereas all or a portion of the life cycle of the other external parasites of the horse occur partially or totally off the animal. Factors helpful in the identification of external parasites, their effects on the horse, and nonpesticide control procedures are summarized in Table 9–2. Although nonpesticide control procedures are quite helpful, and for some external parasites necessary for their control, the proper use of pesticides is more important. The type of pesticides recommended for control of each external parasite are given in Table 9–3, and specific pesticides and fungicides recommended for use on horses are given in Table 9–4.

Pesticides have maximum efficiency only when applied to the horse and surrounding area at the right time. Knowing the right time requires knowing which insects are present. If an external parasite causing a problem can't be identified, a specimen should be collected and shown to someone capable of identifying it, such as a veterinarian or diagnostic laboratory, university, or agriculture extension personnel. These individuals may also have the latest information on the seasonal occurrence of external parasites, species found in a given location, the best or approved methods and materials available for their control, recommended times of treatment, and other useful information on local external parasites.

Two approaches should be taken in controlling external parasites: 1) controlling them in the area where horses are

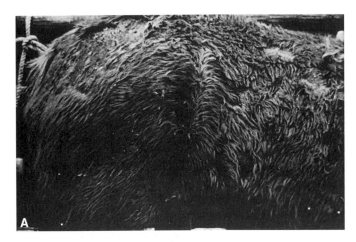
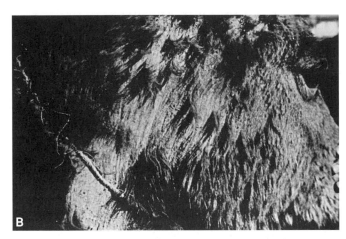

Fig. 9–7(A,B). Hair loss due to itching caused by lice infestation (pediculosis). Lice may also cause blood loss and poor condition. They occur particularly on debilitated horses and, like mites, whose life cycle (like that of fleas) occurs on the animal, but in contrast to other external parasites in which much of the life cycle occurs off the animal, lice are a problem primarily during the winter. See Table 9–3 for treatment and control.

kept, and 2) controlling them on the horse. By doing a thorough job of spraying the area and facilities, many external parasite problems can be minimized or eliminated. A product containing both an insecticide and an insect growth regulator (Table 9-4) not only to kill adults but also to inhibit egg hatching and larval development may be quite helpful or necessary to eliminate heavy infestations. Controlling external parasites on the horse often is more difficult than eliminating them on the premises. The control of many external parasites on the horse frequently requires at least daily application of a pesticide during peak insect season. However, too frequent an application of some pesticides induces a systemic toxic effect. Because of this, pyrethrin insecticides are frequently used for horses. Pyrethrins and other pesticides for control of external parasites are available in many different forms, including dips, sprays, dusts, wipes or smears, injections, rubbers, pour-ons, and feed additives. Horses have a very sensitive skin and may have a skin reaction to the solvents and other ingredients in a pesticide formulation. This occurs most commonly when they are treated with formulations not approved for application to horses, but may occur in some horses treated with approved products. Some formulations may cause burning, blistering, or cracking of the skin. Because of these possible effects, a product not previously used on a particular horse should be applied to only a small area of the horse and used thereafter only if there is no adverse reaction to it in the following 24 hours.

Pesticides can also be toxic to the horse and the people who apply them, and can be destructive to the environment if they are not used and handled in a safe and correct manner. A few precautions to follow when choosing and applying pesticides for the control of external parasites of horses are the following:

1. Use only pesticides recommended and approved for use on horses by the government or competent authority (Table 9-4).
2. Use a formulation of the pesticide that is approved and especially designed for use on horses. In particular, in dipping vats use only those formulations designed specifically for dipping vats.
3. Follow the label directions exactly. The label should contain all the information about dilution, time for retreatment of animals, antidotes for poisoning, methods of disposing of unused pesticide, and other important information.
4. Avoid treating horses in cold, stormy weather; avoid treating stressed, weak, overheated, or sick animals; don't dip thirsty horses.
5. Be sure that spraying equipment is clean, works properly, and provides sufficient agitation to allow for thorough mixing of pesticides.
6. Be aware of safe practices when mixing, applying, or storing pesticides. Do not contaminate feed or water troughs.
7. Know the signs of pesticide poisoning in livestock (and people) to avoid delay in instituting antidotal measures.
8. Dispose correctly of all containers, unused concentrate, and used diluted pesticides to avoid contamination of the environment.

INFECTIOUS-DISEASE PROBLEMS AND VACCINATION PROGRAMS

Preventing infectious diseases in horses requires in addition to a good vaccination program isolating all incoming horses as previously described (Fig. 9-4). On broodmare farms, new horses should not be introduced into the resident population, but instead kept separately. If an outbreak occurs, healthy horses in contact with sick horses should be considered potential incubators and sources of the disease. Because of this, in order to minimize the spread of the disease, no horses should be moved to other barns or sites on the farm. In addition, people working with diseased or exposed horses should either not handle other horses on the farm or should disinfect themselves and change clothes before doing so.

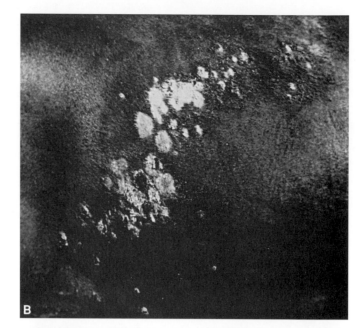

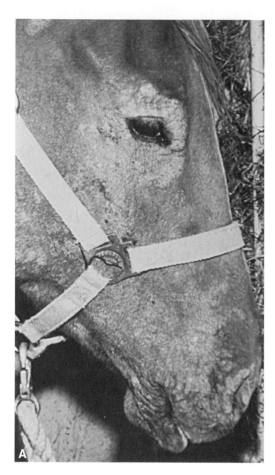

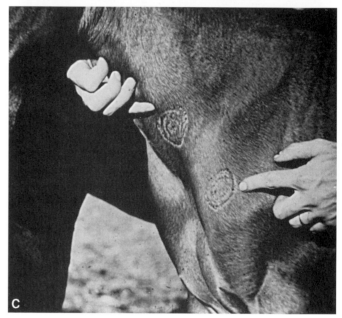

Fig. 9–8(A,B,C). Ringworm (dermatophytosis or girth-itch). Three different-appearing skin lesions, all of which were due to ringworm. Be careful not to use brushes, combs, or tack from an affected animal on another animal, as infection is readily spread in this manner. For diagnosis, treatment, and control see Table 9–2.

A good vaccination program for the control of bacterial and viral diseases, like a good parasite control and feeding program, is an essential aspect in the care of the horse. A good vaccination program will vary depending on numerous factors, including: (1) disease prevalence in that area and farm, (2) degree of confinement, (3) number of horses, (4) what the horses are used for, and (5) frequency of contact with other horses. Because of these and other variables, and the continual development of new vaccines, a vaccination program should be set up that is adapted as needed for each farm, stable, or situation. Regardless of the vaccination program used, all horses on a farm should be on the same program and schedule when possible. This will maximize herd immunity and thus minimize infectious-disease challenge, thus protecting those that may respond poorly to vaccination. Manufacturers' recommenda-

tions for vaccine storage, handling, and administration should be followed to maximize the vaccine's efficacy.

Diseases for which vaccination should be considered include tetanus, encephalomyelitis (sleeping sickness), influenza, rhinopneumonitis (equine herpes virus or EHV), strangles or distemper (strep equi), rabies, anthrax, botulism, equine viral arteritis, salmonellosis, Potomac horse fever, (monocytic ehrlichiosis) and, in broodmares on farms with a high incidence of foal septicemia, Clostridium perfringens type C and D toxoids. A minimum vaccination program for all horses includes tetanus toxoid and encephalomyelitis every spring (Table 9–5). More frequent vaccination and vaccination for influenza, rhinopneumonitis, and strangles are indicated in many situations (Table 9–5).

Acute allergic reactions to vaccines are uncommon but

TABLE 9–2
External Parasites of Horses
Identification, Effects and Nonpesticide Control[a]

External Parasite	Identification	Effect on Horses	Control Procedures
Flies			
Deer flies (Chrysops spp. & tabanids)	1/4–1/2 inch, orangish with dark markings.	Painful bite, blood loss, skin nodules.	Stable horses near dusk & dawn, and allow horses to escape from wooded areas. Hang electric insect light in barn.
Horse flies (tabanids)	1/3–1 1/4 inch, variable color and markings	Painful bite, blood loss, skin nodules.	
Face flies (Musca autumnalis)	Black or orange lateral abdomen, larvae yellow & pupa white. Develop in fresh cattle manure.	Face and house flies feed on mucus from mouth, nostrils, eyes or fresh wounds. Cause intense irritation & are vectors for eye worms (Thelazia spp.)	For face flies separate horses from or treat & feed larvicide to cattle, & for face & house flies use fly bait, trap & electric grid. Dispose of all manure & contaminated forage twice weekly
House flies (Musca domestica)	Yellow lateral abdomen, larvae white & pupa red-brown.	House and stable flies are vectors for habronemiasis or *summer sores* (ulcerative granulomas especially on legs & prepuce during summer	
Stable flies (Stomoxys calcitrans)	Blood-sucking mouth	Especially on legs & abdomen; blood loss, crusts & papules.	Dispose of all contaminated forage, especially hay in pastures.
Horn flies (Haematobia irritans)	3/16 inch cattle parasite that develops in fresh manure.	Feed head down especially on neck, withers, abdomen & ventral midline causing ulcers, crusts, & blood loss.	Control flies on cattle or separate horses from cattle.
Bot flies (Gastrophilus spp.)	See Fig 9–3 (A), page 157.	Oral & gastric irritation, colic, ulcers, rarely perforation (Fig. 9–3, C).	As described in this chapter for "Seasonal Deworming."
Blow flies (Phormia regina & Phaenicia sp.)	Black or green (bronze-like)	Lay eggs in dead tissue which hatch into larvae or maggots.	Dispose of dead animal tissue and general sanitation.
Gnats & Midges			
Black flies, buffalo gnats or Simuliidae	1/16–3/16 inch, black, hump-backed; often in swarms near rivers or ponds.	Especially in ears, bloody crusts & itching, & around nose.	Ear net & petroleum jelly in ears. Stable horses near dusk & dawn; for biting midges, having horses under fans may help. Water management recommended for mosquitoes is helpful for some species of midges.
Biting midges (gnats, punkies, no-see-ums, sand flies, Culicoides, & Leptoconops)	1/32–3/16 inch, black, spots on costal wing border, peak activity evening & dawn at >50°F (10°C) with no breeze.	Painful bite, onchocerciasis (summer, Queensland, sweet, dhobie or muck itch, kasen & Sommerekzem), itching, hair loss & scaling especially at ears, mane, withers, tail or ventral abdomen.	
Mosquitoes	Active in evenings, develop in still water.	Blood loss & itching & transmit encephalomyelitis.	Eliminate standing water. Put pesticides & surfactants on, & minnows in water. Attract purple martin birds.
Maggots & Grubs (Myiasis)			
Maggots (facultative myiasis, screwworms, & black & green or bronze blow fly larvae)	White, short, stubby worms.	Larvae are in dead tissue, screwworms in fresh tissue.	Clean & debride wound & treat it with a residual insecticide.[a]
Cattle grubs (obligate myiasis), (Hypoderma spp.)		Skin nodules with breathing pore, especially in spring & on back.	Surgically remove or give Ivermectin.
Lice			
Chewing & biting lice (Bovicola equi & of poultry)		Chewing lice feed on skin & sebaceous secretions & sucking lice on blood. First on head, neck, mane & tail. If severe, cause anemia & poor condition. See Fig. 9–7 (page 166).	Lice are not transferable between horses & cattle. Separate horses from poultry & nonaffected from affected horses. Groom & give a residual insecticide,[a] twice 2 weeks apart. Some horses seem to be carriers.
Sucking lice (Haematopinus asini)			
Fleas			
Sticktight poultry fleas & Cat fleas (possibly)	Affects horses sharing areas with infected chickens or cats.	Local itching & skin inflammation, and/or possibly anemia.	Same as lice.

(continued)

are a life-threatening emergency requiring prompt administration of epinephrine. Local irritant tissue reactions to vaccines are much more common. These reactions usually resolve without treatment, but oral administration of anti-inflammatory drugs, topical application of warm compresses or drawing agents, and gentle exercise may be helpful. If the neck is affected, the horse may be reluctant to lower its head to eat or drink, and feed and water should be positioned accordingly. Horses that repeatedly react to a vaccine may benefit by prior administration of non-

TABLE 9–2
External Parasites of Horses
Identification, Effects and Nonpesticide Control[a]–(Continued)

External Parasite	Identification	Effect on Horses	Control Procedures
Mites & Chiggers			
Mites (pyemotid & hay, straw or grain itch)		Nonitching papular eruptions especially on neck & withers. People affected also.	Dispose of infected straw, hay, or grain.
Mange mites,			
Sarcoptic mites	Circular with short legs.	Small nodules with hair loss, & a scab develops where they burrow into the skin, especially of head, neck, shoulders, chest, flank & abdomen.	Transmission is by contact so isolate affected horses & their equipment, and treat with Ivermectin.
Psoroptic or scab mites	Oval, longer legs with segmented pedicels.	On skin causing hair loss, papules, moist, bloody crusts at mane, tail & forelock.	
Chorioptic (most common of 3 mange mites)	Same as Psoroptic mites but unsegmented pedicels.	On skin causing scaling, especially on legs.	
Chiggers (red bugs, harvest mites)		Itching papular skin inflammation & crusting especially on head, neck, chest & legs.	Limit access to infected areas and repellants[a] for prevention.
Demodex (follicle mites): D. caballi & D. equi	Minute long-oval shape, short legs with cross-striated abdomen. Both types are rare	D. caballi in eyelid meibomian glands & skin of muzzle. Both cause patchy hair loss & scaling due to mites in hair follicles.	Administer Ivermectin
Ticks			
Soft tick, spinous ear tick	A separate group of ticks attack horses and other animals in different geographical areas.	Local inflammation, edema, pain, infection, & maggot site, especially in ears. Deafness. Meningites. With heavy infestation poor condition, anemia, & fluid in abdomen. Disease vectors including Lyme disease, & tick paralysis.	Examine & groom horse, especially its ears, after it is in tick areas (e.g., woods & brush) & again 5–7 days later. Mow, clear and burn tick-infested areas & apply pesticides in ears, understory, floor & paddock ground.
Hard ticks, many Ixodidae, including Dermacentor			
Ringworm			
Dermatophytosis (girth-itch, Microsporum or Trichophyton spp.)	Growth on dermatophyte culture medium.	Especially in young horses when wet, warm, crowded, & dark, and on girth & saddle area (Fig. 9–8, page 168).	Eliminate source and decontaminate environment. Isolate horse. Clip & wash lesions. Fungicide[a] bath 7 times first day then twice weekly until cured.

[a] For type of pesticides recommended for control of each external parasite, see Table 9–3, and for pesticides and fungicides recommended for use on horses see Table 9–4.

---

steroidal anti-inflammatory drugs, or the use of a different injection site or a different brand of vaccine.

Tetanus

Tetanus (lockjaw) is caused by neurotoxins produced by the bacteria Clostridium tetani, particularly in deep or closed wounds such as puncture wounds, but may occur, due to intestinal infections. This highly fatal disease is a constant threat for all horses as the bacteria are widely distributed in soil and manure. The disease affects all animals, with the horse being particularly susceptible.

Vaccination of all horses for tetanus is recommended, as given in Table 9–5. For horses not previously vaccinated or with an unknown vaccination history, tetanus toxoid should be given twice, 1 to 2 months apart. Protection is attained within 2 weeks after the second injection and may persist, but not necessarily at protective levels, for as long as 5 years. For all horses, yearly revaccination with the toxoid is recommended, as it is following an injury. The broodmare should be given the toxoid prior to breeding and again 1 to 2 months before the expected foaling date. The foal should receive an adequate amount of the vaccinated mare's colostrum and be vaccinated with the toxoid at 2, 4, and 6 months of age.

Tetanus antitoxin is indicated for the injured horse that is not known to have been vaccinated with the toxoid in the past year. It provides immediate protection which lasts for about 2 weeks. Following injury, both antitoxin and toxoid should be administered to unvaccinated horses or those with an unknown vaccination history. Following foaling, both antitoxin and toxoid should be administered to unvaccinated mares and the antitoxin administered to her foal. After receiving the antitoxin, the horse should be revaccinated with the toxoid as described in the previous paragraph.

Administration of tetanus antitoxin, but not toxoid, carries the risk of inducing serum hepatitis 3 to 9 weeks following its administration. Most cases of serum hepatitis,

TABLE 9–3
External Parasites and Type of Pesticides Recommended for Their Control on Horses[a]

Insecticides	Insecticides & Repellents
Flies, face	Chiggers
horn	Flies, black (gnats)
house	deer
Lice, biting or chewing	horse
Maggots	stable
Mosquitoes	Gnats (biting midges, Culicoides)
Fleas	Onchocerciasis
Ticks	Maggots
	Mosquitoes
Repellents	Ticks
Chiggers	
Flies, black (gnats)	**Systemic**
horse	Grubs
Gnats (biting midges, Culicoides)	Habronemiasis (summer sores due
	to house or stable fly larvae)[b]
Premise Treatment	Lice, sucking
Flies, house & stable	Mites
Mosquitoes	Onchocerciasis (Culicoides or
Fleas	biting midge hypersensitivity)[b]
Insect Growth Regulators	**Fungicides**
Flies	Ringworm
Fleas	

[a] See Table 9–2 for Nonpesticide control procedures and Table 9–4 for specific pesticides recommended for horses.
[b] Corticosteroids are helpful in decreasing itching. Tar and sulfur shampoos or sprays formulated for animals are also helpful. Lotions or oily preparations or a sheet covering affected areas to provide mechanical barriers to gnats may be helpful if used before onset of severe itching. Densensitization or hyposensitization is not helpful.

TABLE 9–4
Pesticides Recommended for External Parasite Control on Horses[a]

Insecticides	Repellents
Pyrethroids:	MGK 326 (di-n-propyl isocinchomeronate)
Cypermethrin	Stabilene: butoxypoly-propylene glycol
Fenvalerate	
Permethrin	**Botanicals**
Resmethrin	Pyrethroids
Tetramethrin	
S-Bioallerthrin	**Synergists**
Sumethrin	Piperonyl butoxide
Organophosphates:	MGK 264 (N-oxtyl bicyclo-heptene
Coumaphos	dicarboximide)
Dichlorvos	
Malathion	**Systemic**
Tetrachlorvinphos	Ivermectin (0.2 mg/kg orally)
Organochlorines:	Moxidectin (0.4 mg/kg orally)
Lindane	
Methoxychlor	**Fungicides**
	Bleach (0.5% sodium hypochlorite)
Insect Growth	Captan 3%[c]
Regulators[b]	Chlorhexidine 0.5 to 2%
Methoprene	Enilconazole
	Lime sulfur 3 to 5%
	Providone-Iodine

[a] Categories may overlap, e.g., some pyrethrins are insecticidal, repellent, and botanical. For all, follow product label directions closely. Many sprays require 4 to 8 oz (120 to 240 ml) per horse to give good residual control.
[b] These inhibit egg hatching and larval development which may be necessary to eliminate heavy animal and premise infestations. They are usually combined with an insecticide such as pyrethrin for use on animals and chlorpyrifos for premise treatment (e.g., Siphotrol Plus II House Treatment, Vet-Kem, Zoecon Corp, Dallas, Texas).
[c] 1 oz of 50% wettable powder in 1 gallon of water (10 g/L) of Orthocide (Ortho Products, San Francisco).

even with treatment, are fatal. A proper tetanus vaccination program eliminates this risk, as well as greatly decreasing the risk of tetanus, because antitoxin administration then is not needed or recommended.

Clinical signs of tetanus in affected horses begin following an incubation period of 3 days to several weeks, but usually 1 to 2 weeks. Muscle spasms and a stiff paralysis progressing from the head to the neck, front, and then hind legs occurs. The jaw muscle is the most commonly affected muscle, giving rise to the name lockjaw for the disease. Prolapse of the third eyelid, as well as eyelid retraction, erect ear carriage, flared nostrils, and hyperesthesia, are the most consistent clinical signs. These are usually followed by stiffness, resulting in a sawhorse stance, and reluctance to feed from the ground. The horse may be unable to swallow, resulting in saliva dripping from the mouth and regurgitation of ingested food and water through the nose. Convulsions, muscle rigidity, sweating, and fever may follow. Colic, urine retention, and difficult respiration may occur. About 50 to 75% of affected horses die within 2 to 10 days after the onset of symptoms, usually as a result of an inability to breathe. For those surviving, clinical signs may be apparent for up to 6 weeks, and founder, muscle damages aspiration pneumonia, and decubitus ulcers may occur.

Treatment of tetanus includes early administration of tetanus antitoxin and an antibiotic, and cleaning the infected wound. Tranquilizers may help alleviate muscle spasms, paralysis and pain. Supportive care is very important and should include housing in a dark, quiet stall with padding and thick bedding to minimize injuries. Slings or bales of hay may be necessary to help keep the horse standing or lying on its sternum. Urinary catheterization and frequent manual removal of feces may be necessary.

Equine Encephalomyelitis (Sleeping Sickness)

Equine encephalomyelitis or encephalitis is caused by three antigenically different arbovirus strains: Eastern (EEE), Western (WEE), and Venezuelan (VEE). Wild animals and birds, which are not affected by the viruses, serve as their reservoirs. The viruses are transmitted to horses and people by blood-sucking arthropods, mainly mosquitoes. Disease therefore occurs primarily during the season in which mosquitoes occur. VEE is the only virus of the three that is transmitted from one horse to another. It can also be transmitted by insects to people and other animals. Although it's possible for EEE, neither it nor WEE is transmitted from horses or people to other horses or people; i.e., a horse or person cannot get EEE or WEE, but can get VEE from other horses or people.

Prevention of equine encephalomyelitis is to vaccinate twice, 2 to 3 weeks apart, with annual revaccination 2 weeks to 2 months before blood-sucking-insect season be-

TABLE 9–5
Equine Vaccination Program[a]

Horse	Vaccination History or Foal's Age	Situation	Vaccine to Administer
All yearlings & older	Unvaccinated or unknown	To start program	Tetanus toxoid & encephalomyelitis } twice 1 mo. apart
All yearlings & older	Previously vaccinated	Every spring	Tetanus toxoid & encephalomyelitis[b]
All yearlings & older and performance & show horses	Previously vaccinated	2 weeks before travel & repeated every 2–3 mo	Influenza and rhinopneumonitis (EHV)
Broodmare	Unvaccinated	After foaling	Tetanus antitoxin & toxoid
	Either vaccinated or unvaccinated	{ Before breeding 5–6 mo pg. 7–8 mo pg. } 9–10 mo pg.	Tetanus toxoid { Killed rhinopneumonitis or herpes virus vaccine (K-EHV) K-EHV, influenza, tetanus toxoid & encephalomyelitis
Foals[c]	1–2 days	Unvaccinated dam	Tetanus antitoxin & toxoid
	2–3 mo[d]	All foals[d]	Influenza, rhinopneumonitis, tetanus toxoid & encephalomyelitis
	4–5 mo	All foals	Influenza, rhinopneumonitis, tetanus toxoid & encephalomyelitis
	6–7 mo	All foals	Influenza, rhinopneumonitis, tetanus toxoid & encephalomyelitis
	Every 2–3 mo to 1-yr-old	High-exposure risk foals	Influenza, rhinopneumonitis (EHV)

[a] Other vaccines are available but are recommended only for horses in or going to areas or farms where these diseases have occurred or been a problem. These include equine viral arteritis (state approval may be required), equine monocytic ehrlichiosis (Potomac horse fever), rabies, anthrax, botulism and "Shaker Foal Syndrome" (See Chapter 19), and Clostridium perfringens types C and D.
[b] Encephalomyelitis vaccination may be needed every 6 months in endemic areas where blood-sucking insects are present all year, e.g., southeastern and south central United States.
[c] On farms that have recurrent strangles outbreaks, administer strangles vaccine at 3, at 4, and again at 5 months of age and then annually until 3 to 5 years of age.
[d] Vaccinations are generally uncessary at 2 to 3 months of age for foals receiving ample amounts of colostrum from vaccinated mares.

gins, as summarized in Table 9–5. Vaccines are available that contain all three viral strains, just EEE and WEE, or only VEE. There is increased specific antibody production to all viruses when bivalent or trivalent vaccines are administered. The response to VEE vaccination alone is lower in horses previously vaccinated against EEE and WEE. Vaccination is recommended against all strains to which a horse may be exposed, whether that exposure is from being in an area where that strain has occurred or being exposed to horses (for VEE), or other animals or birds that have been. In the United States and South America, clinical disease due to EEE occurs primarily, but not exclusively, in the east. WEE in the west, and both in the center; whereas VEE, along with both EEE and WEE, occur primarily in Mexico, Central America and northern South America. In 1962 a severe epidemic of VEE occurred in Venezuela and Colombia infecting and killing countless horses, and infecting 300,000 people, over 300 of whom died. The last occurrence of VEE in the United States was in 1971, but an outbreak occurred in Chiapas, Mexico in July 1993.

Foals receiving adequate colostrum from a properly vaccinated mare may have adequate protection until 6 months of age, but it is safer to vaccinate them at 4 months, at 6 months, and again at 1 year of age (Table 9–5). In endemic areas where blood-sucking insects exist (e.g., southeastern and south central portions of the United States), horses should be vaccinated every 6 months, as protective titers

appear to last only 6 to 8 months. During an outbreak, all susceptible horses should be vaccinated.

Clinical signs of all three forms of equine encephalomyelitis, following a 1- to 3-week incubation period, include high fever, absence of feed intake, stiffness, incoordination, a reeling gait, compulsive walking, circling, drowsiness, partial to complete loss of vision, grinding of the teeth, inability to swallow, and in severe cases, hyperesthesia, aggression, excitability, and even frenzy after sensory stimulation may occur. Death generally occurs 2 to 7 days following recumbency. Because of these symptoms, the condition is commonly referred to as sleeping sickness, and occasionally brain fever or blind staggers. For horses that develop these neurologic signs, the mortality rate, even with, treatment, for EEE is 75 to 100%, for VEE 40 to 80%, and for WEE 20 to 50%. VEE may result in a subclinical infection.

Diagnosis of encephalomyelitis may be confirmed by detecting a rise in plasma antibody levels against the disease, or by a virus isolation from the brain. Antibody levels begin increasing before clinical signs, so that the peak levels may already have been reached when the first sample is taken. Diseases that must be differentiated from encephalomyelitis include other viral encephalitides, trauma, liver failure, rabies, moldy corn disease, bacterial meningoencephalomyelitis, equine protozoal myeloencephalitis, and verminous encephalitis.

Treatment of encephalomyelitis is primarily supportive. Phenylbutazone or flunixin meglumine frequently are administered to control fever, inflammation, and discomfort. If convulsions occur, tranquilizers and anesthetic drugs may be administered. Antibiotics may be indicated to prevent or treat secondary bacterial infections. Most cases of EEE, and some cases of WEE and VEE, do not recover completely from neurologic deficits, resulting in persistent incoordination, depression, and abnormal behavior.

Equine Influenza

Equine influenza is a highly contagious acute respiratory disease caused by two distinct strains of virus, type A-1 and type A-2, and an altered form of the A-2 virus. It affects horses of all ages but is most common in horses 2 to 3 years old. It is considered to be the most important viral respiratory-tract disease in horses at training centers, race tracks, and shows.

Prevention of influenza requires frequent vaccination of exposed horses. Vaccination is recommended beginning when foals are 2 months of age, although not vaccinating foals until they are 4 to 6 months old is probably quite adequate for those that received ample amounts of colostrum from mares vaccinated yearly 1 to 2 months before foaling. A second injection should be administered 1 to 2 months after the first vaccination. Repeated vaccinations may be indicated at 2- to 3-month intervals until maturity is reached, depending upon exposure risk. Currently available vaccines contain both type A-1 and type A-2—and some drifted A-2—inactivated influenza viruses. Some horses develop a transient self-limiting fever, decreased appetite and depression following influenza vaccination; it may therefore be best not to vaccinate a horse for influenza within 7 to 10 days of the horse's use in an event.

Clinical signs of influenza begin 1 to 3 days following inhalation of the virus by susceptible horses and are characterized by fever (up to 106°F or 41°C); depression; a dry, harsh often violent cough; decreased appetite; and usually a clear nasal discharge early in the disease. Affected horses are usually depressed, may be reluctant to move, and may have leg edema. Coughing is the most common sign and usually persists for 1 to 3 weeks in uncomplicated cases. In the absence of secondary complications, the respiratory lining regenerates, and recovery occurs in approximately 3 weeks.

The most common secondary complication of viral respiratory diseases, such as influenza or rhinopneumonitis, is the development of a bacterial pneumonia resulting in a persistent, often productive cough, fever beyond the first 4 to 5 days, and a thicker, yellowish-white nasal discharge. Prolonged excessive coughing may predispose the horse to pulmonary emphysema or hemorrhage, and bronchitis. Additional secondary complications that may occur include a sore throat, diarrhea, inflammation and fluid in the thoracic cavity (pleuritis), and heart disease. Few horses are able to return to athletic usefulness after developing pleuritis. Occasionally, in young, old, debilitated, or stressed horses, these viruses may localize in the muscle, causing skeletal or heart muscle damage.

Diagnosis of influenza is generally confirmed by an increasing serum influenza antibody titer in samples taken within 1 to 2 days of the onset of symptoms and another 2 to 3 weeks later, although in recently vaccinated horses, levels in both samples may be high.

Treatment of viral respiratory disease, no matter what disease is responsible—influenza or rhinopneumonitis—is mainly rest and supportive therapy. Early detection of respiratory disease and cessation of heavy work until inflammation has resolved are critical to its successful management. Complete rest for 3 weeks is the most important aspect in the treatment of viral respiratory diseases and prevention of secondary complications. With rest, other therapy may not be needed. Without adequate rest, other treatments are generally ineffective.

Antibiotic administration is also beneficial in protecting the horse against secondary bacterial infection. Nonsteroidal anti-inflammatory drugs, as well as antibiotics, are generally administered, if the fever is severe or persists longer than 3 to 4 days.

Horses with respiratory disease should be immediately isolated and every effort made to minimize their contact with other horses for the first 7 to 10 days of the disease. Separate water, feed buckets, halter, and grooming equipment should be used for each horse. Barn personnel should handle sick animals last, since they may otherwise transmit the viruses to unaffected horses. During an outbreak of either influenza or rhinopneumonitis, all horses not ill should be vaccinated to limit the spread of the disease; however, clinically ill horses should not be vaccinated.

Rhinopneumonitis (Equine Herpes Virus)

Equine rhinopneumonitis is caused by equine herpes viruses type-1 (EHV-1) and type-4 (EHV-4). EHV-4 used to be called EHV-1 subtype 2. Both EHV-1 and EHV-4 can cause respiratory disease in horses. It is reported that these viruses cause 30 to 40% of all respiratory diseases in horses, with most of these being due to EHV-4. EHV-1 may also cause either abortion or a neurologic disease. A high percentage of adult horses are inapparent carriers of both viruses. When they are stressed, clinical or subclinical disease and viral shedding from the respiratory tract, which may infect other horses, may occur.

Rhinopneumonitis (EHV) is a highly contagious disease transmitted by inhalation of infectious aerosols or by direct contact with infected secretions on utensils or in drinking water. Although EHV can spread rapidly among young horses under stressful crowded conditions, it is rarely transmitted between horses in separate but adjacent paddocks or stalls if direct contact is prevented. On breeding farms it may take several months before respiratory disease spreads to all susceptible horses. This provides the opportunity to limit the spread of the disease. However, abortion storms may occur because of spread of the infection before clinical signs occur.

The respiratory form of EHV occurs primarily in young horses in high horse-population density areas. Following a 2- to 20-day incubation period, it is characterized by fever for 1 to 7 days; mild cough; a profuse, clear watery nasal and ocular discharge; and enlarged submandibular lymph nodes. Decreased appetite, depression, and infrequently diarrhea and subcutaneous ventral and leg edema may occur. Occasionally, young susceptible foals may suffer a fatal bronchopneumonia, whereas infections may be subclinical in older, partially immune horses.

Treatment of EHV is the same as described in the previous section for influenza. With proper treatment, secondary complications are prevented and recovery is usually complete within 1 to 2 weeks.

In the pregnant mare, abortion may occur 9 to 120 days, but most commonly 10 to 20 days, following clinical or subclinical EHV-induced respiratory infection or may occur without any prior respiratory infection. EHV-induced abortion most commonly occurs during the eighth to eleventh month of gestation, and is characterized by complete and rapid expulsion of placental membranes and a fresh infected fetus that probably died as a result of suffocation following separation of the membranes. Occasionally a fetus may be aborted as early as at 4 months of gestation and may be severely autolyzed. Abortion may occur in a high percentage of mares on the farm. Less commonly, instead of abortion, infected mares may give birth to a live but weak foal that usually dies of acute pneumonia or pleuritis within the first few days of life. Infections that result in abortions or birth of infected foals often occur at the same time as an outbreak of respiratory disease in young horses on that farm. Affected mares may or may not show any signs of respiratory disease. Aborting mares' subsequent reproductive efficiency is not impaired.

Rarely, EHV-1 may affect the central nervous system of horses of any age. When this occurs, neurologic signs usually begin within 8 to 10 days after respiratory infection and as signs of it begin to wane. There is usually an acute onset and rapid progression over 1 to 2 days of incoordination, frequently with urinary incontinence, a decrease in tail tone, and sphincter paresis with fecal retention, penile prolapse and repeated erections, and variable anesthesia of the perineal area. Although it is usually fatal, mild cases may recover but have a persistent neurologic deficit. Treatment of neurologically affected horses is primarily supportive and depends on the degree of neurologic deficit present. Antibiotic administration is generally not required unless pneumonia or pressure sores occur. Corticosteroids may be administered.

All fetuses, sickly newborn, and suspected respiratory or neurologic cases should be isolated for 3 weeks from other horses, particularly pregnant mares. The environment should be thoroughly disinfected and bedding removed and burned. Fetuses, afterbirth, and dead foals should be submitted to a diagnostic laboratory for diagnosis of EHV. In addition, all newly introduced horses should be quarantined for 3 weeks.

Diagnosis of EHV is based on detecting the antigen or culturing the viruses from nose and throat swabs, or blood obtained as soon as possible after symptoms of the disease are first noted. Diagnosis of all forms of EHV from blood samples is difficult.

The immunity to EHV produced by either natural infection or vaccination is short lived. Antibody titers disappear from vaccinated horses in 3 to 4 months, and from foals in 3 to 4 weeks. Two types of EHV vaccines are available: a modified live-virus (MLV) vaccine and an inactivated or killed viral vaccine. Both provide protection against the respiratory form of the disease. The MLV vaccine may not give good protection against abortion and therefore isn't recommended for pregnant mares. Vaccines containing EHV-1, EHV-4, and three strains of influenza viruses are available (e.g., Fluvac EHV 4/1, Fort Dodge Labs, Fort Dodge, IA 50501).

Vaccination, particularly with a vaccine containing both EHV-1 and EHV-4, is recommended beginning when the foal is 3 months of age (Table 9–5). A second injection should be administered 1 to 2 months later. Repeated vaccinations may be indicated at 2- to 3-month intervals until maturity, depending on exposure risk. Pregnant mares should be vaccinated with the killed-virus vaccine during the fifth, seventh, and ninth months of gestation. Vaccination of pregnant mares is recommended even though 100% protection against abortion isn't achieved; sporadic abortions may occur in vaccinated mares.

Equine Viral Arteritis

Equine viral arteritis (EVA) is caused by a togavirus and affects only equine species. It generally occurs in sporadic but rare outbreaks. The clinical appearance of the disease depends on the individual; in an outbreak, symptoms range from acute death to profound fever, anorexia, depression, leg edema, inflammation around the eyes, nasal and ocular discharge, underline and genital edema, and occasionally skin rashes, diarrhea, and colic. Sometimes clinical signs are the same as those of influenza and rhinopneumonitis (EHV). Infection may result in high rates of abortion at any stage of pregnancy. In contrast to EHV-1, the aborted fetus is often autolyzed and does not usually show the typical arteritis seen in adults.

The long-term carrier stallion appears to play a major role in perpetuation of the virus from year to year. The carrier state hasn't been confirmed in mares or foals. Persistently infected stallions appear to shed the virus only venereally during the chronic-carrier phase of the disease. About 30 to 50% of serum positive stallions are carriers. However, during the acute phase of the disease, and for up to 2 weeks after infection, nasal secretions appear to be the most common source of virus dissemination.

Diagnosis of equine viral arteritis may be made by isolating the virus from nose or throat swabs or blood samples. Viruses may also be cultured from aborted fetuses, urine, and the semen of some affected stallions. An increasing serum antibody titer to EVA in samples taken at the onset of the disease and several weeks following recovery confirms the diagnosis. Treatment and prevention is the same as for the other viral respiratory diseases, influenza, and rhinopneumonitis or EHV.

Vaccination for EVA with a modified live virus vaccine (Arovac, Fort Dodge Labs) has been found to be a safe and effective means of control and prevention. Vaccination of stallions and nonpregnant mares at least 3 weeks before breeding has been recommended. However, vaccination effects may interfere with testing requirements for export; prior approval by the state veterinarian for vaccination may be required. Pregnant mares should not be vaccinated.

Strangles

Strangles (equine distemper or shipping fever) is an acute, highly contagious disease of the upper respiratory tract of horses caused by the bacterium Streptococcus equi. Following a 3- to 8-day incubation period, the disease is characterized by fever, depression, a nasal discharge that becomes thick and yellowish-white, a soft moist cough, and swollen, frequently abscessed, lymph nodes of the throat area (Fig. 9–9). The head and neck are often held outstretched, and the larynx or voice box is painful on palpation. Swelling may be sufficient to cause respiratory obstruction and difficult breathing, giving the disease its name—strangles. In 10 to 14 days the abscesses rupture, expelling a thick yellowish pus either to the outside (Fig. 9–9) or occasionally into the body; rupture into the body may result in death. Other signs include depression, anorexia, and difficulty swallowing. Recovery generally occurs 1 to 2 weeks after abscess rupture or 3 to 6 weeks after the onset of clinical signs. However, in severe cases recovery is prolonged due to chronic anemia and weight loss. Conversely, a milder form of the disease, resulting in a transient fever, moderate nasal discharge, and lymph node enlargement without abscessation, may occur in unstressed horses with some immunity. The disease most commonly occurs in horses 1 to 5 years old; it occasionally occurs in foals, weanlings, and older horses. In compro-

mised foals it can result in "bastard strangles" in which there is widespread lymph node abscessation, pneumonia, septicemia, heart damage, and brain abscesses. Occasionally, particularly in older horses, an allergic reaction may cause the condition referred to as purpura hemorrhagica. This results in widespread spots of hemorrhage on body membranes and subcutaneous edema of varying degrees of severity.

The disease is spread by inhalation or ingestion of infected droplets. This occurs rapidly to a high percentage of susceptible horses. Prevention, therefore, involves isolating both clinical cases and exposed horses from unexposed horses. Nasal shedding of the organism and thus spread to other horses can occur for up to 6 weeks after onset of clinical signs. Strict sanitation measures must be followed to minimize its spread. Stalls and equipment used for infected horses should be disinfected, preferably with a phenolic disinfectant, and not used for at least 4 weeks.

All affected horses should receive good nursing care. Horses suspected of being affected should be isolated, kept warm and dry, and offered palatable, good-quality feed. Antibiotics, fluid therapy, surgical drainage of abscesses, or tracheotomy may become necessary. Once the center of the abscess is sufficiently soft, most will rupture spontaneously, but it may be lanced if necessary. After rupture, the cavity should be flushed regularly with a providone-

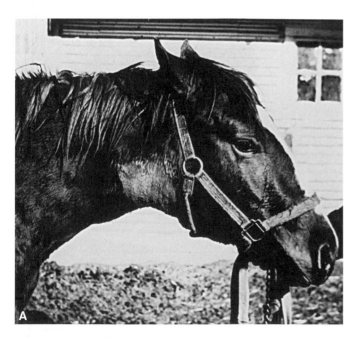

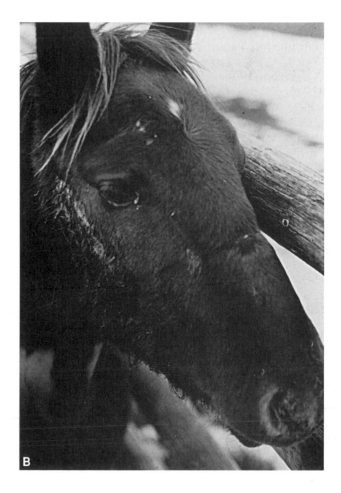

Fig. 9–9. Strangles (equine distemper, or shipping fever). Abscesses and swelling of lymph nodes and throatlatch (A) which may cause respiratory obstruction and thus the disease's name—strangles. Affected horses often stand with their head outstretched (A). In 10 to 14 days abscesses, such as the one to the left of this horse's eye (B), rupture, exuding a thick yellowish pus.

iodine solution until the wound heals. It is essential that affected horses be allowed 4 to 6 weeks to recover before they are put back with others or are gradually returned to work. Complications, such as pleuritis, may be precipitated by too early a return to work. Protective immunity following recovery is short, so an individual can suffer repeated attacks at approximately 6-month intervals.

During an outbreak, there should be strict hygiene to minimize transmission of the disease between horses. In addition, the rectal temperature of all susceptible horses that have been in contact with affected cases should be monitored daily, and isolation and treatment begun at once if it increases.

High doses of antibiotics for prolonged periods (4 to 6 weeks) are recommended for horses with complication sequelae including purpura hemorrhagica, guttural pouch infection, pleuritis, pneumonia, infectious arthritis, encephalitis, and bastard strangles. Antibiotic administration is also indicated in all affected foals. Corticosteroids should be administered to horses with purpura hemorrhagica; phenylbutazone or flunixin meglumine administration may also be helpful for these cases.

Vaccination of either affected or exposed but still clinically healthy horses during an outbreak is of questionable value. In addition, horses incubating the disease may have a severe reaction to the vaccine. Even when given to horses not incubating the disease the vaccine is of questionable value and reactions at the injection site are common. Outbreaks have occurred in herds where the vaccine has been administered repeatedly, but repeated vaccination does appear to decrease the severity and duration of the disease. A single vaccination is probably of no benefit.

Vaccination is indicated on farms that have recurrent outbreaks of the disease. On these farms mares should be vaccinated 3 to 8 weeks before foaling. Foals should be vaccinated beginning at 3 months of age with a second and third injection recommended at 3-week intervals. An additional dose at 6 months of age and thereafter annually for the first several years of life may be indicated. For horses traveling to areas where the disease is known to occur, it may be advisable to begin a 3-dose series at least 8 weeks before shipment. Soreness and, rarely, abscesses may occur at the vaccination site, particularly in older horses.

Potomac Horse Fever (Equine Monocytic Ehrlichiosis)

Equine monocytic ehrlichiosis (EME, equine ehrlichial colitis, or Potomac horse fever) is an acute diarrheal disease of horses caused by the rickettsia Ehrlichia risticii. It is characterized by an acute onset and 2 to 10 days of fever, anorexia, depression, and decreased intestinal sounds. Some horses develop anemia, a decrease in white blood cells, and ventral and leg edema. Most cases develop a severe diarrhea, resulting in dehydration, and in approximately 3% of cases, laminitis or founder. However, up to two thirds of horses with EME develop a subclinical or mild form of the disease. Fetal infection and abortion may also occur. Pregnant mares exposed to EME even

as early as 60 days of gestation, and even if it doesn't result in clinical illness may abort at 6 to 8 months of gestation.

Equine monocytic ehrlichiosis, first diagnosed near the Potomac River in Maryland in 1979, has now been reported in horses in most states as well as in Canada and France. In 1985 and 1986, prior to a vaccine being available, 76% of over 2500 nonclinically affected horses tested in New York state were positive for EME. The clinical disease occurs sporadically in random horses of all ages. It currently is thought to be transmitted by blood-sucking arthropods, although the vector and hosts aren't known. Although EME occurs most often in the summer, sporadic cases have been reported during the winter.

Diagnosis of EME can be confirmed by detecting an increasing serum titer in samples taken at the onset and one to several weeks later using serologic test kits.

Treatment of EME is the administration of antibiotics. If severe diarrhea occurs, fluid and electrolyte replacement may be necessary.

Two vaccinations, one in the spring and a second in mid-to-late summer during peak incidence of the disease, have been recommended for horses in endemic areas or in horses transported to these areas. Vaccination is reported to decrease the severity of, if not prevent, the disease and to be safe for pregnant mares, breeding stallions, and foals over 3 months old. Several vaccines are available commercially.

Rabies

Rabies is caused by a neurotropic rhabdovirus transmitted to horses, people, and other animals from infected secretions, most commonly the bite of a rabid animal. In horses, as in other animals, it produces a rapidly fatal disease, with death within as little as 12 hours or as long as 10 days, but more commonly 3 to 5 days after onset of clinical signs. Some affected horses may be found dead with no signs observed. It should be considered in any horse with a rapidly progressing neurologic disease. The presenting signs of rabies in horses are extremely variable and nonspecific. Initial signs include intermittent fever, a personality change followed by facial spasms or paralysis, lameness, hindleg incoordination or paralysis, teeth grinding, colic, urinary incontinence, and usually depression or stupor with sporadic hyperesthesia or occasionally viciousness toward people, animals, inanimate objects or themselves. Some rabid horses won't eat or drink, but hydrophobia or fear of water is uncommon, and some may continue to eat and drink until near death. When affected horses go down, paddling, convulsions, or coma occur.

Rabies antibody testing of sections of both the cervical spinal cord and brain may be necessary, because testing just the brain of rabid horses may yield negative or equivocal results. Rabies antibody testing is rapid and highly accurate. Confirmation by mouse inoculation may also be performed. Tissue examination for the presence of characteristic intracytoplasmic inclusion bodies (Negri bodies) is less accurate.

No treatment is indicated or of benefit as rabies is invariably fatal. All persons exposed to a confirmed case should promptly contact their physician.

Of the rabies cases confirmed in animals in the United States, 44 of 6975 cases in 1991, and 49 of 8645 cases in 1992 were in horses; 27 of these cases occurred in Oklahoma, Texas, Minnesota, Iowa, and New York. These are also the areas where the highest incidence occurred in other species, but cases occurred in all states except Hawaii. Over 90% of all cases occurred in wild animals (primarily racoons, skunks, bats, and foxes). There were 182, 184, and 290 cases in dogs, cattle, and cats, respectively, in the United States in 1992. In Canada 2377 cases were confirmed in 1992 with 50, 13, 5, 4, and 0% in foxes, cattle, dogs, cats, and horses, respectively. In Mexico 85% of 7111 cases in 1992 were in dogs. Six of 8 cases in people that occurred in the United States from 1981 through August 1993 were acquired from bats. All 8 people died.

Although the incidence of rabies in horses is low, annual vaccination, beginning in foals at 3 months of age, has been recommended in areas where the disease is common in any species of animal. Only vaccines recommended specifically for the horse should be given. Rabies vaccination is not generally recommended for pregnant mares. Vaccinated, but not unvaccinated, horses that are bitten by a rabid animal should be revaccinated at once and kept under observation for 90 days.

Anthrax

Anthrax is an uncommon, rapidly fatal septicemic disease caused by Bacillus anthracis and acquired through wound contamination, primarily from biting fleas, or by ingestion. The bacteria are more prevalent in warm moist climates and in the presence of alkaline soils. Infective spores can remain viable in the soil for many years. Clinical signs include fever, colic, and diarrhea, if the infective organism is ingested. Infected wounds are hot and painful, and edematous swelling of the throat, lower chest, and abdomen may occur. Death generally occurs within 2 to 3 days of the onset of symptoms. Treatment is rarely successful and mortality is high. Carcasses should be buried at least 6 ft (2 m) deep, as flesh eaters can spread the disease.

Vaccination for anthrax is indicated for horses in contact with exposed livestock or pastures. Vaccination is recommended 2 to 4 weeks before the season when anthrax outbreaks are anticipated and again 1 month later. Annual revaccination is appropriate in areas where the disease occurs. Pregnant mares should not be vaccinated because of possibly severe local tissue reaction to the vaccine. Vaccines, which are administered subcutaneously, are frequently associated with local and occasionally generalized systemic reactions.

Equine Infectious Anemia (Swamp Fever)

Equine infectious anemia (EIA) is a worldwide retroviral disease transmitted by blood-sucking and biting external parasites (primarily flies) and blood-contaminated needles or equipment; it can also be passed through the placenta by the mare to her fetus. Because of the prevalence of insect vectors, the incidence of EIA is highest in the southern and eastern United States. Over 80% of cases in the United States occur in the southeast, but there was a recent outbreak in Illinois. An EIA virus-carrier mare may abort or deliver an infected or uninfected foal. Only about 10% of foals delivered from carrier mares are infected at birth, and they remain lifelong carriers. However, foals will become EIA positive if they nurse colostrum from a carrier mare. These passive antibodies should be undetectable by 6 months of age. But if the foal is infected, it will produce EIA antibodies and remain EIA positive.

Clinical signs of EIA are recurrent and include fever, anemia, depression, anorexia, weakness, leg and ventral edema, icterus, and abnormal bleeding. Most recurrences are within 1 year of initial infection. The severity and frequency of the recurring clinical episodes usually decreases with time. Each bout of illness may last a few days to several months. Death of affected horses is uncommon.

Surviving horses become lifelong carriers and a source of infection for other horses. Because of this, horses entering another state and for many horse events must test negative for EIA by a USDA-certified laboratory, usually within the previous 6 to 12 months. The test used is the Coggins or, more recently, ELISA test. Of nearly 1 million blood samples tested in 1991, only 0.277% were positive for EIA antibody. Current regulations require that horses testing positive be reported by the testing laboratory and be freeze branded and kept in quarantine or euthanized. An EIA vaccine is not currently available in the United States but is under development; it will stimulate an immunity distinguishable from antibodies produced by the disease and present in the carrier horse.

DENTAL PROBLEMS AND CARE

Proper dental care is as necessary a part of health care for horses as it is for people. Bad teeth, dental problems, or a sore mouth as a result of dental problems cause numerous detrimental effects, including bit chewing, tongue lolling, abnormal head carriage, head tossing, refusal to accept bit pressure, and stiffness. Some horses may even wring their tails and buck or try to buck. There may be a change in temperament resulting in a sour or mean disposition: their mouth hurts and they are trying to tell you that. You have to pay attention and determine what's wrong, not just conclude that they're being bad and whack them—just as with children. These effects may occur with or without visible abnormal eating behavior, which includes slow eating, reluctance to drink cold water, a decrease in feed intake, tilting of the head when chewing, wallowing the feed around in the mouth before swallowing, and slobbering grain (quidding). Swallowed but improperly chewed feed may cause intestinal impactions and colic. A decrease in feed intake, if sufficient, will cause weight loss, poor physical condition, and impaired performance. There may be excessive slobbering, and the saliva may be blood tinged. If tooth decay, gum disease, or retained deciduous teeth are present, there is often a foul mouth odor, which may be particularly noticeable on the hand following a dental exam. Unlike many other species, horses do not

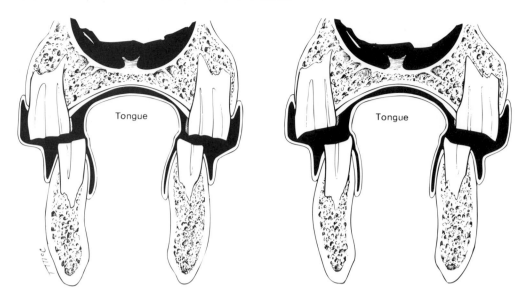

Fig. 9–10. The horse's upper cheek teeth, as shown here, extend as much as one-half a tooth width outside the lower cheek teeth. The teeth wear down where they come in contact with each other, progressing from the shape shown on the left to that shown on the right. The sharp point on the teeth shown on the right may lacerate the cheeks and tongue, making the horse's mouth sore. This should be prevented or corrected by floating the horse's teeth, or filing off these points, with a rasp or float.

shed infected teeth. The tooth remains in place, even when the infection has destroyed the peridental structure. If infection is limited to the tooth root, an abscess may develop causing a hard, bony, painful swelling of the bottom of the jaw bone or on the facial bone over the apex of the tooth. Occasionally, there is a draining tract. If this occurs with an upper cheek tooth, the tract may lead to a sinus, causing a chronic, fetid discharge from the nostril on the affected side.

The most common cause of a sore mouth is irritation or lacerations of the cheeks, tongue, or gums by sharp edges, hooks, or protuberances on permanent or retained deciduous (baby) cheek teeth. The horse's upper-cheek teeth extend as much as one-half the width of a tooth outside the lower-cheek teeth. Chewing wears the teeth where they contact each other, creating points or edges on the outside of the upper-cheek teeth and on the inside of the lower-cheek teeth (Fig. 9–10). These can become quite sharp and damaging, particularly in 2- to 5-year-old horses. Loss of a tooth may also cause problems because the tooth opposite the lost tooth is not worn off and may become too long, hindering chewing. Chewing is also hindered by uneven wear of the teeth. Aged horses often have profound dental abnormalities of wear and need to have large segments of tooth removed to return the dental arcade to a functional state. However, old horse's teeth have little crown remaining in the socket, and therefore, unfortunately, may come out easily during cutting or filing procedures.

The front of the first upper-cheek teeth and the back of the last lower-cheek teeth, particularly in horses with an overbite (parrot mouth or prognathism, in which the upper incisors extend out further than the lower incisors) should be checked carefully for hooks or protuberances. The front hook may interfere with the bit; the back hook may grind into the opposite gum, causing considerable pain. The opposite protuberances develop in the horse with an underbite (prognathia, monkey mouth, or sow

mouth, with the lower incisors extending out further than the upper incisors). The longer an abnormality is present, the worse it gets. Once a horse gets to be 3 to 4 years old, routine dentistry cannot correct most problems of malocclusion, whereas they can if done routinely prior to this age. An overbite, which is the most common malocclusion in horses, can be improved or corrected by initiating treatment with bite plates at an early age.

Dental care should begin by having the newborn foal examined, at which time malocclusions and congenital abnormalities of the lips, tongue, palate, facial bones, jaw bones, and gums can be detected and early treatment begun. The teeth should be rechecked every 6 months for the first several years of life and then annually to identify and correct things such as retained deciduous teeth; maleruption of permanent teeth; extra teeth; injuries and lesions caused by things such as foreign bodies, bits, and grass awns; points and hooks on teeth; malocclusion; abnormal wear; cracked or missing teeth; excessive tartar buildup; and periodontal disease. Many of the severe, often untreatable malocclusions and wear abnormalities seen in older horses can be prevented by regular dental care. Regular dental care also enhances feed utilization and maintenance of body condition and helps minimize gastrointestinal disorders.

A thorough oral exam requires patience. Be sure the halter allows the mouth to be fully open. Backing the horse diagonally into a corner often works well. Many times it is necessary to flush the mouth out with warm water so it can be visually examined. Externally palpate the jaws, mouth and sinus for abnormalities. Visually examine and where needed, palpate the oral cavity including the teeth and under the tongue. The outer edge of the upper cheek teeth can be palpated externally through the cheek, and internally by inserting the hand between the cheek and teeth. The inner surface of the cheek teeth can be palpated by pushing the horse's tongue with the back of the hand to in between the upper-and lower-cheek teeth on one side of the mouth and/or by pulling the tongue out one side of the horse's mouth. This discourages the horse from biting down. Keep the wrist in the interdental space, not between the incisors, and keep the thumb against the roof of the horse's mouth. Using the tips of the fingers, feel for points, sharp edges, hooks or protuberances, missing or damaged teeth, and uneven wear on the side opposite the side the tongue is being pushed to with the back of the hand.

Most sharp edges, points, and protuberances can be corrected by filing or "floating" the teeth or, if necessary, clipping or cutting a tooth (Fig. 9–10). Neither floating nor cutting teeth is painful. The sensitive part of the horse's tooth is deep within the embedded portion of the tooth.

Dental caries or cavities and periodontal disease, although not as common as in people, may occur and are relatively common in older horses. Cavities occur particularly in the second and third cheek teeth. They are often noticed only when there is facial or jaw swelling due to infection. Periodontal disease may result from abnormal occlusion, allowing feed to accumulate in the gums, leading to erosion of the tissue, and finally, tooth loss. The cavity, broken teeth, or periodontal disease may be seen on oral examination. Generally, affected teeth must be removed, the mouth flushed, and antibiotics administered. Occlusal leveling to reduce the overgrowth and malalignment of remaining teeth may be necessary at least every 6 months following extraction of a tooth.

Wolf teeth (first premolars) if not lost on their own are generally removed. Wolf teeth are tight against the first major cheek teeth (second premolars) and are only $\frac{1}{2}$ to $\frac{3}{4}$ inch (1 to 2 cm) long. They are usually present only on the top, but may occasionally also be in the lower arcade. They erupt during the first 6 months of life and are often shed about the same time as the first major cheek teeth behind them (at $2\frac{1}{2}$ years of age), but may remain. Unlike other teeth, the roots of the wolf teeth are short and not anchored deep in the bone; they are therefore much easier to remove. Removal is best done before the horse is 2 years old and preferably between 12 and 18 months of age since the periodontal membrane is more easily broken at this time. Retained wolf teeth can cause dental problems and may be painful when hit by a bit. If broken off, a chronic sore may develop so that a bit can't be used until the sore has healed. Horses with sore wolf teeth may carry their heads to one side or sling their heads to try to escape the pressure from the bit.

The canine teeth (tusks, tushes, bit teeth, male teeth, or fang teeth) are located between the front and middle one-third of the space between the incisors and cheek teeth of mature horses. They may grow too long and strike the opposite gum, making it sore. They should be clipped shorter and smoothed off with a float. Only 20 to 30% of mares, but over 70% of males, have all four canine teeth. A few (20 to 30%) males have only lower canine teeth, and even fewer (6 to 7%) have only upper canine teeth. They erupt when horses are 4 to 5 years old.

Temporary teeth, as they are pushed out by permanent teeth, may stay attached to the gum. These dental caps should be removed, as they interfere with chewing and may lacerate the tongue or cheek. Split or partially detached caps may rotate laterally and become trapped between the cheek and gums leading to ulceration and swelling. Bacteria may accumulate under caps leading to periodontitis. Caps for the 2nd and 3rd cheek teeth (3rd and 4th premolars) are the most commonly retained. Retained caps may also interfere with eruption of the permanent teeth, resulting in maleruption or delayed or arrested eruption and, in the case of lower premolars, deformation and infection in the mandible. Nonpainful bony lumps or protrusions (eruption bumps) may occur on the bottom of the jaw and, less commonly, on the facial bone at the base of the permanent premolars as they push out the temporary premolars. These generally disappear within months after the temporary tooth is lost. If these bumps don't regress within 3 months after the permanent cheek tooth's expected eruption time, as given in Table 9–6, a cap has probably been retained and should be extracted. This is suggested by two large bumps together in the 2- to 4-year-old horse. However, some horses retain these bony lumps for several years even when a cap isn't retained. Horses with retained or loose caps may get feed impacted under the caps, causing excessive salivation and the general symptoms described previously for dental problems in horses. Before a retained cap is removed, it may be best to have any necessary teeth-floating done first.

Age Estimation by Horse's Teeth

An estimation of a horse's age by its teeth is just that—an estimation. Teeth eruption dates are more reliable indicators of age than is teeth wear. In contrast to people and many other animals, the horse's teeth continue to erupt and grow out throughout the horse's life. As each tooth emerges, it is ground down and shaped by the opposing tooth. After teeth eruption is complete, the effects of the amount of wear are the major criteria used in estimating the horse's age from its teeth. As a result, age estimating becomes more speculative with increasing age because of differences in the feed that the horse has eaten and its environment during its lifetime, both of which have an effect on the rate that teeth wear down. A guide to age estimation from teeth is given in Table 9–6 and depicted in Fig. 9–11. Three additional criteria that can be used to estimate a horse's age from its teeth are:

1. As viewed from the side, the angle formed where the upper and lower incisors meet becomes sharper with increasing age.
2. As viewed from the front, the teeth diverge from the mid-line or center of the young horse; they converge in toward the middle or center of the old horse.
3. The six incisors form a semicircle in the young full-mouthed horse and a straighter line in the old horse.

There are many exceptions to all indicators of a horse's age from its teeth. No single criterion should be used.

TABLE 9–6
Age Estimation by Horses' Teeth[a]

Dental Criterion	Center Incisors	Intermediate Incisors	Corner Incisors
Eruption of:[b]			
Deciduous[c]	7 d[d]	7 wk[d]	7 mo[d]
Permanent	2½	3½	4½
In wear	3	4	5[e]
Cups[f] gone on:			
Lower	6	7	8
Upper	9	10	11[g]
Grinding surface shape:[f]			
Round	9	10	11
Triangle	14–16	15–17	16–18
Biangle	17–19	18–20	20–22
Less reliable criteria:			
Dental star[f] appears	8	9	10
Enamel spot[f] gone	12	13	14
Galvayne's groove[h]			10–30[h]
7-year hook[i]			7 & 11–17[i]

[a] All numbers not indicated otherwise are horse's age in years.
[b] All deciduous cheek teeth (premolars) erupt by 2 weeks of age. Canine teeth erupt at 4 to 5 years of age, and permanent premolars (P) and molars (M): P1 (wolf teeth) at 0.5, P2 at 2.5, P3 at 3, P4 at 4, M1 at 1, M2 at 2, and M3 at 3.5 to 4 years of age. The erupted permanent cheek tooth has a rounded double-dome shape on its occlusal surface that is distinctly different from the flat occlusal surface of a deciduous tooth that is in wear. Permanent premolars come into wear about 6 months, and molars 1 year, after they erupt.
[c] Deciduous (baby, milk, or temporary) teeth are smaller and whiter than permanent teeth, have a constricted neck at the gum line, and may have many fine grooves on their lip surface.
[d] Ranges from 1 to 8 days; 4 to 8 weeks and 6 to 9 months for eruption of deciduous incisors 1, 2, and 3 (center, intermediate and corner), respectively.
[e] Age at which horse is first said to be "full-mouthed."
[f] See Figure 9–11 for depiction of cups, grinding surface shapes, dental stars, and enamel spots, which are slightly elevated.
[g] Age at **and above** which a horse is said to be "smooth-mouthed."
[h] A shallow darkened groove on the outside surface running up and down the center of the third or corner incisor. The groove appears from under the gum at 10, is one-half way down at 15, is full length at 20, is one-half way gone at 25, and is gone at 30 years of age.
[i] An overhang at the back of the upper corner incisor that appears at 7, disappears at 8, reappears at 11, and disappears again by 18 years of age.

Using several criteria minimizes major errors from abnormalities or even fraud, in which incisors of an aged horse are drilled and the cavity stained to make artificial cups, referred to as "bishoping."

FOOT CARE

Care of the feet is one of the most important aspects in the care of the horse. Good stall and paddock sanitation is essential to good foot care. Standing in urine and wet manure breaks down the periople, a waxy-like waterproof covering of the hoof wall that minimizes moisture evaporation from the hoof. Moisture loss from the hoof may make it soft or, upon drying, hard, brittle, and subject to cracking and splitting. Standing in urine and feces is also the major cause of thrush and grease heel, or scratches (Fig. 9–12).

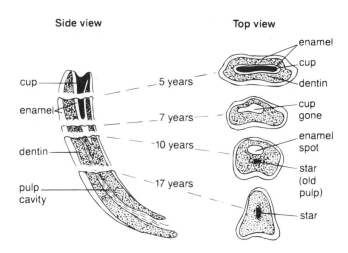

Fig. 9–11. Horse's incisors wear with age. Note the change in tooth shape with age, becoming round at about 10 years and triangular at 17 years of age.

Thrush, a bacterial infection of the sulci of the frog, is characterized by the presence of a black necrotic material with a very offensive odor. The infection may penetrate the horny tissue and involve the sensitive structures, resulting in lameness. Prevention is clean stalls, exercise, and frequent cleaning of the feet. For horses confined to stalls or small paddocks, ideally their feet should be cleaned and inspected daily. Thrush is treated by: (1) ensuring a clean environment and thus eliminating the cause, (2) removing degenerated frog tissue, and (3) cleaning and packing the sulci of the frog with cotton soaked in 10 to 15% sodium sulfapyridine solution daily until the infection is eliminated.

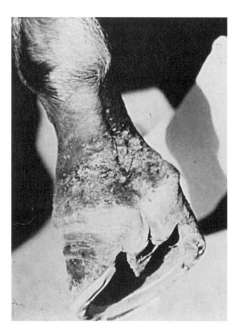

Fig. 9–12. Grease heel, scratches, or mud fever: a bacterial or fungal skin infection that may occur as a result of standing in moist dirty bedding.

Factors that interfere with hoof moisture content besides standing in urine and feces include stabling in dry sand, excessive rasping of the sides of the hoof wall, turpentine, and most commercial hoof dressings. These, like urine and wet manure, may remove periople, allowing loss of hoof moisture content. Factors that enhance proper hoof moisture content include exercise, massaging the coronary band, and in dry climates allowing water troughs to overflow. Exercise and coronary band massage increase blood flow to the foot, which may increase hoof moisture content. The sole may also be packed with mud or wet clay and wrapped with wet burlap if necessary to increase hoof moisture content. To retain hoof moisture, an oil-base hoof dressing can be applied to the wall, heels, frog, and sole. Maintaining proper hoof moisture not only enhances hoof elasticity and minimizes hoof cracking and splitting, but may increase the rate of hoof growth.

Under optimum conditions, the hoof growth rate of nursing foals is approximately 0.6 inches (1.5 cm)/month; of yearlings, 0.5 inches (1.2 cm)/month; and of mature horses, 0.25 to 0.35 inches (0.6 to 0.9 cm)/month. Hoof growth is most rapid during the spring and during recovery from injury (e.g., founder); it is slowest during hot and cold weather. A hoof bearing the most weight grows more slowly, which can cause hoof distortion and shearing-produced cracks. Rapid hoof growth is beneficial in recovery from hoof damage and in maintenance of good hoof structure. Hoof growth can be increased by applying a counterirritant to the coronary band.

Several nutritional factors are claimed to influence hoof growth, most commonly by those selling these nutrients. These include gelatin, various vitamin, mineral, and amino acid supplements (particularly the sulfur-containing amino acids methionine and cystine) and dietary additives. However, none have been shown, in controlled studies, to have an effect on hoof growth if the horse is receiving a diet that meets that class of horse's nutritional requirements. But an inadequate diet will slow hoof growth, and correcting nutrient deficiencies may increase the rate of hoof growth and improve hoof quality. For example, in one study, the rate of hoof growth was one-third slower (0.76 versus 1.15 (cm/mo), and growth rate 80% slower, in weanling ponies receiving about one-third as much feed as those allowed all they would eat of the same diet. However, this severe diet restriction had no effect on hoof strength or elasticity, and little effect on hoof content. Giving 30 g, and then 90 g, of gelatin/100 kg body weight had no effect on hoof growth rate, elasticity, strength, or content.

In contrast, feeding additional biotin or calcium may be beneficial for horses with thin, brittle hoof walls, or hoofs with crumbling of the lower edges of the walls and thin, tender soles, as described in Chapter 17.

The horse should be shod if necessary, but only if necessary. Shoeing, although at times a necessary evil, is often unnecessary. Shoeing interferes with the normal functioning of the foot. Concussion is dispersed by expansion of the hoof at impact, as well as by the digital and coronary cushions. The ability of the hoof to expand and contract aids in pumping blood through the foot. These functions are performed most effectively when the foot is level, balanced, properly aligned with a concave sole, and unshod. However, shoeing may be necessary for the following reasons: (1) to prevent discomfort and/or excessive hoof wear when the horse is used on hard or rocky surfaces; (2) to correct faulty hoof structure or growth, or uneven wear; (3) to complement or assist in correcting the gait; and (4) to aid in gripping hard slick ground or grassy surfaces. It's doubtful that shoes help grip soft ground or hard artificial surfaces. Horses that wear the hoof wall unevenly usually have crooked legs or feet. Keeping the hoof wall level by trimming and shoeing won't correct the fault but may prevent foot interference. If these factors are not present, the horse does not need to be shod. Many cared-for horses are shod that don't need to be, and when shod are not reshod often enough.

The hoofs should be trimmed every 6 to 8 weeks if the horse is shod; if not, the frequency of trimming depends on hoof wear. If shod horses aren't trimmed and reshod often enough, their toes become too long because they grow faster than the heel. After 7 to 9 weeks this is sufficient to alter the horse's gait, which may result in injury and impaired performance. Failure to trim the long toe also leads to contracted heals and corns, or sole bruises, from the heels of the shoe pressing on the sole. Trimming the hoof so that there is a long toe-low heel also causes these problems. The dorsal surface of the hoof-pastern axis should be a straight line (Fig. 6–5). As little as $3°$ off a straight line may cause serious lameness in very upright horses. Intentional lowering of the hoof angle has been used to increase stride length, but studies have shown that it does not do so and that it increases the risk of breakdown in race-horses. Doing the opposite, i.e., raising the heel, is also detrimental, and in contrast to what some have believed, does not reduce the force on that region of the hoof wall. In addition to trimming to maintain a straight hoof-pastern axis, the hoof should land flat or with the heel landing slightly before the rest of the foot. Lameness, stiffness and poor performance are more likely to occur if it does not.

SKIN AND HAIR-COAT CARE

Skin oils, or sebum produced by the skin, normally coat each hair, causing them to lie flat and giving them a shine. Sufficient sebum is necessary to help the hair repel water and to lubricate the skin by forming an oily protective barrier, which also inhibits the growth of harmful microorganisms. But skin oils also increase the adherence of dirt and dust to the hair, dulling its appearance. However, even this dirt and dust is at times of benefit to the horse in absorbing sweat and helping repel insects. These may be the reasons for the horse's desire and tendency to roll in the dirt, particularly following sweating and when insects are bothersome.

Dirt and debris can be removed by brushing, which also stimulates increased sebum production and its distribution over the hair shaft, restoring the coat's natural sheen. Shampooing also removes dirt, but in addition it removes the skin and hair oil, or sebum. The harsher the shampoo, the more sebum it removes and, therefore, the benefit the sebum provides, thus decreasing hair shine and creating a dry skin that is more susceptible to microbial and parasitic invasion. The best shampoos for horses are those sufficiently strong to remove dirt, but sufficiently mild to retain as much of the skin and hair's natural oils as possible. However, even the mildest shampoo, if used too frequently, will remove skin oils and, if the shampoo is not rinsed out well, or is one that does not rinse out of the hair completely, it may leave the hair dry and dull. These effects can be prevented by shampooing only occasionally with a mild shampoo, thoroughly rinsing, and frequently grooming in between. Shampooing could be done, for example, only when a thorough grooming and/or vacuuming isn't sufficient to restore the hair's natural shine. Using a cream rinse or hair conditioner after shampooing, or a shampoo that contains these, may also be helpful.

Hair conditioners are designed to coat the hair shaft in the same manner as sebum. Oils or waxes which tend to leave a greasy residue that contributes to a reaccumulation of dirt are rarely used anymore. Most currently used conditioners are protein-based natural moisturizers such as extracts of aloe vera, coconut oil, and lanolin; some contain optical and fluorescent brighteners. Brighteners, such as silicone, in hair polishing or finishing products may also be applied following shampooing, or a thorough grooming, to give the hair an even brighter shine.

No amount of grooming or grooming product will, however, compensate for hair that isn't healthy to begin with. Chronic illness of any type may decrease production of skin oils, decreasing hair shine. This may occur as a result of any prolonged illness due to an imbalance of any nutrient. In addition, a vitamin A deficiency or excess, or a protein deficiency, will cause a dry lusterless hair coat (Fig. 1-4). This also occurs as a result of a deficiency in the essential fatty acid linoleic acid, which is needed for production of skin oils or sebum. However, in contrast to many other animals, a fatty-acid deficiency doesn't appear to occur in horses.

It is believed by many, but without well-controlled confirmation, that feeding high amounts of fat, particularly those high in unsaturated fatty acids such as linoleic acid, will increase the amount of skin oil or sebum and thus give the hair coat a glossier, shinier appearance. Adding plant oils high in linoleic acid to the horse's diet has been commonly recommended, and many commercially available coat conditioners and supplements contain oils for this purpose. Adding 1 to 2 oz (30 to 60 ml) daily of commonly used cooking oils, such as corn, safflower, or soy oil, to the horse's grain for several weeks has been recommended. However, adding oil to even extremely low-fat experimental diets consumed for a prolonged period has been shown to have no effect on the horse's skin or hair coat. For example, in one study, hair-coat condition improved 1.16 and 1.34 points (on a 5-point scale) in horses receiving and not receiving, respectively; a popular commercial coat conditioner containing oils, vitamins and minerals. What does help improve hair-coat appearance most is frequent and thorough grooming.

RECORD KEEPING

A complete set of records should be kept on every horse from the time it is born until it dies. The records should stay with the horse regardless of the owner or the horse's use. These records should include the following information. Additional information may be needed or desired for different horses in different circumstances.

1. Horse's name, and dam and sire names, breeds, and registration numbers.
2. Identification—sex, color, markings, tattoos, brands, scars, size (height and weight), etc.
3. Breed registry information and papers.
4. Foaling—date, birth rate and problems or lack therefore, everything given to the foal, and procedures used on the foal and by whom.
5. Health Records—when and what's been given and/or procedures performed by whom and with what method of application and specific product name. This should include the following:
   a. Vaccinations.
   b. Dewormings.
   c. Illness and injuries and their treatment.
   d. Dental exam results and care.
   e. Foot care.
   f. Castration.
   g. Diagnostic tests—e.g., Coggins, physical exams, etc.
   h. Allergies.
6. Feeding—date, all feeds and supplements amounts and kind, nutrient content of diet, and weaning.
7. Training—date, by whom, purpose, and performance parameters.
8. Performance Activities—date, event, ridden or shown by whom, results, cost, and winnings.
9. Breeding and reproduction—date, procedure performed, by whom, results, and cost including:
   a. Rectal palpation—ovaries, ovulation, uterus, pregnancy, etc.
   b. vaginal exam.
   c. Caslick's—inserted or opened.
   d. Artificial lighting.
   e. Uterine culture and/or biopsy.
   f. Estrus behavior.
   g. Hormones administered.
   h. Teasing.
   i. Breeding, method, to whom, by whom, date, and weight and body condition score (Table 1-4) at breeding.
   j. Foaling details, including any problems, date, lactation, mare's weight and body condition score (Table 1-4).
   k. Stallion fertility exam, e.g., testicular palpation, semen analysis, libido, etc.
10. Growth rate—weight, height, and body condition score (Table 1-4) at numerous ages.
11. Boarding—date, location, costs.
12. Owner(s)—name, address, when, where, and from whom the horse was obtained.

HOUSING FOR HORSES
Open-Front Sheds

Most horses seem to like being outside, but like shelter from hot weather, cold rains, sleet, and strong cold winds.

Having free access to an open-front or three-sided shelter allows horses to satisfy these preferences. Most horses go in the sheds only for food, for shade, or to get out of cold rain or sleet. Most horses, when they can obtain warmth during cold, and particularly wet, weather, do so. However, they don't seem to be bothered by ordinary snow, rain, or wind, unless the weather is really severe.

The shed should be facing away from prevailing winds and toward the low winter sun. The opening should be at least 10 ft (3 m) high with no barriers. It should be a minimum of 20 ft (6.1 m) deep to provide sufficient shelter from weather extremes. Minimum size recommendations are 100 sq ft (11 sq m) per yearling or younger horse and 120 sq ft (13 sq m) per mature horse. The roof should slope away from the opening. The shed should be located so that water drains away from it. If the roof is metal, which makes them noisy in rain or sleet, they should be insulated so that the noise doesn't drive the horses out. Salt and grain feeders can be built into the back wall of the shed. These sheds are inexpensive to build and maintain, easy to clean, and well ventilated. Their disadvantage is that horses in open sheds tend to fight if fed in the shed. Feeding at the front of a 3 ft wide × 9 ft long × 6 ft high (0.9 × 2.7 × 1.8 m) free stall with solid sides is reported to eliminate this problem. However, most prefer to feed hay outside. Waterers should be away from the shed.

Stalls

Individual stalls are one of the most common housing for horses. Horses kept in stalls can receive more individual attention and be kept cleaner and more presentable, and their feed and exercise program can be better controlled. Horses accustomed to stalls spend more time lying down than when outside. However, horses unaccustomed to stalls may not lie down and, therefore, do not get deep sleep (REM sleep), which may result in a tired horse with an altered personality, behavior, and performance. Although slow-wave sleep occurs in horses both standing and lying down, REM sleep occurs only when horses lie down on their side or sternum with their muzzle touching the ground so that their head is supported.

Stall barns are expensive to build and to maintain. The labor and time involved in cleaning the stalls and caring for the horses are greatly increased. Horses kept in stalls should be exercised at least once daily. This can be accomplished by turning them out in an exercise lot of at least 500 sq ft (46 sq m) per horse for several hours, or a minimum of 30 minutes riding, lounging, or on a mechanical walker. Exercise is important for both the psychological and the physical well-being of the horse. Exercise is important for the maintenance of muscle tone and appetite, and to prevent digestive disturbances.

Individual stalls should be large enough to allow the horse room to move around and lie down. A minimum stall size of 12 ft by 12 ft (3.6 m) is preferred for most horses, although 10 ft by 10 ft (3 m) is adequate for ponies and small horses, whereas 14 ft by 14 ft (4.3 m) is preferred for draft horses, stallions, and mares with a foal. Foaling stalls should be a minimum of 12 ft by 16 ft (3.6 by 4.9 m) and designed so the mare can be observed without disturbing her. Tie stalls should be a minimum of 5½ ft by 11 ft (1.7 by 3.3 m), with a minimum 6½ ft (2.0 m) rear passageway.

The stall interior should be smooth and free of projections. Walls and doors should be high enough to discourage horses from trying to jump or fight over them. A total height of at least 7 ft (2.3 m) is recommended for most horses. Chain link, wire mesh, or bars above 4 to 5 ft (1.2 to 1.5 m) solid walls are preferred to totally solid walls so horses can see each other, be seen more readily, and have more light and ventilation. Studies have shown that horses prefer a light over a dark environment and to know that other horses are nearby. When other horses are not nearby, there are signs of increased stress and restlessness, including 3 times more activity and 10% less time spent eating. Social facilitation appears to be important in maintaining feeding behavior.

Not only do horses prefer a light environment, but increased duration of light is the primary factor that initiates shedding of the winter hair coat and stimulates the mare to begin cycling in the spring. In addition, ultraviolet rays from sunlight are a potent killer of bacteria, viruses, and other microbes, including intestinal parasite larvae. To obtain this benefit, ultraviolet translucent glass or plastic is preferable to normal glass, which blocks UV rays. Ultraviolet rays are also necessary for vitamin D production by the animal. Skylights should make up 10% of the roof area. An exterior stall door and at least one openable window a minimum of 4 ft sq (0.4 m sq) located at least 5 ft (1.5 m) above the floor is recommended. Windows should be free of drafts and either protected with iron bars or heavy wire mesh, or made of high-impact plastic instead of glass.

Two doors for each stall, one into the aisle and the other outside into a run or paddock, are preferred. Each door should have a minimum height of 8 ft (2.4 m) and a minimum width of 4 ft (1.2 m) without any projections. The outside door should be left open when possible to allow the horse free access between the stall and the outside (Fig. 9–13 A,B). Exterior doors on each stall are also an efficient means of improving ventilation, light, air quality, and they provide a fire exit. Sliding doors are safer and more convenient than hinged doors, particularly those inside that open into an aisle (Fig. 9–13 A). If doors are hinged, they should swing out from the stall. Dutch doors are popular (Fig. 9–13 B). A height of at least 4 ft (1.2 m) is preferred for the bottom portion of a dutch door. Open-top doors enhance stable ventilation and light and allow horses to put their heads out into fresh air. This decreases respiratory diseases and helps alleviate boredom and thus stable vices.

The most popular floors for stalls are packed clay. Packed clay provides a firm surface for bedding, is quiet and provides good resiliency and footing when dry. However, it is slippery when wet, laborious to clean, difficult to keep level and sanitary, and doesn't drain well. To maintain sanitary conditions, once yearly the top several inches of clay should be removed and replaced. Drainage frequently can be greatly improved by digging in the floor of the stall several holes a foot (0.3 m) or so in diameter and several feet (1 m) deep and filling them with rocks, gravel and a porous material like lime.

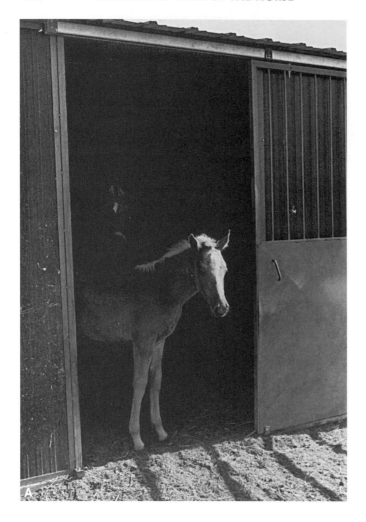

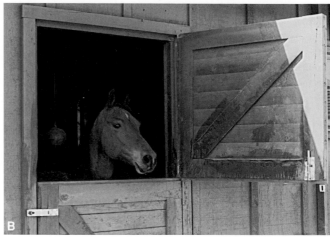

Fig. 9–13. If the horse must be stabled, it is best to have a run from each stall and to leave the box stall door always open to ensure fresh air, decrease dustiness in the stall, and let the horse go in or out of the stall at will. If the stall does not have a run, a double or dutch door to the outside is still preferred as it provides a fire exit, and leaving the top half open provides light and ventilation and allows the horse to put its head out into fresh air. This decreases respiratory disease and helps alleviate boredom and thus stable vices. Sliding doors (A) may be safer and more convenient than hinged doors (B) but don't allow the top half to be opened separately from the bottom.

Concrete floors are durable and easy to clean and maintain sanitary, but are generally the least desirable because they are slick, cold, and lack resiliency. Gravel, limestone, tartan, and asphalt provide a good floor, providing there is adequate drainage. When asphalt (blacktop or macadam) is used, a coarse mix 4 inches (10 cm) thick over a well-drained base allows good drainage and easy cleaning. It is not as slick, hard, or cold as concrete. Tartan is somewhat expensive and hard, but it cleans well and is nonskid, springy and durable.

Rubber flooring, which includes mats and interlocking rubber paving bricks, also provides a firm surface, has good resiliency, and is quiet. If sealed to prevent dirt, manure, and urine from getting under them, the mats or bricks do not have to be removed for cleaning. However, if not well sealed, they must be routinely removed and cleaned, and the stall dried out to prevent a build-up of disease-producing organisms and odors. Good drainage and sand under the flooring material will decrease the frequency that this time-consuming and labor-intensive job is necessary, but it should always be done prior to using the stall for foaling.

Tan bark and sand are soft, providing a good exercise surface, but are hard to clean. Sand must be cleaned regularly and changed occasionally; it is poor as a bedding. Sand is particularly good as an underlayer for the other flooring materials. In all cases it is best to place drainage tile under the floor.

Stable Ventilation

Adequate ventilation is extremely important for stabled horses. All stables contain varying amounts of airborne dust, bacteria, viruses, fungal spores, and ammonia produced from urinary and fecal excretions. These are major causes of respiratory diseases in horses. These airborne particles, and as a result respiratory diseases, increase with decreasing stable ventilation. Respiratory disease may permanently impair young horses' future performance ability and in mature horses is a major cause of impaired racing performance.

Excess ammonia in the air is thought to be a predisposing cause of foal pneumonia and to increase the incidence of eye and respiratory lesions and to decrease growth. What amount of ammonia is acceptable for horses isn't known. Levels as low as 50 ppm are known to have a negative effect on pigs, and 25 ppm on poultry, and it's recommended that levels not exceed 25 ppm for people in the same environment for 8 or more hours daily. A concentration of 50 ppm is the minimum concentration required by most people to detect ammonia, so if you can smell ammonia, its concentration is too high and may be harmful.

Since ammonia in stables originates from bacterial production from fecal and urinary urea, to prevent harmful aerial ammonia levels requires frequent stall cleaning and good ventilation. Sprinkling 1 to 2 lbs (0.5 to 1 kg) of hydrated lime on stall floors following cleaning also reduces ammonia levels. A markedly higher reduction may be obtained by using clinoptilolite instead of lime (Sweet PDZ/Stall Fresh, Tenneco Corp.).

Good ventilation is the major means of preventing recurrent airway obstruction or chronic obstructive pulmonary disease (COPD, which is also referred to as heaves or broken wind)—a disease similar to asthma in people. COPD is the most common cause of lower respiratory disease in young horses and occurs primarily in stabled horses. COPD and exercise-induced pulmonary hemorrhage are two of the major causes of poor performance ability in horses. In one study it was found that only 10% of horses that finished first or second in racing performance had signs of COPD, whereas 39% of those finishing last or next to last did. In the vast majority of cases, COPD is caused by a hypersensitivity or allergy to fungal spores, although grass pollen may be responsible for cases occurring in horses on summer pasture. Fungal spores may be present even in the finest-quality hay and straw. The hay or straw does not have to be visibly musty, although if it is it certainly contains large numbers of fungal spores. Thus, to minimize inhaled fungal spores and, therefore, respiratory diseases, only good-quality feed and bedding that aren't visibly dusty or musty should be used, and stable ventilation must be good. The amount of fungal spores and other contaminants in the air indicates ventilation adequacy. Management of horses with COPD is described in Chapter 17.

For good stable ventilation, there should be a continuous exchange of fresh air to dissipate odors, foul air, and airborne particles, but there should be no drafts. Drafts can be minimized by baffling vents or by covering vents with plastic mesh. This will also prevent the entry of rain or snow. In a stable, 8 air exchanges per hour is recommended and is adequate if clean bedding and hay are used, if not, 14 or more air exchanges/hour are necessary. There are many things that can be done to ensure good ventilation. They include the following recommendations. It is best if the stable is built with its longest side facing the prevailing wind and without major obstructions, particularly upwind in the predominant summer wind direction. Zones of poor natural ventilation are more likely with other orientations or when the wind is not free to hit the building from all directions. There should be no ceiling above the stalls; they are detrimental to natural ventilation. Interior walls also decrease natural ventilation and, therefore, should be minimized both in number and height. Natural ventilation for rooms not at the ends of the barn can be increased with 4 to 8 ft (1.2 to 2.5 m) long exterior wing walls perpendicular to the rooms exterior side wall. They turn the wind into that room, enhancing its natural ventilation.

Barn or stable roof slope should be at least 4:12 with 5:12 to 10:12 preferred. The inside of the roof should be insulated; otherwise, dripping moisture may be a problem in cold weather. Condensation is a tell-tale sign of poor ventilation. Although insulation provides little benefit for warmth within the stable, it does enhance air movement by maintaining a slightly greater temperature differences between inside and outside the stable. Vents that are well distributed throughout the stable are the most important factor in maintaining good ventilation. Under-eave and ridge vents are quite beneficial both in enhancing stable ventilation and in decreasing humidity and moisture that drips from the roof in cold weather. Eave vents located in the soffet should be the equivalent of a 4-inch (10 cm) continuous opening. There should be openings in both end walls of the barn. These may be closed during the winter but opened during the summer, particularly when the wind blows parallel to the barn length.

Ridge vents may be cupolas, dormers, and/or a continuous covered ridge equivalent to a 2-inch (5 cm) slot per 10 ft (3 m) of building width. Cupolas, dormers, or chimneys generally should be 2 ft (0.6 m) square every 16 to 24 ft (5 to 7 m) apart. For foals, a 2 inch by 7 ft (5 cm by 2 m) slot vent in an exterior wall, 20 inches (50 cm) above the floor is recommended except in cold climates. This may decrease respiratory problems in foals that are not at door height or window level during their first critical months of life. A respiratory disease at this age can greatly decrease later racing ability.

It's been recommended that heated barns have a ventilating fan with a capacity of 100 cubic feet per minute for each horse. During very cold weather, only one-fourth of the capacity of the fan is needed. Although a fan may be beneficial in very wide or long barns, or under conditions of climatic extremes, hot or cold, they are unnecessary for most stables. Adequate ventilation can be achieved in most stables by natural forces without mechanical intervention by using vents, windows, and doors as described, which increase interior brightness and decrease operating costs and noise. Although similar during the winter, during the summer, health and growth rate of pigs have been shown to be better in naturally ventilated barns than in those mechanically ventilated. Similar results would be expected in foals. Air filters, ionizers, and spray systems for disinfectants are of little benefit.

Hay and bedding should not be stored in lofts of barns where horses are kept. Doing so greatly increases dustiness and the risk of fire. Cleaning and bedding stalls also increases dustiness; it should be done only while all horses are out of the stable and before exercising the horse. This is important to allow time for dust particles to settle before the horse is reintroduced to the stall.

The temptation to shut all doors and windows during cold weather should be resisted. Cold won't harm the horse; poor ventilation will. It may be best to place a permanent vent above outside stall doors or high in the back wall of any stall that has no outside door to ensure proper air mixing and movement through each stall when doors and/or windows in the stall are closed. Horses tolerate well a wide range of environmental temperatures. When it is especially cold and for horses especially prone to cold, such as young foals and sick or malnourished horses, additional heat may be required. Quartz-halogen heaters work well. The horses may also be blanketed. Particularly helpful are blankets or rugs that inhibit radiant heat loss. Deep bedding also helps but should be quite clean to minimize particulate inhalation.

Bedding

Horses have a strong preference for bedding over no bedding but don't appear to prefer one common bedding over another. In one study, when given a choice, horses spent two thirds of their time on wood chips and one third on bare concrete; they would lie down only on the wood chips, never on the concrete. A similar preference for wood chips over a dirt surface was shown. However, no preference was shown between wood shavings and straw bedding.

Bedding should provide a good cushion for the horse and be absorbent but not dusty, palatable, or abrasive. It should absorb ammonia and odors, provide secure footing, and be easy to clean, readily available, and inexpensive. The many different substances used for bedding vary in these desired properties.

Straw is commonly used. It should be left long, as chopping increases its dustiness. Oat straw may be preferred, as it will absorb about one fourth more water than wheat, rye, or barely straws. Straw is the preferred bedding for foaling mares. **Wood shavings** or chips are more likely to be drawn into the vagina during foaling and are more abrasive; in one study, foal diarrhea was found to be higher when wood shavings, rather than straw, were used. However, wood shavings or chips are preferred over straw for horses with respiratory problems, as they are usually less dusty and may result in lower stable air ammonia levels (Table 9-7). The water-absorption capacity of soft woods is similar to straw and about 50% greater than hard woods. Wood shavings or chips should not contain sawdust, black walnut (Juglans nigra), or bitterwood (Quassia simarouba). Sawdust increases dustiness. Black walnut shavings cause acute founder and lameness, and bitterwood skin eruptions and inflammation around the nose, eyes, anus and the lips, the last causing excessive salivation. Both are described in Chapter 18.

Papers, shredded, chopped, or repulped to a cotton-like texture, are all excellent bedding. They decrease stable odors, are highly absorbent, and give stalls a brighter, cleaner appearance. Repulped paper dries quickly, and is fluffy and comfortable for the horse to lie on. However, if the paper has print on it, the ink can stain the horse. Also there is a noticeable increase in compaction and wetness in areas of fecal contamination and wetness of paper bedding, and they are more labor intensive. Loose paper bedding frequently dislodges from bales in transport and blows from the stables and compost areas. It does decompose in compost piles adequately to a suitable product for fertilizer and tree culture use. Heavy metal concentrations of paper bedding compost from print ink on the paper has been of concern but these concentrations have been found not to be different from straw or wood shavings bedding compost.

As shown in Table 9-7, paper, wood shavings, and a commercial synthetic bedding all result in a low amount of air contamination when used in well-ventilated stalls cleaned and bedded daily. However, air contamination greatly increases when the stall is poorly ventilated, hot, and humid, and even more so when deep-litter bedding is used in a stall of this type.

Peat moss also makes a good bedding. It will absorb 3 to 5 times more water than straw or wood shavings. Horses won't eat it. It's not flammable and is easy to clean. Peat moss, paper beddings, and wood shavings are usually practically free of fungi and actinomycetes when fresh. However, they may cause problems in deep-litter management systems or if they heat up in warm, poorly ventilated stables.

Nonbiological and tissue beddings are very clean and thermally efficient and do not provide a base for fungal growth. **Peanut hulls** are absorbent, but some horses will eat them, and they may attract rodents. **Rice hulls,** in contrast, don't absorb water well and are light and dusty. They have been found in the lungs of horses with respiratory problems and, therefore, are not recommended. **Hay** should not be used for bedding because many horses will eat it and because it is not very absorbent. **Corn stover** has an absorptive capacity in between that of oats and other straws, but it doesn't provide a good cushion and is abrasive. In addition, corn stover should be closely inspected for mold, which may produce mycotoxins that cause moldy corn disease s described in Chapter 19. **Sugar cane residue** is difficult to handle and may be eaten. **Sand** is a poor bedding; it is not absorbent, is abrasive, and is ingested when dropped feed is eaten off it. Over time, ingested sand accumulates in the intestinal tract and may cause sand impaction and colic as described in Chapter 17.

Regardless of the bedding material used, it is important to maintain a dry clean stall to assist in preventing thrush, grease heel, ringworm, respiratory disease, and poor skin and hair coat. Good drainage, clean dry bedding, and frequent cleaning of the stall are necessary. Although important for all horses, this is particularly critical for sick or recumbent horses, especially when due to a respiratory disease and following inhalation anesthesia. Used bedding should not be placed near stables, especially close to vents, as it is a potential source of disease-producing organisms and ammonia. Used bedding is best put in a trailer and removed from close proximity to stables at least every third day.

FENCING FOR HORSES

The many different types of fences vary in a number of criteria important for horses and those who keep them. Plank or rail fencing made of wood or PVC (polyvinyl chloride, or plastic), metal pipe or rod fencing, fencing made from 2 × 4 inch (5 × 10 cm) rectangular mesh woven wire, diamond or V-mesh woven wire, and chain link fencing with a board or metal pipe on top are the safest types of fences for horses. Stock or larger mesh woven wire is less desirable because its wire is smaller and its mesh openings are large enough to allow a horse's hoof to pass through. Wire in a horse fence should be at least 9 gauge. Barbed wire is the least desirable fence for horses. It causes thousands of injuries yearly and should never be used.

A board or a smooth electric wire at the top of the fence helps keep the horse from leaning over it. The electric wire

TABLE 9–7
Bedding Material: Characteristics, Amount Needed and Relative Costs

Bedding Material	Air Contamination Particles		Water Absorption vs Straw	Quantity Needed[c]- lb (kg)/d	Value vs Cost of Straw[d]	Comments
	Released /min	/cu cm of air[a]				
Straw	1490–28,100	167–724	1	14 (6.3)	1	Preferably: long to chopped, oat to others, & for foaling, but not if respiratory problems are present.
Pine sawdust	Probably equal to or greater than straw			100 (45)	0.14	Dusty. Chips & shavings preferred.
Pine shavings	148–873	6–104[b]	1	40 (18)	0.34	Soft wood's water absorption equals straw & is 50% over hard woods.
Oak shavings			0.7	95 (43)	0.15	Ensure no black walnut or bitterwood.
Paper shredded	78	25–100	Greater	44 (20)	0.31	Loose pieces clutter farm. Makes stalls cleaner, brighter, & less odor. Print on it can stain. Increased labor, & compaction & wetness in contaminated areas. Repulped paper is fluffy, comfortable & dries quickly.
Paper chopped			Greater	36 (16)	0.38	
Paper repulped			Greater			
Synthetics[e]	19	1.5	Greater			
Peat moss	Low when clean		3.5			Horses won't eat it, nonflammable, easy to clean.
Peanut hulls			Good			Not recommended.
Rice hulls	Dusty		Poor			Some horses eat them & may attract rodents.
Hay			Poor			Many horses eat it. Not recommended
Corn stover			1			Poor cushion, abrasive, & if moldy, may be toxic.
Sugar cane						
Sand			0			

[a] In well-ventilated stalls, cleaned and rebedded once daily.
[b] Increased to 603 in a poorly ventilated, hot, humid barn, and to 400 to 1223 when deep litter bedding is also used.
[c] Amount used to uniformly bed 12 × 12 ft (3.6 sq m) box stalls containing a pregnant mare, or a lactating mare with foal, with all manure and wet bedding replaced with fresh bedding twice daily.
[d] Considering only the cost of the bedding and the weight/day of the bedding used. For example, if straw costs $40/ton, pine sawdust would need to cost the value given for it times this cost, or 0.14 times $40/ton which equals $5.60/ton, for it to cost the same to use as straw. If pine sawdust costs more than this, it is more expensive to use than straw, whereas if pine sawdust costs less than this, it is less expensive to use than straw. To compare costs between other beddings, divide the value versus straw given for the bedding in question, by the value versus straw given for the bedding to which it is being compared. For example, the value given for shredded newspaper divided by the value given for pine sawdust, or 0.31 divided by 0.14 which equals 2.21. Thus, shredded newspaper's value for bedding as compared to pine sawdust is 2.21, i.e., you could afford to pay up to 2.21-times more for the same weight of shredded newspapers as for pine sawdust.
[e] An absorbent synthetic bedding (Equibed-Melcourt Ind, Tetbury, Gloucestershire, UK).

also helps prevent horses from fighting over the fence, and prevents wood chewing and cribbing. Planks and wire should be placed on the same side of the posts as the horses. This prevents horses from pushing the planks or nails out of the post, where they can injure the horse, and the posts don't stick out from the planks, where they can be bumped as a horse runs by.

Wood plank, rail, or pole fences require considerable maintenance both in replacing boards and in painting, although painting isn't necessary. If painted, be sure to use lead-free paint so as to prevent lead toxicosis (described in Chapter 19). Oak, other hardwoods, and less preferably cedar and southern yellow pine are the best woods for horse fences. Northern white pine, western pine, and Douglas fir are less desirable because horses chew on these woods more than on others. Planks should be at least a full 1 inch (2.5 cm) thick and 5 to 7 inches (13 to 18 cm) wide. A four-board fence minimum is preferred.

PVC or polymer plank or rail fences, although more expensive to install (generally about twice that of a board fence), are basically maintenance free, attractive, and long lasting. PVC fences have guarantees for up to 20 years and a life expectancy exceeding 50. The flexibility of the fence decreases injury, and the rails will not splinter or cut on impact.

Rubber nylon manufactured from belting material and cut into 2 to 4 inch (5 to 10 cm) strips also provides a flexible, safe, attractive, durable, minimal maintenance, relatively inexpensive horse fence. With severe freezing and thawing, however, a rubber-nylon fence has a tendency to loosen. Impactions have occurred in young horses from chewing on and ingesting material from the ragged edges of the belting material. As a result, manufacturers are now more careful of the edges on the material produced.

SUPPLEMENTAL READING RECOMMENDATIONS

1. For dental problems and care there is an excellent section of 9 articles in the Proceedings of the American Association of Equine Practitioners 1991 annual meeting on pages 83 to 150.
2. For all aspects of foot care, including trimming and shoeing, see *Adam's Lameness in Horses*, 4th ed. Edited by Dr. Ted S. Stashak. Philadelphia, Lea & Febiger, 1987.

Chapter 10

FEEDING IDLE AND WORKING HORSES

Feeding Horses for Maintenance or Work 186	Aged Horses 191
Cold Weather Care of Horses 187	Aging-Induced Changes in Horses 191
Hot Weather Care of Horses 189	Care of Aged Horses 192

FEEDING HORSES FOR MAINTENANCE OR WORK

In addition to having trace-mineralized salt and good-quality palatable water always available for all horses, the idle or minimally used horse requires 1.5 to 1.75 lbs of average- or better-quality forage per 100 lbs body weight (1.5 to 1.75 kg/100 kg) daily for maintenance of body weight. Most forages, pasture or hay, contain adequate quantities of all nutrients to meet the idle horse's requirements. No grain or supplements of any type are generally needed. However, some forages may be deficient in phosphorus and mature grass forage may lack protein (Table 10-1).

Many mature grass hay and pasture forages contains only 5 to 7% protein, and some as little as 3%, while 8% is needed for maintenance. In addition, in some areas mature forages contain less than the 0.2% phosphorus needed. Deficiencies of this degree over a few months' time do not cause any noticeable effect on the horse in good body condition. Body reserves are used and will be repleted the next spring when growing forages, which are higher in nutritional value, are consumed. However, in the thin horse whose body reserves are already low or depleted, or in situations where the deficiency is severe or prolonged, this lack of adequate nutrition may be quite detrimental, causing the effects described in Chapters 1 and 2. Both the protein and the phosphorus deficiency can be corrected or prevented by feeding daily 1.5 to 2 lbs (0.7 to 0.9 kg) of a 24 to 30% protein supplement, or by feeding 3 to 5 lbs (1.4 to 2.3 kg) of a 16% protein grain mix. Feeding 3 to 5 lbs (1.4 to 2.3 kg) of alfalfa (lucerne) hay or pellets daily would also correct or prevent the protein deficiency, but may not correct the phosphorus deficiency. The phosphorus deficiency may also be corrected or prevented by feeding a phosphorus-containing salt-mineral mix as the only available salt. A commercially available mix containing 8 to 16% calcium, 8 to 16% phosphorus, and salt, or a mix prepared from equal parts dicalcium phosphate (Appendix Table 7) and salt, may be used. This same mineral mix may be used whether the forage is a grass or a legume such as alfalfa or a clover. The calcium is not needed nutritionally when a legume forage is consumed, and isn't generally needed for maintenance even when a mature grass forage is consumed (Table 10-1). However, both calcium and salt increase the palatability of a phosphorus-containing mineral and help prevent the mineral mix from caking and becoming so hard that consumption is reduced. Because calcium is inexpensive, it adds little to the cost of the mineral mix, and the additional calcium is not harmful nutritionally. However, if a legume is being consumed, the mineral mix can be much lower in calcium than phosphorus, since legumes are high in calcium (Table 10-1). Palatability of the mineral mix and, therefore, its consumption can also be increased and caking prevented by adding 5 to 10% of an oilseed meal, such as soybean meal, or dry molasses to the salt-mineral mix. From 2 to 4 oz (60 to 120 g) daily of the salt-mineral mix may be needed.

For work or use, dietary energy needs are increased. The additional energy needed, up to a limit, can be provided by feeding more forage. If the physical activity is strenuous, prolonged, and frequent, so that energy needs are more than twice that needed when idle, the horse may not be able to consume enough forage to meet its needs. Grain, which is 50 to 100% higher in energy density than forage (Table 10-1) must be fed. However, even when physical activity is not so strenuous or prolonged that grain must be fed, most people like to feed grain when the horse is being used or in training. Feeding the hard-working horse grain is beneficial in meeting its nutritional needs without excessive feed consumption; as a result, excessive gastrointestinal fill is avoided. This is the reason a diet higher in energy density is recommended for the working horse (Table 10-1). Since increasing a diet's energy density decreases the amount of that diet consumed, it also decreases the amount of all nutrients consumed, unless their concentration in the diet is increased equivalent to the amount that the diet's energy density is increased. This is the reason a higher concentration of energy and other nutrients is needed in the higher-energy-dense diet recommended for the working horse (Table 10-1).

A good feeding program for physical activity is to continue feeding the amount of forage needed for maintenance, and to feed as much grain as needed for physical activity. Guidelines on the amount of grain needed for physical activity are given in Table 10-2. Like all amounts of feed recommended, these are only guidelines and will vary with numerous factors, as described in the section on "Energy Needs" in Chapter 1. The amount fed should be adjusted as necessary to maintain optimum body weight and condition. This is generally a moderate body condition as described in Table 1-4. If the horse is too thin, it may not have sufficient body fat as a reserve source of energy for prolonged or frequent physical activity, and will have a lower amount of muscle glycogen. These effects decrease physical performance ability. The time required to finish an endurance race has been found to increase the thinner the horse is below a moderate body condition. But horses

TABLE 10–1
Idle, Worked, and Aged Mature Horses' Major Nutrient Needs in Diet Dry Matter as Compared with That in Feeds[a]

	Digestible Energy Mcal/lb (kg)	Protein (%)	Calcium (%)	Phosphorus (%)
Needed for:				
Maintenance	0.9 (2.0)	8	0.25	0.20
Work & breeding stallion	1.15–1.3 (2.5–2.9)	10–11	0.3	0.25
Aged horse	1.0 (2.2)	10	0.25	0.25
Composition of:[a]				
Legumes (e.g., alfalfa)	1.0–1.1 (2.2–2.4)	15–20	0.8–2	0.15–0.3
Grasses, mature	0.7–1.0 (15–22)	6–10	0.3–0.5	0.15–0.3
Cereal grains	1.5–1.7 (3.3–3.7)	9–12	0.02–0.1	0.25–0.35

[a] For more exact values, see Appendix Table 6 for the specific type of grain or forage being fed; for the most accurate values, have the feed analyzed as described in Chapter 6.

that are too fleshy, with a body condition above moderate, require more feed, both at rest and work, and therefore produce more heat. In addition, excess fat under the skin decreases heat loss. Both factors contribute to heat stress and as a result impair physical performance. Fleshy horses have higher heart rates and respiratory rates, and recover from exercise more slowly than do horses with moderate body condition. Thus, for optimal performance, health, and enjoyment of life for the horse, it is important to feed the amount needed to maintain moderate body weight and condition as described in Table 1–4.

Not only must the proper amount be fed, the horse must also eat the proper amount. If the horse refuses a feed, both the feed and the horse should be closely examined. If no disease, injury, oral or dental problems, or cause of pain, discomfort, or distraction for the horse are found or suspected, the feed may be at fault, particularly if it is refused or eaten poorly by more than one horse and/or if there has been a recent feed change. The feed should be examined, smelled, and tasted. However, many feed-related poisonings and palatability problems require extensive laboratory and/or feeding tests to determine their cause, as described in Chapter 19. A different feed should

be tried. If that feed is eaten normally, this is a strong indication that there is a problem with the refused feed. If it isn't eaten normally, it suggests the problem is with the horse, particularly if it is the only horse affected.

If there has been extensive sweating, inappetence may be due to water and electrolyte deficits, particularly potassium, chloride, and sodium. If this could be the case, give the horse 3 oz (85 g) of a mixture of equal parts common salt (sodium chloride) and "lite" salt (a mixture of equal parts sodium chloride and potassium chloride, available at most grocery stores), 2 to 3 times daily for 2 to 3 days. The salt mixture should be added to a sweet feed or a dampened grain mix to prevent it from sifting out. The most common cause of a decrease in appetite in the hard-working horse, or the horse in training or use, however, is overwork. In this case, work must be decreased sufficiently until appetite returns.

Whether due to inappetence, disease, injury, or any other reason, as a general rule, if there is a break in work or training, the amount of grain fed should be reduced by one-half, beginning ideally with the evening feeding before the break. If the break is for more than 2 to 3 days, don't feed any, or only a minimal amount of, grain during the break. When the break is over, increase the amount of grain fed at a rate of not more than 0.5 lbs (0.2 to 0.3 kg) daily to a maximum of no more than 0.5 lb/100 lbs body wt (0.5 kg/100 kgs) per feeding and to not more than a total of an amount equal to one-half of the total weight of the diet.

More grain than necessary may be fed because it is easier or less expensive to feed grain than hay, or to decrease gastrointestinal fill and, therefore, the weight carried during physical activity. The horse's gastrointestinal tract can hold up to 25 to 30 lbs/100 lbs body weight (25 to 30 kgs/100 kgs) and it takes 50 hours for undigested fiber, which is highest in forages, to pass through the gastrointestinal tract and be excreted. Thus, decreasing gastrointestinal fill can substantially reduce the amount of weight the horse carries. This reduction may be beneficial for short-duration exertion, but appears to be detrimental for long-duration activity. Forage intake increases the amount of water, electrolytes, and energy-supplying nutrients in the gastrointestinal tract and thus their availability to replace those needed for physical activity and loss due to sweating.

The amount of forage consumed should never be less than 0.5 lb/100 lb body weight/day (0.5 kg/100 kgs), and it is safer if it constitutes at least one-half of the total weight of feed eaten. For the horse being used for prolonged physical activity, forage intake should be at least 1 to 1.5 lbs/100 lbs body weight/day (1 to 1.5 kgs/100 kgs) and grain fed as needed for weight maintenance.

COLD WEATHER CARE OF HORSES

Even in cold weather, horses frequently prefer and are better off outdoors. Closed and heated stables are often poorly ventilated. Respiratory diseases are higher in horses kept in poorly ventilated stables than in those kept outdoors, even during cold weather. Horses acclimate to cold temperatures without much difficulty if given the opportunity. The thermal neutral or comfort zone for the horse is

TABLE 10–2
Grain Needed for Physical Activity[a]

Physical Activity	Grain per Hour of Activity	
	lb	kg
Light; e.g., pleasure ride	0.5–1.5	0.2–0.7
Moderate; e.g., ranch work, roping, cutting, barrel racing & jumping	2–3	1–1.5
Strenuous; e.g., race training & polo	4 or more	2 or more
Draft horse field work	1.2–1.6	0.5–0.75

[a] In addition, the horse should consume 1.5 to 1.75 lbs/100 lbs body weight (1.5 to 1.75 kgs/100 kgs) daily of average- or better-quality forage. Adjust the amount fed as necessary to maintain moderate body condition as described in Table 1–4.

usually quite different from that for people. Don't evaluate the horse's environment based on your comfort. The horse, particularly when cold acclimated, is comfortable at temperatures quite chilling to you. However, during cold weather the horse should have access to shelter from wind, sleet, and storms, and during the summer it should have shade available from the hot sun. Trees, brush, or free access to a stable or open-sided shed work well for all seasons.

Horses in severe cold group closely together to provide mutual shelter and body heat. They may all take a run to increase body heat production, then come back together and stand in a close group to share the resulting increased warmth. In the absence of wind and moisture, horses tolerate temperatures down to near 0°F (−18°C) or, with shelter, to even −40°F (−40°C), but are more comfortable at temperatures above 18 to 59°F (−8 to 15°C), depending on their hair coat (Table 10–3). In severe, stormy weather horses stop grazing and will stand with their rear end to the wind. The tail is held close to the dock, allowing it to be blown between the legs and thus shield the hairless area of the perineum, the groin and the inner thighs. The density of the hair coat and the direction in which the hair lies, especially over the hindquarters and back, act as a weather shield so efficient that ice may form on the horse without chilling the skin.

A long, thick hair coat is an excellent insulator and provides the first line of defense against the cold. Its insulating value is lost, however, if it gets wet, which is why it is important to keep horses dry and sheltered from the wind in cold weather. A combination of cold and wind, especially in wet weather, is particularly stressful. Nothing is so chilling to the horse as wind with cold rain, sleet, or snow. The quantity and quality of hair in the mane and forelock are quite important in protecting the horse's ears and eyes from severe cold. A full mane, with natural length and density, can act as a waterproof screen for the head, throat, and neck.

As shown in Table 10–3, beef cattle, and therefore possibly horses, with a dry, heavy winter hair coat are comfortable at effective ambient temperatures down to 18°F (−8°C), and energy needs for maintenance increase only

0.7% for each degree Fahrenheit (0.4/°C) of cold below this temperature. In contrast, the animal with a wet, or a summer, hair coat is comfortable only down to a temperature of 59°F (15°C), and energy needs increase 2.0%/°F (1.1%/°C). Thus, for example, the 1000-lb (454-kg) horse with a dry, heavy winter coat would need only about 16.5 lbs of good-quality hay (allowing 10% for wastage or loss) at effective ambient, or wind chill, temperatures above 18°F (−8°C). But if the wind chill temperature was 0°F (−18°C), 18.6 lbs (8.4 kgs) (i.e., [16.5 lbs × (18°F × 0.007/°F)] + 16.5 lbs = 18.6 lbs) would be needed; 22.4 lbs (10.2 kg) (i.e., [16.5 lbs × (18°F × 0.020/°F)] + 16.5 lbs = 22.4 lbs) would be needed at this wind-chill temperature if the horse had a summer, or a wet, hair coat instead of a dry winter hair coat.

Blanketing the horse is beneficial when the effective, or wind-chill, temperature is less than comfortable (Table 10–3). Above this temperature, however, blanketing is not beneficial—it does not provide increased comfort for the horse. It decreases hair-coat adaptation to the cold and is uncomfortable for the horse during warm periods of the day, particularly sunny ones. Although blanketing the horse does induce shedding earlier in the spring, frequent grooming and an adequate diet may be preferable, as discussed in Chapter 9 (see section on "Skin and Hair-Coat Care").

After the hair coat, the next line of defense against cold is fat; a layer of fat under the skin provides additional insulation against cold. In cold climates, the horse ideally should be moderately fleshy to fleshy (Table 1–4) when cold weather begins. In cold weather, more dietary energy is needed for maintenance of thin than moderately fleshy animals.

Sufficient cold increases energy needs both to maintain body temperature and, at least in cattle, because feed digestibility decreases with decreasing environmental temperature below the comfort temperature. As shown in Table 10–4, energy needs for maintenance are 23 and 47% higher for beef cattle at 30 and at 10°F (−1 and −12°C), respectively, than at 68°F (20°C), and at 10°F (−12°C), these needs are increased an additional 19% by a wind of 10 mph (16 kph).

The more wind speed increases, the more it decreases the effective ambient, or wind-chill, temperature (Table

TABLE 10–3
Effect of Hair Coat on Comfort and Dietary Energy Needs in Cold Weather[a]

Hair Coat	Lowest Comfortable Effective or Wind Chill Temp [°F (°C)][b]	Increase in Energy Needed— %/°F (°C) Below Lowest Comfort Temperature
Dry winter coat	18 (−8)	0.7 (0.4)
Wet or summer coat	59 (15)	2.0 (1.1)

[a] For beef cattle and, therefore, probably similar for horses. However, growing horses' digestible energy intake has been found to increase by only about one-half this amount with decreasing temperature below freezing, i.e., by 0.36%/°F below 32°F (0.2%/°C below 0°C).
[b] Temperature minus the value given in Table 10–5 times wind speed; e.g., at 54°F and a wind speed of 24 mph, the wind chill temperature would be 54 − (1.5 × 24) = 54 − 36 = 18°F (Table 10–5).

TABLE 10–4
Cold Temperature Effect on Metabolizable Energy Needs[a]

Effective Ambient or Wind Chill Temperature °F (°C)	Wind Speed mph (kph)	Increase in Energy Needs (%)
68 (20)	0	0
30 (−1)	0	23
10 (−12)	0	47
10 (−12)	10 (16)	66

[a] For maintenance of beef cattle in moderate body condition with a dry winter hair coat; probably similar in horses.

TABLE 10–5
Wind Effect on Effective Ambient (Wind Chill) Temperature[a]

Wind Speed mph (kph)	Decrease in Effective Temperature	
	(°F/mph)	(°C/kph)
1 to 20 (1 to 32)	1	0.375
20 to 30 (32 to 48)	1.5	0.5
30 to 40 (48 to 64)	3	1

[a] For beef cattle in moderate condition with a dry winter hair coat; probably similar for horses.

10–5). For example, a wind speed of 15 mph would decrease the effective ambient temperature 15°F (1°F/mph of wind speed, as given in Table 10–5), but an additional 15 mph increase in wind speed would decrease the effective temperature twice as much, or an additional 30°F (1.5°F/mph, as given in Table 10–5, times 30 mph = 45°F decrease). These effects of cold on dietary energy needs and, as a result, feed intake during the winter were well demonstrated in the study shown in Table 10–6.

The major effect of cold on nutrient requirements is an increased need for energy. Most data suggest that needs for other nutrients do not change during cold weather. Therefore, the purpose of feeding during cold weather is simply to increase the amount of feed fed. If additional feed is not available to provide the increased energy needed, body weight and condition decrease. The additional feed needed during cold weather is best provided by giving the horse all the forage it can eat without wastage. Forage is preferable to grain, unless the horse is unable to maintain body weight and condition when consuming only forage.

Fiber, which is high in forages and low in cereal grains, is utilized by bacterial fermentation in the cecum and large intestine. Much more heat is produced in bacterial fiber fermentation than in the digestion and absorption of nutrients in the small intestine. Thus, a greater amount of heat is produced in the utilization of forages than in the utilization of grain. This helps keep the horse warm during cold weather.

During cold weather, if the horse is allowed to consume all of the average- or better-quality forage it wants, addi-

TABLE 10–6
Increase in Energy and Feed Needed During the Winter in Colorado[a]

Month	Increase in Energy Needs (%)	Increase in Feed Intake lb/d (kg/d)
Oct	17	3.3 (1.5)
Nov	26	4.5 (2.0)
Dec	31	5.4 (2.5)
Jan	33	5.9 (2.7)
Feb	29	5.1 (2.3)
Mar	26	4.8 (2.2)
Apr	20	3.6 (1.6)

[a] For beef cattle and, therefore, probably similar in horses.

tional dietary energy from cereal grains is not generally needed. However, if the horse is not able to maintain good body condition when eating only forage, grain should be fed. Any cereal grain may be chosen. If the forage consumed is mature grass pasture or hay, it may contain less than the 8% protein needed (Table 10–1), in which case a protein supplement should be fed. If the forage contains 6% crude protein, 0.15, 0.2, 0.3 or 0.4 lbs/100 lbs body weight/day (or kg/100 kg bw) of a protein supplement or grain mix containing 30%, 24%, 18%, or 14% protein, respectively, is needed. Whereas if the forage contains 4% protein, an additional 0.1 lbs/100 lbs body weight (or kg/100 kg) of these feeds would be needed.

Water, ideally at 45 to 65°F (7 to 18°C), should be always readily available. However, ambient-temperature-induced variations in water temperature may not greatly affect water intake unless the animal has bad teeth, resulting in pain when cold water is drunk. Although it is not verified for horses, cattle drink similar amounts of cold and warm water. Cattle and probably horses will consume sufficient snow or crushed ice to meet their needs if snow and ice are available but water isn't. However, in doing so they will reduce the amount of water and feed consumed: cattle will decrease the amount of water consumed from snow and crushed ice by about one-half, and feed consumed by 10 to 20%. The decreased feed intake may result in weight loss, and the decrease in water consumed increases the risk of impaction and colic.

Water consumption may be increased, and as a result the risk of impaction induced colic decreased, by (1) removing ice several times daily if necessary to keep water open, (2) adding a few percent of salt to the grain fed, (3) feeding hot bran mashes, or (4) using a water heater. If an electric water heater is used, the water should be touched daily to determine if the heater is making the water too warm or is shorting out. An electrical short generally will not create enough of an electrical shock to hurt the horse, but it will prevent water consumption. Hot bran mashes are fed by some during the winter; however, they are of little benefit to the horse. They do little to keep the horse warm, and the nutrients they provide can be more easily fed as hay or grain. They may increase water intake, particularly if a water heater is not used.

If the horse is not being used, if possible it should be left unshod during the winter. It may be necessary, however, to trim the unshod hoofs periodically to prevent pieces from chipping off.

HOT WEATHER CARE OF HORSES

Two common situations that often occur in horses during hot weather, particularly when accompanied by a high humidity, are: (1) excess body weight or, specifically, body fat, and (2) the opposite situation: difficulty maintaining adequate body weight. Both decrease the horse's performance ability (as discussed in Chapter 11) and comfort. Several things can be done to prevent or alleviate both and, as a result, their effects.

Although the insulation provided by fat under the skin is beneficial in cold weather, it's a detriment during hot weather. Not only does excess fat decrease the ability to cool the body, it also increases the total amount of dietary energy the animal needs and, as a result, increases feed intake and body-heat production. The overweight horse requires more feed for maintenance than does the moderately conditioned horse. The greater amount of feed consumed to meet this greater need increases body-heat production and in hot weather increases heat stress since the majority of energy provided by the feed eaten is given off as heat. Fleshy horses have higher heart rates, respiratory rates, and plasma lactate concentrations before, during, and after exercise during hot weather than during temperate weather, and higher than do moderately conditioned horses, indicating they have a greater heat load and more heat stress. The greater heat stress is not only quite uncomfortable, it decreases physical performance ability. Nothing is more miserable than an overweight animal without shade or air movement during hot weather, particularly if physical activity is required.

Dietary energy is required for maintaining normal body temperature in both cold and hot environments. The amount of additional energy needed depends on the amount that the effective temperature is above or below the thermoneutral or comfort zone, and varies between individuals and perhaps breeds, as it does in cattle. In Hereford cattle, dietary-energy needs were 14 to 27% higher during the summer than they were during warm-climate fall, winter, or spring, whereas there was no difference between seasons in the energy needed by Brahma cattle in the same environment. Whether this variation occurs in different breeds of horses isn't known, but it emphasizes the differences between individuals. In one study in France, horses metabolizable energy requirements for body-weight maintenance were 9% higher during the summer than during the winter. If feed intake does not increase sufficiently to provide the increased dietary energy needed during hot weather, body weight, milk production, or growth rate will decrease. However, the heat-stressed animal decreases, rather than increases, its feed intake. The decrease in feed intake decreases body-heat production, but both decreased feed intake and the increased energy requirements during hot weather result in weight loss. Because of these factors, it is often difficult to keep the horse, particularly the performance or working horse, at moderate to even moderately thin condition during hot weather.

To maintain feed intake and efficiency of energy utilization, and thus prevent a loss of body weight and condition during hot weather: (1) prevent excess fleshiness, (2) feed a palatable high-energy, low-fiber and adequate but low-protein and if necessary high-fat diet, and (3) provide shade, ideally where there is air movement. Because both shade and air movement are quite beneficial in minimizing heat-induced discomfort and stress during hot humid weather, trees, or even artificially constructed shades on a hill and without surrounding obstructions, are ideal. If sheds or stables provide the only shade, they should be well ventilated, ideally with an insulated high-vented roof to let out and not trap rising warm air. Both ceiling exhaust fans and fans blowing on the horse are beneficial.

A low-fiber and adequate but low-protein diet is preferred during hot humid weather because more heat is produced in the utilization of fiber and protein than in the utilization of other dietary constituents. Ideally, the diet during hot weather should meet the horse's protein requirements (as given in Appendix Tables 1 and 4) but not exceed them by more than a few percent at the most. In addition, particularly for the horse that tends to lose weight during hot humid weather, a palatable high energy-dense diet containing 18 to 26% crude fiber, and 10 to 20% fat in its dry matter is also preferred. A low-fiber, high-fat diet not only decreases the heat produced from that diet, but also increases the energy density of the diet since fiber is low, and fat is high, in energy density.

Because during hot humid weather the horse's appetite, and as a result its feed intake, may be reduced, the diet should be highly palatable to encourage the horse to eat a sufficient amount, and should be high in energy density so that the horse will meet its energy needs even when a smaller quantity is eaten. Both diet palatability and energy density can be increased and fiber decreased by feeding a high-grain, low-forage diet. However, to decrease the risk of colic and founder, grain or a grain mix shouldn't make up over one-half of the weight of the total diet. Corn is a good cereal grain to feed as it is lower in fiber and protein, and higher in fat and energy density, than other cereal grains (Table 4-5). Adding molasses to the grain mix will also increase its palatability for most horses.

Dietary energy density can be increased, and heat produced from the diet decreased, not only by decreasing dietary fiber content, but also by adding fat (plant oil or animal fat) to the diet. Plant oils provide about 3 times more available energy than a similar weight of grain, and 3.5 to 6 times more available energy than a similar volume of grain (Table 4-8). Thus, adding fat to the grain mix increases the diet's energy density. A high-fat diet also decreases body heat production. This not only decreases heat stress but also leaves more of the dietary energy ingested available for body use. For example, in one study, adding fat to the horse's diet decreased their body heat production 14% and resulted in 60% more energy available for physical activity when energy intake remained unchanged. However, because more energy from a high-fat diet is available for body use, less energy from it is needed, which further decreases body heat production and heat stress.

Although the horse can utilize 20% additional fat in its total diet and 30% in its grain mix, adding 10% fat to the total diet and, therefore, 20% to the grain mix, if it makes up one-half of the diet (10% ÷ $\frac{1}{2}$ = 20%), is recommended. This will decrease the amount of grain mix needed for weight maintenance by 25%. One pint of oil per 5 lbs of grain (200 g or 217 ml/kg) results in 20% added fat in the grain. Additional recommendations and information on feeding fat are given in Chapter 4 (see section on "Fat and Oil Supplements for Horses").

As always, but particularly critical during hot humid weather, salt and good-quality, palatable water should always be readily available. Water, sodium, and chloride needs all increase as energy needs and heat stress increase. As the ambient temperature increases from 0 to 100°F (-18 to 38°C), the horse's water consumption increases by as much as fourfold.

In summary, during hot humid weather, particularly for horses that become thinner than desired: (1) ensure that water and salt are always readily available; (2) provide shade and ideally a breeze; (3) keep the horse in moderate to moderately thin condition (Table 1–4); and, (4) feed a diet consisting of one-half grass forage (rather than legumes, which are higher in protein), and one-half grain to which up to 5% molases and 20% plant oil have been added. For the idle nongrowing horse, this would be 0.5 to 0.75 lbs of the grain mix/100 lbs body weight (0.5 to 0.75 kg/100 kg) daily, and for hard work or peak lactation, up to twice this amount with all the forage the horse will consume without waste.

AGED HORSES

The average life span of the horse has been reported to be only 24 years. However, many well cared for horses over 20, and even 25, years of age continue to be actively ridden and/or worked, and to reproduce (both mares and stallions). Although their physical performance ability has certainly slowed, many are ideal starter horses for inexperienced riders. The rule to remember in matching horse and rider is: what one lacks in knowledge and experience, the other should have. The more inexperienced the rider, the more experienced the horse should be and vice versa; the better and more experienced the rider, the less experienced the horse needs to be. The worst error, and unfortunately one often made, is putting an inexperienced rider on a young or inexperienced horse. The next worst error, also commonly made, is putting an inexperienced rider on a horse with bad habits, such as one that is barn sour (doesn't want to leave the barn, stable, or companions), balky, handles poorly, and/or is difficult to catch, bridle, or saddle. As an old saying goes, "If you want to sour your children on horses, get them a sour horse." Because sour, young or inexperienced horses and ponies are plentiful and inexpensive, they are frequently sold to inexperienced people who because of their inexperience fail to recognize these problems. The reasoning being that if the child decides they don't like horses, the buyer isn't out much for a high priced horse, but if the child stays with it, we can get them a better horse. Doing this makes the outcome fairly predictable: the child is going to get frustrated, fearful, and/or have little fun and, therefore, lose interest because the child has been denied the pleasure of enjoying an enjoyable horse. So, if you want to sour your children or yourself on horses, get a sour horse; but if you want them to be sweet on horses, get them a sweet horse. Many older, particularly working or using, horses are truly sweet and will train, tolerate, and baby-sit the inexperienced person. This, and the attachment people often develop for them, makes many older horses one of the most valued horses in many farms or stables.

Aging-Induced Changes in Horses

From birth, horses mature rapidly compared to people, such that the horse at 6 months is equivalent to the 6-year-old child, at 12 months is equivalent to the 12-year-old, and at 2 years is equivalent to the 18-year-old; thereafter, 1 year of the mature horse's life is equivalent physiologically to about 3 years of human life. Therefore, a 20-year-old horse is equivalent in age to a 60-year-old person. Common signs of aging, which for most horses begin to become increasingly noticeable after 20 years of age, include: graying of the hair, particularly around the eyes, temples, and nostrils; sunken hollows above the eyes, greater swaying of the back, increased prominence of the backbone and polls, drooping of the lower lip, and changes in the teeth showing their age (see Table 9–6 and Figure 9–11).

Tumors are more common with increasing age and are present in the majority of horses 20 years of age and older. Skin melanomas are commonly present in the anal and perineal region in gray horses. Nearly 80% of gray horses over 15 years old have benign skin melanomas, but these lesions occasionally are malignant. Thyroid and pituitary adenomas, followed by abdominal fat lipomas, are the most common tumors in other old horses.

Thyroid adenomas are present in about one-third of horses over 18 years of age. None of these tumors have been reported to be either functional or malignant. If they obtain sufficient size, they produce a nonpainful swelling, usually of only one lobe or side of the thyroid gland. Rarely, they become large. They can be removed surgically if desired.

Pituitary adenomas are the next most common tumor in aged horses. They occur primarily in older mares. The pituitary tumor causes excess corticosteroid secretion, resulting in Cushing's syndrome. Clinical signs include excess urination and a responsive increase in water consumption. A long, coarse, shaggy hair coat that may be wavy or curly often occurs and doesn't shed off normally in the spring. The mane and tail are normal. Later in the course of the disease, there may be a noticeable loss of muscle resulting in bony prominences, a swayback or potbellied appearance, and poor condition in spite of a normal or increased appetite. Gradually, lethargy and weakness occur. Often, there is laminitis or founder, and decreased exercise and heat tolerance resulting in excessive sweating with physical activity. Occasionally, affected horses have dilated pupils, vision disturbances, rapid respiration, and decreased heart rate. Estrus cycles may be suppressed or abnormal. Wound healing is slowed and there is an increased susceptibility to infectious conditions, which usually are the cause of death, although some horses with a pituitary tumor do well for years even without treatment. Treatment requires the daily administration of a drug to suppress pituitary adenoma activity. Horses responsive to therapy usually improve in 4 to 8 weeks. Good nutrition, adequate water, attempts to minimize infection, and early treatment of any infectious disease that occurs are also necessary.

Additional health problems, besides tumors that are more common in older horses than in younger horses include arthritis and decreased hepatic, renal, and possibly large intestinal function. Discomfort from arthritis is worsened by excess weight. A decrease in renal or hepatic function decreases the animal's ability to properly metabolize and excrete waste products from excess protein intake. However, the digestibility of protein, phosphorus, and possibly fiber, but not soluble carbohydrates (NFE or starch) or calcium, is lower in the older horse. It appears that the decrease in digestibilities with aging are due to a decrease in large intestinal function.

Care of Aged Horses

One of the most important aspects in caring for the older horse is good dental care. Poor dental health is one of the most common causes of an inability of the older horse to maintain optimum body weight and condition. Older horses may have numerous dental problems, such as uneven tooth wear and sharp points that damage soft tissue, making chewing difficult or painful, or loose, damaged, or broken teeth. These will decrease feed intake. Cold water may cause tooth pain and, therefore, reduced water and as a result feed intake. Thus, the first thing necessary in caring for the older horse is to have the teeth and the oral cavity closely examined and any problems found corrected, as described in Chapter 9 (see section on "Dental Problems and Care").

Every effort should be made to assist the older horse in maintaining optimum body weight and condition (moderate to moderately fleshy, as described in Table 1–4). Once the older horse gets thin, it may be difficult to regain body condition. However, a horse should not be overweight, as obesity causes a number of detrimental effects, as described in Chapter 1.

The feeding program necessary to maintain optimum body weight and condition in the older horse depends primarily on the horse's dental health. If the horse's incisors are damaged, the animal will have difficulty grazing or grasping long-stemmed hay. Pasture or long-stem hay, therefore, should not be depended upon as a major portion of the horse's diet. To determine if there is a problem, watch closely as the older horse eats. If the horse has trouble chewing hay or grazing and this can't be corrected by dental care, or if the horse begins to lose weight, either a chopped, wafered, cubed, or pelleted hay and grain, or a complete pelleted or extruded feed, should be fed. These feeds also work well for the horse that has trouble chewing because of wear or damage to the cheek teeth. However, the old horse may be more prone to choke on pelleted feeds, particularly if they are consumed too rapidly. The risk of choking can be decreased by feeding soft rather than hard pellets or by feeding an extruded rather than a pelleted feed, and by slowing the rate of feed consumption as described in Chapter 4. In addition, all hay and grain fed to these horses should be easy to chew. The hay should be high quality, fine stemmed, and leafy. Not only is this type of hay easier to chew, it is also more palatable and nutritious, and the horse will eat more of it if needed. The grain fed should be processed. Even easier to chew, and therefore more conducive to maintaining body weight in the older horse, is a complete pelleted or extruded feed. Because older horses with dental problems are able to chew these pellets, they can obtain the nutrients needed and are less susceptible to colic, which can occur in these horses due to the ingestion of poorly chewed feeds. If the horse's teeth are sufficiently bad, the complete pelleted or extruded feeds or dehydrated alfalfa pellets may be soaked with sufficient water to make a thick slurry which can be consumed without chewing. The pellets can also be softened, the risk of choke reduced and additional dietary energy for maintaining weight be provided by adding as much as several cups (60 to 120 mL) of fat or oil to the diet daily.

Although 8% protein and 0.20% phosphorus in the diet dry matter is adequate for the mature but not aged idle horse, at least 10% protein and 0.25% phosphorus (but preferably 12% and 0.3% respectively) is recommended for the older horse because of its decreased ability to digest these two nutrients. As shown in Table 10–1, most good-quality forages, pasture or hay, and cereal grains will meet the older horse's nutritional requirements. Mature grass forage, hay or pasture, however, may not contain sufficient protein or phosphorus. Additional amounts of both can be provided by feeding 4 to 6 lbs (2 to 3 kg) of a 16% protein grain mix, 7 to 9 lbs (3 to 5 kg) of dehydrated alfalfa pellets or alfalfa (lucerne) hay, or 2 to 3 lbs (1 to 1.4 kg) of a 30% protein pellet to the 1000- to 1200-lb (450- to 550-kg) horse daily. However, if renal or hepatic function are reduced, as described in Chapter 17, care must be taken not to feed excess protein or calcium because of a decreased ability to metabolize and excrete excess protein waste products and calcium.

Generally, it is necessary to feed older horses by themselves so that they get their feed and are not injured or driven away by other horses. Often the problem causing older horses to lose weight and condition is that younger more dominant horses will drive them away from the feed. After this happens a few times, they will not attempt to obtain feed when other horses are there, and by the time the other horses leave, there may be little feed left for them. Providing a sufficient number of feeders placed in a large circle may alleviate this problem.

Chapter 11

FEEDING AND CARE OF HORSES FOR ATHLETIC PERFORMANCE

Energy Production and Utilization for Athletic Performance	. .	193
Diets and Supplements for Athletic Performance	. . . . . .	195
Dietary Protein for Athletic Performance	. . . .	196
Dietary Fat for Athletic Performance	. . . .	197
Feeding and Supplements Before Athletic Performance	. . . .	198
Water and Electrolytes for Athletic Performance	. . . .	199
Heat Production, and Water and Electrolyte Losses	. . . .	199
Water and Electrolyte Deficit Prevention	. . . .	200
Training to Increase Fitness for Athletic Performance	. . . . .	202
Age to Begin Fitness Training	. . . .	204
Loss of Fitness with Rest	. . . .	205
Fitness Evaluation for Athletic Performance	. . . .	205
Body Weight as an Indicator of Fitness	. . . .	206
Heart Rate as an Indicator of Fitness	. . . .	206
Plasma Lactate as an Indicator of Fitness	. . . .	207
Plasma Enzymes as Indicators of Fitness	. . . .	207
Diseases Due to Athletic Performance	. . . .	208
Exercise-Induced Pulmonary Hemorrhage (Bleeders)	. . . .	208
Heat Stroke	. . . .	210
Anhidrosis (Dry Coat)	. . . .	211
Exertional Myopathy (Azoturia or Acute Rhabdomyolysis)	. .	211
Synchronous Diaphragmatic Flutter (Thumps)	. . . . . .	213
Hypocalcemic Tetany (Tying-up, Cramps or Slow-Onset Rhabdomyolysis)	. . . .	213
Exhaustion and Post-exercise Fatigue	. . . .	214
Colic	. . . .	215
Injuries Due to Athletic Performance	. . . .	215
Foot Injuries	. . . .	216
Muscle Injuries	. . . .	216
Tendon and Ligament Injuries	. . . .	216
Bone Stress Injuries	. . . .	217
Management Summary for Athletic Performance	. . . . . .	218
Selecting the Equine Athlete	. . . .	220
Supplemental Reading Recommendations	. . . .	222

There are three general types of athletic performance or physical activity by the horse:

1. Endurance activity generally of 2 hours or more of low-intensity exertion requiring aerobic energy production. It includes activities such as: endurance races, competitive trail rides, and draft horse, ranch horse, heavily used lesson horse, and heavily campaigned show horse work.
2. Middle distances (0.5 to 2 mi, or 800 to 3200 m) activity for several minutes at an average of 75 to 95% of maximum intensity exertion, requiring both aerobic and anaerobic energy production. It includes most major Thoroughbred and Standardbred trotter racing.
3. Sprint (¼ mi, or 400 m, or less) activity for a minute or less at near 100% maximum exertion intensity, requiring primarily anaerobic energy production. It includes activities such as Quarter Horse racing, barrel racing, rodeo events, and draft horse pulling contests.

These three types of activities are equivalent to the marathon, the 440-yard to 1-mile (0.5- to 2-km) race, and the 100-yd (or 100-m) dash and weight lifting competition for people. Activities such as polo and cutting horse competition require some of all three of these types of activities. Others, such as show jumping, require both middle distance and sprint-type activity. All of these competitive activities and the training for them—and, as a result, the effects, problems, and their management, as described in this chapter—are different in many respects from those of the horse not in training or not competing in athletic events.

For frequent or prolonged physical activity, such as training for and competing in athletic events, the nutrients needed, in their order of importance, are: (1) water, (2) body salts or electrolytes, and (3) those needed for energy. A horse can lose essentially all of its body fat and up to one-half of its body protein, whereas a loss of only about 15% of its body water is fatal. Water is not lost from the body alone, however; electrolytes are lost with it. Extensive quantities of water and electrolytes must be lost during physical exertion to dissipate the large amount of heat produced in the production and utilization of energy necessary for physical activity.

ENERGY PRODUCTION AND UTILIZATION FOR ATHLETIC PERFORMANCE

The only source of energy that can be used directly to produce muscular movement is that derived from the adenosine triphosphate (ATP). As ATP is used, it can be reproduced almost instantaneously from creatine phosphate. But all of the ATP and creatine phosphate in the muscle provides enough energy for only 6 to 8 seconds of maximum muscular exertion. The amount of energy they provide is not affected by either feeding or training. For additional activity, another means of ATP resynthesis is necessary. There are two major means of providing the energy needed for the resynthesis of ATP: (1) glycolysis, which is the anaerobic (an, meaning without, and aerobic, meaning air, and thus anaerobic, meaning without air or oxygen) metabolism of the carbohydrates glucose or glycogen to lactic acid, and (2) aerobic (meaning with air or oxygen) oxidation of glucose, glycogen, fats, or protein to carbon dioxide and water. Anaerobic production of ATP occurs rapidly but can produce only a relatively small amount of ATP. In contrast, aerobic metabolism produces large amounts of ATP, but since oxygen is required, this occurs slowly.

Available amounts of energy from sources in the horse's body, as compared to the amount available from pre-formed ATP, are 5 times more from creatine phosphate, and if there is sufficient oxygen available, 2000 times more from glucose and glycogen, but 17,000 times more from fat. The horse has over 35 times more energy available from the utilization of body fat and protein than from the complete utilization of glucose and glycogen. However, without oxygen, glucose and glycogen are not completely utilized, so that lactic acid instead of carbon dioxide is produced. As a result, over 600 times more energy can be produced from body stores aerobically than anaerobically, i.e., with oxygen than without oxygen.

Thus, anaerobic metabolism produces small amounts of energy rapidly from glucose or glycogen only. These are either depleted, or the lactic acid produced inhibits their utilization, so that only enough ATP can be produced from them for a few minutes of intense exertion. The greater the muscular exertion, the faster this occurs, and the quicker fatigue or exhaustion occurs. For example, the horse can run at top speed for only about 1 min ($\frac{5}{8}$ mile, or 1 km), after which speed decreases because there is inadequate rapid energy (ATP) production by anaerobic metabolism and the slower energy (ATP) production by aerobic metabolism isn't fast enough to provide the energy needed for the horse to run at its top speed. Races of less than 3 minutes duration depend primarily, although not exclusively, upon anaerobic energy production.

With adequate oxygen available large amounts of energy or ATP can be produced slowly, primarily from free fatty acids from fats, but also from glucose, glycogen, and protein, and thus can provide the energy for sufficient ATP production for prolonged activity. However, as the degree of muscular exertion increases, the rate of ATP utilization increases, until it exceeds the rate at which aerobic energy production for its resynthesis can occur, at which time the faster rate of energy production by anaerobic metabolism is required to prevent ATP depletion and a cessation of muscular activity. A heart rate above 140 to 150 beats/min (bpm) is considered to be the anaerobic threshold above which lactic acid is produced faster than oxygen is available for its utilization and thus it begins to accumulate. This occurs at speeds from 2:40 to 5:20 min:sec/mile (5 to 10 m/sec), depending primarily on the horse's physical condition, weight carried, and difficulty of terrain covered. Thus, as exertion intensity increases and performance time decreases, the percentage of energy or ATP supplied by creatine phosphate increases and by aerobic glycolysis decreases, whereas anaerobic energy production is highest at middle-distance or exertion events. This is demonstrated for various equine activities in Table 11-1.

The amount of glycogen and fat stored in the muscle, as well as the rate at which they and oxygen can be utilized, differ with different types of skeletal muscle fibers. As given in Table 11-2, there are three types of muscle

TABLE 11-1
Estimate of Relative Contribution (%) of Different Sources of Energy for Various Equine Activities

Event	Creatine Phosphate[a]	Anaerobic Glycolysis	Aerobic Metabolism
Sprint			
Barrel racing	95	4	1
Cutting events	88	10	2
Racing Quarter Horses (440 yd/400 m)	80	18	2
Middle Distance			
Racing			
Thoroughbreds:			
(0.6 mi/1 km)	25	70	5
(1 mi/1.6 km)	10	80	10
(1.5 mi/2.4 km)	5	70	25
(2 mi/3.2 km)	5	55	40
Standardbreds:			
(1 mi/1.6 km)	10	60	30
(1.5 mi/2.4 km)	5	50	45
Polo	5	50	45
Show jumping	15	65	20
3-day event (cross-country)	10	40	50
Endurance			
Endurance rides	1	5	94
Pleasure & equitation shows	1	2	97

[a] Value probably overestimated, as is anaerobic contribution, because the small amount of creatine phosphate in a horse's muscle can only contribute sufficient energy or ATP for a few seconds of activity unless it is reformed by aerobic metabolism.

TABLE 11-2
Equine Muscle Fiber Types and Their Characteristics

Muscle Fiber Type	I (ST)	IIA (FTH)	IIB (FT)
Contractible or twitch rate	slow	fast	fast
Oxygen utilization ability	highest	high	low
Color	alpha red	beta red	white
Myoglobin content	highest	high	lowest
Fiber size	smallest	middle	largest
Strength or maximum power	least	intermediate	greatest
Glycogen storage content	moderate	high	highest
Glycogen depletion with exercise	fastest	intermediate	slowest
Lipid storage content	highest	moderate	negligible
Blood capillary density	highest	moderate	lowest
Endurance or duration of contraction ability	highest	intermediate	low
Order of utilization with increasing exertion	1st	2nd	3rd
In use for low exertion	Yes	No	No
In use for moderate exertion (HR ≃ 150 bpm)	Yes	Yes	No
In use for high exertion (e.g., sprint, pulling, or after prolonged submaximal exertion)	Yes	Yes	Yes
Percentage of total[a]			
Top endurance horses	40	55	5
Top sprint horses	6	54	40
Heavy hunters	30	35	35
Ponies	20	40	40
Standardbreds	20	50	30
Arabians	20	50	30
Thoroughbreds	12	53	35
Quarter Horses	8	50	42
Man (mid-distance runners)	60	35	5

ST = slow-twitch; FTH = fast-twitch, high oxidative, FT = fast-twitch, low oxidative, HR = heart rate, and bpm = beats per minute.
[a] The Type I percentage muscle fiber is determined primarily by genetics, whereas prolonged training increases the proportion of IIA to IIB fibers, or the ability of Type II fibers to use oxygen and thus decrease the rate of glycogen utilization, lactic acid production, and fatigue.

fibers: type I, or slow twitch (ST); Type IIA, or fast twitch high oxidative (FTH); and Type IIB, or fast twitch low oxidative (FT). With low-intensity exertion and, therefore, low rates of ATP utilization, only ST fibers are used. These are the smallest muscle fibers; allowing good oxygen diffusion into them and have the greatest ability to use oxygen. Because of their smaller size, they have the lowest strength, but because they have the greatest oxygen utilization and the largest amount of fat from which large amounts of energy can be produced, they can continue muscular activity for a prolonged period without becoming fatigued. These then are the muscles for endurance, whereas the larger fast-twitch fibers are the muscles for the strength or power needed by the sprinter or draft horse. This is evident by the difference in the thin appearance of the marathoner to the heavily muscled appearance of the sprinter and weight lifter, or the difference in the appearance of the Arab to the Quarter Horse or draft horse. As might be expected from their appearance, Arabian Horses tend to have greater aerobic or endurance ability than Quarter Horses, whereas Quarter Horses have greater strength and therefore greater speed for short distances.

Speed, like pulling or lifting a heavy load, requires strength. Strength requires large muscles, whereas prolonged activity requires oxygen-utilizing ability, which requires small muscle fibers—not the strength provided by big muscle fibers. Increased muscle size for strength is provided by an increase in both the number and size of muscle fibers, both of which are increased by genetics and strength (speed and weight) training; whereas increased oxygen-utilizing capacity for endurance is influenced by genetics and cardiovascular training. Thus, a horse may have the genetic ability to be good at a particular type of activity, and appropriate training will increase this ability.

The fast-twitch (FT) muscle fibers are large fibers that have high strength but low oxidative capacity because the fiber is high in myofibrils rather than mitochondria, where oxygen is utilized. The reverse is the case for the small slow-twitch (ST) muscle fibers. Because of their large size, oxygen is less able to diffuse into the FT fibers, but they are low in fat, which requires oxygen for its use, and are high in glycogen, which doesn't require oxygen for its use. Thus, the FT muscle fibers can produce energy and high power very rapidly anaerobically, and thus high power, but not for very long before fatigue occurs, since lactic acid is produced and little energy can be produced from glycogen as compared to fat.

These are the reasons sprinters and weight lifters or pullers have high strength but rapidly fatigue, and that the marathoner has low strength but endurance. Regardless of the muscle fibers present, as speed or exertion increases, the nerves activate more muscle fibers, so that at a walk only 10% of muscle fibers are used and all are ST, at a trot 50% of fibers are used and include all the ST and many FTH fibers, and at a full gallop or exertion 100% of all three fiber types are used.

Fatigue, and as a result a decreased ability to continue muscular activity, occurs because of numerous factors whose contribution to causing fatigue varies in different situations. These include the following:

1. Increased muscle lactic acid accumulation is probably what causes slowing toward the end of a race. How rapidly lactic acid increases and thus slowing occurs depends on the amount of exertion or speed and the cardiovascular fitness of the horse. The fitter the horse, the greater its aerobic capacity, the slower the production of lactic acid, and the faster lactic acid is removed from the muscle.

2. Decreased muscle glycogen content needed for energy production. When glycogen becomes depleted, there is insufficient ATP or energy production for a fast pace. There is ample fat available for sufficient energy production for several days at a slower pace. The inability to maintain the initial pace, often experienced by human marathoners at about 20 miles (32 km) into the race, forces them to slow down. This is referred to as "hitting the wall." If the fatigued horse isn't allowed to, or doesn't, slow down, musculoskeletal damage may occur (as discussed later in the section on "Injuries Due to Athletic Performance"). Because fatigue with submaximal exertion is due to glycogen depletion, it can be delayed by increased fitness and feeding to increase glycogen stores and to decrease their rate of utilization. Recovery from submaximal exertion-induced fatigue requires glycogen repletion, which takes up to several days, whereas recovery from maximal exertion-induced fatigue requires repletion of an oxygen debt to return muscle and blood lactic acid to normal, which takes less than a few hours.

3. Water and electrolyte sweat loss-induced deficits and alterations, and increased body temperature may contribute to fatigue when exercise results in excessive sweating. These effects may cause fatigue by decreasing blood volume and blood flow to muscles, thus enhancing the above causes of fatigue, and/or may also cause fatigue by inhibiting energy production or altering neuromuscular excitation, contraction, and relaxation. This cause of fatigue, like glycogen depletion, requires several days for complete water and electrolyte repletion and recovery.

4. Lameness, altering the normal gait and placing abnormal strains on muscles, bones, tendons and ligaments. This cause of fatigue may require weeks, rather than days, for recovery depending on its severity.

The greater the amount of glycogen in the muscle and the slower its rate of utilization, the longer before fatigue occurs. Three procedures to increase muscle glycogen content are: (1) training to increase physical conditioning, (2) feeding diets high in either fat or soluble carbohydrates, such as starch, and (3) glycogen loading. Each of these three methods is described in the following sections of this chapter.

DIETS AND SUPPLEMENTS FOR ATHLETIC PERFORMANCE

The nutrients most needed and likely to be of benefit for the exercising horse are those lost in sweat and those used to provide energy. Those lost in sweat can be best provided by always ensuring that good-quality water and salt (sodium chloride) are easily available at all times. The amount of additional salt needed to replace lost sweat, and the effects, prevention, and treatment of water and electrolyte deficits, are described later in this chapter.

The increased amount of dietary energy needed for athletic training and performance can be provided by increasing the energy density of the diet. This can be accomplished by increasing its fat, protein, or starch, and decreasing its fiber content. Because cereal grains are high in starch and low in fiber, and forages are the opposite, dietary intake of starch is increased and fiber is decreased by feeding a relatively high-grain and, therefore, low-forage diet. However, forage should constitute at least one-half of the weight of the diet eaten. If this amount of forage is not being consumed, the amount of grain fed should be reduced until it is. This amount of forage is needed in the diet to decrease the risk of laminitis or founder; gastrointestinal disturbances, such as colic and diarrhea; and behavioral problems in stabled horses, as described in Chapter 20.

Increasing protein and fat in the diet also increases its energy density, although protein appears to be the least preferred, and fat a preferred, source of dietary energy for athletic performance. As a result, as described in the following sections, a high-fat diet appears to be beneficial, and a high-protein diet detrimental, for both sprint and endurance type of activities.

Increased energy production and utilization needed for exercise increases the need for vitamins A, E, B_1 and folacin. Increased amounts of vitamin E and selenium are needed to prevent tissue damage caused by the increased oxidation needed for increased energy production. The additional amount that may be of benefit can be provided by adding to the diet 1 mg of selenium, or 2 mg of sodium selenite, and 1000 IU of vitamin E per horse daily. Additional selenium can instead be provided by using as the only salt mixes available, ones containing selenium. The additional amount of all of the vitamins that may be needed and beneficial for the equine athlete may be best provided by giving a balanced vitamin supplement. One recommended and used that appears quite good is given in Table 3–5. Whether this or other vitamin preparations are given, the amount should be sufficient to supply the horse's requirements as given in Appendix Table 3.

In addition to a good, balanced vitamin supplement and selenium, adding probiotics, or live yeast cultures, to the diet for horses being used for athletic performance may be beneficial. Although the benefit of feeding probiotics is controversial, some studies in horses showed these products are of benefit for athletic performance. Because of this, and the lack of any harm from doing so, adding a good probiotics product to the equine athletes' diet may be worthwhile. Adding fat or oils to the diet, as discussed previously, and administering sufficient sodium bicarbonate (baking soda) at the proper time prior to sprint-type exertion, but not in conjunction with other types of activity, as discussed later in the section on "Feeding and Supplements Before Athletic Performance," may also be beneficial.

In contrast, there is no indication of any need for, nor any benefit from, giving "blood builders" or hematinics, such as iron or vitamin B_{12}, or from giving vitamin C (ascorbic acid). For a discussion of all of these vitamins and minerals, see the sections on each of these nutrients in Chapters 2 and 3. In addition, in contrast to occasional anecdotal reports, like giving hematinics or vitamin C, there are no good, controlled, or convincing studies demonstrating increased performance or benefit from giving numerous substances promoted and sold as aids to athletic performance. These substances include: (1) MSM (methyl sulfonyl methane, dimethyl sulfone or $DMSO_2$), the oxidation end product of dimethylsulfoxide or DMSO (but without DMSO properties), (2) octacossanol (an alcohol present particularly in wheat germ oil), (3) the enzyme superoxide dismutase (SOD, which is probably destroyed in digestion and absorption), (4) gamma hydroxybutyrate (a free-radical scavenger), (5) gamma oryzanol (a ferulic acid ester proposed as a natural antioxidant that prevents membrane damage during anaerobic exercise), (6) bioflavanoids (a naturally occurring antioxidant that may enhance vitamin C availability), (7) inosine and carnitine (dietarily nonessential amino acids), (8) pangamic acid (sometimes referred to as vitamin B_{15} although it is not a vitamin or even a nutrient), and (9) drugs such as furosemide, amphetamine, and nandrolone. Most of these substances are promoted based on appealing rationales and many testimonials, but not on supporting data from properly conducted trials. When they are evaluated in controlled studies, these and numerous other substances fail to demonstrate any benefit. For example, when the performance times of 58 Standardbreds run 160 times without furosemide and 232 times with furosemide were compared, there was no significant difference although performance times averaged 0.14 second slower when furosemide was given.

Both carnitine and DMG have been used as nutritional supplements for athletes in the hope of reducing lactate accumulation and delaying fatigue. Both, when added to the horses' diet, have been shown to lessen the exercise-induced increase in plasma lactate concentration but neither had any effect on performance. In another study there was no improvement in oxygen transport or reduction in plasma lactate concentration after exercise in horses fed DMG. It was concluded that DMG had no beneficial effects on cardiac or respiratory function or lactate production in the exercising horse.

Dietary Protein for Athletic Performance

There are several disadvantages to using protein for energy. Protein is generally an expensive source of dietary energy compared to carbohydrates; e.g., soybean meal provides less energy than corn, yet costs several times more because it is several times higher in protein content. From 3 to 6 times more heat is produced in the utilization of protein for energy than in the utilization of carbohydrates or fats. This contributes to excess body heat and increased sweat-loss-induced water and electrolyte deficits during exercise. Protein utilization for energy also increases water and electrolyte losses in the urine necessary to excrete nitrogen. The nitrogen removed from protein, when protein is used for energy, is excreted in the urine as urea and ammonia. The increased urinary ammonia in the horse's stall, if not well ventilated, may contribute to increased respiratory disease or impairment (as described in the section on "Stable Ventilation" in Chapter 9).

No studies have shown any benefit, and some have shown detrimental effects during athletic performance from feeding horses diets containing substantially more protein than needed, as given in Appendix Table 1. In one study, heart rate, respiratory rate, and sweating were higher in horses receiving a high-protein diet and performing submaximal long-duration activity. In another study, excessive protein intake was found to increase water intake and urine production, and to decrease the efficiency of digestible energy utilization in horses going 50 miles (80 km) at a medium trot or slow lope. At both high speeds (running at 20 mph, or 9 m/sec) and moderate speeds (fast trot, slow canter, or lope at 11 mph, or 5 m/sec), blood glucose concentration fell more and over a longer period in horses fed a high-protein diet (25%) than in those fed either a high-carbohydrate or a high-fat diet. It is recommended that the protein content of the equine athlete's total diet dry matter be between 10 and 16%, to thus meet, but not greatly exceed, needs.

Dietary Fat for Athletic Performance

In contrast to a high-protein diet, a high-fat diet provides several benefits for athletic performance. These include:

1. Fat increases the energy density of the diet, allowing the horse to consume more dietary energy without a proportionate increase in feed intake. This is also accomplished by increasing grain and decreasing forage intake. However, decreasing forage intake decreases water, electrolytes and energy-supplying nutrients in the intestinal tract; these are beneficial for endurance. In addition, more than 40 to 60% of the weight of the diet as grain increases the risk of colic, founder, diarrhea, exertional myopathy, and, in horses not on pasture, stable vices.
2. Fat decreases the amount of energy used for heat production which
   a. decreases the horse's heat load, and
   b. increases the amount of energy available for physical activity and glycogen storage

   In one study where fat was added to the horse's diet, it decreased the horse's total heat production by 14%, and had no effect on the amount of energy needed for maintenance, thus leaving more energy available for physical activity or for body energy storage in the form of glycogen or fat. As a result, even though the energy intake was unchanged, over 60% more energy was available for physical activity. If this additional energy weren't needed, that much less feed would need to be consumed. This was shown in one study by a decrease in the amount of dietary energy needed for maintenance of body weight in exercising horses when a high-fat diet was fed. This occurred regardless of the horse's body condition or the ambient temperature. The amount of a fat-supplemented diet needed is reduced further be-

cause of the fat induced increase in the diet's energy density.
3. A high fat diet not only decreases both the amount of diet and the amount of energy that needs to be consumed, but if fed for a sufficient period of time, will increase muscle glycogen content. Although it is reported that in one study horses fed a high-fat diet for 3 to 4 weeks had lower than normal muscle glycogen content, this effect did not occur when the high fat diet was fed for a longer period of time. Muscle glycogen content was increased with increasing amounts of added fat, up to 10 to 12% of the total diet, but didn't increase further or began to decrease with 15 and 20% fat added to the total diet.
4. Horses fed a high-fat diet also appeared to have greater muscle glycogen utilization and no change in their blood glucose concentration during anaerobic (sprint-type) activity, whereas during aerobic (submaximal, long-duration) activity, there was less decrease in their blood glucose concentration and there was muscle glycogen sparing. Muscle glycogen sparing isn't necessary or desirable for anaerobic activity, because with anaerobic activity glucose and glycogen are the primary substrates for energy production, whereas with aerobic activity, glycogen sparing helps delay fatigue.

As a result of these effects, high-fat diets have been shown to enhance both aerobic and anaerobic performance activities and to delay fatigue.

A high-fat diet (15% added soy oil) appeared to be better than either a high-starch (40%) or a high-protein (25%) diet for both high-speed (running at 9 to 10 m/sec) or moderate-speed (fast trot, slow canter, or lope at 5 m/sec) exercise. On the high-fat diet, the blood glucose concentration decreased less and for a shorter duration. At high speed, muscle glycogen use and plasma lactate concentration were both substantially lower than when the horses were consuming the high starch, low-fat (3%) diet. Whereas in two other studies muscle glycogen levels before exercise were substantially higher in horses fed high-fat diets (65% grain with versus without 10% added animal fat), and were similar following high-speed, short-duration activity. Thus, there was greater glycogen utilization during this activity which, as the investigators suggest, may enhance performance that requires primarily glycogen utilization for anaerobic energy production. This suggestion was supported in other studies where it was found that horses fed high-fat diets ran faster at a constant heart rate, and faster before their plasma lactate concentration began to increase sharply and reached 4 mM/L, than did horses fed non-fat supplemented diets. When Thoroughbred horses were fed a fat-supplemented diet, 14 of 15 had faster race times, and when in moderate or moderately high body-fat condition, utilized significantly more glycogen than when in moderately low body-fat condition. These studies emphasize the benefit of both fat supplementation and maintaining the horse at moderate to moderately high body-fat condition for maximum Thoroughbred race performance.

In addition to anaerobic activity, increased muscle glycogen in horses fed high-fat diets has also been shown to be effectively utilized for aerobic or endurance-type activity. Horses fed a diet with 10.5% added fat were able to trot for about 35 minutes before their heart rate reached 160/min; this heart rate was reached after only 20 minutes in horses fed a diet with no added fat. Cutting horses fed high-fat diets were found to work harder than those fed a conventional diet. Full metabolic adaptation to a high-fat diet has been shown to be achieved in 11 weeks, but not 6 weeks. Fat-supplement sources, and procedures for feeding them, are described in Chapter 4.

FEEDING AND SUPPLEMENTS BEFORE ATHLETIC PERFORMANCE

Prior to athletic performance, procedures to increase muscle glycogen, referred to as glycogen packing or loading, have been utilized, most often in people. This is accomplished in people by decreasing or stopping exercise and increasing carbohydrate intake during the 2 to 3 days before a race. An even greater increase in muscle glycogen content, but one no longer recommended because of numerous problems associated with it, can be obtained by first decreasing muscle glycogen by decreasing carbohydrate intake while continuing strenuous anaerobic exercise for 2 to 4 days before beginning the glycogen loading phase. Similar regime's increase muscle glycogen in horses, but, in contrast to people, appear to provide little or no benefit. However, impaired racing performances due to low muscle glycogen levels, and improvement in performance by increasing nonfiber carbohydrate intake (feeding an additional 2 lbs, or 0.9 kg of corn daily) for several days before a race, has been reported. Too much of an increase in grain intake, however, may cause founder and predispose to exertion myopathy. These risks are decreased by increasing grain intake slowly and by dividing it into several small meals.

In contrast to a possible benefit from increased grain intake during the last few days and up to 4 to 5 hours before a race, increased grain intake within a few hours or less before a race is detrimental. Blood glucose and insulin concentrations peak 2 to 3 hours after the horse eats grain, but not after forage. These effects decrease fat utilization and worsen the fall in blood glucose during exercise, which decreases both endurance and speed. The type of cereal grain or forage fed doesn't appear to matter, as there is no difference in these effects between different cereal grains (barley, corn, oats, and a sweet feed were evaluated) or between chopped, cubed, pelleted, or long-stemmed hay. In contrast to feeding grain within less than 4 hours before a race, feeding grain before this period, and feeding small amounts of grain periodically during endurance-type activity, is not only not harmful but may extend the time before fatigue or exhaustion occurs.

Feeding 3 to 5 lbs (1.5 to 2 kg) of grain 4 to 5 hours before, and allowing free access to forage and water up until endurance-type activity begins, is recommended. The ingested grain will provide needed energy and, by 4 to 5 hours, the increase in blood glucose and insulin concentrations it induces will have returned to normal; they will therefore not be present to decrease fat utilization or exercise. Water and forage intake maximizes the amount of water and electrolytes in the gastrointestinal tract, and thus their availability to replace those lost during prolonged exercise. These are important for prolonged submaximal activity, as the horse's endurance capacity is limited by their loss. Low-forage–high-grain diets, which decrease gastrointestinal water and electrolyte storage, have been found to correlate with increased risk of failure in endurance racing.

In contrast to allowing and encouraging water and forage intake before endurance activity, not allowing forage intake for a period prior to all types of physical exertion has been recommended to decrease gastrointestinal fill and, therefore, the weight the horse must carry. This amount may be quite substantial, as the horse's gastrointestinal tract can hold an amount equal to as much as 25% of its body weight. Thus, gastrointestinal fill is certainly an added weight handicap for the horse, which offsets the benefit it provides as a storage source of water, electrolytes, and nutrients. The benefit of this nutrient storage source, however, offsets the detriment of added weight for endurance-type activity, but not for short-duration maximum- or near-maximum intensity activity. For races of several minutes duration or less, there is no need for or time to absorb nutrients from the gastrointestinal tract.

It has also been theorized that feeding before exercise may be detrimental because it will increase blood flow to the gastrointestinal tract and away from the skeletal muscle. However, it has been shown that although feeding before exercise did result in a higher blood flow to the gastrointestinal tract during exercise, blood flow to the skeletal muscle was also higher, not lower, as compared to ponies fasted for 24 hours prior to exercise. The fed ponies' heart rates and cardiac outputs during exercise were also higher than in the fasted ponies.

Administering sodium bicarbonate (baking soda) prior to maximum exertion of a few minutes or less, such as races of 1.5 miles (2400 m) or less, may be beneficial. The sodium bicarbonate buffers the high amount of lactic acid produced with the high amount of anaerobic glycolysis this type of activity requires (Table 11-1). Buffering the lactic acid produced allows greater glycogen utilization to occur, which permits greater exertion and prolongs fatigue, and thus enhances performance. These effects and benefits have been shown in several studies. However, the proper amount of sodium bicarbonate must be given at the proper time to be beneficial and not harmful, and it is illegal to give it at many tracks and events.

A dosage of 0.3 g/kg bodyweight has only a moderate effect, and administration of 0.4 g/kg only 1 hour before racing has been shown to not improve performance. Peak blood buffering capacity does not occur until 2 to 6 hours, after administration of sodium bicarbonate by stomach tube. A dosage of 0.4 g/kg has been found to be more effective than 0.2 g/kg, and as effective as 0.5 g/kg, but with less detrimental effect. Giving 1 g/kg results in a major and potentially deleterious increase in plasma sodium and decreases in plasma potassium, chloride, and calcium concentrations. These electrolyte concentration alterations are the same as those induced by heat stress, sweating, and furosemide administration, and, therefore, a combination of these factors would exacerbate these potentially deleterious alterations.

Thus, 0.4 to 0.6 g/kg body weight of sodium bicarbonate (200 to 300 g, 7 to 10 oz or about one half of a 1-lb box of baking soda/1100-lb or 500-kg horse), dissolved in several quarts (liters) of water and administered by stomach tube 3 to 6 hours before an event requiring primarily anaerobic type exertion (Table 11-1), may enhance performance. More than this amount should not be given, and it should not be given before primarily aerobic or endurance-type activity (Table 11-1); doing so is of no benefit and is likely to be harmful because of the electrolyte alterations it induces. Adding sodium bicarbonate to the feed instead of giving it by stomach tube may not be effective. At least in one study, horses would not eat the amount needed when it was added to 4.6 lb (2.1 kg) of grain-mix.

Red blood cell transfusions (blood doping, boosting, or packing) is another procedure that has been used to try to enhance athletic performance. Although it may increase human endurance, its benefit is slight, and in dogs, it appears to be detrimental, causing increased blood viscosity, which results in increased resistance to blood flow, decreased cardiac output, and decreased blood return to the heart, which were greater the higher the dogs hematocrit. Although the effect of red blood cell transfusions on horses' athletic performance has not been determined, it quite likely would be even more detrimental for them than for dogs, because splenic contraction in horses during exercise results in a high hematocrit and blood viscosity.

WATER AND ELECTROLYTES FOR ATHLETIC PERFORMANCE

Heat Production, and Water and Electrolyte Losses

About 75 to 80% of energy used in the body is given off as heat. Energy utilization and, therefore, heat production greatly increase during exercise. Even at gentle exercise (a trot, canter, or lope at 9 to 11 mph, or 4.2 to 5 m/sec), heat production increases 10 to 20 times that produced at rest, and during sprinting it can increase 40 to 60 times. Without heat loss, this would increase the horse's body temperature to a life-threatening level above 106°F (41°C) within 4 to 6 minutes. Even at 50% of exertion capacity, the horse's body temperature without cooling would approach the critical level after 10 minutes. Fortunately, with normal heat dissipation, these increases in body temperature do not occur. The heat produced in the body, which during exercise is produced primarily by the muscles, is transported by the blood to the skin and, to a lesser extent, the respiratory tract, where it can be dissipated. The greater the increase in body temperature and, therefore, cooling need, the more blood is shunted to the skin. This may contribute to fatigue, as it decreases oxygen delivery to the muscle, which would increase glycogen utilization and lactic acid production and decrease lactic acid removal.

The evaporative cooling of sweat accounts for about 55 to 60%, and evaporative cooling from the respiratory tract about 25%, of heat dissipation by the horse. Evaporative cooling occurs even at ambient temperatures above the horse's body temperature, but is greatly impaired as the humidity increases. In contrast, the remaining 15 to 20% of heat dissipation by the horse is primarily by convection, but only if the ambient temperature is less than the horse's body temperature. Both evaporative cooling of sweat and heat loss by convection are enhanced by air movement over the body, which occurs when the horse is moving or there is a breeze, and both are impaired with increasing ambient temperature and humidity. When the sum of the ambient temperature in degrees Fahrenheit and the percent relative humidity combined are under 130, heat loss for horses or people should not be a problem. When the sum exceeds 150, especially if humidity contributes over 50% of the sum, heat loss is severely compromised; and when the sum is over 180, little heat dissipation can occur. Neither equine nor human competition or exertion should occur when the value is over 170, and at values between 150 to 170 they should be done with caution. Heat loss is further impaired in the poorly conditioned horse, the fleshy horse, and the horse that still has its winter coat. Not only is heat loss decreased, but heat production is greater for a similar amount of exercise the poorer the horse's physical condition. In one study, rectal temperature increased 50% more in unfit than fit horses following the same amount of exercise.

The evaporation of 1 liter of sweat dissipates 580 kcal of heat, which is the amount of heat produced by 7 to 8 minutes of trotting or loping at 5:30 to 6:40 min:sec/mile (9 to 11 mph, or 4.2 to 5 m/sec). Horses' sweat contains protein, whose concentration decreases after the early stages of sweating. This protein has detergent-like properties that help disperse sweat droplets into a thin film along the hairs; this helps evaporation. This is the reason horse's sweat lathers. With prolonged or frequent sweating, this protein becomes depleted, resulting in a more watery sweat, more likely to run off the horse instead of evaporating and thus cooling the animal. Evaporated cooling from sweat, and thus the efficiency and benefit derived from sweating, also decrease with increasing humidity. As a result, a horse that is only slightly wet with sweat may be losing more heat by rapid evaporation of its sweat than one that has sweat running off it. Wiping sweat off is counterproductive, as it prevents its evaporative cooling effect; putting water on the horse and/or enhancing evaporation enhances cooling.

The horse's maximum sweating rate is 10 to 15 L/hr and is 6.5 to 9 L/hr at endurance racing speeds (trotting or loping at 4:20 to 6:40 min/mile, or 4.2 to 5.8 m/sec). Thus, as shown in Table 11-3, an extensive amount of body water is lost during athletic performance by the horse resulting in up to a 50 (qt) sweat loss, an amount equal to the horse's total blood volume. If not replaced, this would result in 7 to 11% dehydration or decrease in body weight. From 12 to 15% dehydration is fatal. The effects of moderate dehydration in horses are probably similar to those in people, in which it has been shown that physical performance is impaired with fluid losses that decrease body weight by only 2 to 4%. A dehydration-induced decrease in blood volume decreases blood flow to both the muscles and the skin. Decreased blood flow to the muscles decreases muscle performance and leads to fatigue or exhaustion. Decreased blood flow to the skin decreases heat dissi-

TABLE 11-3
Weight Loss by Horses Due to Athletic Competition[a]

Event	Weight Loss[b]	
	Lbs.	Kg
Thoroughbred galloping or breezing	10–16	4.5–73
Standardbred 1 mile (1.6 km) race	12–33	5.5–15
Field Hunters 3 hrs fox hunting	24–100	11–45
After phase D of endurance day in a 3-day	40 ± 18	18.4 ± 8.3
event and 18 to 24 hrs later	12 ± 25	5.5 ± 11.4
50 mile (80 km) endurance race	65–110	30–50

[a] Greater the higher the environmental temperature and humidity, the poorer the condition of the horse, and the more the exertion required.
[b] 90% of which is water.

pation both by decreasing heat transport to the skin and by decreasing sweating, which increases the risk and onset of heat stress or exhaustion.

Sweating results in the loss of not only water but also sodium, chloride, potassium, and lesser amounts of calcium and magnesium, and if excessive, may result in a significant body deficit of these electrolytes. At similar sweating rates, the horse will lose 3 times more sodium and chloride and 5 to 10 times more potassium than do people. However, plasma sodium and potassium concentrations generally remain within the normal range. But, particularly with exhaustion, a significant decrease in plasma potassium may occur. Decreased sodium concentrations may also occur due to sodium losses, followed by partial replacement of the water deficit by drinking. However a decrease in chloride is the most consistent plasma concentration alteration in profusely sweating horses. Calcium and magnesium concentrations also tend to fall with excessive sweating, whereas phosphate concentration tends to increase as a result of phosphate release from muscles upon physical exertion.

A sweat-loss-induced decrease in plasma chloride concentration results in alkalosis. Alkalosis inhibits respiration, resulting in a decrease in carbon dioxide excretion and in oxygen intake and thus oxygen's availability for energy production. This contributes to glycogen depletion, lactic acid accumulation, inadequate energy production, and consequently fatigue or exhaustion. Oxygen availability to the tissues is decreased further by inadequate tissue perfusion due to electrolyte depletion and dehydration-induced decrease in blood volume, and an increase in blood viscosity.

A decrease in plasma potassium concentration decreases muscle strength and tone. It and a sodium deficit also decrease appetite and thirst, which decrease water and food intake necessary to correct the deficits and the energy depletion.

These acid-base and electrolyte alterations as a result of endurance-type activity-induced sweat losses are opposite to what occurs with anaerobic sprint-type exertion at speeds near or above 2:40 min/mile (10 m/sec). The anaerobic exertion-induced increase in lactic acid production tends to cause acidosis and an increase in the plasma potassium concentration. Potassium, along with phosphorus

and cellular enzymes such as creatinine kinase and alkaline phosphatase, are also lost from the muscle in response to strenuous exertion. Following exercise, the plasma potassium concentration returns to normal within 4 to 5 min, whereas it takes from 40 to 70 minutes for the plasma lactate concentration to return to normal.

A decrease in the plasma calcium concentration following extensive sweating by the horse is generally accompanied by a decrease in plasma magnesium concentration. This decreases, and if sufficiently severe, causes anxiety, increased neuromuscular excitability resulting in muscle twitching, increased muscular tension (particularly of the extremities), incoordination, synchronous diaphragmatic flutter (thumps), and hypocalcemic tetany or tying up, as described later in the section on these diseases.

The presence of dehydration can be detected clinically by: dryness of the mucous membranes and eyes, and decreased jugular vein distensibility, rate of capillary refill, and skin elasticity. However, physical performance is reduced prior to any indication of dehydration. Dehydration of 4 to 5% (i.e., a 4 to 5% water-loss-induced decrease in body weight) or greater can be detected by delayed recoil of a fold of pinched-up skin, which is best observed in the skin over the shoulders. The skin over the neck is looser so when pinched, it stands up more readily, making it a less accurate indication of hydration. In the normally hydrated horse, a pinch of shoulder skin should return to its original position within 1 second, and capillary refill time should be less than 3 seconds. Both become increasingly delayed with increasing dehydration. With further dehydration, additional effects become noticeable, including sunken eyes, dry mouth, dry feces, and decreased urine volume. The plasma protein concentration and hematocrit are increased. The hematocrit of the dehydrated, exhausted horse used for endurance activity is generally, but not invariably, greater than 45 to 50% and may be up to 60%. The hematocrit seldom exceeds 45% unless the horse is dehydrated. Treatment of these effects, which result in fatigue and exhaustion, are described in the section on "Diseases Due to Athletic Performance" later in this chapter. A number of things may be done to minimize exercise-induced water and electrolyte deficits and, as a result, help prevent decreased performance, fatigue, and exhaustion.

Water and Electrolyte Deficit Prevention

In contrast to many nutrients, there are no body stores of water or electrolytes other than those carried in the gastrointestinal tract. Any excess absorbed is rapidly excreted in the urine. Thus, body water and electrolyte deficits cannot be prevented by giving them before they are lost. But severe deficits can be prevented by replacing them as they are lost. To do this, salt (sodium chloride), like water, should be always available for the horse to consume as much, as often, and whenever it wants.

All feeds are low in sodium and below that needed to meet the frequently sweating horse's needs (Appendix Table 2). Many feeds contain even less sodium than that needed to meet the nonsweating horse's needs. For the frequently or profusely sweating horse, loose salt may be preferred, as some horses may not lick enough from a block.

Horses need 125 g of sodium and 175 g of chloride (318 g, or 11 to 12 oz of salt) per day of excessive sweating. The horse will consume the additional amount of salt needed if it is available. If it isn't, this amount, or appropriately lesser amounts for shorter-duration or less-profuse sweating, should be added to the grain mix at each feeding for 1 to 2 days afterward. This amount of salt should not, however, be continually present in the grain mix fed. Over 15 lbs (7 kg) of a grain mix containing 4% salt would be needed to provide the amount of salt lost from a full day of excessive sweating. However, since workouts and, therefore, excessive sweating do not occur daily, and because consumption of excessive amounts of sodium is detrimental, it is recommended that if salt is added to the grain mix it not exceed an amount equal to 0.5% of the total diet.

Adding excess salt to the horse's diet increases water and potassium excretion. This, particularly in conjunction with excessive sweating-induced potassium losses, may cause a harmful potassium deficit resulting in a low plasma potassium concentration, decreased performance, excessive urination, and mild dehydration. The potassium deficit is worsened by a high-grain-low-forage diet which is low in potassium, as potassium is low in grains is (0.3 to 0.5%) and high in forages (1 to 3%). At least 0.2% potassium in diet dry matter is adequate for the horse at rest, whereas 0.6% is needed during periods when sweating is frequent or profuse. The horse needs from 5 up to 13 lbs (2.3 to 6 kg) of forage daily to provide this amount of potassium.

Before beginning endurance-type activity, the gastrointestinal tract should contain as much water and electrolytes as possible. The gastrointestinal tract contains an amount of water and electrolytes equal to 6 to 10% of the horse's body weight (8 to 12 gal, or 30 to 50 L, in the 1100-lb, or 500-kg, horse). The amount is increased by the consumption of forage, and is decreased by the consumption of grain and a complete pelleted feed. Thus, both water and forage consumption before, and as frequently as possible during, endurance activity is beneficial in preventing dehydration and electrolyte deficits. To encourage drinking during prolonged competition, the horse should be offered water frequently during training. It has been noted that horses that drink little during endurance races, particularly races that are long, difficult or during hot humid weather, are less likely to finish the race, or more likely to finish slowly, than horses that drink sufficiently during the race to prevent excessive dehydration. Thus, the horse's learning to drink during prolonged activity is a helpful aspect of training.

Particularly during and following exercise, cold water is preferred over warm water, as it helps cool the horse and is emptied from the stomach, and thus absorbed, faster. Drinking even large amounts of cold water during exercise does not lead to colic or any other detrimental effects, and in contrast may be quite beneficial.

During endurance activity, if the temperature and humidity are high (if °F + % humidity exceeds 150) and it is more than 1 to 2 hours between watering places, carrying a couple of gallons (8 L) of water and giving it to the horse in a hat or collapsable pail between otherwise available watering places may be warranted. If doing this in competition is anticipated, it should be done during training to encourage the horse to drink. Feeding a small amount of grain as a source of glucose, and replacing electrolyte losses, during endurance activity may also be beneficial for some horses. Giving electrolytes is of little benefit unless sweating and, therefore, electrolyte losses, are fairly high. As has been shown in people, and is quite likely valid in horses, drinking a glucose-electrolyte-containing solution delays fatigue and improves performance more than water during endurance activities. Providing horses water, sodium, potassium, chloride, and glucose or grain during extended work in hot weather has been shown to increase water consumption, thus decreasing dehydration and does seem to enhance their aerobic performance capacity and delay fatigue.

The major electrolytes in the 6.5 to 9 qts./hr of sweat the horse loses at endurance speeds may be replaced by giving the horse 3 oz (6 level tablespoons or 85 g)/hr of a mixture of equal parts common salt (sodium chloride) and "lite" salt. This should be given just before, every 1 to 2 hours during, and after endurance activity by mixing it into about 1 qt (1 L) of grain mix containing molasses. The molasses in the grain keeps the salt mixture from sifting out. The grain mix not only serves as a vehicle to get the horse to eat the electrolytes needed, it also provides glucose. Following its consumption, water should be offered. Consumption of the grain and the electrolytes stimulates drinking, as does their benefit in preventing a decrease in the plasma sodium concentration which inhibits thirst.

"Lite" salt, or low-sodium salt, is one-half sodium chloride and one-half potassium chloride. It can be purchased at most grocery stores. Instead of "lite" salt, an identical mixture can be prepared by mixing 3 parts sodium chloride and 1 part potassium chloride, although potassium chloride is generally less readily available and more expensive than "lite" salt. Either salt mixture, however, is an economical way to provide the major electrolytes lost in sweat.

The salts should not be added to the horse's drinking water, as they will decrease most horses' water consumption and, therefore, are counterproductive. In addition, if added to the horse's water, they prevent the horse from compensating if intake of any of the electrolytes is more than that needed. Providing that water is available for the horse to drink to satiety, there is little or no risk of giving too much of the salt or electrolyte mixture recommended. Whether giving them is of benefit depends on the amount of sweating-induced losses. Thus, giving electrolytes as recommended, whether needed or not, will not be harmful; if not needed, they won't be of any benefit, but if needed, they may be quite beneficial and, therefore, are recommended in situations where there is prolonged, profuse, or frequent sweating.

Feeding a high-fat diet and good physical conditioning, (both of which decrease body heat production), cooling the horse, and minimizing or avoiding the factors that cause or predispose to hyperthermia, as discussed later in this chapter in the section on "Heat Stroke," are also quite helpful in minimizing sweating and, therefore, water and electrolyte deficits.

TRAINING TO INCREASE FITNESS FOR ATHLETIC PERFORMANCE

Much of a horse's ability is genetic. However, the genetic ability the horse is born with may be altered greatly by life's experiences, one of which may be training. Training has many effects that alter a horse's behavior and physical ability. These include: (1) mentally and physically learning what, when, and how to do, and (2) improved physical fitness to do what it is trained to do. Optimal training enhances both the horse's desire and its ability to improve its performance. In contrast, inadequate, excessive, or improper training will decrease either or both the horse's desire and its ability to improve and maximize its performance.

Factors that affect performance include:

1. Motivation or desire to run and win. This may be a true competitive desire or it may come from knowing as a herd animal that danger is coming from the rear, which makes the horse want to be in front. In either case, it can generally be enhanced by encouragement from a rider or driver, and inhibited by pain, insufficient oxygen intake, fatigue, and excess body temperature, as well, undoubtedly, as numerous psychologic factors.
2. Sprint speed or strength ability (i.e., increasing anaerobic capacity), which is affected by conformation, muscle strength, and neuromuscular coordination. Factors such as properly warming up before a race, and shoeing, can also affect sprint speed or strength ability.
3. Physical fitness for decreased fatigue; i.e., increasing aerobic capacity.
4. Durability to not "break down" from physical exertion.
5. Biomechanical skills or neuromuscular coordination.
6. Ability to minimize exertion induced increase in body temperature, i.e., thermoregulation ability.

Training can influence all of these factors to varying degrees. The importance of training on improving these factors depends on the horse and the type of athletic activity for which the horse is being trained, although for nearly all types of activity, training to enhance durability is beneficial. For example, show jumping requires training of biomechanical skills as well as enhancing both aerobic and anaerobic capacity. In contrast, for endurance racing an improvement in cardiovascular and respiratory function for increased aerobic fitness or stamina is the major aim, whereas for sprint or strength events such as Quarter Horse racing or draft horse pulling contests, training should emphasize improving anaerobic fitness, speed, and muscle strength. Training that increases physical fitness that enhances performance ability does so in many ways. These include training effects that: (1) increase muscle size or strength, contractile speed, and endurance; (2) increase skeletal, tendon, and cartilage strength and flexibility; (3) improve thermoregulation with decreased water and electrolyte losses; (4) increase oxygen intake, delivery, and utilization capability; and (5) increase the rate of energy production and utilization.

Exercise increases aerobic capacity by increasing: (1) the percentage of oxidative muscle fibers and the oxidative capacity of individual Type IIB fibers, (2) muscle capillarity; (3) blood volume; (4) red blood cells release of oxygen to the tissues, and (5) muscle mitochondria. Increased muscle capillarity enhances carbon dioxide and lactic acid removal and oxygen delivery by allowing for a greater blood flow and shorter distance for diffusion into and out of the muscle fibers. Increased capillarity, or size of the vascular compartment, requires an increase in blood volume which also occurs as a result of training. Training increases the horse's plasma volume 25 to 35%, with 90% of the increase occurring in the first week of training. The ability of the muscles to use the additional oxygen is increased by an increased proportion of high oxidative muscle fibers (I and IIA) and oxidative enzymes in Type IIB muscle fibers, and by an increase in muscle mitochondria, which is where oxygen and fat utilization for energy production occur.

Training at speeds that maintain a blood lactate concentration of 4 mM/L is considered to be optimal in enhancing both aerobic and anaerobic metabolism needed for middle-distance (Table 11–1) racing performance. In most horses, this speed produces heart rates of about 190 to 220 bpm and corresponds to about 80 to 85% of the horse's maximal speed. Running at this speed for 2 to 5 furlongs (400 to 1000 m) or incorporating short sprints into a fartlek routine, increases heart and lung capacity to deliver oxygen to the muscle, which is probably the limiting factor for aerobic capacity in highly conditioned race horses. For other horses, the most limiting factor for aerobic capacity is probably the rate at which the muscles can utilize oxygen, which can be doubled with training by long, slow-distance exercise (i.e., galloping continuously for long distances at a speed that maintains the heart rate at 140 to 150 bpm).

Training to improve physical condition increases exercise capacity not only by increasing the rate at which oxygen can be delivered and utilized and, therefore, that energy or ATP can be produced without using glycogen or producing lactic acid, but also by increasing the amount of glycogen that can be stored in muscle and by increasing the use of fat as an energy source, thus sparing glycogen. These effects delay glycogen depletion and lactic acid accumulation, and as a result delay fatigue and exhaustion. Two procedures (besides training for increased physical fitness) used to increase muscle glycogen content, or delay its depletion and lactic acid accumulation during physical exertion, are feeding diets high in either soluble carbohydrates (starch from cereal grains) or fat, and glycogen loading. Both were discussed previously in the sections in this chapter on "Dietary Fats for Athletic Performance" and "Feeding and Supplements Before Athletic Performance."

A training program should consist of three parts: an initial stage, a developmental stage, and a maintenance stage. In horses, the cardiovascular and muscular systems respond rapidly to incremental increases in their workload or training with significant changes being produced in only a few weeks. In contrast, supporting structures such as bone, cartilage, ligaments, tendons, and hooves adapt more slowly over a period of several months. Consequently, early improvements in the horse's cardiovascular and muscular systems allow exertion sufficient to cause injury to these supporting structures. To prevent this, the early stages of training must be kept at levels of exertion below what the horse is able to do. To do this the initial stage of training for any type of competitive event should be long, slow/distance (LSD) workouts for at least 1 month for mature horses sufficiently fit for competition without injury the previous season to as long as 3 to 12 months for the young horse in first year of training. The objective of the LSD training phase is to prepare the horse to cope with 45 to 60 min of easy exercise at a walk, trot and canter, at an average speed of 4 to 5 mph (6 to 8 km/hr), including 2- to 3-min periods of cantering at moderate speeds of 10 to 12 mph (16 to 18 km/hr). This type of exercise is performed 3 times a week, alternating with schooling days. By the end of the LSD phase of training the horse should be able to gallop up to 6 mi (10 km) in 20 to 24 min and maintain a heart rate of near 140 bpm. The initial stage of LSD training increases the horse's suppleness, mobility, and adaptation to saddle and rider, or to pulling a sulky. It strengthens structural components, decreasing the occurrence and risk of training and racing injuries, including stocking-up, bucked shins, splints, bowed tendons, carpal bone chips, fractures, etc. Bone, tendon, and ligament strength increase with exercise that loads these structural components. Both the number of repetitions and the intensity of load factors increase their strength. Long, slow-distance, or aerobic exercise also increase the horse's cardiovascular ability, but do little to improve anaerobic performance ability. As a result, long, slow-distance exercise will not help make a slow horse run fast. But increasing aerobic or oxygen utilization ability by long, slow-distance exercise will help all horses maintain a faster speed longer, which for distances of more than about $\frac{5}{8}$ mile (1000 m) may increase the speed that distance can be run. It's major benefit and necessity, however, is to prevent the exertion induced injuries described later in this chapter that occur so commonly in training and competition.

The second or development stage of training is for the development of the cardiovascular system and muscles specific for the future competitive event desired. There should be a good balance between high-intensity and prolonged duration, with this balance depending on the type of competitive performance event for which the horse is being trained. The more intense the exertion, the more important high-intensity, speed, or anaerobic training is; the less intense the exertion, the more important duration or aerobic training becomes. It is the intensity of competitive exertion that is important, not the duration of exertion or event. For example, although the speed of show jumping is slow and the duration long, this event requires very intense exertion, and therefore the use of anaerobic metabolism. Draft horse pulling competition is another example of slow activity which requires maximum, intense exertion, whereas Quarter Horse racing is an example of maxi-

mum intense exertion for speed. Both require strength and anaerobic energy production. Thus, the development stage of training for the show jumper and the draft pulling horse—like the Quarter Horse sprinter, cutting, rodeo event, and barrel racing horse—should emphasize training to increase anaerobic capacity (i.e., speed and strength). For endurance sports, training should concentrate on just that: i.e., endurance to increase aerobic capacity. For middle-distance events, such as Standardbred trotter racing and Thoroughbred racing and jumping, both anaerobic and aerobic work must be done. Thus, the development stage of training should be exercise in performing the same task as planned for future competition. This is necessary not only for conditioning all parts of the body used for that type of competition, but also for neural learning of the task for neuromuscular coordination to perform that task most efficiently. Neural learning may account for a large proportion of the improvement from training.

For high-intensity exertion or sprint strength training, a thorough warm-up is followed by running the horse several times at near maximum speed for about 200 m (1 furlong), with complete recovery to a heart rate of near 70 bpm in between each sprint. Complete recovery will take about 10 min, depending on the horse's fitness. Running uphill also increases strength and thus sprint speed. Although these high-intensity sprint workouts are beneficial in increasing anaerobic capacity, they should be limited to once every 3 to 5 days depending on the number of sprints and their duration, to prevent musculoskeletal injuries. Barring severe or clinically apparent tissue damage, short anaerobic sprints require about 48 hours for recovery, while long-duration anaerobic and aerobic exercise can require 3 to 7 days for recovery. In contrast, with lower-intensity exercise (at heart rates below 150 bpm), the horse can work out 5 times a week. Usually it is best to vary the intensity of work between sessions.

Anaerobic capacity, the essence of raw speed, is a genetic characteristic that may perhaps not be greatly improved with training. But even in a quarter-mile (400 m) race, some aerobic metabolism is used, with its use increasing as the distance increases. Sprint training increases lactic acid buffering and increases oxygen intake and utilization, thus delaying fatigue and allowing the horse to maintain a faster speed throughout the race. Such horses appear to finish fast at the end of the race, whereas in actuality what is happening is that other less-fit horses are slowing down while the fit horse is maintaining its speed.

For all types of equine competitive activities, for maintenance training during the competition season, shorter duration (one-half), but near competition-intensity workouts, may be best for the fit horse to maintain fitness and optimum performance ability.

For middle-distance or traditional racehorse developmental training, the procedures currently used by most trainers include trotting and a slow lope or canter over a distance longer than the actual race distance. This is done every day. In addition, 2 to 4 times per week the horse is given a single sprint or breeze at about $\frac{3}{4}$ speed for 35 to 65 seconds going 3 to 5 furlongs (600 to 1000 m) followed by a cool-down. Interval training may be used by some racehorse trainers to try to increase performance.

Interval training refers to a series of two to six sprints at a fast lope or gallop from one-half to full speed for 1 to 8 furlongs (200 to 1600 m), with walking or trotting in between sprints until the heart rate decreases to 100 to 150 bpm. As this wide variation in interval training methods indicates, the best method varies with stage of training, its specific purpose, and the horse's response to it. Each individual horse being interval trained should be evaluated daily and its training regimen continually revised, as indicated by the horse's performance and response.

When beginning interval training, sprint duration will be longer and the number of repetitions fewer than as fitness develops. Interval training should be done only every 4 days to allow full recovery, with lower-intensity exercise on the days in between. A compromise between interval and conventional training is often used in Thoroughbred race horses. After warm-up, horses are run at moderate to high speed for a short duration with rest periods in between each run. For example: 4 runs of 3 furlongs at 45 seconds each with a 3:30-min recovery period between each run.

For interval training to increase stamina, initially it may be best to run fast enough to increase heart rate to 180 to 200 bpm, then with increasing fitness increase speed enough to increase the heart rate above 200 bpm. The duration of recovery should be sufficient to allow the heart rate to decrease to around 110 bpm. If the heart rate exceeds what is expected for that particular stage of the training, or if it takes longer for the heart rate to decrease, this indicates that the workout is too stressful and no further work intervals should be done. An unexpectedly high heart rate during warm-up or recovery may also be an early warning that something is wrong, in which case the horse should be examined thoroughly for a problem.

A variation of interval training is fartlek training, which is unstructured alternating periods of slow work and fast work generally below maximum speed but maintained until the horse begins to tire. It helps alleviate boredom for both horse and rider and is useful for both endurance and eventing horses, particularly for those that have an intermittent pattern of energy expenditure, such as polo, combined driving and eventing.

The basic idea of interval training is that it allows more intense work for a longer total duration than if that work were continuous, and that it requires a more frequent recruitment of a higher percentage of muscle fibers and lactate production. This allows adaptation, which increases aerobic metabolism capacity, thus decreasing reliance on anaerobic metabolism.

An increase in aerobic capacity or stamina, however, is not beneficial for sprint-type activities. Increased aerobic capacity is associated with decreased muscle size to allow increased oxygen movement into the muscle fiber, but a decrease in muscle size decreases its strength and, therefore, its rapid acceleration ability needed for sprint-type events. Sprinters, therefore, need training programs that build maximum strength, not maximum stamina. You cannot train for both, nor will an individual horse be good at both. This is why most horses have a certain distance at which they perform best, and why true sprinters cannot be stayers and vice versa. Interval training, therefore, appears to decrease maximum early speed. But it does appear to allow the horse to maintain a fast speed longer and to race well more frequently, both of which are of benefit for middle-distance-type events. Interval training has been shown to substantially delay fatigue as compared to what is obtained by long, slow distance work-outs. In one study, although the differences weren't statistically significant, the average speed of four noninterval-trained Thoroughbred racehorses was faster at the first furlong (220 yds, 1/8 mile, or 200 m), but the average of the four interval-trained horses was faster for each of the next 4 furlongs, and for the 5 furlongs was 0.66 sec faster, which is equivalent to the interval-trained horse's winning by about 11 yards (10 m) in a 5/8-mile (1600-m) race. Regardless of the benefit of interval training and of long, slow-distance training, some contend that because both take much more time, management and, therefore, cost than conventional training, they may not be practical for some horses (e.g., horses raced in claiming races).

For endurance training, emphasis should be placed on the development of aerobic metabolism capacity. To do this, the following training regimen has been recommended. Begin with walks and easy trots of 6 to 8 miles (10 to 13 km) or 30 to 60 minutes 3 times a week for 3 or 4 weeks. Increase to 10-mile work-outs during the second month, but at the same pace of 6 to 8 mph (10 to 13 kph) 3 to 5 times per week. Work-outs should last an hour or more with a heart rate of 80 to 100 bpm. Rest is indicated for a few days to a week if there are any signs of stiffness, soreness, or swelling, or if the heart rate is higher than it has been previously. The heart rate may be used as an indication of appropriate training level. At 10 minutes after beginning exercise, a heart rate of 60 ± 4 bpm indicates a good training level, 48 ± 4 indicates that you can increase training intensity, and 72 or greater indicates that you should decrease training intensity. Others feel that it is best to train at a slow gallop sufficient to maintain the heart rate at 140 to 150 bpm beginning with 10 minutes daily and increasing this gradually to 20 minutes 5 times per week. Following the third month of training, if no stiffness or soreness has occurred, then once or twice a week include two, gradually increasing to four, short sprints that increase the heart rate to 180 to 210 bpm for 40 to 60 sec. In between each sprint, walk to allow the heart rate to recover to 80 to 110 bpm. Ideally this should be continued for 3 to 6 months before competition begins. In the final 2 weeks before the endurance event, the overall intensity of the workout is decreased, although one moderate ride should be taken.

Age to Begin Fitness Training

It appears that beginning exercise conditioning to increase physical fitness when the horse is 18 months of age, but not much younger, is beneficial. Four-year-old Standardbreds exercised since 18 months of age had higher percentages of oxidative muscle fibers and oxidative enzymes in their muscles than those that were not given forced exercise until 3 years of age. These same results have also been obtained in Thoroughbreds and Quarter Horses. However, no metabolic benefit is obtained from forced exercise training prior to 18 months of age. Horses not given forced exercise until 18 months of age appear to catch up within a few months to the metabolic advantages obtained by forced exercise prior to this age.

Loss of Fitness with Rest

In horses—in contrast to people, who lose muscular adaptation to fitness training within a few weeks—the effects of training to increase fitness are maintained even after several weeks to months of rest, as may be necessary in the management of illness or injury. No decrease in fitness was observed in physically fit horses following 5 weeks of rest, and there is little loss of cardiovascular fitness during 6 months of paddock rest. Training effects on muscle oxygen utilization ability are maintained for 5 to 8 weeks. However, in non-sprint-type events requiring high levels of aerobic energy production, significant reductions in peak oxygen intake capacity can occur with as little as 2 weeks of inactivity. Based on results of this type, it's been suggested that horses taken out of training for less than 4 weeks can return to initial levels of cardiopulmonary fitness with 2 to 3 weeks of retraining, but that longer periods of inactivity may require 6 to 8 weeks of retraining to attain maximum cardiopulmonary fitness. This or a longer period of retraining to bring the horse back to the same level of training it was at prior to an interruption in training of even as short as one to several weeks may be necessary to prevent stress-induced tendon, ligament or bone injuries, such as bucked shins. A rule of thumb is to allow a week of reconditioning for every week off, but this should be modified as indicated in the individual by such things as too rapid a heart rate for the situation or any soreness or stiffness.

FITNESS EVALUATION FOR ATHLETIC PERFORMANCE

There are two major reasons that the physical fitness of the equine athlete should be closely monitored: (1) so the progress of training can be determined, which is necessary so training procedures can be altered as indicated; and (2) so overtraining, lameness, soreness, respiratory problems, or any other illness, injury or dysfunction can be readily detected and appropriate measures taken to prevent and minimize their severity and effects. Training and performance are stressful and may result in musculoskeletal injuries and suppression of the immune system. Suppression of immune function predisposes to infectious diseases, particularly respiratory diseases.

Overtraining or overuse so that the horse doesn't have sufficient time to recover from exertion may not only result in physical damage decreasing the horse's ability, but may also suppress the horses desire and, therefore, effort. Overtraining or overuse may be indicated by two different blood tests. One is a persistently low ratio of the white blood cell types neutrophils/lymphocytes. An intermittent or transient decrease in this ratio is normal following physical exertion, but if it is persistently low, it suggests overuse-induced stress. The second blood test suggesting overuse is an increase in the plasma activity of the liver enzyme gamma-glutamyltransferase (GGT) to more than twice nor-

mal. About 30 days of small-paddock or pasture rest is often sufficient to allow the horse to recover from overtraining or overuse without losing a significant amount of previously achieved fitness.

Physical problems requiring rest are also common in the horse in training or competition. The most common causes of inadequate performance are: (1st) musculoskeletal pain, most commonly from multiple, not single, sources; (2nd) upper respiratory dysfunction, such as from laryngeal or pharyngeal muscle problems; and (3rd) lower respiratory dysfunction, such as bronchitis and exercise-induced pulmonary hemorrhage. From 60 to 90% of all Thoroughbreds in training and competition are reported to develop major lameness problems. Most, if detected prior to being visibly evident, such as by heart rate monitoring during exercise and recovery, will respond to an appropriate rest period with no permanent detrimental effects and minimal loss of training and competing time and fitness. Early detection and treatment of respiratory dysfunction also minimizes its detrimental effects and their duration.

Observing a horse before, during, and after workouts, including its respiratory patterns, gait, day-to-day progress, and overall performance as compared to other horses are routinely used subjective indicators of fitness or problems. The time it takes to cover a specific distance is also commonly used a gradual decrease being indicative of training progress, and an increase being indicative of a problem. However, there is a poor correlation between speed for a short distance (5 furlongs, or 1200 m, or less) and that achieved for a longer distance. A more precise indication of training progress and increased fitness is a decrease in either the plasma lactate concentration or the submaximal heart rate that occurs at any specific workload sufficient to increase them above resting levels. Thus, fitness and training progress can be assessed by determining either: (1) the amount of increase in either the plasma lactate concentration or the submaximal heart rate that occurs with a specific amount of exercise, or (2) the amount of exercise (speed, or duration at a certain speed) necessary to reach either a certain plasma lactate level or a certain submaximal heart rate. Typically, the amount of exercise that results in a plasma lactate concentration of 4 mmol/L or a heart rate of 200 bpm is used as an indication of physical fitness. The amount of exercise necessary for either to occur also increases with increasing age from 2 to 5 years, at which age they plateau until 8 years of age before beginning to decrease.

The heart rate 5 minutes after exercise has stopped is also a meaningful indication of the horse's degree of physical fitness. In contrast, neither resting nor maximum heart rates, rate of decline in plasma lactate concentration following exercise, body temperature, plasma activities of muscle enzymes, respiratory rate, or any blood parameters prior to exercise, including hematocrit, blood hemoglobin concentration, or red blood cell number, volume, or hemoglobin concentration or sedimentation rate, or any number or proportion of white blood cells is a meaningful indicator of the horse's physical fitness.

The hematocrit at rest in hot-blooded horses is generally 32 to 46%, and in cold-blooded horses 26 to 32%. It tends to be lower in sprint than endurance horses because endurance horses perform more aerobic work, which stimulates increased red blood cell production. The hematocrit in some fit sprinters may be as low as 32%. It may be decreased by many tranquilizers and is increased by anything causing splenic contraction, which includes excitement, stress, or physical activity.

Body Weight as an Indicator of Fitness

A frequently overlooked but meaningful indication of physical fitness affecting racing performance is the horse's weight. Horses, like all athletes, have an optimal performance weight. Thoroughbred racehorses' optimal racing weight has been found to be within a 16-lb (7.3-kg) range. It was found that performance is more likely to be adversely affected when the horse is below its optimal weight than when it is above it. For most horses, optimal physical performance weight is at moderate body condition as described in Table 1–4. Below this condition, body energy-source nutrients, including muscle glycogen, are reduced before, as well as after, exercise. This decreases both endurance and sprint-type performance ability. However, above-moderate body condition is also detrimental because: (1) muscle glycogen content is not increased, (2) there is excess weight to carry, and (3) the dissipation of exercise-induced heat production is impaired, which increases sweating-induced water and electrolyte losses and body temperature. Most horses' ideal racing weight is the same when they are 3 year olds as when they were 2 year olds. The average weight loss by Thoroughbreds during a race is about 9 lbs (4.1 kg). Those that perform well the next week gain this weight back within 48 hrs.

Effects on, and methods for obtaining, the horse's weight are given in Chapter 6.

Heart Rate as an Indicator of Fitness

Of all the means of assessing physical fitness, measuring heart rate response to exercise and recovery is the easiest to do and the most meaningful. Numerous on-board heart rate monitors are available to measure heart rates during both exercise and recovery. These include Equistat Heart Rate Computer (Equine Biomechanics and Exercise Physiology, Inc., Unionville, PA), Hippocard (Speedtest Thoroughbreds, Inc., Ontario, Canada), and VMAX (Equine Racing Systems, Vevay, IN). The heart rate during recovery can, of course, easily be obtained by listening to the heart or counting the pulse. The pulse may be taken at the maxillary or facial artery on the inner aspect of the lower mandible just in front of the jaw, immediately before the artery crosses under and to the outside surface of the mandible. In most horses, the normal resting heart rate is 30 to 45 bpm; about 80 when walking; 120 to 140 when trotting; 160 to 200 when cantering, loping, or swimming; and over 200 when galloping. At about 210 bpm, the heart rate begins to plateau to its maximum of 220 to 250 bpm, which varies among individuals.

As people become more physically fit, their resting heart rate decreases. This occurs because there is an exercise-induced increase in heart strength which increases stroke volume (SV), allowing cardiac output (CO) to be maintained at a lower heart rate (HR) (since CO = HR × SV).

However, unlike people, stroke volume in horses changes little with exercise, so change in heart rate is the only significant means of changing cardiac output. As a result, although some horses' resting heart rate decreases somewhat with increased fitness, this doesn't occur to any significant degree in most horses. Nor does increased fitness affect most horses' exercising or their maximum heart rate by any significant amount. However, there is a direct correlation between increasing physical fitness of the horse and both (1) a faster speed, or longer duration at a certain speed, that can be obtained before a pre-plateau heart rate (up to 210 bpm) is reached; and (2) a faster decline of the heart rate following exercise. Both of these factors are reliable indicators of the horse's degree of physical fitness. The heart rate at 5 minutes after exercise stops appears to be the most useful criterion.

When no change occurs in either the pre-plateau heart rate reached during, or the heart rate at a specific time after, successive bouts of running at a specific speed for a specific time (or any other identical bouts of exercise intensity and duration), either: (1) the intensity of the training program should be increased if further cardiopulmonary fitness is wanted, or (2) the horse has reached its maximum level of cardiopulmonary fitness, and increasing the intensity of training is unlikely to be beneficial. To distinguish between these two possibilities, the intensity or duration of the training program should be increased. If the heart rate at a given speed does not continue to decrease, or if the speed at a given heart rate (or percent of maximum heart rate) does not continue to increase, it indicates the horse has reached its maximum level of cardiopulmonary fitness. Changes in plasma lactate concentration before and after exercise can also be used to measure physical fitness, but doing so is technically more difficult than measuring the heart rate.

The heart rate is increased not only by exercise but also by fatigue, apprehension, anxiety, discomfort, or pain from any cause, and by any respiratory dysfunction or difficulty. Because of this, any lameness, soreness, or respiratory difficulty generally, before it is sufficiently severe to be seen, can be detected by an increase from the previous day's or exercise's effect on the heart rate. In addition, the amount of increase in the heart rate is proportional to the severity of the pain or respiratory difficulty. However, because of the wide variation in each individual horse's heart rate, these increases can be detected only by comparing each horse's heart rate when not in pain or with a respiratory problem to its heart rate when affected. In addition, the effect these problems have on enhancing the exercise-induced increase on heart rate decreases rapidly following exercise, so that, although it may be evident at 1 minute, it may not be evident at 5 minutes following exercise.

Lameness-induced increases in heart rate during exercise are greater at trotting than at faster speeds, since pain has a greater psychological effect at lower-intensity exertion. However, following exercise, the greatest percentage increase in heart rate as a result of lameness occurs the faster the exercise speed was.

Monitoring the heart rate within the first minute and again at several intervals following a fast workout, and comparing it to that obtained previously on the same horse, provides the best opportunity of detecting any lameness or soreness the earliest. Less diagnostic but, perhaps helpful, is the recommendation that fit Thoroughbred horses' heart rates after exercise should return to 45 bpm or less: (1) within 20 min after a trotting-induced increase in heart rate to greater than 100 bpm, (2) within 40 min after a galloping-induced increase in heart rate to greater than 180 bpm (2 mi, or 3200 m), or (3) within 60 min after a breezing-induced increase in heart rate to greater than 210 bpm (3 to 5 furlongs, or 600 to 1000 m). If a horse's heart rate exceeds these values, or is higher than it was following the same workout done previously, the horse should be examined carefully for evidence of musculoskeletal or internal pain, or a respiratory problem. If no cause for the higher heart rate is found, yet it is elevated even more following the next workout, the training should be lessened or stopped to allow recovery. Doing so will quite likely prevent the problem from becoming more severe and result in less loss of training and competition time. This, as well as a measure of physical fitness and, therefore, appropriate training, rest, and competition, are valuable benefits of and reasons for always monitoring the horse's heart rate response to exercise or recovery.

Plasma Lactate as an Indicator of Fitness

The amount that the plasma lactate concentration ($[lac]_p$) increases with exercise, or conversely the speed or exertion that increases the horse's $[lac]_p$ to a certain level is one of the best indications of the horse's physical fitness or endurance capacity. The less the increase in the $[lac]_p$ with a specific degree of anaerobic exercise, or the greater the exercise speed or duration before a specific $[lac]_p$ is reached, the more physically fit the horse. Changes in peak lactate concentration after exhaustive exercise is also indicative of peak anaerobic power and endurance. However, fitness has no effect on the resting $[lac]_p$ or its rate of decline following exercise. These effects are well illustrated by the results of the study shown in Table 11–4. The rate of decline in the $[lac]_p$ following exercise, although not affected by physical fitness is hastened by physical activity as shown in Table 11–5.

The plasma lactate concentration ($[lac]_p$) increases hyperbolically as a horse's speed or degree of exertion increases. The speed at which the $[lac]_p$ first begins to increase is called the lactate or anaerobic threshold. This occurs in most horses at a heart rate above 140 to 150 bpm and at 50 to 60% of maximum oxygen consumption. At a heart rate of 170 to 220 bpm and greater than 90% of maximum oxygen consumption most horse's $[lac]_p$

TABLE 11–4
Physical Fitness Effects on Quarter Horses' Plasma Lactate Concentration (mM/L)

	Unconditioned	Conditioned
Pre-exercise	0.6	0.9
After 5 min of exercise	3.0	1.1
After 10 min of exercise	4.5	1.5
After 15 min of exercise	20	10

TABLE 11–5
Postexercise Physical Activity Effect on the Horse's Plasma Lactate Concentration (mM/L)

Physical Activity	20 Min	30 Min
	Following a 2-min run	
Standing	12	9
Walking	9	5
Slow trot	5	2

reaches a concentration of 4 mM/L and begins to increase sharply with small increases in speed or exertion. This is referred to as the onset of blood lactate accumulation (OBLA). Both are indicative of aerobic or endurance capacity and have been shown to be closely correlated to people's performance in marathon races, but to have poorer correlation for middle-distance events which require more anaerobic capacity. The OBLA, which is more commonly used in horses than is the lactate threshold, has been shown to be well correlated to Standardbred trotter racing performance and to physical fitness. When the speed at which the OBLA occurs plateaus, the horse has probably reached its maximum endurance capacity fitness. The OBLA is obtained by three to four bouts of running the horse at different speeds for 2 to 3 minutes, or at the same speed for different lengths of time, and taking a blood sample after each run to determine at what speed or for what duration at a specific speed, the plasma lactate concentration first exceeds (4 mMl/L).

The exercise-induced increase in the $[lac]_p$, like the exercise-induced increase in the submaximal heart rate, is increased not only by decreased physical fitness but also by the following factors:

1. Increasing body temperature due to:
   a. increasing ambient temperature and/or humidity
   b. decreased sweating due to water and electrolyte deficits or anhidrosis
   c. excess body fat or hair coat
2. Increasing age over 8 years of age
3. Increasing pain or soreness from any cause
4. Increasing impairment to respiratory gas exchange due to, for example:
   a. exercise-induced pulmonary hemorrhage
   b. respiratory disease
   c. laryngeal hemiplegia (paralysis of one side)
   d. increased head flexion
5. Pre-exercise furosemide administration
6. Genetic or developed inferiority for the exercise performed and, therefore, increasing work necessary to perform it.

Plasma Enzymes as Indicators of Fitness

Monitoring the plasma activities of enzymes released from damaged or working muscles (CPK, AST, or LDH), like monitoring the heart rate, is useful as an indicator of soreness or muscle damage that may inhibit performance which it can detect before impaired performance is seen. The measurements, however, are of no benefit in assessing the horse's physical fitness. Early in training, creatine phosphokinase (CPK), aspartate aminotransferase (AST, AAT, or SGOT) and gamma-glutamyltranspeptidase (GGT) tend to be elevated; they decrease later in training and then remain relatively constant unless there is an increase in exercise intensity, or muscle or liver damage from some other cause. Thus, if exercise intensity has not increased, even a small increase in these enzymes activities should be considered significant and its cause determined or appropriate rest or treatment given. CPK increases within 6 hours following muscle damage and begins to return to normal by 24 hours, whereas AST will remain elevated for up to 7 days following muscle damage. An increase in alkaline phosphates is indicative of intestinal or skeletal damage, whereas an increase in sorbitol or succinate dehydrogenase or gamma-glutamyltranspeptidase (GGT) indicates liver damage. These enzymes should not increase to any significant extent regardless of the severity of exercise. However, plasma GGT activity may increase to more than twice normal as a result of overtraining or overcompetition. When this occurs, although the horse may appear normal and perform well in training gallops, racing performance is likely to be reduced. In one study, winnings were only one-half as much during that and the following racing season in horses with increased liver or muscle enzyme activity during the last one third of the racing season. This emphasizes the importance of not overtraining or overcompeting the horse.

DISEASES DUE TO ATHLETIC PERFORMANCE

Numerous diseases occur during, and while training for, athletic performance. Diseases due to water and electrolyte losses and inadequate energy production—such as heat stroke, anhidrosis, synchronous diaphragmatic flutter, hypocalcemic tetany, the tying-up syndrome, exhaustion, and post-exercise fatigue—occur most commonly with prolonged or frequent physical activity, although some, such as exertional myopathy, may occur within a few minutes of even minimal exercise. Other diseases due to athletic performance, such as exercise-induced pulmonary hemorrhage, are uncommon with endurance activity, occurring most commonly with sprint and middle-distance-type exertion. The most common diseases and injuries due to athletic performance, and their causes, clinical signs, times of occurrence, and prevention are summarized in Table 11–6.

Exercise-Induced Pulmonary Hemorrhage (Bleeders)

Blood in the airway is present in from 40 to 85% of horses following fast strenuous racing with the incidence increasing with age. However, pulmonary hemorrhage sufficiently severe to cause bleeding from the nose occurs in only 0.5 to 2.5% of horses following strenuous sprint-type racing. The intensity of the exercise, not the distance covered, dictates the likelihood of pulmonary hemorrhage. Although most commonly reported in horses participating in flat racing, it is also reported in those engaging in 3-day events and polo; it rarely occurs in endurance racing or in other species of animals. In about 80% of horses affected, it recurs repeatedly during or following race training or competition.

The cause of exercise-induced pulmonary hemorrhage (EIPH) is unknown and may differ in different cases. Most believe that it occurs secondary to either upper or lower airway obstruction from any cause, and that the greater the obstruction, the less exertion required for EIPH to occur. Airway obstruction may be caused by previous damage to the lungs from viral or bacterial respiratory diseases (such as rhinopneumonitis and influenza) heaves or chronic obstructive pulmonary disease (COPD), or the migration of intestinal worm larvae through the lungs as described in Chapter 9. Airway obstruction may also be caused by a narrow width between the jaws within the throat latch, resulting in a narrow laryngeal opening, laryngeal paralysis, tumors, a displaced soft palate, and excess flexion of the head at the neck which can reduce airway passage by as much as one-half. It's been reported that the majority of Thoroughbred and Standardbred racehorses have both narrow jaws and some degree of laryngeal paralysis, which increases resistance to air movement, impairing performance and predisposing to EIPH. (See section later in this chapter on "Selecting the Equine Athlete.")

Regardless of the cause, both pulmonary hemorrhage and pulmonary disease decrease athletic performance ability. The presence of both together more severely affects racing performance than either by itself. Although neither one or even both together, prevents a horse from winning, they sure decrease the chances.

If pulmonary hemorrhage is sufficiently severe, affected horses may have a distressed or anxious expression, cool out slowly, cough occasionally, and swallow frequently when hemorrhage is occurring. Coughing following racing is not a dependable sign as it may be initiated by a variety of irritating stimuli, such as inhaled particles of any type. Frequent swallowing following exercise is a more consistent sign and is often the first indication of EIPH noted by astute observers. Difficult respiration doesn't commonly occur, and in only a few is EIPH sufficiently severe to cause a bloody nose. Other causes of bleeding from the nose, that should be considered include guttural pouch disease, nasal tumors, and hematoma.

In severe cases, EIPH may cause sudden death with or without bleeding from the nose. Thus, the absence of a bloody nose doesn't rule out pulmonary hemorrhage as a cause of sudden death during or immediately following exercise.

EIPH is confirmed by finding blood in the airway following exercise. This may be done by endoscopic observation of the airways one-half to several hours after exercise, or by microscopic examination of fluid aspirated from the trachea. Increased density of the upper posterior aspect of the lung is also evident on radiographs if there has been sufficient recent pulmonary hemorrhage.

Treatment is usually not required or given. In most horses, hemorrhage ceases soon after exercise, and blood is usually cleared from the airway within 6 hours. A few horses continue to bleed into the airways for several days to weeks. These horses are often afebrile, listless, and dull, and eat little. They usually are anemic. Such horses should

TABLE 11–6
Diseases and Injuries Due to Equine Athletic Performance

Disease or Injury	Major Cause	Clinical Signs	Time of Occurrence with Exercise	Prevention
Exercise-induced pulmonary hemorrhage (Bleeders)	Airway constriction	Frequent swallowing, poor performance, blood in airway, and rarely, from nose	During sprint to middle distance racing and immediately following	Minimize respiratory disease by minimizing dust, and by good vaccination and parasite control throughout life
Exertional myopathy (Azoturia, or acute rhabdomyolysis)	Unknown	Muscle spasms, cramps, stiffness, reluctance to move, and colic	Usually within first 10 to 15 minutes of exercise	On rest days decrease grain and don't confine; warm-up slowly; do not move horse if it occurs!
Tying-up, cramps, or hypocalcemic tetany	Excess sweating, stress, and/or muscle energy depletion			For hypocalcemic tetany, also avoid high-calcium diets, e.g., alfalfa.
Fatigue and exhaustion	Energy, water, and electrolyte deficits	Slow pulse recovery, flaccid muscles, decreased feed and water intake, often hyperthermia	Usually during or after prolonged physical exertion	For all 6 diseases or conditions, feed adequate forage; train to increase fitness; decrease exertion; rest more often; and give grain, electrolytes and water just before, during and after physical exertion
Synchronous diaphragmatic flutter (Thumps)	Excess calcium, potassium, and chloride losses	Flank movement in synchrony with heartbeat		
Postexercise fatigue	Potassium deficit	Fatigue for days		
Colic	Excess sweating	Intestinal atony and pain		
Heat stroke	Hot and humid, overexertion, anhidrosis, poor fitness, and dehydration	Decreased performance and sweating, and increased temp., and heart & respiratory rates		For heat stroke, also cool the horse
Anhidrosis (Dry coat)	Sweat gland exhaustion	Decreased sweating, and heat stroke effects	Any time	Keep in cool environment
Foot injury	Trauma	Lameness and foot pain	Any time	Shoes or protective boots; good hoof care
Muscle injury	Overexertion	Stiffness, pain & heat in affected muscle	Any time, often early or in fatigued horse	Increased fitness; good warm-up; decreased exertion when tired
Tendon & ligament injury	Overexertion	Heat, swelling & pain, ± lameness	During fast work but signs occur later	
Bone stress injury	Overuse	Focal pain & swelling ± lame & poor performance	Increases after repeated use & decreases with rest	Decreased frequency of exertion

be evaluated closely for concurrent pulmonary disease and, if present, treated accordingly. Assistance in correcting the anemia by giving hematinics is also indicated.

Numerous things have been tried to prevent EIPH in previously affected horses. In spite of anecdotal reports of their benefit, in controlled studies the administration of citrus bioflavonoids or vitamins C or K (for a discussion of this see the sections on these vitamins in Chapter 3), or inhalation of water-vapor-saturated air, cromolyn, or numerous other substances have been found to be ineffective. In one study, administration of the bronchodilator ipratropium by nebulization into a nasotracheal tube passed into the pharynx 1 hour before exercise prevented EIPH 17 of 18 times in two horses who were repeatedly affected when it was not given. In contrast, administration of the diuretic furosemide (Lasix) appears to have no effect in preventing EIPH. Although furosemide administration before exercise is currently the most popular method used

to prevent or decrease EIPH, numerous studies have shown no decrease in the recurrence of EIPH following furosemide administration at various dosages.

Regardless of furosemide's effect on EIPH, its administration 2 to 4 hours before a race has been thought to improve racing performance. However, variable effects of furosemide on racing times of horses both with and without EIPH have been reported. Some have found better and others poorer racing times following furosemide administration.

Since the cause, occurrence, and severity of EIPH appear to be related to the prior and current occurrence of clinical or subclinical respiratory disease and possibly to parasitic migration through the lungs, emphasis for the prevention of EIPH should be on prevention of respiratory diseases and minimization of parasitism. Prevention of respiratory diseases is important not only to assist in preventing EIPH and its effect on decreasing athletic performance ability, but also to decrease the direct effect respiratory disease itself has on decreasing athletic performance ability. Thus, for top athletic performance ability, respiratory disease and damage by viral diseases, intestinal parasites, and poor stable ventilation must be prevented as discussed in Chapter 9.

Heat Stroke

Heat stroke occurs most commonly during hot, humid weather in poorly conditioned, overexerted horses. It generally occurs during strenuous activity over short periods, or in the later stages of endurance activity, but may occur in nonexercising horses confined to hot, poorly ventilated quarters, particularly during transport. Other factors that predispose to excess body temperature with exercise and, therefore, that should be avoided when possible, include the following:

1. Inadequate heat acclimatization due to a sudden weather change or recent arrival to a hotter or more humid climate. The time required for heat acclimatization by the horse is unknown. In people—who, like horses, the major means of cooling is sweating—most of the acclimatization occurs within 4 to 7 days and is complete after about two weeks. During acclimatization, the sweating rate may double. However, some horses cannot acclimatize, and increased demands for sweating lead to sweating fatigue and a decreased ability to sweat (anhidrosis).
2. Stabling in a cool barn most of the day with exposure to a hotter environment only during exercise. This is thought to predispose to heat stroke but help prevent anhidrosis.
3. Not allowing the horse to drink, eat, rest, and/or cool off following transport before beginning exercise.
4. Excitement or nervousness before or at the beginning of exercise, which is a more common problem in young or inexperienced horses.
5. Dehydration before and during exercise, which is worsened by:
   a. furosemide administration, which causes the same water and electrolyte losses and alterations as excessive sweating.
   b. a low amount of water and electrolytes in the gastrointestinal tract as a result of either low forage or water intake or both before or during prolonged exercise.
6. Poor physical fitness, which results in increased heat production with exercise.
7. Excess fleshiness or hair coat, which decreases heat loss. For the horse with excess hair, clipping may be indicated to enhance heat dissipation.
8. Anhidrosis.
9. Overexertion.

The horse's performance isn't greatly decreased until its body temperature is quite high. Initially, the overheated horse may have a relatively bright appearance. However, if the excess body temperature persists, the following signs occur:

1. Depression, weakness and a refusal or inability to continue exercise.
2. Decreased sweating.
3. The skin may be hot and dry or, because of decreased peripheral blood flow due to dehydration and the maintenance of blood flow to the muscles to continue exertion, the skin may feel cool even though the horse is overheated.
4. Rectal temperature is elevated, often to 104 to 110°F (40 to 43°C), and doesn't fall below 102°F (39°C) within 10 minutes of rest. If the horse is greatly fatigued, anal sphincter tone is absent, resulting in an erroneously low rectal temperature.
5. There is a persistent markedly increased heart rate and respiratory rate.
6. In severe cases the horse may progress to ataxia, collapse, convulsions, coma, and death.

Panting (increased respiratory rate with a decreased depth or tidal volume) occurs to enhance evaporative cooling. As a result, the respiratory rate may be over 200 breaths per minute and exceed the heart rate. However, panting also occurs in the horse that isn't overheated following, but not during, exercise, particularly during hot, humid weather.

If the rectal temperature remains above 104°F (40°C), muscle damage, synchronous diaphragmatic flutter or thumps, a lack of gastrointestinal movement, colic, renal failure, brain disorders, founder, and death may occur. At a temperature of 111°F (44°C), tissue protein is broken down although death is imminent at temperatures above 106°F (41°C).

Early recognition and treatment of overheating are necessary to prevent these harmful effects. There are two aspects of treatment, both of which are needed as quickly as possible: (1) cooling the horse, and (2) water and electrolyte administration to correct the dehydration and electrolyte losses and alterations that occur due to excessive sweating, as described later in this section for the exhausted horse.

The horse should be moved into the shade in a well-ventilated area, preferably in a breeze or using fans if needed and available. Air movement is quite helpful in enhancing evaporative cooling of water, which should be sprayed over the horse's entire body ideally in a fine mist. If a hose is unavailable, the horse's coat should be continually soaked by pouring buckets of cool or cold water over the horse or sponging the horse down. If ice is available, it should be placed over the large veins of the head, neck and legs. Ice water enemas may be used in an emergency. Alcohol rubdowns may not be beneficial as they may cause too rapid a cooling of the body surface, stimulating vasoconstriction and retention of deep body heat.

In many instances, heat stroke can be prevented by avoiding the factors that predispose to it. Conditions that avert overheating include keeping the horse physically fit, acclimatized, not over moderate body condition (Table 1-4), and clipped, if necessary; feeding a diet containing at least one-half forage; giving and encouraging water, forage, and electrolyte intake before, during and after exertion; slowing the horse down during unfavorable conditions;

and cooling the horse when it is hot. The horse may be cooled during rest stops by the procedures described above and by having the horse stand in water whenever possible, even up to the body being totally submerged. However, if the water is too cold, it may cause peripheral vasoconstriction and slow down cooling. It has been feared that cold water on the major muscle masses may lead to cramping of these muscles and, therefore, should be avoided. However, there appears to be little evidence that this occurs or at least is a recognized problem.

Anhidrosis (Dry Coat)

Anhidrosis is a decreased ability to sweat in response to overheating. It generally develops gradually over time. Most affected horses initially have a normal sweating response but gradually develop a failure to sweat. As a result, anhidrosis is most likely to develop after months or years of the horse's being in a tropical climate. Less commonly, the onset may be acute. It develops in about 20% of racing horses and 6% of all horses in areas with protracted periods of hot, humid weather, and is relatively uncommon in areas of low humidity, even though these areas may be hotter. It occurs both in horses native to temperate regions and moved to more tropical areas, as well as those that have always been in tropical areas. Exhaustion and gradual degeneration of the sweat glands due to continuous stimulation by a hot, humid environment appear to be responsible for causing anhidrosis. Hypothyroidism has been suspected but not found to be present in affected horses in one survey.

The first and sometimes only things noticed in horses affected by anhidrosis are poor performance, hard breathing after exercise suggesting a respiratory disease, and/or a poor hair coat. The horse's decreased ability to sweat may or may not be noticed. Additional clinical signs are the same as for heat stroke. Affected horses may prefer to stand in the shade and near or in water. Failure of the rectal temperature to fall below 102°F (39°C) within 10 minutes after exercise is highly indicative that anhidrosis is present in horses training in tropical climates. Long-term effects of anhidrosis include a dry, sparse hair coat, excessive skin scaling, focal and generalized hair loss, decreased appetite, and impaired performance.

Anhidrosis can be confirmed by sweat response to the administration into the skin of several concentrations of epinephrine or terbutaline sulfate. Although numerous treatments have been used, the only effective treatment is movement to a more temperate climate or into an air-conditioned or cool stable with fans. Some horses regain their sweating ability after relocation, but anhidrosis generally recurs if the horse returns to a tropical climate. The likelihood of recurrence can be determined by light microscopic examination of the sweat glands 6 weeks after affected horses are taken to a cooler climate.

Adding electrolytes—4 oz (120 g)/day of lite salt (a mixture of one-half sodium chloride and potassium chloride)—to the feed will relieve some of the signs in about half of the cases. You should ensure that all horses, and particularly those that do, or need to, sweat frequently or excessively, always have free access to good-quality,

palatable drinking water and loose salt so they may consume as much of both as often as they want. Loose salt may be preferred, as some horses with extensive repeated sweat losses may not lick enough from a salt block. Not instead of, but in addition to, having loose salt available, salt may also be added to the horse's diet, generally as 0.5% of the total diet dry matter (which would be 0.5% divided by the fraction of grain mix in the total diet added to the grain mix). In addition, their diet should be low in grain and consist of at least half forage to ensure adequate potassium intake.

Prevention of anhidrosis is reported to be provided by cool or air-conditioned stables, although a cold environment except during exercise is thought to predispose to heat stroke. Horses should be physically fit before summer begins. Starting training when environmental temperatures are already high may predispose to anhidrosis. Horses with anhidrosis that are rested through the hot summer months may compete without problems in the cooler months of the year or when moved to a cooler environment. They seem to resume sweating once nighttime temperatures cool.

Exertional Myopathy (Azoturia or Acute Rhabdomyolysis)

Equine exertional myopathy is a disease affecting the skeletal muscles, or those used for movement, and the muscles of the heart, which occurs shortly following the beginning of exercise, although it has been observed rarely in resting horses. It is referred to by several names, including: azoturia, paralytic myoglobinuria, Monday morning sickness, overstraining disease, myositis, set-fast, and type A exertional, sudden-onset, or acute rhabdomyolysis. Like type B exertional or slow-onset rhabdomyolysis discussed later, it may also be referred to as tying-up syndrome. The incidence is higher in fillies, but there are no sex differences in the incidence in mature horses.

The cause of exertional myopathy is unknown. The explanation most often given is that the high amount of muscle glycogen stored during rest is, upon exercise, converted to lactic acid more rapidly than it can be removed, resulting in levels high enough to cause muscle damage. There is doubt as to the validity of this cause. Numerous other explanations have been offered but currently appear to have even less supporting evidence than this. These include defective muscle metabolism, low levels of blood calcium, hypothyroidism, selenium/vitamin E deficiencies, and potassium deficiency at the muscle. There is no evidence indicating that a dietary deficiency of selenium, vitamin E, or any other nutrient is involved.

Regardless of the cause, exertional myopathy most commonly occurs within a few minutes to an hour after beginning exercise following 1 or more days of rest, particularly when a high-grain (40% or greater) diet has been fed and the horse has been confined so that little or no exercise was received. These factors increase the amount of glycogen in the muscle, particularly in the physically fit horse. Little exercise may be necessary to induce the disease. The more strenuous the exercise, without beginning physical activity slowly, generally the sooner following the onset of exercise the condition occurs. The condition may also occur from excessive struggling associated with restraint, or from colic, or following general anesthesia, particularly when general anesthesia is prolonged. A rare, severe, and often fatal atypical myopathy has been reported in horses on pasture with no history of sudden exertion. In these horses, the muscle protein myoglobin is lost from damaged muscles and is excreted in the urine, giving it a coffee-colored appearance.

In mild cases of exertional myopathy, there may be only a slight stiffness, shortened stride, or change of gait, or decreased athletic performance. In more severely affected horses, muscle cramping and twitching occur. The largest muscle masses are generally the most severely affected and are stiff, swollen, firm, and painful to the touch. Although it is usually the croup, loin, and thigh muscles that are most severely affected, the forelegs alone or in combination with other muscles may be involved. Usually, myopathy is generalized and affects both sides, but uncommonly it may be localized or only one side may be affected. Due to pain, affected animals often have a tucked-up appearance, sweat profusely, have a stiff, stilted gait, and are reluctant or unable to move. Muscle tremors and increased heart and respiratory rates occur. In severe cases these signs are followed by the horse going down and death.

In mild cases with only subtle lameness or inadequate athletic performance, laboratory changes may be minimal. In more severe cases, muscle enzymes—such as AST (SGOT), CPK, and LDH—and muscle myoglobin and phosphorus concentrations in the blood are elevated due to muscle damage. The myoglobin is excreted in the urine. If sufficient quantities are excreted, it gives the urine a coffee-colored appearance, and cause renal damage. The horse going down or the appearance of dark-colored urine indicates a grave prognosis.

Anything that increases muscle glycogen deposition or rate of utilization, or decreases circulation to the muscle, predisposes to the occurrence of exertion myopathy. These include: (1) genetic predisposition to any of these factors, which appears to be important in some cases; (2) poor physical conditioning, which decreases circulation to the muscle; (3) good physical conditioning, which increases the amount of glycogen stored in the muscle and the rate that it can be mobilized; (4) high energy intake, particularly from cereal grains, during a period of rest, which increases muscle glycogen deposition; and (5) failure to begin physical activity slowly in order to increase muscle circulation. It appears that each time an animal is affected, the more likely the condition will recur, and that anxious, nervous, or hyperactive horses may be more prone to recurrent episodes.

Exertion myopathy must be differentiated from overexertion, heat stroke, colic, founder, tetanus, soreness from castration, spinal cord damage, neuromuscular disease, back injury, vitamin E-selenium deficiency myopathy, acorn toxicosis (see Chapter 18), monensin toxicosis (see Chapter 19), and Lyme disease. Diagnosis is based on the history, clinical signs, physical exam, and elevated CPK and AST activities in the plasma.

Affected animals should not be moved since this is likely to worsen the condition. Mild cases may recover with no treatment if they are not moved, either walked or in a trailer. If moved even a short distance, the condition may become severe, resulting in death regardless of the treatment given. Horses that are down should not be forced to rise but assisted to rise as soon as possible. The horse should be kept warm, dry, out of drafts, and well bedded. If the horse is down, it is important to ensure that adequate urination is occurring. Warm compresses on the muscles, and muscle massage to increase muscle circulation are helpful. From 2.5 to 5 gallons (10 to 20 liters) of fluid should be given intravenously, and 2 to 2.5 gallons (8 to 10 liters) of a nutrient-electrolyte fluid given by stomach tube are helpful and recommended in severely affected cases. Oral fluid administration should be repeated as needed. In addition, water should be easily available for the horse to drink. Bicarbonate should not be given unless the plasma bicarbonate concentration is low, which is rarely the case. Fluid administration may be necessary and beneficial until the urine is free of pigmentation.

Drugs to control pain and anxiety and to decrease muscular activity may be helpful. However, tranquilizers generally should not be administered until after adequate fluid therapy as some may induce shock. Shock is frequently present in severe cases. The B vitamins, thiamine and pantothenic acid administration may be helpful.

Following recovery, an injection of vitamin E and selenium may help minimize tissue damage. Only minimal amounts of hay should be given for 2 days, and there should be no grain fed or exercise given until plasma activities of muscle enzymes have returned to normal. This will generally require 2 weeks or longer. Exercise prior to this time may cause further muscle damage. Return to normal exercise and feeding should be gradual. The horse should be turned out into a small paddock for at least several days before riding or lunging exercise is begun.

To prevent the exertion myopathy that occurs soon after exercise, one should avoid as many of the factors that predispose to it as possible. Steps one should take include: (1) a regular exercise program without any complete rest days; (2) decrease confinement and allow more frequent exercise; (3) feed more hay and less grain, or don't feed any grain, particularly when the horse isn't being used; (4) don't feed grain for at least 6 hours before strenuous exercise; and (5) begin physical activity slowly and increase it gradually. Although a vitamin E or selenium deficiency is not responsible for causing or predisposing to exertion myopathy, giving these nutrients may be beneficial in preventing its recurrence because of their effect on stabilizing cell membranes. Adding 1 oz (30 g) of brewers' yeast as a source of B vitamins to the horse's diet daily may also be helpful, although there are no studies indicating its benefit.

In horses that are repeatedly affected, thyroid function should be determined, as thyroid supplements may be helpful in preventing recurrence if thyroid function is low. Adding 2% sodium bicarbonate (baking soda) to the diet dry matter was reported to be effective in preventing repeated recurrence of exertional myopathy in one case. However, feeding bicarbonate does not help prevent exertion myopathies in most affected horses and may even aggravate its occurrence. Any benefit obtained from sodium bicarbonate may be as a result of the sodium, not the bicarbonate, as in two horses with repeated occurrence of exertion myopathy, adding 2 to 3 oz (60 to 90 g) of sodium chloride (common salt) to their diet helped prevent recurrence. Giving phenytoin (Dilantin) for 1 to 2 months has been found to prevent recurrence of episodes of exertion myopathy in some horses.

Synchronous Diaphragmatic Flutter (Thumps)

Synchronous diaphragmatic flutter (SDF), or "thumps," results in movements of the horse's flanks, (generally on both sides but, occasionally on only one side), and rarely, a hind leg, in synchrony with each heart beat. Although SDF itself is not serious and will subside with rest, it indicates that electrolyte alterations are present and, therefore, is grounds for elimination from a competitive event.

SDF occurs during or following excessive sweating, severe diarrhea, colic, or prolonged surgery or general anesthesia. It has also been reported in racehorses following furosemide (Lasix) administration, which induces the same water and electrolyte losses and alterations as excessive sweating. It may also occur due to blister beetle ingestion (see Chapter 19) or lactation-, transit-, or, stress-induced decrease in the plasma calcium concentration. It occurs as a result of a decrease in the plasma concentration of calcium, and often of magnesium, potassium, and chloride. These alterations increase the irritability of the phrenic nerves. As a result, the electrical activity that occurs when the heart beats stimulates these nerves where they pass over the heart. The diaphragm, which is stimulated by these nerves, then contracts with each beat of the heart. It may become sufficiently violent to produce an audible thumping sound; hence, the descriptive term for the condition, "thumps." The condition is generally transient in mild cases. Intravenous calcium administration results in prompt alleviation of clinical signs.

SDF is a recurrent problem in some horses. Providing water and electrolytes as described previously in this chapter for "Water and Electrolyte Deficit Prevention" will help prevent SDF. Not feeding a diet providing excess calcium, such as alfalfa, may also be beneficial in preventing a fall in the plasma calcium concentration and its effects, as described for the prevention of tying-up. It has been reported that some horses with chronic recurring SDF may have alterations of the phrenic nerve. Injury or scar tissue subsequent to pneumonia or pleuritis are potential but unproven causes of refractory cases of SDF.

Hypocalcemic Tetany (Tying-up, Cramps or Slow Onset Rhabdomyolysis)

Horses with tying-up syndrome have muscle twitching and cramping. Generally, they have anxiety or decreased sensory awareness, abnormal facial expression, and stiffness or incoordination (particularly of the hind legs), resulting in a stiff, stilted gait and a reluctance to move. Additional signs that may occur include a raising of the tail head, muscular tremors, sweating, increased respiratory rate and difficulty with flared nostrils, increased heart rate and abnormal rhythm, teeth grinding, and a difficult or inability to chew or swallow. This may result in the loss of saliva and make passing a stomach tube difficult. If the condition progresses, the horse will go down within less than 24 hours, tetanic convulsions will develop, and death will occur within 48 hours after the onset of clinical signs.

It's because of these clinical signs that the condition is often referred to as "tying-up syndrome" or "cramps." These symptoms are similar to those due to exertion myopathy. However, as indicated in Table 11-6, exertion myopathy occurs early after the onset of physical activity, whereas tying-up does not occur until after prolonged activity and, as a result, generally sweat losses and stress.

The major cause appears to be a decrease in the plasma calcium concentration, although muscle fiber energy depletion and a decrease in the plasma magnesium concentration may also be causative factors. All may occur as a result of a number of prolonged physical exertion-induced effects. These include losses in sweat and possibly urine, and stress-induced inhibition of intestinal calcium absorption and mobilization from bone.

These factors, even without calcium losses from the body, may result in a decrease in the plasma calcium concentration sufficient to induce what has been referred to as stress tetany or transit tetany when it occurs due to prolonged stress and lack of calcium intake during transit. However, most often both prolonged stress and excess calcium losses from the body, either in milk or sweat, are responsible for causing a decrease in calcium sufficient to result in clinical symptoms. When this occurs in the pregnant, foaling, or lactating mare, it is referred to as lactation tetany or eclampsia. Some muscle fibers may also become energy depleted following prolonged submaximal or endurance-type activity. Energy is necessary not only for muscle contraction but also for muscle relaxation. Muscle energy depletion is the reason rigor mortis occurs following death. Relaxation occurs following rigor mortis due to muscle fiber autolysis.

A definitive diagnosis is made by finding a low plasma calcium concentration. However, generally a tentative diagnosis is made based on clinical signs, a history of prolonged exertion or stress, and response to treatment.

Treatment of hypocalcemic tetany is to administer intravenously calcium-, magnesium-, and dextrose-containing solutions, and analgesics. Additional water and electrolytes should generally be administered as described later in this section for exhaustion and postexercise fatigue, as these conditions, or the factors that cause them, are also generally present to varying degrees.

Prevention is the same as that described previously for preventing water and electrolyte deficits due to prolonged exertion and sweating. An additional factor that may be helpful in preventing tying-up syndrome is not feeding a diet high in calcium for at least 2 to 3 weeks prior to when the syndrome may occur, such as before endurance-type activity or foaling and lactation. Excess calcium intake decreases parathyroid hormone secretion, vitamin D activation, and intestinal calcium absorption. As a result of these effects, when a large amount of calcium is suddenly needed to replace that lost in sweat or milk, there is a decreased ability to increase intestinal calcium absorption and calcium mobilization from the bone fast enough; consequently a decrease in plasma calcium concentration occurs. This has been well demonstrated as a cause of, and a low-calcium diet as being beneficial in preventing low blood calcium after calving. It is also quite likely the basis for reports that endurance riders have found that feeding high-quality alfalfa sometimes results in a tendency to tie-up, and that horses fed diets high in calcium have more frequent occurrences of synchronous diaphragmatic flutter, which also occurs as a result of a low plasma calcium concentration. Alfalfa contains 3 to 7 times more calcium than needed (Table 10–1). A low-calcium diet is one consisting of a grass forage, any cereal grain with no added calcium, and no mineral mixes containing calcium. Feeding alfalfa, or a high-calcium diet, beginning immediately following periods when a low plasma calcium concentration may or has occurred, however, is beneficial in its prevention or treatment.

Exhaustion and Post-Exercise Fatigue

Fatigue or exhaustion occur as a result of a body deficit of either or both energy, or water and electrolytes. Early signs of a horse about to become fatigued include:

1. A slight imprecision of gait and/or change in breathing pattern. As fatigue occurs, stride speed and length are decreased and the duration of foot contact with the ground increased and non-contact duration decreased. The horse may appear to lift itself higher with each stride to lengthen the duration of inhalation which occurs as the front legs in cantering, loping, or galloping move forward and are not bearing weight.
2. Sleepiness and/or glassiness of the eyes, droopy ears, and behavior, although this can be normal in some horses,
3. A capillary refill, or skin rebound time of 2 seconds or more,
4. A heart rate recovery to a specific rate delayed by 2 to 3 minutes more than is usual for that particular horse,
5. A loosening of the stool, or absence of gut sounds,
6. The sweat becoming thick, sticky, or scanty.

The heart rate recovery index is an excellent means of identifying the horse with incipient fatigue. It is obtained by taking the heart rate and generally, although not necessarily, waiting until it is less than 64/min, having the horse led at a brisk trot out about 125 ft (40 m) and back to you. Take the heart rate again one minute after the horse started the jog out (25 to 35 seconds after the horse gets back to you). The fit, healthy horse's post-jog rate will be equal to or less than its pre-jog rate. With simple fatigue, the horse's post-jog rate may be 10 to 15% higher than its pre-jog rate. If exhaustion, colic, or muscle problems are developing, the horse's post-jog rate may be 20% or more higher.

The heart and respiratory rates of the exhausted horse are similar to those of the nonexhausted horse during and initially following exercise, but in the nonexhausted horse, these decrease more rapidly following exercise. In the fit, healthy horse, the heart rate should fall to less than 55 bpm and the respiratory rate to less than 25 breaths per minute (unless ambient temperature and humidity are high) within 20 to 30 minutes following exercise. If the heart rate doesn't fall to less than 60 bpm within 30 minutes following exercise, or to less than the pre-jog rate at 1 minute after beginning a 250-ft (75- to 80-m) jog, the horse should probably not continue exercise or endurance competition. In the United Kingdom, but not the United States or Australia, the horse is also not allowed to continue if the respiratory rate is over twice the heart rate after a 30-minute rest. However, respiratory rate is indicative of fatigue or exhaustion only if it is both rapid and deep. A deep or gasping respiratory rate after 5 minutes of rest is of concern, whereas a rapid, shallow respiration may be a means of evaporative cooling, not fatigue.

Exhaustion is generally present if, within 10 minutes after exercise, (1) the rectal temperature doesn't fall to less than 102°F (39°C), and (2) the heart rate is greater than 70 and the respiratory rate is greater than one-half the heart rate. Increased body temperature occurs because dehydration and electrolyte deficits decrease sweating, and the sweat becomes sticky rather than watery. Affected horses are extremely depressed and lethargic, often with little interest in food or water despite a dietary energy need and dehydration. The failure of a hard-worked horse to eat and drink is the hallmark of exhaustion. Varying degrees of muscle energy depletion, overheating, low plasma calcium, potassium, and chloride concentrations, and electrolyte deficits may be present. These may result in a dilated anus (resulting in an inaccurately low rectal temperature), occasional colic, heart irregularities, muscular cramping or twitches, renal failure, and synchronous diaphragmatic flutter as complications of exhaustion. An increased hematocrit and plasma protein concentration due to dehydration, and an increase in muscle enzyme activities and phosphorus concentration in the plasma due to muscle exertion and damage are frequently present in exhausted horses.

Treatment should be prompt and aggressive. Early treatment is often important in producing a rapid recovery without complications. If severe signs are not evident, orally administered fluids along may be adequate. From 6 to 10 L may be given by stomach tube and repeated every 30 to 60 minutes as needed. If diarrhea does not occur, fluid, preferably nonalkalinizing, is best. A fluid for orally replacing sweat losses may be prepared by adding one level teaspoon (5 g) of both sodium chloride (table or common salt) and "lite salt" (which is one-half sodium chloride and one-half potassium chloride, and can be purchased in most grocery stores), plus 2 packages (2 oz or 60 g/pkg) of jam and jelly pectin (which is primarily glucose), made up to about 1 gallon (4 L). Fluids given orally offer the advantage of speed and convenience and are less expensive than giving fluids intravenously, but shouldn't be used in horses that are unable to stand.

In the severely dehydrated or affected horse, or if there is no improvement within 1 to 2 hours following oral administration of fluids, fluids should be given intravenously.

If the horse's rectal temperature is 102°F (39°C) or greater, the horse should be cooled as described previously for heat stroke. The horse should be moved as little as possible during treatment. Exhausted horses may look deceptively well after an hour or so of intensive, appropriate fluid administration. But ongoing monitoring and treatment may be needed for several days to prevent relapse, founder, and/or death. Prolonged transportation should be avoided for at least 12 to 24 hours following successful therapy. Transportation is associated with considerable muscular activity, which impairs recovery and increases the risk of harmful effects. The horse should be rested for several weeks afterward. Three ounces (85 g) of a mixture of equal parts common salt and "lite" salt should be added to the diet twice a day for several days.

Post-exercise fatigue is closely associated with exhaustion, but occurs after rather than during physical activity. It is characterized by the horse that, for as long as several days after prolonged physical exertion, is depressed and lethargic, has flabby muscle tone, often stands with its head hanging, and has little inclination to eat or drink. Gastrointestinal motility is decreased or absent. Often there is renal shutdown. Hepatic and gastrointestinal dysfunctions, myopathy, synchronous diaphragmatic flutter, and founder may develop. Most affected horses have a marked decrease in their plasma concentration of chloride, potassium, and, sometimes, calcium. Although a number of factors, including an energy deficit, may be present, frequently the major cause is a body potassium deficit. Most cases are due to a failure to give exhausted horses adequate fluid and electrolytes following prolonged endurance-type activity.

Treatment of postexercise fatigue is correction of electrolyte and acid-base alterations. Doing so is frequently complicated by the presence of renal shutdown, which should be alleviated by fluid and electrolyte administration, as described previously for the exhausted horse, before attempting to correct the potassium deficit. A potassium deficit may be corrected by adding "lite" salt to the diet as described above. Prevention includes better physical conditioning, and rest, water, electrolytes and carbohydrates (grain) during prolonged or frequent strenuous physical exertion.

Colic

Abdominal pain or colic may be either the predominant or a minor symptom of any of the previous conditions occurring as a result of excessive sweating-induced water and electrolyte losses. It occurs as a result of a lack of gastrointestinal motility. It frequently occurs the evening after prolonged exercise. Treatment should be prompt, aggressive, and similar to that described for exhaustion, including giving fluids orally. Generally, fluids given orally will be absorbed and are quite beneficial. However, no more should be given if by several hours following their administration it is found that, when a stomach tube is inserted, a large amount of fluid is still present in the stomach. Analgesics as needed to control pain are also indicated.

In horses competing or in full training, colic may also occur in response not to fluid and electrolyte losses but to minor changes in routine. This may be due to alterations in nervous control of the gastrointestinal tract, decreasing its motility. A decrease in its motility results in gastrointestinal gas or feed-induced distention, which causes pain and colic. Travel, stabling in strange surroundings, and unfamiliar routines prior to competition or during training may induce these alterations, resulting in acute colic. Treatment to decrease pain should be instituted, even though the drugs necessary may make the horse liable for disqualification because their administration is not permitted prior to competition. If treatment is withheld, the horse may hurt itself sufficiently to be detrimental to its competitive performance.

INJURIES DUE TO ATHLETIC PERFORMANCE

Numerous injuries resulting in lameness occur during athletic training, competition, and work. According to one survey, lameness accounted for nearly 70% of all training days lost, with over one-third of racehorses in training developing lameness which prevented training. Two-year-olds had the highest rate of affliction with more than one-half becoming lame during training or racing. Delaying training and racing until a later age is the most optimum means of decreasing exertion-induced injury in young horses. However, this is economically unfeasible unless there are major changes made in the racing industry, which is unlikely. Feeding zeolite during growth, as described in Chapter 4, appears to be a safe and effective means of decreasing the risk of exertion-induced injuries in young horses.

The most common injuries due to athletic performance are those summarized here, and in Table 11-6, in which there is injury to the feet, muscles, tendons, ligaments, or bones that results in lameness. A conclusive diagnosis of the cause of a lameness can often be obtained by physical examination, diagnostic anesthesia, radiography, or more recently, ultrasonography, all of which provide physical information on the tissue examined. However, in some cases a diagnosis cannot be obtained using these procedures. In these cases, scintigraphy, which provides physiologic rather than physical information, is frequently quite helpful, particularly when used in conjunction with the physical information-providing procedures. However, currently scintigraphy is not widely available.

Diagnosis, of course, is a necessary prerequisite for successful therapy. One of the most commonly used forms of therapy for injuries resulting in inflammation is physical therapy. Many different kinds of physical therapy are used—cold, heat, ultrasound, and magnetic being the most common. Cold therapy is generally applied in the first 24 to 48 hours after an injury to decrease swelling, hematoma formation, inflammation, and possibly pain. A compression bandage after cold therapy is unnecessary, and because of its insulating effect, may be counterproductive.

Heat therapy is generally applied after the first 48 hours following injury. Heat increases circulation and metabolic rate, enhancing healing and resorption of swelling, but also increases capillary permeability and, as a result, edema and toxin absorption. Applying a compression wrap after either heat or ultrasound therapy may be beneficial in enhancing their effects by decreasing heat loss and heat-induced edema.

Ultrasound causes cell vibrations, producing a deep heating effect without greatly increasing skin temperature. An intensity of 1.0 W/cm^2 has been found to be more effective than 0.5 or 1.5 W/cm^2 on lower leg flexor tendons of horses. Ultrasound therapy has been reported to increase healing rate of skin, muscle, ligaments, tendons, and bone. Magnetic therapy produced by a pulsating electromagnetic field appears to be of little benefit in increasing skin temperature.

Foot Injuries

Even in endurance racing, lameness is reported to be the most common reason for not finishing, with the foot being most commonly affected by the following injuries:

1. Sole bruises, corns, or subsolar hematoma due to trauma. These injuries can be detected as pain with hoof testers or by palpation, or as a red-brown discolored area.
2. Puncture wounds.
3. Demineralization of the third phalanx, or most distal bone of the leg, as a result of chronic bruising, persistent corns, founder, navicular disease, puncture wounds, or other causes of inflammation.
4. Laminitis, or founder, due to trauma.
5. Cracks in the hoof wall.

Two procedures, besides shoeing, that may be helpful in preventing these problems include:

1. Padded shoes, which should be filled between the pad and sole of the foot to prevent rocks from entering. Padded shoes help protect and decrease trauma to the sole, but may over time tend to weaken the horse's sole and hide disease conditions that may develop.
2. Protective boots used without regular shoes and which cover the entire foot. These may give better footing and traction and can be easily and repeatedly put on and taken off, but some may come off during competition.

Muscle Injuries

A common injury due to athletic performance in horses and people is muscle-tendon strain, commonly referred to as a pulled or torn muscle. This may occur anytime as a result of overexertion. It commonly occurs if the horse isn't fit, sufficiently warmed up, or allowed to or doesn't slow down when it becomes fatigued. Muscle inflammation, edema, and sometimes hemorrhage may occur and tendons may be involved. Damage is most often at the distal muscle-tendon junction and not in the muscle belly. In the horse, croup or caudal thigh muscle-tendon units are most commonly affected.

When croup muscles are affected, the horse may be stiff, drag its hind toes, and take short strides similar to horses with stifle problems. Caudal thigh-muscle damage may cause a hip hike or hoof slap gait similar to horses with

fibrotic myopathy. Pain is usually elicited by firm pressure over the area, which is warmer than nonaffected areas. A creatine phosphokinase (CPK) activity of 1000 to 30,000 IU/L 6 to 12 hours after training or competition is indicative of localized exercise-induced muscle damage, whereas levels above 50,000 IU/L are more indicative of generalized muscle damage such as with exertional myopathy.

Treatment of exertion-induced muscle injuries is directed at decreasing pain and enhancing healing while minimizing muscle atrophy and the formation of adhesions which may limit future muscle range of motion. Massage is helpful in accomplishing these objectives, and may be provided by hand, ultrasound, localized low-amperage electric current, or low-power cold lasers. Electric current stimulates nerve endings, causing muscle contraction. Although this helps decrease muscle edema and can prevent or break down muscle adhesions, contraction of damaged muscles may be painful; electric current must therefore be applied gently and with a low current. If the current is too strong, it may cause further damage and pain. With ultrasound, which is more commonly used, sound waves vibrate the muscle fibers, increase muscle temperature, and relax muscle tension, which may enhance healing. These effects may also be produced with low-power cold lasers which emit infrared spectrum light pulses. Regardless of how the muscle is massaged, nonsteroidal anti-inflammatory drugs are commonly administered. The horse with muscle damage initially should be rested and kept in a small paddock but not confined to a stall. When clinical signs are alleviated, the intensity but not duration of work should be greatly decreased from that prior to the injury, and long, slow warm-ups and cool-downs should be used. Several months are usually required for complete recovery, without which recurrence is common. Even in severely injured muscles, low-force exercise is indicated. Complete rest may prolong recovery, but excessive exertion increases the risk of additional injury.

Tendon and Ligament Injuries

Tendon and ligament injuries in horses are common with high-intensity sprint to middle-distance athletic activity (Table 11–1). In one survey it was found that 13% of competing racehorses suffered a tendon injury. The injury most frequently occurs during the latter part of a fast or strenuous workout or performance as the horse tires, and is most common in horses under-conditioned for the amount of exertion required. The role of inadequate fitness is emphasized by the finding that one-half of these injuries occur during the final stages of preparation for racing and in the first several races. Clinical signs of the injury often aren't apparent for 1 to 2 days or more afterwards.

Bowed tendon, or tendonitis, is one of the most common tendon and ligament injuries. The front legs, are most commonly affected, hind legs injuries also occur frequently. Swelling of the affected flexor tendons or ligaments and the surrounding soft tissue occurs, and can be detected on physical or ultrasonographic examination. The term bowed tendon refers to this swelling on the back side of the leg, below the knee or hock, which causes a "bowed out" appearance. Heat and pain upon palpation are usually evident. Lameness occurs in about one-half of affected horses. If injury is severe, an abnormal angulation of the leg, such as a dropped fetlock or subluxation of the pastern, may occur. Lameness without tendon or ligament swelling is generally not due to tendon or ligament injury. Ultrasonographic measurement of increased size and a relative loss of echogenicity of lesions compared to surrounding tendon tissue may indicate the presence of an injury before clinical signs occur, or the presence of an injury too mild to be clinically evident. This finding allows early rest and rehabilitation, thus minimizing the injury and the recovery period necessary.

Treatment of tendon or ligament injuries includes stall rest with hand walking, cold water hydrotherapy, application of ice and poultices, and administration of anti-inflammatory drugs. Although support wraps are also frequently used and may be beneficial in reducing edema formation after acute injury, they do not provide fetlock support during convalescence of injuries, nor do they assist in preventing injury by reducing strain, at least not that on the suspensory ligament during standing or walking. In contrast, strain on the suspensory ligament can be reduced most by cast support and about one-half as much by dorsal fetlock support splints. Increasing hoof wall angle is harmful for the treatment and prevention of suspensory ligament injuries.

Two to 3 months after most tendon and ligament injuries, walking and jogging for progressively longer periods of time can be initiated; doing so helps stimulate healing and increases tendon strength. The majority of horses can successfully return to competition if given adequate time for healing. Because the horse may appear clinically sound but still have substantial tendon or ligament injury, ultrasonographic evaluation may be helpful in indicating when healing is sufficient that rehabilitation, and later when use, can begin.

The more severe the injury, the longer required for recovery and the greater the chance of recurrence of the injury. Nearly one half of competing racehorses that develop bowed tendons have bowed previously. Although tendon strength increases with rest and healing following injury, it does not return to preinjury levels. At 6 months following injury, the tendon still contains a weaker type of collagen fibers. Even at 14 months, although normal collagen fibers are present, they are smaller in diameter than normal, resulting in decreased tendon strength. Surgical techniques to speed tendon healing and compensate for scar tissue inelasticity have had variable results.

Bone Stress Injuries

Athletic performance and training may result in stress-induced bone injuries. These occur when bones are subjected to repeated episodes or severity of stress that exceeds their ability to adapt to it. A program of gradually increasing stress is vital to allow bone remodeling for the prevention of bone stress injuries. Even short interruptions of one to several weeks in training increases the risk of stress-induced bone injury. Preventing this may require several weeks of training to bring the horse back to the same level of training it had before the interruption. Short-distance high-speed workouts two to three times weekly have been reported to be helpful in decreasing the incidence of one of the most common bone stress injuries—bucked shins.

Bucked Shins are due to microfractures and inflammation of the periosteal membrane covering the front of the foreleg cannon bones, or less often, those of hindlegs. Bucked shins occur in 70% of Thoroughbreds that begin race training. Other common sites affected by injuries of this type include the third carpal bone, the proximal and distal sesmoids, and the third phalanx. Less commonly, the distal femur and proximal humerus may be affected.

The incidence of bucked shins is about twice as high, and occurs with fewer miles of fast work training on a dirt track than on either a wood fiber surface or a grass (turf) track. The highest incidence of bucked shins occurs in 2 year-olds, after their first race, and most often, both legs are affected or the left front only (the leg on the inside of the turns). Susceptibility to bucked shins decreases with increasing maturity, during which time, bone size, stiffness, and strength are all increasing.

The characteristic history of bone stress injuries is leg pain, associated with repeated activity and relieved by rest. Over time the pain develops earlier and with increasing intensity resulting in acute or chronic single leg or bilateral lameness. If bilateral or multiple regions are affected, there may be a gradual onset of poor performance without obvious lameness. Focal tenderness, swelling and radiographic changes may or may not be evident. Affected horses usually exhibit pain on limb flexion or palpation of the affected bone. The most consistent and earliest means of diagnosis is scintigraphic studies (bone scans) indicating increased radioisotope uptake by the damaged bone, and also muscle.

The sooner stress-induced bone injuries are diagnosed and rest is instituted, the shorter the rehabilitation time necessary. Treatment most often given for bucked shins is cold therapy for the first 2 days, administration of an anti-inflammatory drug for 1 to 2 weeks, and reduced intensity, controlled exercise until soreness is gone, or preferably until scintigraphic bone scans are normal, which may require anywhere from 1 to 6 months. This should be followed by a gradual return to training, ideally with scintigraphic monitoring. Stall rest is not indicated unless lameness is severe, as rest will decrease bone remodeling and result in a recurrence of the condition as soon as exercise is resumed. Too rapid a return to too high a level of exercise will also result in recurrence.

Fractures of the first phalanx and the third metacarpal or cannon bone condyle are another common bone stress injury due to athletic performance. Often, the lameness fractures of the condyle it induces resolves with rest, providing it is diagnosed and rest provided before fracture displacement occurs. An external compression casting boot may provide adequate immobilization of the fetlock and prevent displacement of these fractures. It may be used both as an immediate post-injury external stabilization device and as a replacement for casting. It also is useful for the immobilization required for treatment of deep lacerations of the flexor tendons or suspensory apparatus, since it can be easily removed and reapplied allowing regular treatment of the wound.

Fractures of the Splint Bones (2nd and 4th metacarpal and metatarsal bones) are also relatively common in racehorses. Fractures of their distal portion usually occur as an acute exertional injury without the skin being broken. Generally they can be treated successfully by surgical removal of the fracture fragments with little effect on athletic ability. In contrast, fractures of the proximal portion of the splint bones is usually, but not always, caused by external trauma, with many bone fracture pieces and an open skin laceration. Swelling and lameness occur. Wound management and administration of a broad spectrum antimicrobial are usually necessary. Stall confinement may be adequate if the fracture doesn't involve the joint and isn't displaced. For others, open reduction and internal fixation are frequently necessary.

Carpitis and Carpal (Knee) Bone Fractures are also relatively common injuries of horses in sprint to middle-distance race training and competition, especially as they near competitive speeds for the first time, on dirt tracks or with unnatural shoeing. In contrast, they are uncommon in horses involved in other athletic activities. Training and subsequent strengthening of soft tissue support elements and the carpal bones help prevent their injury. If training proceeds faster than adaptation, carpitis, pain and lameness occur. This is commonly encountered early in training. Chip or slab fractures of the carpal bones may occur, particularly with sprint racing.

Carpitis-induced lameness is characterized by a bilateral stiff-legged paddling-type gait that minimizes knee flexion. A few weeks of reduced exercise, generally in conjunction with anti-inflammatory medication, when carpitis first begins is usually adequate. If exercise is not reduced, carpal fractures commonly occur and surgery will be required.

MANAGEMENT SUMMARY FOR ATHLETIC PERFORMANCE

For the horse in training or used for athletic performance the following factors are recommended:

1. Minimize respiratory dysfunction throughout the horse's life by always:
   a. maintaining the horse in a minimum-dust environment. Ensure proper stable ventilation (see Chapter 9) and feed only good-quality forage containing as little dust and as few fungal spores as possible (see Chapter 4).
   b. maintaining a good internal-parasite control program (see Chapter 9).
   c. maintaining a good vaccination program, particularly for influenza and rhinopneumonitis (see Chapter 9).

2. Have salt (preferably loose rather than block salt when sweat losses and, therefore, needs are high) and palatable good-quality water always readily available.

3. Have forage, like water and salt, available for the horse to eat all it wants without waste. At least 1 to 1.5 lbs of forage/100 lbs (1 to 1.5 kg/100 kg) body weight daily should be consumed. If the horse is not eating this amount, decrease the amount of grain fed. Depending on the amount of physical activity, generally from 3 to 9 lbs (1.5 to 4 kg) of grain should be fed. No more than 5 lbs (2.3 kg) of grain should be fed at a single feeding.

4. Adding up to 10% plant or vegetable oil to the total diet beginning at least 6 and preferably 10 weeks before athletic performance of any type may be of benefit. This may be done by adding 1 cup (8 oz) to each 2 to 3 lbs of grain fed (1 cup/2 lbs, or 250 ml/kg, of grain mix if 40% of the weight of the total diet is the grain mix, and 1 cup/3 lbs, or 167 ml/kg, of grain mix if 60% of the diet is a grain mix).

5. Each individual horse's optimal performance weight should be determined and maintained. For most horses, this is at moderate body condition as described in Table 1-4.

6. Dietary protein should be from 10 to 16% and other nutrient levels as given in Appendix Tables 1, 2, and 3, for working horses, those with frequent or excessive sweating, or in use and training for athletic performance. This may be done by feeding any cereal grain and either a grass or legume forage, whichever is available in the best quality with the least dust and fewest fungal spores.

7. Providing additional amounts of vitamins A, E, B_1 (thiamine), and the B vitamin folacin by adding a balanced vitamin supplement, such as that given in Table 3-5, to the grain mix may be beneficial. Adding (1 mg) of selenium (2 mg, of sodium selenite) to the horse's grain daily, or instead using a selenium-containing trace-mineralized salt as the only salt available, may also be of benefit.

8. Adding a good quality live yeast culture to the grain mix so that it constitutes 1% of the total diet may be beneficial. Thus, if grain constituted 40% of the diet, 1% divided by 0.40 or 2.5% yeast culture added to it would result in its constituting 1% of the total diet.

9. The following or similar training regimens to increase physical fitness should precede competitive performance:
   a. Begin by gradually increasing the intensity and duration of long slow distance (LSD) training, maintaining the heart rate at 140 to 150 bpm. Do this 5 days/week for at least 1 month, and longer for the young horse in its first year of training.
   b. Follow this by training specifically for the future competitive event desired. For example:
      (1) For middle-distance racing, run the horse at speeds that produce a heart rate of 190 to 210 bpm (about 3/4 speed) for 400 to 1000 yards or meters. Gradually increase from 2 sprints to 4 sprints per workout interspersed by walking, until the heart rate falls to 80 to 110 bpm. This should be done only every 3 to 4 days. On other days, trot and slow lope or canter the horse over a distance longer than the actual race distance anticipated.
      (2) For high-intensity speed or strength exertion, run the horse several times at near maximum

speed for a short distance (1 furlong, or 200 meters), allowing complete recovery to a heart rate of near 70 bpm in between each sprint. Do this once every 3 to 5 days depending on the individual horse's response to training. Use LSD workouts on the other days.

(3) For endurance racing, increase workouts from an initial 6 to 8 mi (10 to 13 km) to 10 mi (16 km) at 6 to 8 mph (10 to 13 kph) and a heart rate of 80 to 100 bpm 3 to 5 times/week. Occasionally speed may be increased sufficiently to increase the heart rate to 140 to 150 bpm for about 10 minutes. After the third month of training, once or twice a week include two, increasing to four, 40- to 60-second sprints to increase the heart rate to 180 to 210 bpm, followed by walking until the heart rate falls to 80 to 100 bpm.

c. During competition season, shorter-duration (e.g., one-half) but near competition-intensity workouts may be best.

10. The horse's heart rate at 1 and 5 minutes following, and ideally during, exercise should be monitored as an indication of fitness and of any problems. If the rates are above the preceding workouts of identical intensities for that horse, the horse should be examined for a cause of pain or respiratory dysfunction and workouts decreased or stopped until recovery.

11. Beginning 2 to 3 days before competitive performance and for 1 to 2 days afterward, feeding an additional 2 lbs (0.9 kg) of grain daily may be beneficial.

12. Ensure adequate time for recovery from transportation and new surroundings, feed, and water. Long-distance air travel is particularly stressful as it causes a disruption of an individual's biological clock or rhythm. In people this may result in weariness, occasional disorientation, and sometimes headaches and intestinal upsets. It seems likely that it would adversely affect some horse's performance. Because transportation stress varies between individuals and increases with increasing distance of transport, no specific time for recovery can be given. The horse should have a margin of 2 days after it is considered to have recovered from 7 or more hours of air transport before competition. However, trailering for up to 2.5 hours has been shown to have no affect on sprint racing times run immediately after trailering, and it did not differ, nor did indications of stress, whether the horse was facing forward or backward in the trailer. In contrast, others contend, but without supporting data, that having the horse face backward, or opposite to the direction of travel, is safer, more comfortable, less strenuous, and less stressful, and is preferred by the horse. In addition, most horses eat and drink poorly for a day or more when their surroundings are changed, even when their feed and water are not changed. The following procedures may help minimize this if it is a problem.

a. Add to the drinking water a small amount of vinegar, molasses, or other flavor that the horse prefers for several weeks before leaving home and then at new locations to mask changes in the taste of the water. However, even if this is done, or even without a water change, intake by most horses decreases the first day their surroundings are changed but increases the next day to compensate for the previous day's decrease.

b. Take feed from home, and gradually increase the proportion of the feed from the new location.

c. Don't add anything new to the diet for the first few weeks at a new location.

d. Clean nose-rubbing spots in the new stall, preferably with a phenolic disinfectant.

13. The night before and the day of athletic competition at maximum or near maximum exertion for several minutes or less (sprint and middle-distance races), don't feed any forage but allow free access to water. In contrast, for endurance-type athletic competition, allow and encourage the horse to eat all the forage and drink all the water, preferably cold, that it will at all times before and as often as practical during competition.

14. Giving 0.4 to 0.6 g/kg body weight of sodium bicarbonate (7 to 10 oz or about one half of a 1-lb box of baking soda/1100-lb or 500-kg horse) in several quarts (liters) of water by stomach tube 3 to 6 hours before maximum exertion of a few minutes or less, such as races of 1.5 miles (2400 m) or less, may be beneficial but may be illegal. Giving more than this or any at all prior to primarily aerobic or endurance type activity won't be beneficial and may be harmful.

15. Prior to a workout or competition of any type, warm the horse up for 10 to 20 minutes by walking for several minutes then slowly trotting for 8 to 15 minutes (shorter the higher the ambient temperature and humidity and the fleshier and poorer the condition of the horse). Warming the horse up stimulates a splenic contraction-induced increase in hematocrit and increases body temperature. Increasing body temperature 1°F (0.6°C) increases oxygen delivery to the muscle. Increased body temperature also increases fat mobilization and muscle neuroreceptor sensitivity and speed of impulse. Horses warmed up prior to exercise tend to have lower plasma lactate and higher free fatty-acid concentrations before and after exercise than horses not warmed up prior to exercise. Thus, the warmed-up horse has greater amounts of oxygen available to the tissue and/or increased fat utilization, both of which spare glycogen and decrease lactic acid production during exercise. Warming up is also beneficial, particularly for sprint-type activities, because it decreases exertion-induced damage to muscle fibers. Mechanical walkers are beneficial for warming the horse up and cooling it down but are probably of little benefit in training to enhance cardiovascular or muscle development.

16. Following a race or workout, the horse should be cooled down by walking for 1 to 2 minutes until it recovers its wind, then trotted slowly for 20 to 30 minutes, and finally walked for 10 to 30 minutes. This helps remove lactic acid from the muscle (Table 11–5) and as a result helps prevent post-exercise

muscle soreness. Muscle soreness decreases muscle strength and as a result performance.

17. Additional factors that may be of benefit for endurance-type activity include the following:

a. Four to 5 hours before endurance competition, feed 3 to 5 lbs (1.5 to 2 kg) of grain.

b. Feed 1 to 1.5 lbs (1 qt, or 0.5 to 0.7 kg) of sweet feed within 5 to 10 minutes before and every 1 to 2 hours during endurance competition. Water consumption or wetting the horse's mouth with water may be necessary, however, before the horse will eat. Horses salivate while chewing and cannot moisten their mouth at will as people can. Horses with a dry mouth will often stand playing with a wisp of forage in their mouth in an attempt to stimulate salivation and wetting of their mouth before they will eat.

c. If the temperature and humidity are high (°F + % are over 150), or the horse is not accustomed to a high temperature and humidity, giving water and electrolytes and cooling the horse in the following manner may be of benefit.

(1) Add 3 oz (85 g) of a mixture of equal parts common salt (sodium chloride) and "lite" salt (equal part sodium and potassium chloride) to each feeding of sweet feed fed as described in (b) above.

(2) If it is more than 1 to 2 hours between watering places, carry a couple of gallons (8 L) of water and, before each feeding of sweet feed and electrolytes, offer it to the horse. At least allow the horse to wet its mouth if dry to encourage consumption of the feed.

(3) Add 3 oz (85 g) of the salt mixture to the grain twice daily for 2 days following prolonged, profuse, or frequent sweating.

d. To encourage feed, electrolyte, and water consumption during competition, offer these nutrients during training workouts.

e. Cool the horse when practical with water (poured or sponged on, or ideally, sprayed in a fine mist) and, when possible, by standing the horse in the shade, water, and a breeze.

SELECTING THE EQUINE ATHLETE

Many different factors affect a horse's performance ability. Some of these can be assessed or measured before performance or maturity; some not until afterward. The results of any one or two of any of these factors is unlikely to be very indicative of performance ability. For example, a horse with major conformational faults is unlikely to be a top performer no matter how good all other factors are. Conversely, a perfect conformation is of little benefit for performance if the horse has a low respiratory-gas exchange ability, or a low cardiac output or heart capacity. Just as a chain is only as strong as its weakest link, the horse's performance will be limited by the poorest parameter that affects its performance ability. Thus, a horse with favorable values for all of the factors affecting performance ability is likely to be a better performer than one with

better values for some parameters but worse values for others. However, unlike a chain in which all of the links are of equal importance to its strength, there is a wide variation in the value or importance of the numerous factors necessary for athletic performance and, therefore, their effect on performance ability. The factors that appear to be the most important, that is, that have the highest correlation with the horse's racing performance, are: (1) conformation, (2) oxygen intake ability, (3) gait, (4) heart size and heart rate capacity, and (5) proportion of muscle fiber types in the hamstring muscles (middle gluteal muscle, which is the largest muscle of locomotion in horses and is active at all exercise intensities).

Because many of these and other factors important for performance ability are inherited to varying degrees, one of the most important selection criteria for performance ability, and the one most widely used, is the performance of the sire, dam, and most important, their offspring or progeny. Progeny information is probably the most relevant of all the information that can be compiled on a horse; no amount of pedigree information or the horse's own performance record is as indicative of a horse's potential for producing certain qualities in its progeny. For horses with no progeny record, the records of its close relatives, such as brothers or sisters or half-brothers or sisters, will give some indication of that horse's breeding potential. In horses, heritability of most traits of importance for athletic ability is quite high. As shown in Table 11–7, the heritabilities for speed and stride length are quite high and nearly identical, indicating their close relationship; i.e., speed depends to a great extent on stride length, which in turn depends to a great extent on the height and weight of the horse, the next highest heritability traits. Unfortunately, fertility heritability is quite low; fortunately, that has no effect on athletic performance.

There is of course no assurance that the factors that correlate with performance ability will be inherited by a specific individual, or that any individual won't be an outstanding performer even though there is little parental or sibling indication of that ability. However, the odds of outstanding athletic ability are certainly greatly increased by outstanding athletic performance of the dam, sire, and

TABLE 11–7
Estimation of Heritability Traits in Horses

Trait	Heritability*
Stride length	0.68
Speed	0.67
Height	0.61
Weight	0.57
Intelligence	0.53
Conformation	0.41
Fertility	0.10

* 1.0 would be a trait always inherited, and 0, a trait for which there is no relationship between its occurrence in parents and their offspring or progeny, i.e., a trait that may or may not occur in both, but does so entirely by chance.

their other progeny. This is well indicated by statistics on Thoroughbreds that indicate that regardless of pedigree, stakes winners bred to stakes winners produce 10 to 12% stakes winners, whereas stakes winners bred to non-stakes winners produce only 2 to 3% stakes winners, and non-stakes winners bred to non-stakes winners produce only 0.5 to 1% stakes winners. Statistics such as these are the basis for the old adage of "breed the best to the best and hope for the best," which is quite valid for the breeder. But once you have a live, healthy horse, many criteria are helpful in selecting which horses are most likely to be the best rather than just hoping for the best. The more of these criteria evaluated, the more indicative the results will be as to the horse's ability.

Conformation and oxygen intake ability are two of the most important criteria for a horse's athletic performance ability, and both can be evaluated readily without any equipment or specialized procedures.

One of, if not the most limiting factor to a horse's athletic ability appears to be its maximum oxygen intake capacity (VO_2max). Maximum oxygen intake capacity is highly reproducible within an individual horse, but there is more than a 50% variation between horses, indicating a wide range of aerobic capacity and, therefore, a means of determining differences in aerobic performance ability between horses. Although a horse's VO_2max can be measured, an indication of it can be determined much easier by assessing: (1) the width between the jaw bones within the throat latch, and (2) the degree of muscle wasting and loss of tone in the larynx caused by recurrent laryngeal neuropathy. A horse so afflicted by laryngeal neuropathy or hemiplegia as to have clinically evident symptoms is referred to as a "roarer" or "whistler" due to the noise it makes on inspiration during and following intense, often exhaustive exercise.

It's been stated that up to 95% of both Thoroughbreds and Standardbreds suffer varying degrees of recurrent-laryngeal neuropathy, and that 50% have a narrow throat; both qualities appear to be inherited. Laryngeal neuropathy occurs primarily in horses over 15-3 hands (160 cm) tall; it is rare in those less than 15-0 hands (152 cm). Both it and a narrow throat increase resistance to air movement, which decreases oxygen intake capacity, causing a decrease in oxygen in the blood and tissue during exertion. This not only decreases the muscles' ability to produce and utilize energy, thus impairing athletic performance, but it may also affect the brain, making the horse's decision to decrease performance more important to the horse than its desire to win. Although cerebral blood flow is maintained in short-duration moderate to severe exercise, with prolonged exhaustive exercise there is a pronounced blood vessel constrictive-induced decrease in blood flow to the brain, which would decrease cerebral oxygen availability unless there is a sufficient exercise-induced increase in blood oxygen content. Thus, an unobstructed supply of oxygen intake is a fundamental requirement for maximum racing performance.

Although even clinically affected horses with recurrent laryngeal neuropathy have no respiratory problems at rest, when exercising up to 10 times, but generally about 2.5 times, more effort is required to move air in and out of the lungs. Although increased expiratory effort may further interfere with respiratory gas exchange by causing exercise-induced pulmonary hemorrhage (EIPH), all or nearly all of the increased effort occurs during inspiration.

Recurrent laryngeal neuropathy is present at an early age, and its effects increase with age. A great majority of stakes winners are reported to be among the 5% of racehorses that have little or no recurrent laryngeal neuropathy and have exceptionally wide jaws. It's also been shown that 2-year-old Thoroughbreds with the best throats (least indications of laryngeal neuropathy and widest jaw) showed the most improvement as 3-year-olds; conversely, those with poor throats tended to show only marginal improvement or performed worse as 3-year-olds.

A diagnostic test that measures the response time, or latency of the laryngeal reflex, which is triggered by a gentle slap on the horse's back, can be measured by tiny electrodes placed at the larynx and recorded on a computer. This procedure has been developed as a means of grading the degree of recurrent laryngeal neuropathy. The greater the neuropathy, the longer the latency and the greater the impairment for respiratory gas exchange during exercise. A comparison between right and left sides of the larynx may also be helpful, as the less laryngeal neuropathy present, the closer they are to equal and the shorter their latency times for this reflex. Because recurrent laryngeal neuropathy is present at birth or soon after, this test permits early detection of the degree of impairment. This test is also useful for the diagnosis of cervical vertebral malformation or wobblers' syndrome, which causes the complete loss of the laryngeal reflex on both the left and the right sides. A portable unit for measuring this reflex is available (Electrolaryngograph, General Analysis, Inc., Jeffersonville, PA 19403).

The most common treatment for recurrent laryngeal neuropathy in the past has been surgical removal of the linings of the laryngeal ventricles (roaring operation or laryngeal ventriculectomy) with the expectation that, when they heal, the resulting scar tissue will pull the vocal cords out, increasing airway size and correcting the fault. In the majority of cases this doesn't occur, but it does decrease the roaring noise. More recently, a laryngeal prosthetic operation (or laryngoplasty) to tie the left arytenoid cartilage back out of the way is used; it does improve air flow and pressures to near normal. A new procedure using nerve-muscle pedicle grafts to repair the diseased nerve has been developed and may alleviate the impairment with minimal postoperative complications.

Heart strength and size are also important factors for athletic performance; the longer the race or duration of athletic performance, the more important they become. The maximum heart rate is an indication of heart strength. The more a horse can increase its heart rate, the greater its athletic ability. A horse's maximum heart rate closely correlates with its maximum oxygen intake capacity (VO_2max) and how fast it can run.

It also has been shown that there is a significant correlation between increasing heart size and both middle-distance and endurance racing, but not sprint, performance. Although heart size, like other performance selection criteria, is only one aspect of a particular system and, therefore, by itself may not be indicative of performance ability, a large heart or heart score is one of many factors necessary for top physical performance. An indication of heart size can be determined by heart score and by echocardiography.

Heart score is measured from a horse's electrocardiogram (EKG). However, an accurate measurement is difficult to obtain and is one reason for sometimes disappointing results. Heart size and left ventricular scores can best be measured directly by echocardiography.

Inborn gait characteristics appear to be a major factor in determining a horse's speed ability. Gait analysis, which includes the timing of gait, the overlap of stance phases, and the stride frequency and length at various speeds, can be measured by video or cinematic techniques. Computer analysis of this data can be used to characterize the horse's gait. This done at 12 to 14 months of age currently appears to some to be the single most promising selection method criterion indicative of future racing performance, although this has yet to be confirmed. Gait analysis, however, like muscle-fiber typing analysis, requires individuals and laboratories experienced in and doing these specialized techniques.

As shown in Table 11–2, breeds that excel at endurance-type activity (Heavy hunters and Arabians) have 20 to 30% and some over 40% slow-twitch muscle fibers (Type I, which have long contraction duration ability), as compared to only 6 to 10% in Quarter Horses, who have a greater percentage of fast-twitch muscle fibers (Type IIB, which have explosive strength but short contraction duration ability). Quarter Horses are a breed bred and raised for their ability to run a short distance (one-quarter of a mile or 400 meters) very fast, but are not known for their endurance ability. Thus, horses with the greatest proportion of slow-twitch fibers would be expected to be the best endurance-type athletes, and those with the greatest proportion of fast-twitch low-oxidative fibers, the best sprint-type athletes. However, there appears to be little correlation between the proportion of fiber types and the horse's athletic ability at different types of events. But a horse with 40% slow-twitch muscle fibers will never be a sprinter of much consequence, and, conversely, one with only 8% slow-twitch fibers will never be an endurance athlete of much consequence, regardless of how good their other athletic parameters may be.

The reasons there is a poor correlation between the proportion of different muscle fiber types and the horse's ability at different types of events lie in the numerous other factors that are of greater importance, including airway opening size, desire to win, heart size and capacity, and anatomic proportions and coordination. The desire to win is difficult to assess prior to competition. However, indications of airway opening size and anatomic parameters affecting the horse's gait can be evaluated as described above. These appear to be such major factors in determining ability to run that they supersede the importance of muscle-fiber distribution.

An additional factor worth considering in selecting a horse for either athletic performance or show activity is its sex. If they are not to be used for breeding purposes, geldings and even spayed (bilateral ovariectomized) mares are sometimes preferred to eliminate undesirable sexual activity behavior and aggressiveness. However, extreme aggression exhibited by mares toward other horses or people is rarely corrected by spaying. But decreasing estrus behavior is generally beneficial for both athletic and show performance because it promotes more consistent behavior. Following spaying, some mares maintain mild, but generally not objectionable, signs of estrus. The surgery may be performed either through the vaginal wall or the abdominal wall. The vaginal approach may reduce postoperative recovery time and expense. An alternative to spaying to minimize estrus behavior, yet to retain the mare's future reproductive ability, is the continual oral administration of progestins. This practice is fairly expensive over a long term.

SUPPLEMENTAL READING RECOMMENDATIONS

Equine Fitness: The Care and Training of the Athletic Horse by Drs. DH Snow and CJ Vogel. (Publisher: David & Charles, Inc., North Pomfret VT 05053, 1987; 270 pp, 6 × 9 inches.) An excellent book on this topic. Both authors are veterinarians, Dr. Snow being one of the world's leading researchers and authorities on equine exercise physiology, and Dr. Vogel, a practitioner involved in the application and use of this research. As a result, although not a referenced text, the material covered is factual, relevant, applicable, and described in an understandable, logical, easily read manner. All of these attributes are in direct contrast to much that is written and many books on these topics. Coverage of feeding and nutrition is minimal and relatively superficial; however, coverage of other topics is good and includes: anatomy, movement, and energy utilization; the musculoskeletal, cardiovascular, respiratory, and temperature regulatory systems; training, and drugs, with all emphasizing athletic performance by the horse. Because it is written for the nonveterinarian, or the individual without a knowledge of physiology, it contains much information well known by those with a knowledge of physiology, but it relates this information to the equine athlete and contains much information of interest and benefit to all who own, care for, or are involved in conducting research on horses used for athletic performance.

The Fit Racehorse by Tom Ivers, (Esprit Racing Team, Ltd., P.O. Box 38206, Cincinnati, OH 45238, 1983, 300 pp, 6 × 9 ½ inches. This is the classic on interval training by someone who has and does make his living training racehorses. It should be read by all who own or are involved with the care or use of horses for athletic performance. Before embracing interval training, it is best to be familiar with what is given in Drs. Snow and Vogel's book (described above). The authors' brash and outspoken style makes the book quite enjoyable and often humorous, which enhances and emphasizes much important and useful information quite well. Mr. Ivers correctly debunks, and in contrast to many, adds little to the multitude of myths involved with feeding, caring for, and using horses, some of which are so old they are widely repeated, accepted, and used with little evidence supporting them, and even when, for some of these myths, there is extensive evidence refuting them. Generally, it is not so much that those that practice and perpetuate these myths refute this evidence, but instead that they are simply not familiar with it. Books such as those by Drs. Snow and Vogel and Mr. Ivers, as well as this book, are of help in increasing awareness of what is or is not supported by currently available evidence.

"**Adams' Lameness in Horses**" edited by Dr. Ted S. Stashak is a (Williams & Wilkins, Baltimore, MD, 1-800-638-0672), 906-page, 8 ½ × 11 inch, 4th edition, 1987 book. This is the classic on this topic written by some of the foremost experts on each topic covered. It covers causes, treatment, and diagnosis of lameness as a result of not only athletic performance, which are summarized only in this text, but also numerous other causes of lameness, as well as functional anatomy of locomotion, the relationship between conformation and lameness, foot trimming and shoeing, gaits and methods of therapy.

For veterinary judging of equine endurance events, see the **American Association of Equine Practitioner's Annual Proceedings,** pages 793 to 843 (1991) and their "**Guide for Veterinary Service and Judging of Equestrian Events**" (1991), and the "**AERC Veterinarian's Handbook**" (1982) from the American Endurance Ride Conference, Auburn, CA.

Chapter 12

BREEDING STALLION FEEDING AND CARE

Feeding Breeding Stallions 224
Exercise for Breeding Stallions 224
Breeding Evaluation of Stallions 224
Breeding Stallion Usage 225

Castration 226
Masturbation 226
Supplemental Reading Recommendations 227

FEEDING BREEDING STALLIONS

The same feeding programs given in Chapter 10 for idle and working horses apply to breeding stallions. Breeding does not require an increase in any nutrient except those needed for energy. The increased energy needed for the act of breeding itself is small. However, the increased physical activity that may be associated with breeding, such as pacing and nervousness, increases dietary energy needs by an average of one fourth to one third above that needed by the idle horse for maintenance (Appendix Table 4). The amount of increase is variable among individuals, but varies little with the number of mares bred. The proper amount to feed is that necessary to maintain a moderate body condition (Table 1–4).

During breeding season, some stallions' appetite may be reduced, and weight loss may occur. Feeding a diet high in quality, palatability, and energy density, and if possible turning the stallion out on green grass pasture for at least a few hours daily, will help prevent this. Up to a maximum of 0.75 lbs/100 lbs body wt (0.75 kg/100 kg) daily of a grain mix containing molasses, high-energy-dense grains such as corn, and even to 10 to 20% added fat or oil if necessary may be fed. However, the amount of grain mix fed and/or its energy density should be reduced if the stallion becomes too high-spirited to handle, or if its body condition increases above moderate. More often, most stallions' body weight decreases a few percent during breeding season.

The breeding stallion should be fed a diet similar in nutrient content to that of the exercised or working horse (Appendix Tables 1, 2, and 3). Vitamin C and E supplements are occasionally used to enhance the stallion's reproductive performance or ability. However, numerous studies have shown that giving vitamins C or E, even in large doses, is of no benefit for this purpose, as described in sections on these vitamins in Chapters 2 and 3. If feeding a vitamin supplement is desired, or if one wishes to ensure that the stallion's diet contains a sufficient amount of all vitamins for optimum health and reproductive ability, giving a balanced vitamin supplement providing additional quantities of all vitamins without excessive amounts of any, such as described in Table 3–5, is best. Giving a vitamin supplement of this type may be beneficial in some situations, as described in Chapter 3, and even if not needed will not be harmful.

EXERCISE FOR BREEDING STALLIONS

Most have considered exercise helpful in maintaining the breeding stallion's appetite and libido. Although exercise increases feed consumption, even moderate, nonfatiguing exercise has been shown to decrease the stallion's libido. The exercised stallion, however, is easier to handle and displays less excessive energy when taken from its stall.

Decreasing or eliminating exercise is unlikely to transform a stallion with poor libido into one with excellent libido. However, less sexually aggressive stallions' libido may gradually increase over a period of time by decreasing or eliminating regular exercise, and by increasing their dietary energy intake, providing these procedures don't result in excess body weight or condition. Conversely, hard-to-handle stallions may become easier to control if placed on a regular exercise program and if their dietary energy intake is decreased.

BREEDING EVALUATION OF STALLIONS

The breeding stallion should be evaluated for breeding soundness: (1) before purchase, (2) before each breeding season, (3) to estimate the number of breedings or inseminations that can be made during a season, (4) anytime lowered fertility is suspected, (5) anytime it would be desirable to increase the number of mares to be bred, (6) when abnormal sexual behavior is observed, and (7) when the stallion is suspected of harboring a potential disease-producing organism. In addition, the stallion's reproductive performance should be monitored continuously with respect to the percentage of pregnancies per service, number of breedings or inseminations per pregnancy, and pregnancy rate (%) by month and by cycle.

At least two ejaculates of semen collected with an artificial vagina 1 hour apart should be evaluated for semen quality; or, to determine daily sperm output, an ejaculate obtained once daily for 7 to 8 days should be evaluated. After 3 to 7 days, spermatozoa reserves are depleted and sperm output becomes stable at the quantity that stallion is capable of producing. Sperm output is normally about 50% lower in the second than in the first ejaculate taken 1 hour apart; it is also lower in semen obtained during the winter than in that obtained during late spring and summer. The number of spermatozoa produced is helpful in predicting the number of mares that can be booked to that stallion if artificial insemination is being used. In contrast to what many stud managers believe, the volume of ejaculate doesn't affect fertility; it is instead the number of sperm in that ejaculate, which is unrelated to semen volume. Also in contrast to common belief, a stallion's sexual behavior, or speed and vigor of mounting and copulation, is not indicative of his fertility.

In addition to semen evaluation, total scrotal width should be measured and testicular tone evaluated. The number of spermatozoa that a stallion is capable of producing is directly related to the size of the testes. The average total scrotal width of normal stallions of light horse breeds of all ages, taken early in the spring, is 85 to 130 mm (3¼ to 5 inches). If the scrotal width is less than 80 mm (3⅛ inches), it is recommended that the stallion not be used even though its seminal characteristics are normal. Stallions with small testes are potentially poor producers of spermatozoa, and testicular size is probably highly heritable, as it is in other species. Breeding a stallion that has one testicle not in the scrotum also is not recommended, as this characteristic may be heritable. Stallions with both testicles retained are not fertile. Those with a retained testicle sooner or later often exhibit abnormal sexual behavior.

In addition to size, testicular consistency or tone is important. A stallion with either soft mushy or excessively hard testes is potentially a poor producer of spermatozoa and generally has abnormal seminal characteristics. Abnormal testicular tone can indicate testicular degeneration or fibrosis. However, stallions may have testes of normal size and consistency and yet not produce any viable spermatozoa. Thus, some type of seminal evaluation must be performed if fertility is to be ensured. In addition, swabs of the stallion's urethra, urethral diverticulum, prepuce, and semen should be checked for blood and potential disease-producing bacteria. If any are present, the stallion should not be used for breeding. Blood in the semen makes it sterile and is most often due to bacteria-induced inflammation of the urethra, trauma, or habronemiasis ("summer sores") on the urethral process. A couple of weeks of sexual rest and broad-spectrum antibiotic administration is generally successful in alleviating bacterial inflammation of the urethra. In those that don't respond, surgery may be indicated.

BREEDING STALLION USAGE

Spermatozoa first appear in a stallion's ejaculate at 11 to 15 months of age, and stallions may be put into breeding service as young as 2 to 3 years of age. However, spermatozoa production, but not fertility of the spermatozoa produced, is generally lower the younger the stallion. Fertility evaluations should be done on all stallions to determine how the stallion and/or its semen should be used to obtain maximum reproductive efficiency. Regardless of semen quality, young horses should be used sparingly as overuse may lead to poor breeding behavior and/or disinterest. Although the percentage of live foals born per breeding season decreases as the age of mature mares increases, the age of the mature breeding stallion appears to have no effect on the live-foal percentage, which averages 58% in Thoroughbreds.

Anabolic steroids or testosterone should not be given to stallions that are to be used for breeding. These androgens decrease sperm production and have no beneficial effect. Restoration of normal sperm production requires a minimum of 2 months following cessation of their administration and, in many instances, may require considerably longer. Administration of androgens will not restore potency of impotent stallions. In addition, androgen administration can result in decreased liver function and premature closure of bone growth plates in young horses, thus decreasing their mature size. They do not promote an increase in the growth, muscling, or performance of the horse in good condition, even though these are the reasons for which they are generally given.

The stallion is limited by both its sex drive and its spermatozoa production in the number of mares it can effectively breed. Breeding too frequently will deplete the number of spermatozoa and, therefore, reproductive efficiency, but in contrast to popular belief, doesn't result in the ejaculation of immature spermatozoa or a reduction in the fertility of individual spermatozoa. Since spermatozoa production by the normal stallion is a relatively continuous process unaffected by ejaculation frequency or semen removal, if a stallion must be used several times a day, it is best to space the breedings evenly over time. This will give the last mare bred the maximum opportunity to conceive. However, for most stallions, sex drive is more limiting than spermatozoa production. Once sexually satiated, the stallion may refuse to breed or may exhibit abnormal sexual behavior. Most mature stallions can be used for breeding once daily 6 days a week, or twice a day 3 to 4 days a week. The sex drive of a "well-adjusted" stallion will generally remain as high on a daily breeding or collection schedule as on a schedule of once per week.

For breeding, most stallions normally approach a receptive mare with a flexed, extended, trotting-type gait while making repeated throaty sounds. He smells the mare's perineum and shows flehmen or flaring (fully extends his head and neck, contracts his nostrils, raises the upper lip and takes shallow breaths). Usually, after repeatedly nipping the mare's hindquarters and sides for several minutes, the penis is fully erect. Most stallions will then make one to three false mounts without foreleg gripping of the mare's flanks or pelvic thrusting movements before intromission is attempted. When the stallion is securely mounted, repeated thrusting pelvic movements are made to locate the mare's vulva and achieve intromission. Once intromission is attained, the head is lowered so the mouth rests against the mare's crest or alongside her neck. Biting of these areas may occur. In some cases this can be severe. After several pelvic thrusts, ejaculation begins, usually 10 to 15 seconds after intromission. Pelvis thrusting stops just before ejaculation and commonly tail flagging occurs (a series of up and down motions). About 30 seconds after copulation began, most stallions have achieved ejaculation and dismount.

A frightening early or repeated experience, such as falling because of slippery footing, banging the head on something overhead when breeding indoors, or pain such as from a severe kick from a mare or excessive roughness or discipline during breeding or teasing, may reduce the stallion's libido or make him afraid to mount and copulate. If this occurs, patient training, often with a change in handlers, breeding site, and/or methods used, which allow the stallion to breed without being hurt or frightened, will usually resolve the problem. However, stallions should be trained so that they do not endanger people or the mare.

During teasing, the young stallion should be allowed to be more aggressive than normal. After he learns how to breed mares, overaggressiveness can be corrected. Continuous teasing of mares, without the stallion's being allowed to breed, results in a decline in most stallions' sexual arousal and response in about 2 weeks.

For maximum use of a stallion in an artificial insemination program, with a minimum amount of labor, it is recommended the stallion be collected every other day and that all mares in standing heat for 2 days or longer be inseminated. More frequent collections will not increase the number of spermatozoa obtained as only so many are produced and available, and the number produced is not altered by ejaculation or collection frequency. It is recommended that at least 400 to 500 million progressively motile spermatozoa be used per insemination. The first ejaculate of fertile stallions contains an average of $12 \pm 9 (\pm SD)$ billion spermatozoa, of which about $55 \pm 15\%$ are progressively motile. Thus, the average fertile stallion's first ejaculate contains sufficient spermatozoa to breed 12 to 20 mares, but may contain substantially more or less depending on the stallion, the frequency of ejaculation, and the time of the year.

Testicular size and sperm output, but not motility, are significantly affected by the time of year. Total scrotal width, seminal volume, and number of sperm per ejaculation increase 15 to 20%, 40%, and 50%, respectively, from mid-winter to late spring and summer. Since the number of spermatozoa per ejaculate is the most important seminal characteristic in relation to fertility, with the possible exception of motility, semen obtained early in the breeding season is only about one-half as good as that obtained during peak normal breeding season. But, since season doesn't affect the percentage of progressively motile spermatozoa or their chemical characteristics, on a per sperm basis season probably doesn't affect fertility. However, because fewer spermatozoa are produced, and because sex drive is lower from fall to spring, fewer mares can be bred during this time. Plasma testosterone and total androgen concentrations, and libido in the stallion are lowest in the winter and highest in the spring. As with mares, artificial light beginning an hour before sunset to increase total light to 16 hours daily beginning 2 to 3 months before the desired breeding season will increase the stallion's fertility (both the spermatozoa per ejaculate and libido), but the effects are less pronounced than in the mares. If most mares are to be bred by natural service early in the season and are put under artificial lighting, it may be worthwhile to do the same for the stallions.

CASTRATION

There are many reasons for castrating stallions. Geldings are easier to care for and haul, less prone to injury, and may be kept with other horses. Some stallions' physical performance also tends to be or become lazy or inconsistent. Stallions are also castrated to alleviate objectionable sexual behavior and aggression. Postpubertal castration is effective in eliminating this behavior toward people in 60 to 70% of the cases, and toward horses in 40% of the cases.

The colt can be castrated anytime from birth on, when the testicles are descended into the scrotum. Both testes should be descended into the scrotum from 30 days before to 10 days after birth. Starting at about 12 months of age, the testes grow and develop rapidly and begin to produce spermatozoa. The stallion is, of course, incapable of reproduction before this age. Puberty is generally reached around 18 months of age.

Tetanus toxoid should be given and sweet clover hay or haylage not fed for 2 to 5 weeks before castration. The newly gelded horse may be allowed with mares 1 week following castration without fear of his successfully breeding a mare. It is unlikely that pregnancy will occur in a mare bred by a former stallion after the first 2 days following his castration. The occurrence or number of, ejaculations following castration does not appear to hasten the disappearance of spermatozoa from the ejaculate and, therefore, does not change this recommendation. Stallion behavior or libido usually subsides in 4 to 6 months but may last for a year.

From 20 to 30% of geldings continue to exhibit stallion-like aggressive behavior toward other horses, and 5% show this behavior toward people. It has been thought that this occurs if improper castration (referred to as a "proud cut, rig or false rig" horse) leaves residual tissue thought to produce testosterone (epididymis and sufficient vas deferens), because the resulting testosterone produced would induce this behavior; however, this theory has been disproved. The epididymis does not produce testosterone or play a role in the maintenance of sex drive. It has been found that about one half of horses with male sex drive in the absence of testes in the scrotum do not have elevated plasma testosterone levels and, therefore, testes; whereas the other one-half do, indicating that they are cryptorchids with a retained testicle in the inguinal canal or abdominal cavity. The retained testicle produces testosterone, causing the stallion-like behavior even though it does not produce viable sperm and, therefore, won't impregnate a mare. The cryptorchid horse can be detected by finding an elevated plasma testosterone or estrone sulphate concentration, and its stallion-like behavior can be corrected by removing the testis. However, in others, stallion-like behavior is maintained without a testis and with very low plasma testosterone concentrations. Only time and training may be of benefit in alleviating stallion-like behavior in these geldings.

MASTURBATION

Stallions and some geldings masturbate by bringing the erect penis into contact with the abdomen and thrusting repeatedly. It has been assumed, although there is little data to support this assumption, that masturbation by the stallion depletes semen reserves and sexual energy, thus limiting fertility. As a result, an array of management schemes and devices such as brushes, cages, and stallion rings, which slip over the head of the penis and prevent erection, have been employed to prevent masturbation. However, studies indicate that masturbation is normal behavior, may occur shortly following breeding, and should not be discouraged in horses. Spontaneous erection and masturbation also occurs in geldings, but at about one-half the frequency as in stallions. It is reported to occur with equal frequency and duration in stallions with various levels of libido and breeding activity, and in both free-roaming bachelor, solitary, and harem stallions, as well as intensively managed stabled stallions. It appears to reflect contentment rather than frustration or boredom. Ejaculations occur in less than 1% of observed episodes of masturbation by stallions.

Some contend that there is little evidence supporting the notion that masturbation is associated with or leads to infertility in stallions, or in any way impairs the health or performance of horses. However, some report that there have been stallions in which frequent masturbation and ejaculation were associated with low libido and fertility, and that some of these may show improvement in fertility and breeding behavior when masturbation is prevented by using a stallion ring. However, in general, there appears to be no relationship between fertility and occurrence or frequency of masturbation. In addition, stallion rings may cause damage to the penis, resulting in blood in the semen, which makes it infertile. As a result, stallion rings are not recommended.

SUPPLEMENTAL READING RECOMMENDATIONS

Equine Reproduction by Drs. Angus McKinnon and James L. Voss (Lea & Febiger, Malvern, PA 19355-9725, PA 1992). One of the most current books and the best information available on this topic. A comprehensive coverage of the diagnoses and treatment of reproductive disorders in the mare and stallion.

Diseases and Management of Breeding Stallions by Dickson Varner, James Schumacher, Terry Blanchard and others. (American Veterinary Publications, Goleta, California 93117). A 349-page referenced text which gives a detailed review of reproductive anatomy and physiology, a step-by-step explanation of management of breeding stallions, semen handling, and preservation, castration, sexual behavior, and diseases of breeding stallions. The information given closely follows and expands on the Society for Theriogenology's "Manual for Clinical Fertility Evaluation of the Stallion."

Management of the Stallion for Maximum Reproductive Efficiency, II by BW Pickett, RP Amann, AO McKinnon, EL Squires, and JL Voss. (Animal Reproduction and Biotechnology Laboratory, Colorado State University, Fort Collins, CO 80523, USA, 1989). An excellent 126-page booklet containing some of the best information from one of the leading equine reproduction research centers. However, it like the booklet recommended below, it is at times frustrating reading because of its lengthy descriptions of the procedures and results of a multitude of individual research studies. It covers 1. anatomy and physiology, 2. spermatogenesis, 3. testicular size, 4. age, 5. frequency of ejaculation, 6. sexual behavior, 7. effect of anabolic steroids, 8. seminal characteristics of normal and abnormal stallions, and 9. hemospermia.

Procedures for Collection, Evaluation and Utilization of Stallion Semen for Artificial Insemination by BW Pickett, EL Squires, and AO McKinnon (Animal Reproduction Laboratory, Colorado State University, Fort Collins, CO 80523, 1987). In addition to the collection and evaluation of semen, this 125-page booklet covers temperature effects; mechanics of artificial insemination (AI); effects of and frequency of AI on fertility; duration of estrus effect on fertility; influence of AI volume and sperm number on fertility; effect of seminal extender, storage time, and temperature on fertility; semen freezing; bacterial control in semen; and physical facilities, supplies, and equipment for AI.

Chapter 13

BROODMARE FEEDING AND CARE

Vaccination and Internal-Parasite Control Programs for Broodmares	229
Feeding Broodmares	230
Feeding Nonlactating Mares Not in Their Last Trimester of Pregnancy	232
Feeding Mares During the Last Trimester of Pregnancy and Lactation	232
Nutrition Effects on Mare Reproduction	232
Dietary Protein and Energy Effects on Reproduction	232
Vitamin and Mineral Effects on Reproduction	233
Nutrition Effects on Mare's Milk Production and Composition	234
Nutrition Problems in Broodmares	234
Mare's Estrous Cycle	235
Estrous Cycle Inducement of Mares	237
Prebreeding Examination of Mares	237
Breeding Mares	237
Foal-Heat Breeding	238
Diagnosing Pregnancy and Fetal Viability in Mares	238
Abortion Inducement in Mares	239
Twinning in Mares	240
Supplemental Reading Recommendations	241

Like all horses, but particularly critical for broodmares and breeding farms, records should be kept on each mare. As described in Chapter 9, these records should be complete and thorough, but not overly complicated or detailed. If the records are not easy to use, they won't be kept up and, as a result, will be of little use. But the records must be sufficiently complete to indicate where each mare is in her reproductive cycle; what has been done, by whom, and with what results; and what needs to be done, by whom, and when. Maximum reproductive results and health of the mares and their foals cannot be obtained with anything less. Breeding records, teasing and palpation records, and health records are necessary to attain maximum productivity. Breeding records should include mare identification, breeding dates and to whom, health comments, and expected and actual foaling dates. Health records should identify the date and description of all health care.

Well-managed breeding farms should attain or exceed the following reproduction parameters.

1. A foaling rate (percentage of live foals born) of 70 to 80% in mares bred or on pasture with a stallion.
2. Estrous cycles per conception of 1.43 or less.
3. A 45-day pregnancy rate of 88 to 97%.
4. A pregnancy loss below 13%.

Mares have the lowest reproductive efficiency of domestic farm animals, with only 55 to 60% of those bred annually in the United States producing live foals. The major reasons for this low reproductive performance are poor reproductive management, uterine infections, and irregular estrous cycles. Many things can be done to alleviate these factors and thus improve the mare's reproductive performance.

VACCINATION AND INTERNAL-PARASITE CONTROL PROGRAMS FOR BROODMARES

As described in Chapter 9, optimum vaccination and parasite control programs for broodmares, as for all horses, vary according to regional and farm disease prevalence, economics, and managerial practices and preferences. The goal is to prevent infections and parasitic diseases not only in the mares but also in their foals. This is accomplished by maximizing colostral antibodies and minimizing internal parasites passed to the foal.

Generally all broodmares should be given tetanus toxoid before breeding, and rhinopneumonitis (EHV) killed-virus vaccine at the 5th, 7th, and again at the 9th month of pregnancy, at which time influenza, encephalomyelitis, and another tetanus toxoid injection should be given. In endemic areas or on farms previously affected, giving the broodmare the following vaccines 1 to 2 months before foaling may be beneficial and should be considered: (1) strangles (Streptococcus equi), (2) Clostridium perfringens, to prevent septicemia in newborn foals, (3) Salmonella typhimurium, (4) equine monocytic ehrlichiosis (Potomac horse fever), and (5) Clostridium botulinum type-B or botulism toxoid to prevent shaker foal syndrome. Botulism toxoid should initially be given three times 1 to 3 weeks apart with the last dose 2 to 4 weeks before expected foaling. A single annual booster vaccination is adequate in subsequent years. Anthrax and rabies vaccinations are not recommended for pregnant mares.

In addition to vaccination for immunization against infectious diseases, the mare should be on the farm and in the area where she will foal no later than 1 month prior to her expected foaling date. This allows her to be exposed to, and thus develop an immunity against, infectious organisms in that environment. As a result, the foal can obtain through the mare's colostrum a passive immunity against these potentially disease-producing organisms.

For internal-parasite control, the mare should be on the same control program as the other mature horses on that farm, as described in Chapter 9. Most dewormers may be safely given to pregnant mares. However, benzimidazole dewormers are not recommended during the first trimester of pregnancy. Organophosphate dewormers, carbon disulfide, or purgatives are not recommended past midgestation as they can induce abortion. It is common practice not to deworm mares during the last 1 to 2 months of pregnancy to avoid the deworming from being blamed for any problems encountered in the mare at foaling or in the

TABLE 13–1
Feeding Programs for Broodmares

Type of Forage Consumed	Amount of Grain Mix Needed (lbs/100 lbs body wt/day)[a]	Salt-Mineral Mix Preferred
Nonlactating mares before last trimester of pregnancy:		
Any type of average or better-quality forage (≥8% protein)	0	Trace-mineralized salt
Last trimester and during lactation:		
Legume, e.g., alfalfa	0	Salt + calcium + phosphorus[b]
Grass, green or early cut (≥11% protein)	0	Salt + calcium + phosphorus[b]
Mature grass hay or pasture (<11% protein)	0.5 to 1[c]	Trace-mineralized salt

[a] Or kg/100 kg body weight/day needed when all of the forage the mare will eat is available and she is at or above moderate body condition (Table 1–4); if she isn't, sufficient grain should be fed so ideally she is moderately fleshy at foaling time. If necessary, sufficient grain should also be fed to ensure that she doesn't lose weight during lactation.
[b] Containing 8 to 16% of both calcium and phosphorus, such as equal parts of trace-mineralized salt and dicalcium phosphate (Appendix Table 7). Feed as the only salt available or add 3 to 4 oz (90 to 120 g) daily to a grain mix. From 5 to 10% dry molasses may be added to the mineral mix to increase its free-choice consumption.
[c] A grain mix containing at least 16% protein, 0.8% calcium, and 0.6% phosphorus should be fed, e.g., as given in Table 4–10.

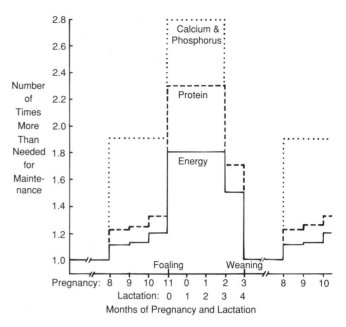

Fig. 13–1. Broodmares' nutritional needs.

foal. In addition to being on the regular farm deworming program, foaling mares should be given deworming medication the day of, or within a few days after, foaling and before they join other mares and foals. Threadworms (Strongyloides westeri), which are passed to the foal in the mare's milk and cause respiratory and intestinal damage, can be prevented by giving an effective dewormer (e.g., an avermectin) to the mare the day of foaling and to the foal at 2 to 3 weeks of age (see Chapter 9).

FEEDING BROODMARES

Mares are classified as maiden (never bred), as barren (never pregnant), pregnant or in foal, and as lactating. Their nutritional needs can be met using the two feeding programs summarized in Table 13–1. Feeding of maiden and barren mares is the same as for other nonpregnant, nonlactating horses. The other feeding program needed is for mares during their last 3 months of pregnancy and throughout lactation, during which time the amount of feed needed increases and then should be decreased in preparation for weaning.

Embryonic development and fetal growth require no additional nutrients through the first 8 months of pregnancy. Nutritional needs are the same as for the nonpregnant nonlactating horse. But fetal growth greatly accelerates during the last 3 months of pregnancy, increasing the mare's nutrient requirements. Her requirements are further increased during milk production. The mare's dietary energy needs increase progressively 10 to 20% during the last trimester of gestation and 80% during lactation (Appendix Table 4). As a result, mares will eat more if the feed is

available. If more feed or energy is not consumed, this may decrease her milk production and reproductive efficiency as described later in this chapter. However, simply feeding more may not be adequate. As depicted in Figure 13-1, the amount of additional protein, calcium, and phosphorus needed for fetal development and milk production is greater than the amount of additional energy needed. As a result, the percentage of these nutrients needed in the diet increases to the amounts shown in Table 13-2. Therefore, simply increasing the amount fed of a diet just adequate for an earlier period (e.g., early gestation) will not provide the additional nutrients needed, resulting in the effects described in the following sections of this chapter.

For the different feeding programs, and to feed and manage optimally and economically, broodmares should be put into the following groups:

1. Nonlactating mares to be bred, e.g., maiden mares.
2. Nonlactating mares in the first 8 months of pregnancy and barren mares. Geldings not in hard use or training may be kept with these mares.
3. Mares in their last trimester of pregnancy.
4. Lactating mares.
   a. Any mares at or below moderate body condition (as described in Table 1-4) may be kept with the lactating mares. As with lactating mares, they should be fed more than other mares so they will gain weight prior to being bred. Maiden mares just off the show or racing circuit may be in this situation. These mares have often been eating as much as 12 to 15 lbs (5.5 to kg) of grain-mix daily plus free-choice hay, yet continue to be thin. Upon retirement for breeding they should continue to receive all the good quality forage they

TABLE 13-2
Broodmares' Major Nutrient Needs in Diet Dry Matter versus That in Feeds

	Digestible Energy Mcal/lb (kg)	Protein %	Calcium %	Phosphorus %
Needed during:				
Last 3 months of pregnancy	1.0–1.1 (2.3–2.4)	11	0.50	0.35
Lactation	1.1 (2.4)	13	0.50	0.35
Nonlactation and before last 3 months of pregnancy	0.9 (2.0)	8	0.25	0.20
Composition of:*				
Legumes (e.g., alfalfa)	1.0–1.1 (2.2–2.4)	15–20	0.8–2.0	0.15–0.3
Grasses, growing	0.9–1.1 (2.0–2.4)	10–20	0.3–0.6	0.2–0.4
Grasses, mature	0.7–1.0 (1.5–2.2)	6–10	0.3–0.5	0.15–0.3
Cereal grains	1.5–1.7 (3.3–3.7)	9–13	0.02–0.1	0.25–0.35

* For more exact values, see Appendix Table 6, for the specific type of grain or forage being fed. For the most accurate values, have the feed analyzed as described in Chapter 6.

will consume plus 0.5 to 0.75 lbs/100 lbs (0.5 to 0.75 kg/100 kg) body weight daily of a 12 to 14% protein grain-mix, depending on their body condition, so they are above moderate body condition (Table 1-4) and gaining weight entering the breeding season.

b. Some like to separate lactating mares for teasing and breeding from those already bred or not to be rebred.

Additional groups may be formed if warranted. For small herds, individual rather than group feeding may be more practical. Separating mares into these groups, or individual feeding, is beneficial for the safety and nutrition of the foals, and so that special consideration can be given to the needs of open and pregnant mares, those that need to gain or maintain weight, and the nutritional differences shown in Table 13-2 for each of these classes of horses. In addition, as with all good feeding programs, the amount fed should be varied as needed. The mare's body weight and condition are the best indicators of the amount of feed needed. The mare should be moderately fleshy but not fat at foaling and fed as much as needed to maintain this weight at least until weaning. The amount of feed needed to accomplish these goals is higher with harsher climates, more work or exercise, and more milk produced, as indicated by how fast the foal is growing.

For mares to maintain body condition during pregnancy, their weight must increase by an amount equal to the foal's birth weight plus the weight of the placenta and fluids. This is about 9-12% of the mare's weight, with two-thirds of it gained in the last trimester. Thus, the 1100-lb (500-kg) mare should gain a total of 100 to 130 lbs (45 to 60 kg) during pregnancy, with 0.75 to 1 lb. (0.35 to 0.45 kg) gained daily during the last 90 days of pregnancy. If the mare's weight increases more or less than this, her body condition must increase or decrease accordingly.

If the mare is provided sufficient feed, she will consume enough to attain the desired body condition, i.e., to store body fat during pregnancy for utilization late in pregnancy and during lactation. When pregnant mares are allowed to self-regulate energy intake with good-quality forage sufficient in dietary energy and protein content to meet the mares' requirements (Table 13-2), they will consume enough to store body fat for later utilization when energy needs increase. No grain, protein, or mineral supplements need to be fed if forage quantity and quality are adequate.

If grain is fed, care must be taken not to get the mare too fat, i.e., to a body condition score of greater than 8 (Table 1-4). Although severe obesity doesn't appear to affect the pregnant mare, the duration of pregnancy, placental weight or passage, foaling ease, or reproductive efficiency, it may decrease the mare's milk production and as a result her foal's growth rate. Obesity's lack of effect on foaling ease in mares is in contrast to what is frequently postulated and stated. Obesity does lead to labor complications and dystocia in women and heifers, but not in horses or mature cows. However, the broodmare should not be kept above moderate or moderately fleshy body condition (Table 1-4) year round, as doing so may be detrimental, as discussed in Chapter 1 (see section on "Dietary Energy Excess"). If the mare is excessively overweight (i.e., has a body condition score greater than 6 to 7, Table 1-4), a weight reduction program as described in that section should be instituted. This should be done during the period from 2 weeks before weaning until the last trimester of pregnancy, but not prior to breeding, nor during the first trimester of pregnancy, nor early in lactation. Weight loss during these periods may decrease reproductive efficiency and milk production.

In addition to obesity and weight loss, excess thinness at foaling may decrease the mare's milk production. But if the mare that is thin at foaling is allowed sufficient feed to gain weight following foaling, she will increase her milk production to a level similar to that of heavier mares at 1 month of lactation. Lactation alone requires nearly a doubling in energy intake. This, added to the amount needed for weight gain, greatly increases the amount the mare must consume. However, shortly after foaling, the mare and foal are often taken to the stud or breeding farm. Along with lactation and mothering, the mare now is in new, strange surroundings with feed and water different from that to which she is accustomed and which she, at least initially, may not consume well. If she doesn't consume, or isn't fed, a sufficient amount, she not only won't gain weight, she may lose weight. In either case, the thin mare's ability to come into heat, ovulate, settle, and maintain pregnancy is decreased. In addition, her colostrum and milk production, and as a result, her foal's immunity and growth rate, are likely to decrease. The birth weight of the foal, however, appears to be little affected by its dam's weight gain or loss during pregnancy, or her body weight at foaling, whether she is obese or thin.

Feeding Nonlactating Mares Not in Their Last Trimester of Pregnancy

The barren mare and the nonlactating mare during the first 8 months of pregnancy should be fed the same as the mature idle and working horse, as described in Chapter 10.

Feeding Mares During the Last Trimester of Pregnancy and Lactation

As shown in Table 13-2, if an average or better-quality legume, or grass cut or grazed at an early stage of maturity, is being consumed, this forage will generally provide sufficient dietary energy and protein, as well as other nutrients, to meet the mare's needs during both the last 3 months of pregnancy and throughout lactation (Fig. 13-2) No grain or protein supplement is needed, provided that there are ample amounts of these high-quality forages for the mare to eat all she wants.

During the last 3 months of pregnancy and lactation, however, all forages generally are lower in phosphorus content than that needed, and grass forages generally do not provide sufficient calcium to meet the mare's needs (Table 13-2). To prevent these deficiencies, allow the mare free access to a salt-calcium-phosphorus mineral mix as the only salt available, as described in Table 13-1. From 2 to 8 oz (60 to 240 g) per mare may be needed daily, but with a mineral mix containing 10% or more of both calcium and phosphorus, 3 to 4 oz (90 to 120 g) is generally sufficient. If grain is being fed, this amount of the mineral mix may be added to the grain. If the grain does not contain molasses, it will generally be necessary to dampen the grain when the mineral mix is added to prevent the minerals from sifting out. If mature grass pasture or hay is being consumed, in addition to more calcium and phosphorus, more protein and dietary energy are generally

needed by the mare during the last 3 months of pregnancy, and particularly during lactation, than these feeds provide.

To determine if the forage being consumed meets the mare's needs, it may be analyzed as described in Chapter 6. If the forage contains adequate energy but not protein, about 2 lbs (1 kg) of a 25 to 30% protein supplement will provide the additional protein needed. If the forage doesn't contain adequate protein or energy density to meet the mare's requirements, a grain mix similar to that shown in Tables 4-9 and 4-10 is needed; or it can be formulated as described in Chapter 6. Along with all the grass forage she will consume, 0.5 to 1 lb/100 lbs body wt/day (0.5 to 1 kg/100 kg/day) of the grain mix should be fed as needed to have each mare moderately fleshy at foaling and to avoid weight loss during lactations, or if she is at less than moderate condition at foaling, so that during lactation she gains sufficiently to reach this condition (Table 1-4). Fat or oil may be added to the diet as described in Chapter 4 (Table 4-8) if desired. Adding fat to the diet is particularly beneficial if increased dietary energy for weight gain is needed.

After 3 months of lactation, if grain is being fed, decrease the amount by one-half, and 1 to 2 weeks prior to weaning stop feeding grain. For at least 2 weeks following weaning don't feed any grain, and if possible, decrease the forage fed to 1.5 to 2 lbs/100 lbs (1.5 to 2 kg/100 kg) body weight daily. This helps decrease the mare's milk production, which is beneficial in getting the foal to eat more solid feed and in decreasing excessive mammary gland distention and, as a result, the mare's discomfort following weaning. Other procedures recommended for weaning are described in that section in Chapter 15.

As described in the following section, if the mare's nutritional needs during pregnancy and lactation are not met, she may lose body weight and condition, and both her reproductive efficiency and milk production may be reduced. A progressive depression and elevation in blood lipids may occur, primarily in pony breed mares, when their dietary energy needs are not met.

NUTRITION EFFECTS ON MARE REPRODUCTION

Dietary Protein and Energy Effects on Reproduction

Inadequate dietary energy or protein intake may prevent ovulation, or, if ovulation and fertilization occur, may result in early embryonic death. A failure to ovulate is the major effect of a protein deficiency in mares. Mares just above moderately fleshy condition (Table 1-4) have also been shown to have greater follicular activity than thinner mares, and feeding them a low-energy diet reduced the number that ovulated. Weight loss early in pregnancy also decreases embryonic vesicle size and increases early embryonic loss. Even without weight loss, thin mares have longer intervals between foaling and ovulation, require more cycles/conception, have lower conception rates, have increased early embryonic death, and have lower plasma luteinizing hormone concentrations during diestrus than do mares that are at or above moderate body condition.

Regardless of the mare's body condition, weight loss seems to decrease reproductive efficiency. This is quite likely the reason that, if a mare or filly isn't bred shortly

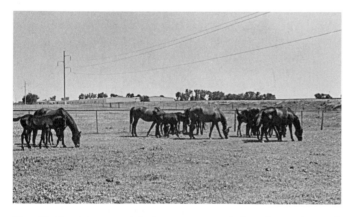

Fig. 13-2. Mares and foals on pasture. A lot of exercise and play is important for good bone and muscle development by the growing horse. Lack of exercise predisposes the foal to contracted flexor tendons. In addition, good, green growing pasture containing ample quantities of forage, along with a salt-mineral mix containing 8 to 16% of both calcium and phosphorus (Appendix Table 7), available for free-choice consumption as the only salt, will meet all of the lactating mare's nutritional needs.

after she leaves training, or the show or performance circuit, it may take quite a long time before she does become pregnant. Following training or the show circuit, most horses lose condition while they adapt to their new environment. This is generally accentuated by their being changed from a stable to a paddock with other horses. If the other horses have been together, there is already an established order of dominance within the herd; as a result, a new mare, especially one without herd experience, may be injured when suddenly placed with the group. To prevent injury and loss of condition, and as a result a decrease in reproductive efficiency, the mare or filly leaving training or the show circuit should be kept stabled and fed individually so she maintains her body weight until in foal. She should be gradually reduced from a high-grain to a primarily forage diet. Before put with a herd, it may be helpful to put her with just one other horse for several days to allow the two to become "buddies." Leaving her and the horses she is put with unshod, and providing ample room to circle, run away, and not get in an area where they can't get away, decreases the risk of injuries.

In summary, the major effects of dietary protein and energy intake on the mare's reproductive ability are the following:

1. Inadequate dietary protein, even with adequate energy or feed intake for body weight maintenance, decreases reproductive efficiency, perhaps primarily due to a failure to ovulate.
2. Mares who are thin (with a body condition score below 4, Table 1-4) at breeding time will have normal-weight foals but low reproductive efficiency and increased early embryonic losses if they do become pregnant.
3. Increasing energy intake prior to breeding (flushing) is beneficial for the thin mare, but not for the mare at or above moderate body condition (Table 1-4).
4. The mare that is losing weight, regardless of her body weight with respect to her optimum, has reduced reproductive efficiency. Weight loss by the pregnant mare doesn't appear to affect the foal's birth weight, but may decrease the mare's colostrum and milk production, thus decreasing the foal's passive immunity and growth rate.
5. For maximum reproductive efficiency, the mare prior to breeding should be moderately fleshy or heavier (have a body condition score of 6 or greater, Table 1-4) and be fed to maintain this weight. Even a moderate body condition (score of 5.0) is only marginally acceptable, particularly for the lactating mare, as the body fat that may be needed for stress and lactation won't be available.
6. Even excess obesity (a body condition score above 8, Table 1-4) during pregnancy doesn't appear to affect pregnancy, foaling ease or the foal's birth weight, placental weight or passage, or the mare's reproductive efficiency, but it may decrease subsequent milk production and as a result the foal's growth rate.

Vitamin and Mineral Effects on Reproduction

The occurrence, effects, diagnosis, treatment, and prevention of a deficiency or excess of each vitamin and mineral are described in Chapters 2 and 3. Vitamins and minerals that affect reproduction, the fetus, and the neonate are mentioned here as a reminder. To ensure adequate but not excessive intake, the broodmare's diet should contain the amounts of each vitamin and mineral indicated in Appendix Tables 2 and 3. If there is any doubt as to the adequacy of vitamins in the diet, or to ensure adequate vitamin intake, a balanced vitamin supplement such as that given in Table 3-5 should be given. In addition, trace-mineralized salt, which in selenium-deficient areas (Fig. 2-4) should contain selenium, should be fed free-choice as the only salt available, or added to the grain mix as 0.5% of the total diet.

A vitamin E and/or selenium deficiency occurs most commonly in foals at birth to one month of age, and as a result of inadequate selenium intake by the dam during pregnancy or inadequate selenium and/or vitamin E intake during lactation. Although vitamin E levels are low in mature forage, pasture or hay, and a vitamin E deficiency impairs reproduction in many species of animals, this effect has never been reported in horses and there is no evidence to indicate that giving vitamin E, even in large amounts, to horses on low vitamin E diets helps resolve reproductive problems in horses or in any way increases their reproductive efficiency or libido.

An iodine deficiency, and more commonly a toxicosis, occurs in horses, or is recognized in horses, most often in newborn foals as a result of either inadequate or excessive iodine intake by their dams. Affected foals may be born dead or alive but weak, and may have an enlarged thyroid gland or goiter (Fig. 2-6) and angular leg deformities. Although a manganese deficiency, like one of vitamin A, greatly impairs reproductive efficiency in many species, this has never been reported or known to occur in horses. A prolonged and severe phosphorus deficiency is also thought to decrease reproductive efficiency in other herbivores but not in horses.

Although a clinically occurring vitamin A deficiency is not known to impair horses' reproductive ability, it will decrease the amount of vitamin A secreted into the colostrum and therefore available to correct the deficiency the foal is normally born with because of minimal transplacental vitamin A transfer. If a vitamin A deficiency persists, it predisposes the foal to increased risk of infectious diseases, particularly respiratory and diarrheal diseases. In contrast to vitamin A, inadequate amounts of its precursor, beta-carotene, does impair the mare's reproductive ability. Injecting mares not grazing green grass with beta-carotene has been reported to increase their reproductive efficiency. Because of this, beta-carotene injections, as described in the section on "Beta-Carotene Effect on Mare Reproduction" in Chapter 3, and adding 50 IU of vitamin E daily to the diet for 6 weeks prior to breeding, and throughout pregnancy, has been recommended for mares not grazing green grass, particularly for the mare that has had previous reproductive problems.

NUTRITION EFFECTS ON MARE'S MILK PRODUCTION AND COMPOSITION

Mares fed a sufficient amount of a nutritionally adequate diet produce amounts of milk equivalent to 3 to 4% of their body weight/day for the first 2 months of lactation, slowly decreasing to 2% by 5 months. The amount of milk produced varies little with duration of lactation during the first 45 to 60 days, but its nutrient content decreases steadily throughout lactation.

The effect of nutritional deficiencies on the amount and composition of the mare's milk depends on her body condition. Mares with adequate body reserves will draw upon those reserves and not decrease the amount of milk produced, even when fed only 70 to 80% of the amount of feed needed. However, once body reserves are sufficiently depleted, milk production, but not composition, decreases. Mares with either inadequate energy or protein intake for a sufficient period of time, or without sufficient body reserves—i.e., with a body condition score of less than 4 (Table 1-4)—have reduced milk production; as a result, their foals' growth rate is decreased.

Excess dietary energy intake, like inadequate energy intake for mares at moderate or heavier body condition, appears to have little effect on the amount of milk produced; its major effect is on the mare's body condition and weight. But excess, like inadequate, energy intake if sufficient for a prolonged period of time will decrease the amount of milk produced. Obese mares, with body condition scores near 9 or above, appear to have reduced milk production, as their foals grow more slowly than those of nursing mares with body condition scores of 5 to 7 (Table 1-4). Excess energy intake, in contrast to what has been speculated, doesn't increase milk fat, energy, or protein content, but instead decreases them slightly.

Nutrient intake, above or below that needed, appears to have minimal effect on milk composition. Wide variations in the mare's calcium and phosphorus intakes have been shown in some studies to have no effect on their concentrations in the milk. In other studies, although dietary phosphorus had no effect on milk phosphorus content, calcium concentration was 40% lower in milk from mares receiving one-third the amount of dietary calcium needed, but milk calcium concentration was not different in milk from mares receiving up to 2.5 times more calcium than needed, than it was in those receiving just adequate dietary calcium. There appears to be no correlation between the amount of inorganic potassium, zinc, copper, magnesium, and iron ingested and the amount in the milk. In contrast, milk iodine and possibly selenium concentrations directly correlate with the amount of each of these minerals consumed, as described in Chapter 2.

In summary, variations in the amount of most nutrients ingested by the mare do not affect their concentrations in her milk. The major effect of variations in energy intake is on the mare's body condition, not the amount of milk produced or its composition. The objective of feeding programs for the lactating mare, therefore, is to keep her at the desired body condition, rather than to try to influence her milk production or composition.

NUTRITION PROBLEMS IN BROODMARES

A summary of nutritionally related problems that occur primarily in broodmares is given in Table 13-3. Poisonous plants and feed-related poisonings as discussed in Chapters 18 and 19, respectively, may affect all horses, and not just broodmares. However, some, such as fescue toxicosis, occur only in broodmares and growing horses. Care should be taken that fescue hay or pasture-forage is not consumed during the last trimester of pregnancy unless it is known to be endophyte free. Infested fescue consumed during this period may cause abortion, prolonged gestation, a thickened placenta resulting in difficult foaling, a decrease or absence of milk production, and the birth of weak or dead foals. The mare also should not consume sorghum forage, sudan grass, Johnson grass, Sudex, or other sorghum-sudan grass hybrid forages. All produce a substance that may be converted to cyanide (prussic or hydrocyanic acids). As described in Chapter 18, sufficient cyanide causes incoordination and bladder paresis in all horses, and may cause pregnant mares to abort or give birth to foals with fused joints. A number of additional plants that may cause the production of foals with physical defects (i.e., are teratogenic) are listed in Table 18-11.

There has been concern that transport of mares early in pregnancy may increase the risk of abortion, but studies have refuted this. However, prolonged transport, exertion, or stress from any cause, particularly during late pregnancy and lactation, may result in a sudden decrease in the horse's blood calcium and magnesium concentrations. This condition is described in the section on tying-up or hypocalcemic tetany in Chapter 11. The likelihood of this occurrence is greatly increased by a decrease in, or absence of, feed intake during this period.

A progressive depression associated with an increase in

TABLE 13-3
Nutritionally Related Problems in Broodmares[a]

Effect	Cause	Treatment or Prevention
Incoordination & bladder paresis, Late abortion, or birth of weak or dead foals	Cyanide	Don't feed sorghum–sudan grasses (Chapter 18)
Prolonged gestation, thickened placenta, difficulty foaling, no milk produced	Fungus in fescue	Don't feed fescue during last 3 mo of pregnancy (Chapter 19)
Progressive depression, coma, and death, generally in late gestation or lactation, primarily in ponies.	Inadequate feed intake and high blood lipids	Ensure adequate good-quality feed intake
Muscle tremors, incoordination, collapse, and colic-like signs.	Low blood calcium and magnesium, usually with transit or stress	Give calcium & magnesium intravenously & increase magnesium intake

[a] See Table 18-11 for plants whose ingestion results in the birth of offspring with physical defects.

blood lipids (hyperlipemia) may also occur during lactation or late pregnancy, when energy needs are high but intake for any reason is low. This may occur as a result of inadequate feed quality or availability, or secondary to inadequate feed intake as a result of inappetence or inability to consume food. Inadequate feed intake is most often due to the horse's being sick or having esophageal or gastrointestinal damage or obstruction. Hyperlipemia secondary to not eating may occur in any horse from one day of age to old age, and in any body condition, but occurs most often in thin horses. However, as a primary disease, not secondary to the horse's not eating, hyperlipemia occurs most frequently, and is a classic problem in obese ponies during late pregnancy, in lactation, and transit, but may occur in nonobese, nonlactating, nonpregnant ponies or horses.

Clinical hyperlipemia, whether primary or secondary, results in inappetence, a failure to drink, a rapid loss of body condition, fever, a progressive drowsiness, dullness and lethargy to a profound depression, muscle quivering or twitching, colic, incoordination, diarrhea, fluid accumulation along the underline or in the abdominal cavity, coma, and death. Blood plasma will have a markedly milky appearance.

Hyperlipemia occurs because a negative energy balance results in peripheral body-fat mobilization at a rate faster than it can be utilized. Ponies, particularly when obese, have excess fat for mobilization and may be fairly slow in utilizing it. Excess lipids are deposited particularly in the liver, kidneys, heart, and skeletal muscles. Liver and kidney function are impaired, and death may result from acute liver failure.

Hyperlipemia is difficult to treat. Over one half of severely affected animals die. However, if detected early and nutritional support is adequate to meet the animal's caloric requirements with a low-fat diet, recovery may occur. Because affected horses won't eat, tube feeding is necessary until appetite and sufficient feed intake return, which usually takes 1 to 3 weeks.

Prevention of hyperlipemia includes ensuring the intake of adequate quantities of good-quality feeds, particularly during the later stages of pregnancy and throughout lactation, especially for obese ponies. Preventing pony mares from becoming more than moderately fleshy (Table 1–4) is also helpful in preventing this condition.

MARE'S ESTROUS CYCLE

Mares are considered to be seasonally polyestrous, having regular estrous cycles throughout the spring and summer (long days) and becoming anestrus (no cyclic activity) during late fall and winter (short days), although anestrus can occur at all times of the year. This is apparently the typical estrous cycle for wild and nonstabled mares. Many stabled or domesticated mares exhibit estrus (heat), or sexual receptivity, throughout the year, but most ovulate only during the spring and summer, whereas some may ovulate at each estrus and, therefore, have a true polyestrous cycle. Ovulation without signs of estrus (silent heat) also occurs (about 3% of the time), especially early or late in the estrous cycle season and during the winter.

The onset of estrus is gradual, beginning with the mare's becoming more active, decreasing her feed intake, and she may become more aggressive toward other horses. At first she may react to a stallion more aggressively than she did when in anestrus. Gradually, she may not object to a stallion's sniffing and biting. Frequent urination while in the presence of a stallion or gelding is common. A few days prior to estrus, the stallion's advances are tolerated for a while. Then the mare will show diestrous (interval between estrus) behavior: moving away from the stallion and/or squealing, striking, kicking, laying her ears back, and annoyedly switching her tail, and sometimes just acting indifferent. Gradually these aggressive acts or this indifferent behavior is delayed or lessens.

When in estrus, the mare will remain calm in the stallion's presence, turn her hind quarters toward the stallion, spread her hind legs, and lower her pelvis to allow the stallion to mount. The tail is held up and often shifted to one side. Frequent urination occurs followed by rhythmic opening and closing of the labia (winking). She may also have a mating facial expression, with ears turned back but not flattened, as if listening for the stallion, and with her lips slack. She may seek out the stallion if she can. These signs gradually decrease during the 1 to 2 days following ovulation.

Certain mares do not develop all these signs of estrus, or they develop different intensities of specific behaviors. Some may reject the stallion even though ovulation occurs, and then show an entirely different behavior the next estrous period. Some aspects of estrous behavior occur in 2 to 10% of pregnant mares, most often during the 3rd to 4th weeks of pregnancy and in those carrying female foals. This may be due to sufficient estrogen production by the female conceptus. However, most pregnant mares, including those showing some estrous behavior, won't allow physical contact or mounting by the stallion.

Teasing by controlled exposure of a mare to a stallion is a commonly used, excellent, and for breeding farms necessary, management practice to increase the signs and detection of estrus. Although a low plasma progesterone concentration is helpful in confirming estrus, particularly in mares with silent heat, the most common, practical, and accurate means of detecting estrus in the mare is by exposing her to a male horse, generally an active stallion, and observing her behavior. The same person should observe the mare when she is teased so that subtle changes in her sexual behavior are recognized. The teaser stallion should be aggressive and enthusiastic, but controllable and not excessively rough on the mare. Mares that are indifferent to a stallion should be teased with a second stallion, preferably at another location. Draft mares may not respond to teasing except to a draft stallion. Teasing should be done daily. This is particularly necessary for mares that are currently in estrus and being bred, so that it may be determined when they go out of heat and, therefore, when breeding should be stopped. Teasing is also necessary for mares that have been bred and out of heat for 14 days or more to determine whether they come back into estrus. If they do not, they are probably pregnant, which then should be confirmed by a pregnancy examination.

Another procedure requiring less labor is to place a stallion in a small sturdy pen in the center of the mares' paddock. Mares in heat will generally approach the stallion, stand next to him, and exhibit mating behavior. However, a dominant mare may keep mares lower in dominance away from the stallion. Once dominance is established, subtle threats replace overt aggression; so the mares need to be observed carefully to detect that one mare is not preventing another from approaching the stallion.

If anabolic steroids have been given, as they occasionally are in an attempt to improve growth and/or performance, estrus and ovulation will be suppressed and early embryonic mortality increased. These adverse effects are reversible with time but may result in the loss of a breeding season. In addition, anabolic steroids when given to horses in good condition are ineffective in enhancing their growth, muscular development, or athletic performance. They do cause stallion-like behavior, and increase biting and kicking behaviors in fillies. The more dominant the filly, the greater these behaviors, regardless of the amount of anabolic steroid administered. Although these fillies develop ovarian follicles, these follicles regress and don't ovulate.

During the breeding season, the mare's estrous cycle is 21 ± 2 days, with 2 to 9 days, averaging 6 to 7 days, of estrus, although the duration of estrus can range from 1 to 37 days, causing a similar variation in the length of the estrous cycle. Prolonged estrus is common, particularly in draft breeds. In addition, during transition from winter anestrus to normal estrous cycling in the spring, it is not uncommon for estrus to last for 20 to 30 days without the development of a preovulatory follicle resulting in ovulation. Split estrus also occasionally occurs, particularly during the transition from anestrus to estrus. With a split estrus, the mare exhibits little estrus behavior for 1 to 2 days during an estrus period generally lasting 4 to 5 days longer than normal. Ovulation normally occurs during the last 1 to 2 days of estrus, and if there is a split estrus period, during the second part of the period. The estrous cycle, follicular development, and ovulation are under the control of the various hormones shown in the graph in Figure 13-3.

Sufficient daylight results in increased secretion of follicle-stimulating hormone (FSH) and luteinizing hormone (LH). FSH stimulates ovarian follicle growth and estrogen production by the follicle. The first surge of FSH (Fig. 13-3) may prime several smaller follicles to initiate their development. FSH, in combination with LH during late estrus or early diestrus, may be responsible for final maturation and ovulation of the preovulatory follicle. As the preovulatory follicle develops, the concentration of estrogen increases, with the peak occurring during mid- to late estrus—approximately 24 hours prior to the LH peak. Estrogen stimulates the brain to induce sexual receptivity; causes positive feedback in the hypothalamus and pituitary resulting in the secretion of LH, and increases uterine, cervical, and vaginal secretions conducive to mating and sperm transport.

LH peaks from the day of ovulation to 2 days after. It is apparently responsible for final maturation of the preovulatory follicle, induction of ovulation, and initiation of corpus luteum (CL) formation. Following ovulation, the CL forms and secretes progesterone, which prevents a new follicle from developing. If pregnancy doesn't occur, prostaglandin F_2-α (PGF_2-α) produced by the uterus stimulates regression of the CL; as a result progesterone secretion decreases, allowing the development of a new follicle, estrogen secretion, estrus, and ovulation, which normally occurs 19 to 23 days after the previous ovulation. However, if pregnancy occurs, the embryo secretes an antiluteolytic substance that prevents uterine release of PGF_2-α; as a result the CL is maintained and grows. Equine chorionic gonadotropin (eCG), also referred to as pregnant mare serum gonadotropin or PMSG, produced by fetal-tissue-origin endometrial cups from day 40 to 140 of pregnancy, apparently stimulates the formation of secondary CL, which are necessary for the production of sufficient progesterone to maintain pregnancy until the placenta begins to produce progesterone later in pregnancy (about day 80 to 100 of pregnancy in the mare) (Fig. 13-3).

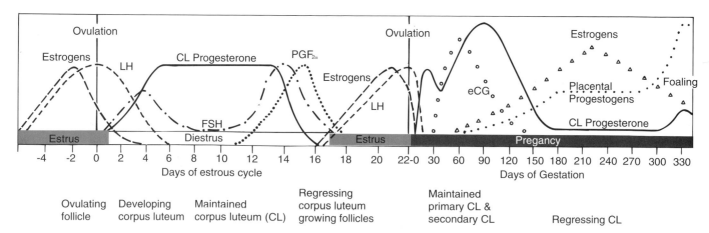

Fig. 13-3. Hormone levels and corresponding ovarian activity during the mare's estrous cycles and during pregnancy. LH = luteinizing hormone; FSH = follicle-stimulating hormone; PGF_2-α = Prostaglandin F_2-α; eCG = equine chorionic gonadotropin or pregnant mare serum gonadotropin (PMSG): CL = corpus luteum.

ESTROUS CYCLE INDUCEMENT OF MARES

Unfortunately, the physiologic or natural breeding season of horses does not coincide with the breeding season set by the horse industry. The assignment of a January 1 birth date for all foals born in a given year has forced those wanting to produce foals that will sell or can compete most successfully on the show circuit and athletically as 2-year-olds to adopt means to hasten the onset of the breeding season. The most effective method of inducing early estrous cycling and ovulation has been artificial lighting to provide a total of 16 hours of light, beginning 2 to 3 months prior to the desired breeding season. Lights should be turned on 30 minutes before sundown every day. The mare won't cycle properly if light duration is inadequate, excessive or erratic. Alternatively, turning on lights for 2 hours beginning 8 to 10 hours after dark is also effective. A minimum of 2 footcandles of light is required. The light is adequate if a newspaper can be easily read in any corner of the stall or pen. A 200-watt light bulb is sufficient for an average-size stall. The lights may be incandescent or fluorescent. Artificial lighting is of benefit for both nonlactating and early lactating or foaling mares. Mares foaling early may enter anestrus if not placed under artificial lights. Estrous inducement by hormone administration is also common. A combination of both lights and hormone administration may produce the best results.

An alternative to using lights to induce estrus and ovulation early in the calendar year or breeding season that has been tested but found ineffective is feeding the serotonin-precursor and amino acid tryptophan.

PREBREEDING EXAMINATION OF MARES

Prior to breeding the mare, the external genitalia should be inspected for evidence of discharge. The vulvar labia should close properly, and a line drawn from the anus to the clitoris should not tilt out by more than $10°$ from vertical. If air is aspirated into the vagina (windsucking) when the vulvar labia are spread, a Caslick's operation should be done. Windsucking can be detected by placing the flat of one hand on each vulvar lip and gently parting them while listening for the sound of aspirated air. Windsucking is the major predisposing cause of vaginal infections in mares. A Caslick's operation, as well as any abnormalities that can be surgically corrected, such as cervical lacerations, urine pooling, and an opening between the rectum and vagina, should be corrected as soon as possible rather than just prior to breeding season.

A rectal examination of the mare's reproductive tract and ovaries, and after confirming that the mare is not pregnant, an examination of the vestibule, vagina, and cervix by either inserting a vaginal speculum or a fiberoptic scope, are recommended to detect any abnormalities or problems. In maiden mares, an imperforated hymen or rarely a persistent medium septum may occasionally be identified by a vaginal exam. The thin hymen membrane, which is just inside the vestibule, should be removed. It can be tough and, if not removed, may result in trauma, pain, and fright upon breeding. A persistent medium septum is a strong membrane partition which divides the vagina and causes considerable problems at foaling. It should be removed well in advance of breeding to allow time for healing. If the mare has had a Caslick's operation, it may be necessary to open what was surgically closed, at least partially, and to insert a breeding stitch to prevent its tearing open farther for natural service, but not for artificial insemination. Before foaling, of course, it should be opened completely.

BREEDING MARES

Most feel the mare should not be bred until she is at least 3 years of age, as occurs naturally with wild mares, and should be first bred before she is 10 years old. Many draft breed fillies are not sexually mature at 2 years of age, especially those that are large for that breed. Increased sexual maturity is thought by some to be indicated by increasing size when usually the opposite is true. Barren mares over 16 years of age are the least fertile, and 6- to 15-year-old foaling mares are the most fertile. The average maximum breeding life of the mare is 18 to 22 years of age.

Common methods used to breed mares include pasture breeding, hand mating, and artificial insemination. Embryo transfer may also be used to get the mare pregnant. Pasture breeding involves turning the stallion into the pasture with the mares to be bred. This requires little labor and relies on the stallion to select mares to breed. Problems with this method include the threat of disease transmission and injury to the stallion, mares, or foals. Pasture breeding is generally used by farms breeding fewer than 30 mares per season. It is not recommended for problem mares. When pasture breeding is used, mares with foals should not be put with the stallion until their foals are several weeks old. Stallions may attack and even kill foals, particularly during the foals' first weeks of life or foals sired by other stallions. How stallions know which foals were sired by another stallion isn't known, but they seem to know.

All other breeding methods require more labor and management. Proper teasing and timely breeding are essential for acceptable conception and foaling rates using procedures other than pasture breeding. Timely breeding entails insemination near ovulation. The ovum retains maximum viability for about 12 hours, and the stallion's sperm normally retains maximum viability in the mare's reproductive tract for at least 48 hours, although this varies from 1 to 5 days with sperm from different stallions. Because mares ovulate near the end of estrus, the most fertile time for breeding is just before the mare is about to go out of heat—thus the recommendation and tradition of breeding mares every other day beginning after 2 or 3 days of estrus until the mare goes out of heat. This essentially ensures that viable spermatozoa are present in the mare's oviducts, where fertilization occurs, at ovulation. The number of breedings can be decreased to one by breeding just prior to ovulation, as determined by rectal palpation or an ultrasonograph. The fertilized ovum passes down the oviduct and enters the uterus 5 to 6 days after ovulation.

The advantages of hand breeding include a better likelihood of pregnancy in problem breeders and greater use of the stallion on a large number of mares. This latter factor is maximized using artificial insemination. Depending on the fertility of the stallion, 20 to 40 mares may be inseminated on a given breeding day. Artificial insemination can also eliminate contamination in problem mares, prevent spread of venereal diseases, provide many more pregnancies in a given season (which can prove the stallion's potential as a sire earlier), and protect the stallion, mare, and foal from injury. In addition, in the future, artificial insemination in conjunction with procedures for separating sperm by sex may allow breeding to obtain either colts or fillies. Although not currently (1994) available for horses but being developed, a kit for separating bull's sperm by sex is available commercially (from Inno Vet Inc., West Palm Beach, FL); it reportedly allows breeding for either bull or heifer calves with more than a 90% reliability. Embryo transfer is an additional procedure that is available and allowed by some breed registries, but not by others.

Disadvantages of hand mating include greater labor and reliance on people's ability to choose the best time for breeding. People are less capable in this respect than stallions. This may be part of the reason for lower conception rates in some breeds on some farms.

Regardless of the breeding method used, the success of breeding is highly dependent on the level of fertility of both the mares and stallions. The stallion's fertility may be estimated by his physical attributes and semen quality, as described in the section on "Breeding Evaluation of Stallions" in Chapter 12. Some physical attributes to consider include general health, musculoskeletal soundness, behavior or "manners," libido, genital health, and testicular size and tone. One or several semen ejaculates should be evaluated.

FOAL-HEAT BREEDING

Foal heat, or the mare's first estrus following foaling, occurs in 45% of mares by 9 days, 93% by 15 days, and 97% by 20 days postpartum. Although conception rates are 11 to 33% lower in mares bred at foal heat than those bred later, embryonic losses are not different. There are several advantages of breeding at foal heat. The major ones are: (1) if successful, it results in a foal born earlier the next year, which is of benefit for show, sale, and performance of the foal prior to 3 years of age; (2) a more consistently occurring estrus and ovulation compared to subsequent heat periods; and (3) an additional heat period in which to breed. Mares foaling in the northern hemisphere in January or February, and not under lights, if not bred and settled in foal heat may not form ovulating follicles and may fail to show heat again for several weeks, or even months. To avoid this, and because of the advantages, many breeding farms feel compelled to breed on foal heat. The longer after foaling before the mare ovulates, the higher the pregnancy rate. Because of this, progesterone may be given following foaling to delay the occurrence of foal heat and thus increase the likelihood of conception.

It has been shown that 24-hour removal of the nursing calf from the cow increases release of her luteinizing hormone (LH) and the occurrence of estrus and, therefore, has been used to enhance early breeding. These effects have also been demonstrated in mares when foals are removed the day of foaling, but not when removed 3 to 4 days after foaling.

Criteria that mares should meet in order to be bred during foal heat include:

1. Delivery of their foal without significant difficulty.
2. Passing of placenta within 3 hours of foaling, without any abnormalities.
3. A live, strong healthy foal that nurses within 1 hour.
4. A cervix, examined at the beginning of foal heat, that is free of bruises and abnormal discharges.
5. At the beginning of foal heat, a uterus that is significantly reduced in size and without fluid accumulations, as determined by rectal palpation or ultrasonography.

Uterine fluid decreases fertility and, therefore, should be removed or breeding delayed. Normally, the lining of the mare's uterus is repaired, the uterus involuted, and uterine fluid absent by the seventh day after foaling. The mare's ovaries should be palpated at least every other day beginning with the onset of foal heat until ovulation occurs. Palpation, ultrasonography, and teasing provide the most accurate predictions of foal heat conception.

DIAGNOSING PREGNANCY AND FETAL VIABILITY IN MARES

All mares should be examined for pregnancy as soon after breeding as detection is possible (15 to 25 days), and again at 30 to 35, 50 to 55, and 70 to 90 days of pregnancy. This is helpful so if the mare is not pregnant, or loses her pregnancy, she can be rebred as soon as possible. Clinically undetectable embryonic loss prior to 90 days, and most often before 35 days, of pregnancy occurs in 8 to 15% of pregnancies, but may be double this in some groups of mares. In contrast, abortions after the fourth month of pregnancy usually account for only a small fraction of total fetal losses. Early embryonic losses can be minimized by (1) being as sanitary as possible in evaluating and treating the mare's reproductive tract and for breeding or insemination, (2) vulvar suturing if indicated, (3) good nutrition, (4 & 5) good parasite and vaccination programs, and (6) the administration of progestins when indicated. Ovulation occurred an average of 10, 13, and 21 days after pregnancy loss occurring during weeks 2 to 4, 4 to 6, and 6 to 8, respectively, which may be soon enough that the mare can be rebred that breeding season. When this is done, nearly 70% of these mares become pregnant, although 40% will also lose their second pregnancy.

Because of a possible failure to conceive or early embryonic losses, the testing program for estrus detection should be continued until pregnancy is confirmed. Each mare found not to be pregnant should receive a thorough examination and any problems found treated prior to the next breeding. Neither the cessation nor the occurrence of estrus confirms that the mare is or is not pregnant. A failure to return to estrus following breeding, although suggestive, doesn't confirm that the mare is pregnant, just as a recurrence of estrus suggests but doesn't confirm that she is not pregnant. A mare may not show estrous behavior for many reasons besides pregnancy; conversely, up to 10% of pregnant mares will show some aspects of estrus early in pregnancy.

Pregnancy can be diagnosed using the following procedures:

1. Ultrasonography using high-quality equipment is 98% accurate in diagnosing pregnancy by 10 to 15 days following conception. Fetal viability, as indicated by fetal heart beat, can be detected by day 22 to 28 by ultrasonography.
2. Rectal palpation by a skilled examiner can detect pregnancy by increased uterine and cervical tone as early as 14 to 17 days after conception, although accuracy this early is less than adequate. A more accurate diagnosis can be made once the embryonic vesicle is sufficiently large (1 to 1.6 inches, or 2 to 4 cm) that it can be palpated, which is at day 20 to 25, and even greater accuracy can be attained by waiting until 30 days. Rectal palpation, particularly after 25 to 30 days following conception, is the most rapid and economical method of detecting pregnancy except in mares that can't be palpated, such as those that won't allow it, are too small (ponies and miniature horses), or which have had previous rectal tears.
3. An elevated plasma progesterone concentration is present in pregnant mares by 16 to 25 days following conception. However, since progesterone is produced by the corpus luteum, its persistence will cause a similar increase in plasma progesterone for up to 90 days following estrus, even in the absence of pregnancy. An increase in the mare's plasma progesterone concentration is also useful in detecting "silent heats" or behavioral anestrus, as it increases by 2 to 4 days following ovulation (Fig. 13-3). It is also helpful in detecting mares in which early fetal resorption or abortion occurs due to inadequate progesterone. An attempt to prevent this, with varying degrees of success, may be made by administering progestins.
4. Gonadotropin (eCG or PMSG) can be detected in the blood from 40 to 120 days of pregnancy, but because it is secreted by the endometrial cups it will be present even if the fetus is lost at 35 days of gestation or later.
5. An elevated serum, urine, milk, and fecal estrone sulfate and total unconjugated estrogen concentrations can be detected and are indicative of both pregnancy and a viable fetus from day 90 to foaling. However, mares with ovarian cysts, nymphomania, or chronic genital disease may have urinary estrogen concentrations similar to that associated with pregnancy.

Thus, as summarized in Table 13-4, pregnancy and fetal viability can be confirmed earliest using ultrasonography followed by skilled rectal palpation. Serum estrone sulfate and total conjugated estrogen concentrations are accurate in detecting both pregnancy and fetal viability following the 3rd month of gestation to foaling. Although pregnancy can be detected earlier by plasma progesterone and eCG (PMSG) assays, neither are indicative of fetal viability. Al-

TABLE 13-4
Reproductive Changes Occurring in the Mare

Days After	Occurrence
Estrus Begins	
6 (2 to 9)[a]	Estrus ends, with ovulation occurring in the last 1 to 2 days
Ovulation	
2 to 3	Plasma progesterone increases above 2 ng/ml
Estrus Ends	
15 (6 to 25)	Estrus begins again, thus completing a 21- to 22-day (18 to 25 d)[a] estrous cycle.
Conception	
10 to 15 on & 22 to 28 on[b]	Pregnancy can be detected and fetal heart beat can be monitored ultrasonographically
14 to 17 on[b]	Pregnancy can be detected by skilled rectal palpation, although a more confirmatory diagnosis can be made after day 20 to 25
16 to 25, to 150	Plasma progesterone is above 2 ng/ml, which may also occur in the nonpregnant mare with a retained corpus luteum
35 on[b]	Most mares at breeding farms can be sent home with instructions for pregnancy exam immediately upon arrival and again at 70 to 90 days of pregnancy
45 to 120, peak at 60	eCG (PMSG) is detectable even if the fetus dies after 35 days of pregnancy
90 on[b]	Serum, urine, milk, and fetal estrone sulfate are increased if fetus is alive
120 on[b]	Plasma estrogen is increased more than twofold if fetus is alive
180 on[b]	Abdomen noticeably increased in size
270 on[b]	Fetal movement and dropped croup and flank detectable

[a] Average (range)
[b] On to foaling

though pregnancy using high-quality ultrasound equipment can be accurately diagnosed as early as 10 to 15 days following conception, it may be more practical to wait until approximately 18 to 20 days, thus eliminating the examination of mares that return to estrus at the normal time. One exception would be mares that have a history of twinning. If the equipment is available, these mares should be examined ultrasonographically at day 12 to 15 after ovulation to most effectively allow manual destruction of one embryo (as discussed in the following section on "Twinning in Mares").

ABORTION INDUCEMENT IN MARES

Abortion may be wanted because of inadvertent breeding, undesirable season, age of stallion, use of the mare, or twinning. Abortion cannot be induced during the first 5 days of pregnancy. The best time to induce abortion is during the second week of pregnancy. The preferred method during the first trimester is intramuscular injection of a prostaglandin. During the 2nd through the 5th weeks of pregnancy, a single injection is usually sufficient. However, if the mare doesn't return to estrus within 5 days, a second injection is needed. This method is highly effective with few, and only minor, side effects, such as sweating and mild colic. If pregnancy is ended after the 5th week of pregnancy, return to normal cycling and fertility is unpredictable; therefore, rebreeding that season may not be possible. Prostaglandin injections daily for 3 to 5 days are necessary and highly effective in inducing abortion during the 5th to the 12th weeks of pregnancy.

Uterine lavage, infusion, or crushing the fetus by rectal palpation during the 2nd through 5th week of pregnancy are also effective in inducing abortion. However, the mare may not return to heat for 3 to 4 weeks. If fetal expulsion doesn't occur within 24 hours of uterine infusion, it should be repeated. After the 11th week of pregnancy, if prostaglandins are not used, abortion should be done by removing the fetus manually and infusing a sterile isotonic saline solution, which may expedite placental expulsion. Inducing abortion after the first trimester may be accomplished, but is not recommended because of the risk of uterine damage, retained placenta, difficulty in passing the fetus, founder, and other complications. Administration of corticosteroids, prostaglandins, or oxytocin during the second trimester generally will not successfully induce abortion.

TWINNING IN MARES

About 3.5% of Thoroughbred and 1% of Standardbred mare pregnancies are with twins. The predisposition for twinning is highest for Thoroughbreds and lowest for pony breeds. From 39 to 94% of twin pregnancies result in the abortion or stillbirth of both fetuses. Only 8% of twin foals born alive live more than 2 weeks. Most twin pregnancies that go beyond 50 days of pregnancy result in abortion between 8 and 10 months of pregnancy. These mares often have a higher incidence of retained fetal membranes, do not recycle, and may be difficult to get pregnant during the same or subsequent breeding season. Twinning is second only to placental and uterine infections as a cause of equine abortion, with twinning accounting for about one-fourth of all equine abortions.

Twinning in the mare occurs as a result of multiple, usually double, ovulations, and not the splitting of one fertilized ovum, as in some species. The double ovulations usually occur within 48 hours of each other. Generally there is a single continuous estrus for both ovulations, not a split estrus.

When multiple pre-ovulatory follicles are detected by rectal examination of the ovaries, or more consistently detected by ultrasonographic examination, procedures most often used to try to prevent twinning are either (1) not breeding that estrus period, or (2) breeding once only at 12 to 24 hours after the first ovulation, in the hope that only the ovum from the second ovulation will be viable. In an attempt to ensure ovulation of the second follicle, HCG may be administered. However, none of these procedures appear to greatly lower the percentage of double-ovulating mares that twin. In contrast, a single-estrus double ovulation provides an improved opportunity for getting the mare pregnant and, therefore breeding should not be withheld.

Ultrasonography can detect twinning as early as 12 to 14 days after conception. Prior to ultrasonography, twin pregnancies were detected by rectal palpation of bilateral enlargements in the uterine horns, a single enlargement larger than normal, or two corpora lutea on the mare's ovaries. However, many twin pregnancies are missed by rectal palpation (false negatives), whereas many false positives are obtained ultrasonographically due to the presence of tumors or lymphatic cysts.

When a twin pregnancy is detected, there are several options. Doing nothing will result in 60 to 65% of mares aborting both twins and 5 to 10% aborting one twin by day 42 of pregnancy. Thus, doing nothing may be the best procedure unless the twin pregnancy is past 50 days. If it is, it may be best to induce abortion of both foals as described in the previous section.

Procedures that may be used to try to abort one embryo and maintain the other include the following:

1. Manually rupturing one embryo vesicle by rectal palpation. When done on days 12 to 16 or 23 to 31 after breeding, this is rapid and relatively nontraumatic to the uterus. However, sometimes both embryos are lost. If embryonic vesicle rupture is done after 35 days of gestation, the chances of success are lower and the mare may not return to estrus for several weeks, which may prevent rebreeding that season. If abortion of neither embryo occurs using the manual procedure, both can be aborted by giving prostaglandin as described in the previous section and the mare will recycle without losing much time in the breeding season.
2. One embryo can be removed surgically, although the remaining embryo also frequently is lost. Surgical intervention to remove one embryo is most successful when they are fixed in opposite uterine horns.
3. Reducing feed intake on a temporary basis has been reported to convert 60% of twin pregnancies to single pregnancies. However, given the consequences of allowing twins to progress to term, a 60% chance of success would not be acceptable for most owners.
4. Injection of potassium chloride into one of the fetus's heart using ultrasound guiding has been reported to result in 56% success when it is done after 115 days of pregnancy, compared to 12% success when done prior to this time.

In summary, the best management for twinning appears to be the following:

1. Breed the mare regardless of the possibility of multiple ovulations.
2. Twelve to 16 days after breeding, if ultrasonographic equipment is available, examine mares with a history of twinning or those with more than one detected ovulation. If twin pregnancy is present, manually isolate and repture one embryonic vesicle at that time. Monitor the viability of the remaining embryo.
3. If ultrasonography is not available and a twin pregnancy is present, don't intervene unless it is 30 days or more since conception. If it is, give prostaglandin to terminate the pregnancy. If rebreeding is not desired or practical, induction of abortion can be delayed to as long as 70 to 80 days of pregnancy.
4. When twin pregnancy is detected late in gestation,

it may be possible to allow one fetus to be carried to term by giving progesterone. Udder development and lactation during mid- or late gestation are often the first observable clinical signs, and are highly indicative of twin pregnancy. Rectal palpation at this time may reveal a soft cervix and relaxed pelvic area consistent with impending abortion. Treatment beginning at first evidence of early udder development, lactation, and impending abortion consists of administering progesterone up until 2 weeks prior to expected foaling time; after which a live foal concurrent with a mummified fetus will generally be delivered. Although the live foal is likely to be small, most will nurse and develop normally. If progesterone is not given, birth of a premature foal too young for survival is likely.

SUPPLEMENTAL READING RECOMMENDATIONS

Equine Reproduction by Drs. Angus McKinnon and James L. Voss (Lea & Febiger, Malvern, PA, 1992). One of the most current and complete references, and the best information available on this topic. It provides comprehensive coverage of the diagnoses of and treatments for reproductive disorders in the mare and stallion.

Management of the Mare for Maximum Reproductive Efficiency by BW Pickett, EL Squires, AO McKinnon, RK Shideler, and JL Voss (Animal Reproduction and Biotechnology Laboratory, Colorado State University, Fort Collins, CO, 1989). An excellent 136-page booklet containing some of the best information from one of the leading equine reproduction research centers. Reading is at times frustrating because of lengthy descriptions of the procedures and results of the multitude of individual research studies, unless you are interested in these details. It covers the following, all in regard to the reproducing mare: anatomy and physiology, function and use of hormones, anabolic steroids, estrus detection and rectal palpation, reproductive examination, endometritis, artificial insemination, management of the pregnant mare, pregnancy diagnosis, twinning and early embryonic death, and embryo transfer.

Equine Reproductive Ultrasonography by AO McKinnon, EL Squires, and BW Pickett (1988). Available from the Reproduction and Technology Lab, Colorado State University, Fort Collins, CO. A 59-page booklet that covers: principles, procedures, equipment and normal ultrasonographic anatomy and artifacts; growth and development of the normal fetus; management of twins and early embryonic death; uterine pathology; follicular dynamics preceding and during ovulation; formation and development of the corpus leteum; and ovarian abnormalities.

Collection and Transfer of Equine Embryos by EL Squires, VM Cook, and JL Voss (1985). This 39-page booklet covers management of donors, selection and management of recipients, synchronization of estrus and ovulation in donor and recipient mares, embryo recovery and identification, surgical and nonsurgical embryo transfers, superovulation in mares, freezing equine embryos, and registration of foals from embryo transfer. Available from the Animal Reproduction Laboratory, Colorado State University, Fort Collins, CO, 80523.

Chapter 14

MARE AND FOAL CARE AT FOALING

Gestation Length in Mares 242
Preparations for Foaling 242
Predicting Foaling Time 243
Inducing Foaling 244
Foaling 245
Behavior of the Mare and Foal After Foaling 246
  Maternal Aggression by Mares 248
Neonatal Foal Care 249
  Respiratory Assistance for Foals 249
  Umbilical Care for Foals 249
  Imprint Training 251
  Stool Passage Enhancement for Foals 252
  Antibiotics, Nutrients and Intestinal Inoculant Administration
    to Foals 253

Foal Immunity Attainment, Determination, and Enhancement 254
  Mare's Colostrum 254
  Assessing Foal's Passive Immunity 256
  Treatment of Inadequate Passive Immunity 257
Signs of Illness in Foals 258
Foal Pneumonia 258
Foal Diarrhea 259
Hernias in Foals 261
Leg Abnormalities in Foals 261
  Weak Flexor Tendons (Dropped Fetlocks) 261
  Knee Swelling 262
  Curbed Hocks 262
Mare Care After Foaling 262
Mare Injuries in Foaling 262
Supplemental Reading Recommendations 263

GESTATION LENGTH IN MARES

The length of pregnancy in most mares is usually 330 to 345 days, although it can vary from 310 to 387 days, and it is not unusual for a mare to go as long as 1 year. Gestation length is reported to average 15 to 20 days longer in Belgian, but not other, draft mares, and in mares bred to jacks, and in jennies bred to stallions. Most mares repeat their gestation schedule but tend to foal about 5 days earlier than their first foaling, 5 to 10 days later as they get older (past 12 to 18 years old) and to go 5 to 10 days longer for the birth of colts than fillies. The length of every pregnancy should be a part of each mare's record, and any marked variation from her expected gestation length should be investigated.

Any birth at less than 320 days is premature. Birth at less than 300 days or at more than 375 days is not usually compatible with life. Gestation over 365 days may rarely produce a large foal, which may cause difficult birth, but more commonly, will result in a foal that is small for its gestational age and that poorly tolerates the stress of delivery and the first few weeks of life. Frequently, foals born prematurely have been infected prior to birth or have been poorly nourished by an inadequate placenta. Thus, foals born either early or late are at an increased risk for the development of many problems after birth.

Neither gestation length nor foaling difficulty is affected by excess body weight of the mare, but gestation may be lengthened 4 to 10 days in severely malnourished mares. It may be prolonged by as much as 2 months in mares consuming endophyte-infested tall fescue hay or pasture (see Chapter 19). In contrast, gestation length may be as much as 10 days short without affecting the foals' birth weight in mares exposed to long day length (16 hours), by artificial or natural light, during the last several months of pregnancy.

PREPARATIONS FOR FOALING

Mares should be on a good feeding program as described in Chapter 13 and on good internal-parasite control and

vaccination programs as described in Chapter 9. In addition, mares should be at the intended foaling location at least 1 month before their anticipated foaling date. This allows them to become acclimated to that location and its procedures, and to produce antibodies to organisms indigenous to that area for subsequent transfer to the foal in the colostrum for the foal's protection against these organisms. If this is not done, disease incidence is increased. For example, in one study, diarrheal diseases were 63% higher in foals born to mares recently brought to farms for foaling than it was in foals born to resident mares on these farms.

Mares may be foaled on pasture or in a box stall. In either case, if the mare has had a Casick's closure of the vulva, it should be snipped open with a pair of sharp clean scissors a few days to a week before her expected foaling date. The mare either on pasture or in a stall should be watched closely day and night when foaling is imminent. Foaling of domestic mares most commonly occurs at night, and the mare and her newborn foal, for at least the first few days to weeks after foaling, should be separate from other mares. If this is not done, other mares may occasionally take over from the mother, who may not feel too good or vigorous for at least the first few days after foaling. In addition, if pasture breeding is to be used, the mare and foal should be kept away from stallions other than that foal's sire for at least the first few weeks of the foal's life. Stallions may attack and even kill foals sired by other stallions, particularly during the foal's first few weeks of life. This rarely occurs with older foals and is not known to occur to foals sired by that stallion.

Foaling in a good, clean, well-drained pasture minimizes the foal's exposure to disease-producing organisms and, as a result, infectious diseases. However, confinement to a box stall for foaling may be needed to protect the newborn foal from inclement weather, and so that the mare and foal may be more closely observed and assistance given if foaling or fetal difficulties or distress occur. Although assistance at foaling is needed in only a small percentage of cases, when it is needed, it may be necessary in order to save either or both the mare and foal. Serious foaling difficulty is reported to occur in 2% of Thoroughbred and more than 5% of draft horse births. An additional 3% of Thoroughbred mares require assistance and 3% of Thoroughbred foals require assistance at birth to ensure survival. Thus, help is required in 8% or less of Thoroughbred births and maybe other light horse breeds, and more often in draft mares. Two thirds of abortions, stillbirths and deaths of foals soon after birth were due to noninfectious causes, with complications at birth causing suffocation being the most common. Delayed delivery or prolonged foaling time in mares unattended at the time of foaling was usually considered to be a factor and, therefore, careful monitoring at foaling and help when needed may greatly reduce these losses. Being present at foaling also makes it possible to (1) test the mare's colostrum to ensure its antibody or immunoglobulin level is adequate to provide sufficient immunity for the foal, (2) provide the foal umbilical care, (3) ensure stool passage, and (4) begin desensitization or imprint training of the foal.

If the mare is not to be foaled on pasture, a foaling stall should be used. Ideally the mare should be kept in the foaling stall during at least the last week of pregnancy so she becomes accustomed to it and in case foaling occurs sooner than expected. However, during the day she should be placed in a large paddock or exercise area to help prevent edema. Stocking up and fluid accumulation along the underline is not uncommon in confined mares in late pregnancy. Decreased confinement or 15 to 20 minutes of handwalking twice daily will prevent or result in marked regression of this edema.

The foaling area should be warm, dry, clean, free of sharp and protruding objects, and of a size adequate for the mare and foal. A foaling stall for light horse breeds should be at least 14 ft (4.3m), and preferably 16 ft (4.9 m), square, with walls solid from the floor to at least 4 ft (1.2 m) high. Prior to the expected foaling date, the stall should be thoroughly cleaned, which includes sweeping, scrubbing with an anionic detergent, rinsing with steam or a pressure-water hose, and disinfecting twice, allowing drying after each application. All feed buckets, managers, and waterers should be included. Disinfectants are effective in killing disease-producing organisms only when used on a clean surface. Raw wood and concrete block surfaces are difficult to clean and disinfect adequately because of their porosity. Cleaning and disinfecting them is much easier and more effective if raw wood surfaces are cleaned, knots and holes filled with a wood filler, and two to three coats of marine-quality varnish or polyurethane applied. Concrete blocks after a thorough cleaning should be painted with two coats of enamel. Phenolic compounds are the disinfectants of choice and can be recognized by the -phenol or -phenate ending of the compounds given in the list of active ingredients on the label. Examples of phenolic disinfectants include: Tek-Trol (Bio-Tech Ind, Atlanta, GA); 1 Stroke Environ (Calgon-Vestal Labs, St. Louis, MO); and o-Syl and Lysol soap (National Labs, Montvale, NJ). Phenolic and iodophore compounds are active in the presence of organic matter and kill even rotaviruses, which

are the most resistant of the commonly encountered disease-producing organisms. Iodophores are useful for handwashing disinfection, but are not commonly used to disinfect stalls. Quaternary ammonium compounds, recognized by the -ammonium chloride ending of the active ingredient names, are often used in human hospitals, but are less effective on a farm. Both quaternary ammonium compounds and bleach are readily inactivated by organic matter. Pine oil may be used for its pleasant odor, but it is not an effective disinfectant. Formaldehyde is commonly used to fumigate swine and poultry units and kills germs even in the presence of organic matter, but is highly toxic and has noxious fumes, making it impractical for routine horse farm use. However, a contact time of at least 18 hours with formaldehyde or ammonia is the only known way to disinfect against the coccidia, Cryptosporidia. The role of these coccidia in foal diarrhea is questionable as they can be detected in both normal and diarrheic foals. The effectiveness of disinfection can be checked by culturing swabs or Rodac plates from the cleaned stall. Rodac plates are contact plates used to assess microbial population after cleaning. These procedures are quite helpful in preventing infectious diseases in the foal. In one report, the incidence of foal diarrhea was reduced nearly 40% using these procedures.

Dirt or clay floors should be limed before and between foalings. Unsealed rubber flooring should be removed so both surfaces can be cleaned and disinfected, and so the dirt, clay, or sand beneath it can dry and be limed before the rubber flooring is put back in the stall. Fresh bedding should be put in the stall between each foaling. Straw bedding is preferred over wood or peat shavings, as shavings are more easily drawn into the vagina during foaling, are much more abrasive, and are associated with a higher incidence of foal diarrhea.

PREDICTING FOALING TIME

The signs of approaching foaling time are given in Table 14–1. Most mares do not show all the signs, and some may not exhibit any signs at all. Sometimes all outward signs fail. Some mares will show all the classic signs of being ready to foal but won't do so for days or weeks. Maiden mares particularly may not begin milk production or have noticeable udder development prior to foaling. The problem in predicting the time of foaling is complicated by the wide variation in-gestation length, which may vary by 6 to 7 weeks. Two test procedures that assist in most accurately predicting the time of foaling are changes in rectal temperature and changes in the calcium concentration of mammary secretions.

A daily variation of about 0.2°F (0.1°C) in rectal temperature occurs in mares, with the lowest temperature occurring late morning and the highest between 10 p.m. and midnight. If a record of the mare's rectal temperature is kept, and it shows that the temperature failed to be higher in the evening than that morning, she will probably foal that night or the next. This does not seem to be affected by the ambient temperature. However, a false positive (a lower evening temperature without foaling within 36 hours) may occur as often as 40 to 50% of the time.

During the last several weeks of pregnancy, sodium and

TABLE 14–1
Signs and Stages of Foaling

Signs and Stages		Usual Time of Occurrence
Distended udder (minimal in many maiden mares)		2–4 weeks before foaling
Dropping of the abdomen (more with age), followed by relaxation evident on each side of tailhead		1–3 weeks before foaling
Teats fill with a clear, watery secretion		4–7 days before foaling
Secretions become cloudy and wax-like and cover end of nipples (waxing-over), and calcium exceeds 320 ppm (8 mM/L)		1–4 days before foaling
Vulva becomes loose, soft, and relaxed and no evening drop in rectal temperature		$^{1}/_{2}$–$1^{1}/_{2}$ days before foaling
Foaling stage 1	Stop eating; pacing, restlessness, lying down and getting up which helps get foal into position for birth. Tail switching, sweating and frequent urination. If disturbed, mare can delay progression for many hours.	Begins 2–5 hrs before delivery and 2–3 hrs before water breaks
	Membranes rupture and several gallons of fluid are expelled. Mare now can no longer delay foaling.	30–60 min before delivery
Foaling stage 2*	Amnion, forefeet soles down, then nose appears. If not, provide help. Mare usually standing.	5–15 min after fluid expelled. If over 20–30 min, help needed.
Foaling stage 3*	Most mares lie down, and labor using abdominal effort begins.	15 min or less before delivery
Foaling stage 4	Expulsion of the placenta (fetal membranes)	15–90 min after delivery

* Some define stage 2 as what is given here as stages 2 and 3, which then makes expulsion of the placenta stage 3.

chloride concentrations decrease in mammary secretions, while calcium, magnesium, potassium, phosphate, citrate, lactose, and protein concentrations increase. These changes are gradual except for calcium. When the calcium concentration, with or without magnesium, exceeds 400 ppm (10 mM/L), the mare will foal within an average of 3.6 nights, and one half of all mares will foal within 48 hours. For some, however, it may be as long as 16 days. Thus, the calcium concentration in the mare's milk more reliably indicates when she is not going to foal than when she is going to foal: i.e., if it's not above 400 ppm (10 mM/L, or 40 mg/dl), she isn't going to foal soon, whereas if it is, she is going to foal anytime within the next 2 weeks and most likely within the next 2 to 4 days. If mammary-secretion calcium or total hardness increases weeks prior to the expected foaling date, premature foaling or still birth is likely to occur. An additional criterion indicative of im-

pending foaling is when the mammary-secretion concentration of potassium exceeds that of sodium.

Calcium and magnesium concentrations can be measured using water hardness test kits or those adapted and sold specifically for predicting when foaling will occur. These include Titrets Calcium Hardness Test Kit (CHEMetrics, Calverton, VA) and Merckoquant Total Water Hardness Test Strip (EM Science, Mickleton, NJ, or E. Merck, 6100 Darmstadt, Germany), which measure calcium only, and Predict-A-Foal Kit (Animal Healthcare Products, Vernon, CA) and Sofcheck Water Hardness Test Strip (Environmental Test Systems, Elkhart, IN), which measure calcium plus magnesium concentrations. Those that measure calcium only may be the easiest to interpret and give the most consistent results. To conduct the milk calcium test, add 6 parts distilled water to 1 part milk, mix thoroughly, insert the test strip for several seconds, remove and shake off excess liquid from the strip, wait about 1 minute, and read the results. Accuracy depends on preventing calcium contamination by using distilled water, and rinsing everything used following washing with tap water followed by distilled water.

The best procedure for ensuring that someone is present at foaling would appear to be the following:

1. At about 320 days of pregnancy, or when udder size begins to increase, begin monitoring either the mare's mammary-secretions' calcium concentration once daily or her rectal temperature each morning and evening.
2. If the mare's rectal temperature is not being monitored, begin doing so each morning and evening when her milk calcium exceeds 300 ppm 7.5 mM/L or when a color change has occurred for the first time in two or more zones of the four-test-zone Merckoquant Test Strip.
3. When her evening temperature is equal to or less than her morning temperature, hourly observations are indicated, particularly if she is showing outward signs of impending parturition (Table 14–1) and her mammary-secretions' calcium concentration exceeds 400 ppm 10 mM/L or a color change has occurred in three or more zones of the four-test-zone Merckoquant Test Strip.

INDUCING FOALING

The mare may be induced to foal at a predetermined time to minimize the amount of time necessary to monitor the mare; to ensure that someone, or that veterinary assistance, is present during foaling; or because of problems such as a history of premature placental separation, prolonged pregnancy, uterine paralysis, rupture or impending rupture of the mare's prepubic tendon, pelvic abnormalities, or other potential causes for foaling difficulty, hydrops amni ("dropsi"), colic, painful skeletal disease that becomes more severe as pregnancy nears full term, or for preventing neonatal isoerythrolysis (a disease in which the foal's red blood cells are destroyed by antibodies in its dam's colostrum).

Some have reported high success rates, while others

report incidents of foal loss and other problems when foaling is induced. Improper foal presentation for delivery, inadequate milk production, weak foals, foals with reduced resistance to infectious conditions, retained placenta, or premature placental separation during delivery (predisposing the foal to suffocation), are complications that may be encountered following induction. Because of these potential problems and complications, inducing foaling is discouraged unless there is a compelling reason for it or there is a wide margin of safety for both the mare and the foal. Problems and complications may be minimized or eliminated and foaling induction utilized successfully by paying careful attention to the following prerequisites for induction.

Except for conditions in which inducing foaling is indicated for the well-being of the mare, the major objective of inducing foaling is to increase the chances for the safe delivery of a live healthy foal. To do so it is recommended that **all** of the following criteria be met before foaling is induced.

1. Fetal age greater than 325 and preferably 330 days of pregnancy. However, in one study, only 3 of 10 foals whose birth was induced at 320 days of gestation survived, one induced at 318 days survived, and none of 69 others induced at 280 to 319 days of gestation survived. Knowing that at least 330 days of gestation have passed is not by itself an adequate prerequisite. This alone is not sufficient; some foals are not ready for birth by even 340 days of gestation.
2. There is adequate mammary gland development. The udder should be well developed, the nipples filled, and the secretions changed from clear and watery to a smokey-to-grey color and a more viscous or thicker concentration. These are indications of the mare's readiness to produce colostrum and milk.
3. Relaxation on each side of the mare's tailhead and of the perineal area has occurred.
4. The mare's milk calcium concentration is elevated.

    An elevated milk calcium concentration is a very helpful indicator and precaution that foaling may be safely induced. Ideally, the milk calcium carbonate concentration should be 200 ppm (5 mM/L or 20 mg/dl) or greater (by Titrets Kit) or the calcium concentration (with or without magnesium) should be above 300 ppm (7.5 mM/L) (a color change has occurred in two or more zones of the four-test-zone Merckoquant Strip).

FOALING

There are three or four stages in foaling, depending on whether what some consider as stages 2 and 3 are considered separate or combined. Knowing these stages of foaling and their durations, as summarized in Table 14–1, helps alleviate unnecessary anxiety and disruptive and occasionally harmful interference during normal delivery, and when help should be provided. During foaling, do not try to help; stay away and out of the mare's sight as much as possible, unless there is trouble.

Over 80% of mares foal between evening and dawn. So most foals are up and going by morning, which is probably an inherent protection mechanism in the wild. The first stage of foaling usually begins 2 to 5 hours before delivery and lasts 1 to 4 hours, although the mare can delay it for much longer. It begins with the primiparous mares in a herd seeking isolation if possible; whereas multiparous mares may remain with the herd. The mare stops eating and becomes restless; she paces and lies down and gets up repeatedly. It is important that she be allowed to do this, as it, and the initial uterine contractions which are occurring, assist in getting the foal into proper position for delivery. The uterine contractions cause mild signs of colic such as tail switching, sweating, and frequent urination. These signs may be transitory and intermittent. When these signs begin to occur, wrap the tail (or it may be easier to put it in a tube sock taped at the top around the tailhead) and wash down the perineal area with a mild soap and disinfectant. This will decrease infectious diseases in the foal. If the mare has a Caslick's closure of the top of the vulva, it should have been opened previously, but if not, snip it open with a pair of sharp, clean scissors. Following this, leave the mare alone but watch her, preferably from where she cannot see you. The mare can delay progression of foaling for probably as long as 10 hours at this stage. Continued uterine contractions force the chorioallantois or "water sac" through the cervix, dilating it until the "water sac" breaks, expelling 2 to 5 gallons (8 to 20 L) of fluid.

In the second stage of foaling, continued uterine contractions force the white, glistening amniotic sac, with the foal's foot inside, through the cervix, further dilating it. If instead of the white, glistening amnion, a reddish velvety membrane appears, it is the prematurely separated chorioallantois or placenta. This means that the placenta has separated and the foal is no longer receiving oxygen; it must be delivered quickly or it will suffocate. The placenta should be ruptured immediately and delivery assisted. However, if nothing appears at the vulva within 20 to 30 minutes after the water breaks, this generally indicates that the foal is breech (coming butt first, which occurs in 2% of cases) or in a transverse dorsal presentation (withers coming first, with head and legs down and usually to one side). The foot normally should appear covered by the amnion with its heel and sole down. If the heel and sole are up, this generally indicates that it is a back leg and, therefore, that the foal is being delivered backwards.

From the moment the water breaks until the amnion is visible at the vulva usually takes 10 to 15 minutes and occurs with the mare standing. If there is an indication of abnormal presentation, or the amnion is not visible within 20 to 30 minutes after the water breaks, the veterinarian should be called. If veterinary assistance must be awaited, walk the mare and keep her standing to delay foaling.

In the third stage of foaling, most mares lie down and exertional labor using abdominal effort begins. However, 3 to 10% of mares will deliver the foal while standing. Both of the foal's feet should appear with their heels and soles down and with one foot 4 to 6 inches (10 to 15 cm) behind the other. If the distance is greater than this, there is a chance that one elbow is caught on the mare's pelvis. Normally the foal's nose should become visible and be near its knees; if it is not, this may indicate that the foal's nose is down and caught on the brim of the pelvis or that its head is turned back. Once a foot is showing, there should be progress within 5 minutes. The feet will generally rupture the amnion. After the foal's shoulders are expelled, the mare may rest for 2 or 3 minutes. Continued uterine contractions and abdominal effort normally deliver the fetus, completing the third stage of foaling in about 15 minutes or less after intense exertional labor using abdominal effort begins.

If there is any variation from normal presentation or duration, veterinary help should be sought. Get the mare up and walk her—this could correct a minor abnormality in presentation such as a caught elbow. Getting the mare up is generally necessary to, and greatly assists in, correcting an abnormal presentation, such as a leg or legs, or the head, back.

Difficulty in foaling, in contrast to calving, particularly heifers, in over 95% of the cases is a result of abnormal presentation, position or posture of the foal or twinning, and not of a fetus too large for the mare's pelvic opening. Of these, the great majority are positional or postural problems involving the head or forelegs which can be resolved by experienced individuals when detected early. More difficult foaling problems are uncommon and include combined neck and foreleg flexion, total shoulder flexions, posterior presentations and its variations, transverse presentations, contracted or malformed foals, and anterior presentation with one (hurdling) or both (dogsitting) hind feet drawn up into the birth canal under the chest. If the foal is dead, dismembering it may be the best treatment to avoid risk to the mare from a cesarean; however, a cesarean may be necessary in some cases.

The last or fourth stage of foaling is the expulsion of the placenta or afterbirth. This usually occurs 15 to 90 minutes after delivery of the foal. Occasional cramping pains, like a mild colic, may occur during placental expulsion, and for a few hours afterwards, due to continued uterine contractions. Before the placenta is expelled, some mares become frightened by the hanging fetal membranes and kick at them, occasionally injuring the foal. If the placenta is retained beyond 4 to 6 hours following foaling, treatment is indicated (see section on "Mare Care After Foaling" later in this chapter).

BEHAVIOR OF THE MARE AND FOAL AFTER FOALING

The normal and common behavior and activities of the mare and foal and their time of occurrence after foaling are summarized in Table 14-2. The mare after delivery usually remains lying down for 5 to 30 minutes. This serves three purposes: (1) to rest following the exertion of foaling, (2) to allow the foal to orient itself to its new environment, and (3) to allow continued umbilical cord attachment. Continued attachment of the umbilical cord allows the foal to receive as much as 1.5 qts (1.5 L) of blood from the placenta during the first several minutes following birth. Although this additional blood isn't necessary, it is helpful.

TABLE 14-2
Mare and Foal Activities after Foaling

Behavior	Usual Time of Occurrence
Foal lifts and shakes head	$\frac{1}{2}$–3 min after birth
Foal sits up, i.e., rolls from side onto sternum	1–10 min after birth
Umbilical cord breaks	3–13 min after birth
Foal sucks fingers placed in its mouth	2–20 min after birth
Pupils respond to light and startle reaction to light flash[a]	10 min after birth
Foal moves ears and head, following sound	10–40 min after birth
Mare stands (3 to 10% don't lie down to foal)	5 to 25 (average 10 min) after foaling
Placenta passed	15 to 90 min after foaling
Foal stands	15–180 min after foaling (fillies average 40, colts 65)
Foal walks well	3 to 9 min after standing
Foal seeks care, approaches and follows mare	10 to 20 min after standing
Foal nurses mare and passes meconium (first stool)	$\frac{1}{2}$–6 hrs and usually 1–2 hrs after birth, or 30–90 min after standing
Continued defecation by foal	Once in 10 hrs, increasing to 3–5 times/day
Foal lies down	$\frac{1}{2}$ to $1\frac{1}{2}$ hrs after nursing
Foal drowsy and sleeps, usually on its side	80 to 100 min after nursing
Foal stretches, trots, gallops and grooms itself	4 hrs after birth
Foal first urinates	3–15 hrs after birth; average 6 for colts, 10 for fillies

[a] An anxious, excited foal may not exhibit these reactions.

Following foaling, either before or after standing, the mare may initially sniff the foal nostril to nostril in the normal response to a strange horse. But many mares, particularly those with their first foal, usually don't concentrate on the foal until they have completely investigated the fetal fluids and membranes. This behavior should not be discouraged, as it is thought that the mare identifies the fetal fluids as hers and subsequently identifies the foal as hers because it smells like these fluids. In contrast to many species, the mare rarely eats the fetal membranes. The membranes should not be removed for the first 2 hours after foaling. Following her investigation of the fetal fluids and membranes, most mares will smell and lick the foal. But in contrast to many species, mares lick their foals for the first few hours only. This grooming is beneficial for the development of the maternal-neonatal bond and shouldn't be interfered with. If the foal is lethargic, the mare may strike it gently with her forefoot. A stillborn foal is eventually pawed more forcefully by the mare as she attempts to rouse it or make it move. Mares will voluntarily leave their dead foal after a day or so.

Most neurologically normal foals will sit up within 3 minutes following birth and will suck fingers placed in the mouth 2 to 20 minutes following birth. Using foreleg and neck movements, the foal will struggle to free itself from the membranes and its mother. During these movements and the ensuing creeping forward, the umbilical cord usually breaks and the hind legs are pulled free of the mare and membranes. Once free, these withdrawal movements stop. Mares commonly view this foal activity while lying on their sternum and occasionally may nicker quietly.

Most foals will stand within 15 to 180 minutes following birth. This averages about 60 to 70 minutes for colts and 40 to 55 minutes for fillies. It isn't affected by birth weight, although it tends to be faster for pony breeds. It may take as much as 2 hours of effort for the foal to stand. Most will fall several times during the effort. Don't try to get the foal up or help it. Trying to help exhausts the foal. In addition, it is important that a foal not be lifted by its chest or abdomen as this may fracture its ribs or damage internal organs. If the foal must be moved, pick it up with an arm under its rump and the other arm under its chest in front of its forelegs. If the foal doesn't stand by 3 hours of age yet appears normal, assistance may be given by extending its front legs in front of it, lifting its hind quarters, and helping it maintain its balance. The quicker the foal stands and nurses the better. Although you can't make the foal nurse, helping it up and aiming it in the right direction, if necessary, may be helpful.

The foal's initial standing stance is wide-based, and the first steps are exaggerated and short-strided. The soft collagenous pads over the soles of the foal's feet rapidly become shredded and are lost, which makes walking easier. Within 3 to 9 minutes after standing, most foals walk with relative ease, and, no matter how unsteady and uncoordinated, search for the mare's udder. This search may be misdirected, leading to an attempt to suckle nearly anything encountered, particularly anything under an overhang such as the mare's body. The foal should be allowed to find the udder unassisted, as this helps imprinting and recognition by both the mare and the foal of each other. Both successful nursing and the passing of meconium (fetal feces) usually occur at 1 to 2 hours of age but may take place from $\frac{1}{2}$ to 6 hours. About 5% of foals need help nursing, and about 2% need help passing their first stools. To pass stools some straining is normal, but prolonged straining may indicate impaction. Following passage of stools, repeated defecation occurs about once every 10 hours and increases in frequency with age to 3 to 5 times daily. Urination first occurs at an average of 6 hours of age by colts and 11 hours of age by fillies, and thereafter a dilute urine is excreted 4 to 10 times per day.

The foal's difficult task of lying down will generally be accomplished shortly following nursing, although some foals will fall asleep while they are standing if they haven't mastered lying down, and may fall down if they go into deep sleep. Drowsiness and sleep occur 1.5 to 4 hours, averaging 3 hours, after birth, for an average duration of 7 minutes. After sleep, the foal will stand and nurse again. Most foals will have nursed twice by the time they are 2.5

hrs of age. Frisky play movements may occur as early as 2 hours, and galloping at 6 to 7 hours of age. Thus, by the end of its first day of life, or most commonly by the first morning of its life, the foal will be self-grooming, galloping, grazing, urinating, and defecating—all the functions of a normal adult. For the first several weeks, most foals will nurse for one-half to 2 minutes 18 to 24 times per day and lie down on their side and sleep for 15 to 30 minutes 20 to 25 times per day. The foal spends about one-third of its time lying down during the first 2 months of life (as compared to 5 to 10% for adults). Even the first day of life the foal on pasture with its dam spends 6 to 9% of its time grazing, with this increasing to 23% by 1 to 8 weeks of age and to 40 to 50% by 21 weeks. Excessive human interference can hasten or delay the occurrence of these normal behavioral activities.

The mare and foal's investigation of each other or the placenta should not be disturbed, as this is necessary for their bonding. Maternal imprinting is necessary for the mother to identify her newborn as an individual to be cared for, protected, and allowed to nurse. Foal imprinting enables it to identify its mother as the specific individual to follow and stay near. The critical period for the foal's recognition and acceptance of its dam is longer than that of the dam for her foal. Foals do not learn to follow their dam to the exclusion of any other large moving object for the first 1 to 2 weeks of life, and as a result are more easily separated from their dams than when older. But the foal will begin to nuzzle the mare's head and forequarters and to follow the mare and take shelter beside or behind her by 1 to 3 hours of age. Different species have different protective behavior tactics. Fawns and kids hide, calves and lambs lie together in groups, and foals and mares stay close together. During the first week of life the foal spends 85% of the time within 3 ft (1 m) of its mother, 94 to 99% of the time within 15 ft (5 m) of her, and rarely is more than 30 ft (10 m) from her. As the foal becomes older it begins to wander farther and spend more time away from its mother. Although there is some variation among individual foals, in contrast to an old horseman's myth, colts are not more independent than fillies; i.e., these activities and distances are not different between colts and fillies.

Foals identify their dam by both smell and sight but not by sound. Foals cannot readily distinguish one mare's neigh from another and regularly will approach the wrong mare if she is neighing. Because of this, foals with quiet mothers take longer to find them. Sight, smell, and sound are all important to the mare in identifying her own foal—not just smell, as some have thought. Even when smell is blocked, the mare can identify her foal, although it does take her longer. Mares also respond more to the sound of their own foals. Foals neigh when they are separated from the dam, and nicker when they are asking for care and attention. Neighs probably are highly individualized, making it easier for the dam to recognize her own foal.

Stretching or pandiculation, which is an indication of well-being and therefore important to note, generally first occurs after the foal's first sleep, or at about 4 hours of age. Thereafter foals stretch during sleep, typically after sleeping, and during lying down as well as when standing.

The healthy foal stretches 20 to 40 times the first day of life with this increasing to 40 to 100 times/day during the 3rd to 5th day of life. This frequent stretching is needed and beneficial in straightening tendons and stiff joints after their 11-month period in the womb, in ensuring that all major parts of the body are extended and exercised, and in assisting the foal in its athletic development. Because of frequent stretching, minor degrees of contracted tendons in foals are self-corrected during the first week of life. Stretching occurs as a brief exercise performed casually when the foal is relaxed and undisturbed, and thus requires a quiet peaceful environment.

Play behavior is also beneficial for the foal's athletic and social development. Because of this and the benefit of exercise, the mare and foal with no problems should be placed on pasture of sufficient size to allow the foal to run and play with other foals by 1 week after foaling. Even the day-old foal will show sudden bursts of playful, solitary leaping, running, and bucking, which progresses to mock fighting and chasing among colts, and simple solitary running among fillies. Although fillies don't play as much as colts, they tend to groom one another more.

Self-grooming is standard behavior among foals, as are biting and scratching. The absence of much tail may be the incentive for some foals' standing head to tail with the dam; her fully grown tail offers insect-chasing benefits. The flehmen response (curling the upper lip), which is seen more often in colts than fillies, occurs most frequently during the colt's first month, probably in response to the mare's first heat or estrus following foaling.

Foals, like other young of most species, including people, show that play is an important business and a necessary part of life. Play is important for both exercise and socialization for foals as they grow. It functions as a means of physical development and of practicing adult behavior skills that are beneficial later in life for a wide range of activities. Play is valuable for the development of normal behavior. In all of the various play activities there is the single emotion of pleasure, whereas in nonplay activities there are numerous emotions: anger, fear, and others. Horse play is a good demonstration of play as a purely kinetic activity. For foals, 75% of kinetic activity is in the form of play.

Foals in groups gradually change from being primarily aware of and with their mothers, to being primarily with their peer group, but do form peer groups even in the first week of life. As the need for self-maintenance increases, peer group activities change from play and rest to primarily grazing. The foals move between their peer group and their mothers in various activities. As a result of these activities, their primary social bonding is in kinship groups. All of this is, of course, quite similar to what should and generally does occur with children as they grow and mature.

Maternal Aggression by Mares

Maternal protective aggression directed toward other horses particularly, but also toward other animals or even people, is normal in the first few days to week following foaling. Even when the foal is considerably older, some mares remain protective, particularly when the foal is lying down. Thus, if it is necessary to approach a mare and foal when the intensity of the mare's protective aggression is unknown, it is best to wait until the foal stands up. Protective aggression is helpful not only in protecting the foal from harm from other animals, but also in preventing it from following other horses or animals. Protective aggression when the foal is not lying down usually decreases within a few days following foaling; however, some mares may show extreme protectiveness until they become pregnant again or the foal is weaned.

Even good mothers normally take aggressive actions against their foal as it gets older and too rough, particularly if they have a painful udder. This aggressive behavior includes threatening signs such as laying the ears back, squealing, switching the tail, bunting with the head, making a smacking noise with the mouth, and threatening to or actually biting or kicking the foal. This normal maternal aggression is uncommon toward foals under a month of age, but it increases as the foal gets older and may be a part of natural weaning. This aggression toward the older foal, in which the foal is not harmed, is normal, but, abnormal if the mare pursues and repeatedly bites or kicks the foal.

Normal aggression is most commonly caused by a painful udder. It occurs most often prior to the first suck in any nursing bout and when the foal repeatedly pushes or bunts the turgid udder; once the mare is aggressive toward it, most foals will either begin sucking or quit pushing hard. Some will briefly interrupt their nursing, less commonly return the aggression against the mare, and least commonly stop that nursing bout. Once the foal stops bunting the udder and begins to nurse, aggression toward it normally decreases or stops.

Excessive abnormal aggression toward the foal (usually biting) when it tries to nurse is the most common behavioral problem in foaled mares. Less commonly, a mare may not take aggressive action against the foal but will not allow it to nurse. Even less commonly, a mare may attack her foal when it is not trying to nurse, for example, when it comes between her and her feed. Others may attack their foal whenever it stands, but not when it is lying down.

Abnormal maternal behavior occurs most commonly in young, often nervous mares with their first foal; causes are unknown. Lack of experience, hormonal imbalance, stress during foaling, or lack of contact with the foal during the sensitive period for bond formation may be factors. Pain and stress can interfere with maternal behavior. Too much disturbance by too many people and having other horses nearby increases the risk of maternal rejection and aggression toward the foal, particularly by first-foaling mares. Free-ranging mares can withdraw from the herd to foal if they desire. Because stalled mares can't do this, they may be aggressive against horses in adjacent stalls, especially stallions. Frequently, the mare that is aggressive toward her neighbors may displace the aggression onto her foal. A nervous mother may also attack her foal if it looks, tastes or smells different: e.g., if it is seen wearing a halter or blanket which it hasn't been wearing previously, or if the foal's odor changes as a result of a clinical treatment or procedure.

To assist in preventing maternal rejection and aggression toward the foal, the following procedures prior to, during, and for at least 2 days after foaling are helpful: (1) the mare should be isolated from seeing, smelling, or hearing other horses as much as possible; (2) her contact with people should be minimized (number of people, instances, and duration, particularly with those with whom she is unfamiliar); (3) nothing should be done to change the foal's appearance or smell; and (4) the placenta should not be removed from the stall for at least 2 hours after foaling.

If the aggression may be due to a change in the foal's appearance, this should be corrected; if it may be due to a change in the foal's odor, the new smell can be masked by applying mentholated ointment to both the mare's nostrils and the foal's head and perianal area. Sometimes the aggression stops if the mare and foal are turned out of the stall. The freedom to wander from her foal while in a large paddock or a pasture will alleviate aggressive behavior by some mares. When this is done, however, someone should be present to protect the foal if necessary. Another approach is to turn the mare and foal out with other horses. Faced with other horses, she may begin to protect her foal.

The safest and most successful technique for getting a mare to accept a foal is to restrain her until she accepts and allows the foal to nurse. Procedures for doing this are described in Chapter 15 under "Nurse Mares" for orphan foals. If the mare can be forced to accept the foal, the aggression usually diminishes and is replaced by normal maternal behavior. However, this may take up to 3 weeks, and some mares will not accept their rejected foal. Thus, as with most problems (behavioral, nutritional, infections, traumatic, or parasitic), procedures to minimize risk of the problem's occurring is always best, or, as an old saying goes, "An ounce of prevention is worth a pound of cure."

NEONATAL FOAL CARE

All interference or "help," no matter how well intentioned, should be avoided unless necessary for the health of the mare or foal as summarized in Table 14-3. Foaling should take place where the mare can't see people or other animals, including horses, or ideally even hear them unless she is accustomed to the sounds. Thus, foaling should be observed from a location where the mare can't see or hear the observer. Videocameras work well, allow one person to watch several mares, and are commonly used to observe foalings on many breeding farms. It is important to watch the mare and foal until both are on their feet and moving fairly steadily. Make sure that when the mare attempts to get up following foaling the foal is not where she can step on it. Frequently the mare will lie down and rest for 15 to 60 minutes after foaling.

Respiratory Assistance for Foals

The fetal membranes generally are pulled off the foal's head during delivery. If the membranes remain on the foal's nose after its chest has been expelled, they should be taken off so that it can breathe. If the foal doesn't breathe within 5 minutes following expulsion of its chest or, if delivered backward, its hips, permanent brain damage or death will occur.

If the foal or amniotic fluid are stained yellow brown, material should be gently suctioned from the upper respiratory tract, ideally before the foal takes its first breath. If vacuum suction equipment isn't available, a soft tube on a large syringe can be used. The yellow brown stain is due to stools passed by the fetus in utero, usually because of fetal suffocation due to compression of the umbilical cord. Fetal gasping in utero can draw fluids and stools into the upper respiratory tract. Following birth, this material is drawn further into the respiratory tract when breathing begins. This causes aspiration-induced pneumonia, unless the material is removed prior to the foal's first breath.

Respiratory assistance, if needed, should be provided in a step-wise fashion as summarized in Table 14-4. If the foal does not breathe within 30 seconds following delivery, place it upright, on its chest or sternum with its head and neck extended, remove material from the mouth and nostrils and briskly rub its back and sides with a dry towel. This helps stimulate respiration. Setting the foal upright on its chest is helpful because respiration is easier and more efficient from this position than it is when the foal is lying on its side. If not excessive, fluids not removed by chest compression during birth can be removed from the nasal cavity by stripping the nostrils with the thumb and forefingers. Stimulating the inside of the nostrils or the ear canal with a straw, and flexion and extension of the limbs, may be helpful in initiating breathing efforts. Although usually not necessary for normal-birth foals, the hindquarters may be raised to help drainage if necessary. Elevation should be only 1 foot or so (one-third meter) as excess elevation increases abdominal pressure on the diaphragm and, therefore, may be detrimental. Suction if available may also be used. A small, soft, rubber or latex tubing on a 60-ml syringe may be used. Excessive negative pressure and prolonged pharyngeal and tracheal aspiration should be avoided because these remove oxygen and can be detrimental. Suction should be applied for only a few seconds at a time and only during withdrawal of the tubing from the airway. If breathing doesn't occur within an additional 30 seconds, or 60 seconds of birth, close the foal's opposite nostril and lips, inflate the lungs by blowing into one nostril until the chest rises, then release both nostrils. This initial inflation, or a few short puffs, may be all that is necessary to get breathing started. Next check the quality of the peripheral pulse, the heart rate, the color of the membranes, and the capillary refill time. If the foal doesn't begin breathing on its own within 2 minutes after a few short puffs to inflate its lungs, establish a respiratory rate of 20 to 30 breaths per minute until the foal begins to breathe normally. If pulse, heart rate, respiratory rate, membrane color, and capillary refill time aren't normal, or the foal is unable to remain sitting up on its chest, veterinary assistance should be obtained.

The foal's normal respiratory rate is 60 to 90 breaths/min at birth, and is higher in colder conditions. It decreases to one-half this rate by 1 to 2 hours of age. The heart rate should be at least 60 beats/min, increasing to 80 to 130 after the first 5 to 10 minutes of life.

Umbilical Care for Foals

Allow normal activity of the mare and foal to break the umbilical cord without interference. If the umbilical cord

TABLE 14–3
Care of the Foal at Birth

Time after Birth	Procedure
	Respiratory Assistance
At birth	Leave both mare and foal alone unless assistance is needed, then give only the help necessary. Make sure the membranes are off foal's nose. If foal or fluid is yellow brown stained, gently aspirate material from upper respiratory tract before the foal's first breath.
	If not breathing:
30 sec	• Place foal on sternum with head and neck extended, clear mouth and nostrils, and rub down with dry cloth.
60 sec	• Inflate lungs (mouth to nostril while holding other nostril and mouth closed).
75 sec	• Inflate lungs 20 to 30 times/min until breathing begins. If it doesn't, treat as outlined in Table 14–4.
	Umbilical Care
15 min	If it hasn't broken, break it at its constriction by twisting it.
15–30 min	Soak umbilicus in a non-tissue-damaging disinfectant solution twice daily for 3 days.
	Imprint Training
15–60 min	Begin desensitization after umbilical care and before the foal stands.
	Stool Passage Assistance
Within 2 hrs	Give gently 1–2 pts (½–1 L) enema of soapy water or 4–6 oz (120–180 ml) of a commercial nonirritating enema solution.
When in discomfort	Give 4% acetylcysteine enema and 2 oz (60 ml) of mineral oil and/or castor oil orally.
	Passive Immunity Determination and Enhancement
	Wash mare's udder with disinfectant solution, rinse, and dry.
	If colostrum immunoglobulin (Ig) G concentration is:
Before nursing & foal is <12 hrs old	>3000 mg/dl or specific gravity >1.060 it is adequate, but if it is 1000–3000 mg/dl (sp gr 1.050–1.060) give foal 10–12 oz (300–360 ml), and if it is <1000 (sp gr <1.050) give foal 24 oz (700 ml) of colostrum containing ≥7000 mg IgG/dl (sp gr ≥ 1.090).
After nursing and foal is 6–10 hrs old	Measure foal's plasma IgG concentration. If it is: 200–400 mg/dl give 10–12 oz (300–360 ml), and if it is <200 mg/dl give 24 oz (700 ml) of colostrum containing ≥7000 mg IgG/dl (sp gr) ≥1.090).
After nursing and foal is >18–24 hrs old	If foal's plasma IgG concentration is: <400 mg IgG/dl give intravenously sufficient Ig to increase it to >400, or if stressed >800. Initially 20–40 ml of plasma/kg or 200–500 mg IgG/kg is suggested.
	Placenta
When passed	Examine to determine if it's all there.
4 hrs	If not all is expelled, veterinary treatment of the mare is recommended.
	Give Foal
Day 1	Tetanus antitoxin (1500 IU) and tetanus toxoid if it is not known that the dam was given toxoid in last trimester. Give a second imprint training session on day 1 or 2.
	Deworm Mare
	With ivermectin to prevent Strongyloides westeri larvae transmission to the foal through the mare's milk.
	Housing and Exercise
Day 2 on	Put normal foal with dam out on paddock or pasture as much as possible but keep separate from the other mares for at least the first several days.

is broken too quickly (within less than a few minutes of birth), blood may squirt from the foal's umbilical stump. In the majority of cases, the amount of blood lost is small; but if blood loss does occur when the umbilical cord is separated, the cord should be pinched closed with the fingers and held for 1 to 2 minutes. During this time, the artery constricts and the cord can generally be released without further loss of blood. If bleeding persists, however, an umbilical clamp or sterile, nonabsorbable ligature can be put around the end of the stump and removed in 6 to 12 hours.

If the umbilical cord hasn't broken by itself by 15 minutes after delivery, find the constriction in it, which is usually about 1 to 2 inches (3 to 5 cm) from the foal's abdominal wall, grasp the cord with one hand on each side of the constriction, then twist and pull it apart. Be careful not to pull on it from the foal's abdomen. Cutting the cord results in excessive hemorrhage from the umbilical stump and

possibly in urine leakage from the stump. In contrast, the elastic muscular walls of the two umbilical arteries generally result in prompt, prolonged constriction of the umbilical stump when it is separated by stretching.

Following umbilical cord rupture, soak the stump for several seconds in a 2% tincture of iodine, a 1% povidone-iodine, or a 0.5% chlorhexidine solution. This should be repeated twice daily for the next 3 days—once is not adequate. A strong (7%) tincture of iodine solution is quite damaging to the tissue and should not be used. Avoid getting iodine on the foal's abdominal wall or thighs as it can irritate and damage the skin. Evaluate the stump daily for signs of infection (moistness, reddening, heat, swelling, or pus discharge), abscess, and urine leakage. If these don't occur, the umbilical stump dries up in less than 2 days. A failure to follow these procedures, or a dirty environment at the time of birth, greatly increases the risk of umbilical infection ("navel ill"). An infected umbilicus is a major

TABLE 14–4
Foal Respiratory Stimulation and Assistance

I. Establish Patent Airway
  1. Clear and remove membranes from over nostrils.
  2. Place foal on sternum, head outstretched with rear end elevated.
  3. Strip fluids gently from nostrils with fingers.
  4. Tickle inside of nostrils to induce sneezing.
  5. Gently suck fluids from mouth and pharynx using a bulb syringe or suction tube.
II. Stimulate Respiration
  Rub with towels and flex limbs.
III. Note the following:
  Heart rate (normal over 60/min), respiratory rate (normal over 60/min, decreasing to near 30 by 1 to 2 hrs of age), reflexes, mucous membrane color, and capillary refill time, and changes in these parameters over a several-minute period.
IV. Administer Oxygen
  1. Inflate lungs by putting your mouth to foal's nostril.
  2. If respiration doesn't begin, inflate lungs 20 to 30 times/min, and
  3. If foal is breathing but respiratory or heart rate are less than 60/min or foal is unable to remain on its sternum, obtain veterinary assistance.

portal of entry for infectious organisms, resulting in septicemia, joint infections (joint-ill), abdominal cavity infections (peritonitis), internal abscesses, and pneumonia. These conditions, even with treatment, often result in death of affected foals. Even if the affected foal survives, its future health and performance ability may be impaired. Umbilicus infection, and as a result these effects, are prevented by proper umbilicus care as described.

Imprint Training

Imprint training permanently desensitizes the foal to handling and other external stimuli, and sensitizes the foal to respond appropriately to human requests. Imprint training can make handling easier for the rest of the horse's life, enhance later training, decrease injuries to both the horse and the people associated with it, and increase responsiveness to stimuli which will later enhance performance and pleasure for both the horse and its handler in working together. Through imprint training, the foal can be taught not to fear or respond inappropriately to touch anywhere on its body, loud or strange noises, or fluttering or whirling objects, and will respond in the manner desired to touch or pressure. But the foal can learn what to fear as quickly as what not to fear so it must not be hurt or scared. Little restraint, a low-voiced comforting murmur, and scratching should be used.

Imprint training of foals ideally should start within a few hours following birth. There is only a narrow period of opportunity in which desensitization can be quickly and easily accomplished: for example, for ducklings from 7 to 22 hours following hatching. Prey species, such as foals, ducklings, calves, lambs, etc., as soon after birth as possible must be able to perceive danger and flee it in order to maximize their chances for survival. Thus, very soon following birth they must be able to determine if a stimulus is or is not something to fear. In contrast, non-prey species, such as carnivorous animals, do not need to be able to flee immediately following birth and are born unable to see,

hear, or flee. Their imprinting period is delayed until they are more mature—e.g., in puppies between 6 to 12 weeks of age.

Some have feared that beginning imprint training of the foal at birth may interfere with normal bonding between the foal and its dam. This, however, does not appear to be a problem, at least in the vast majority of cases of gentle well-mannered mares. It does require that the mare be brought in from pasture for foaling and that she be gentle and well mannered. In addition, when approaching the mare and foal, always greet the mare first. When working with the foal, have the mare haltered and facing the foal. Injury to the foal, mare, or person may occur if the mare becomes aggressively defensive of the foal, or later in trying to get her to accept the foal, if she rejects it. If the mare is not gentle and well mannered, and this has not been corrected before foaling, it is probably best not to begin imprint training until the foal's second day of life.

For a short time following birth the foal will apparently bond simultaneously with its dam and with one or more persons handling it. It then appears to consider people dominant but nonthreatening and nonfearful. This is the ideal relationship between a horse and people. The horse must be submissive if it is to work with us, but that submissiveness should be created by dependency on and trust in a dominant leader (people), and not by fear. In contrast to what some have believed, bonding of a foal to people will not result in a spoiled pet that is indifferent to stimuli that allow it to race or perform well. To the contrary, imprint training will teach the foal good manners and increase its responsiveness to stimuli that will later improve its performance.

It is recommended that the initial training session begin after disinfecting the umbilical cord, but that care be taken not to interfere with the mare's smelling and licking of the foal or the placenta. Begin by rubbing the foal dry with a towel and by gently but rapidly rubbing each area to be desensitized until the foal is oblivious to it. This is indicated by calm resignation, relaxation, and a sleepy expression. Continuing this procedure on each area until this response is obtained is important. If you stop the procedure while the foal is struggling, it will be taught escape behavior instead of being permanently desensitized to handling or touching that area. You cannot overdo stimulus of an area, but you *can* underdo it. Desensitize the foal to noises, motions, and touch anywhere on its body, including body openings. The initial session to do this takes about an hour. It and shorter subsequent periods are quite likely the most effective and valuable time anyone will ever spend with that horse.

Any number of patterns may be followed in desensitizing the foal. The following may be helpful. Start at the poll, next the ears, then insert a finger into the ear canals, next the face, followed by the underside of the upper lip, the mouth, the tongue, and both nostrils. All of this takes 10 to 15 minutes. Next do the eyes, neck, chest, saddle area, and all four legs, including repeated flexing of each joint. Tap the bottom of each foot 50 to 100 times. Do the rump, tail, area between the hind legs, including the genitalia, udder region of the filly, perineum, and anus. Rub a running electric clipper all over the foal's body, especially around the face and ears (without cutting any hair). Even though desensitized to the sound of one kind of clipper, later in life the horse may still be frightened the first time it hears another kind. Rub the entire body with a piece of crackling plastic. Take lots of time. Watch for habituation, as indicated by relaxation, before any stimulus is stopped. If desired, you can desensitize the newborn foal to gunfire, whistles, loud music, flapping flags, whirling ropes, hissing sprayers, and recorded noises such as dogs barking.

A second desensitization session should be done on the first or second day following birth. It is imperative that the foal not learn to escape when being handled, so it is best to have an assistant hold it. Stand the foal nose to nose with its dam to allay apprehension for both. Quietly test all areas previously desensitized. If an area is not adequately desensitized, repeat the process. Standing beside the foal, reach around it and clasp your hands together under its chest. Rhythmically squeeze and relax until desensitization occurs. This will later prevent the horse from being "cold-backed" or "cinch-bound." Desensitize the foal to additional stimuli, such as flapping blankets, running water from a hose, going through and standing in belly-deep running water, livestock, dogs, etc. The foal should experience in a small way whatever people may want it to tolerate when it is older. At several days of age, load the mare and foal in a trailer and take them for a short ride. Each session should not exceed 15 minutes but can be repeated several times a day if necessary. Twice-daily sessions are generally adequate.

Following desensitization, the foal should be sensitized to certain responses, beginning with moving its hind end when requested. Standing beside the foal, put one arm under its neck so it can't move forward. With the other arm, reach over its back and poke a finger into its flank on the other side of you. To escape the pressure, the foal will eventually move toward you and away from the pressure of your finger in its flank. When it does so, even slightly, immediately relieve the pressure. Be sure you are standing away from the foal enough to allow it room to move its hind end toward you and away from your finger pressure. Wait 20 to 30 seconds and repeat the stimulus, immediately rewarding even the slightest movement away from your finger by stopping the pressure. Most foals learn with 3 to 5 repetitions to move whenever they feel pressure on their flank. Don't ask for more than one step in the first training session, but do both sides. In a day or so, when the response is consistent, you may then ask for a second step and later a third.

Next, put a well-fitting halter on the foal. Remove it after the training session to avoid accidents. Working with an assistant in a well-bedded stall, gently pull the halter to one side. The assistant should prevent the foal from moving forward, back, or to the opposite side. Eventually, in order to maintain balance, the foal will move in the direction its head is being pulled. When it does, even slightly, immediately quit pulling. Proceed just as described previously for training the foal to move its hind end until the foal can be circled both ways. Gradually expand the circle until the foal is leading in a circle. After several sessions the foal will be leading. If desired, a loop of rope behind the foal's rump can be used to encourage forward movement. It also helps if initially the foal is encouraged to lead toward its dam. By one week of age, if the mare can be ridden, lead the foal while riding the mare in a small corral or paddock.

Stool Passage Enhancement for Foals

Meconium—dark green, brown to black, tarry stools formed prior to birth—normally begins to be passed without difficulty within one-half to 6 hours, and usually within 1 to 2 hours, after birth, or one-half hour after standing. In most foals, all meconium has been excreted by 24 to 48 hours of age, although some may take 96 hours. Masses of meconium often are quite firm, sticky and large, resulting in various degrees of constipation and pain upon defecation. As a result, impaction of the meconium and an inability to pass it without assistance occurs in about 2% of foals. This occurs more commonly in colts than fillies because the inside diameter of the colt's pelvis is smaller, making it more difficult for the colt to pass meconium. Foals born after 340 days of pregnancy also appear to be more prone to meconium impaction.

Meconium impaction results in signs of mild colic, which become evident 6 to 24 hours after birth, and include repeatedly getting up and down, straining with an elevated tail and arched back, switching the tail, squatting, and frequent attempts to defecate and urinate. It is the most common cause of abdominal discomfort in neonatal foals. The offending impaction sometimes can be felt by digital rectal palpation, which should be done only with a well-lubricated finger. However, sometimes the impaction is in the small colon instead of the rectum and cannot be palpated. A distended colon may become evident even before abdominal distention. In some foals the urachus may reopen as a result of straining to defecate. If the meconium impaction is not relieved, the signs of abdominal pain become more severe. The foal may roll or lie on its back, become more restless, and nurse intermittently and less frequently with increasing duration of impaction, leading to dehydration. If not relieved, depression, sweating, and ultimately death occur.

Clinical signs of meconium impaction are similar to those of a ruptured bladder. However, symptoms of a ruptured bladder usually are not apparent until 48 to 72 hours after birth (instead of 6 to 24 hours, as they are with meconium impaction), and urine can be obtained from the abdominal cavity. Other causes of colic in the young foal include small intestine displacements, and occasionally gas distention and diarrhea due to acute enteritis, such as that caused by Clostridium perfringens. However, intestinal displacements rarely occur in the first few days of life and result in much more acute and severe signs. Clinical signs of developmental anomalies of the intestinal tract, such as the absence of a colon or anus, or ileal innervation, also resemble meconium impaction. However, with the absence of a colon or anus, signs generally don't occur until the foal is 2 to 3 days old and tend to be less severe. The absence of ileal innervation, or lethal white foal syndrome, occurs in white foals born to overspotted horses (ventral portion of the body is spotted white, and the dorsal aspect of the body is a dark color). Inguinal and diaphragmatic hernias may also cause abdominal pain in young foals. Inguinal hernias occur in colts and are characterized by enlargement of one or both sides of the scrotum. Despite their rather common occurrence, inguinal hernias usually don't cause symptoms and self-correct within the first few weeks of life. Foals with congenital diaphragmatic hernias usually have difficulty breathing.

To prevent meconium impaction, an enema should be given within 2 hours of birth. Most commonly it is given 15 to 30 minutes after birth, following umbilical care. The enemas most commonly used are warm, mild, soapy water (1 to 2 pints, or $\frac{1}{2}$ to 1 L) or commercially available enema solutions. The enema solution should be given very carefully to prevent rectal trauma or perforation. The newborn foal's rectal walls are frail and easily damaged. The enema tube should not be advanced more than 10 to 12 inches (25 to 30 cm) into the rectum, and the fluid should flow by gravity.

If the meconium isn't passed or clinical signs occur, enemas may be repeated at 4-hour intervals, and 4 to 8 ounces (120 to 240 ml) of mineral oil and/or 2 ounces (30 ml) of castor oil may be given orally by way of a stomach tube. If no response occurs after two to four enemas, a commercial Fleet enema may be used, but it should not be repeated more than twice. Oral laxatives are almost always effective in relieving impaction when administered before intestinal motility has been decreased by gas distention and persistent colic. Even in refractory cases, repeated enemas and oral laxatives are safer than attempting to remove the meconium with the finger or a surgical instrument. Surgery is rarely necessary to relieve the impaction; it is only necessary if the impaction is not responsive to persistent medical therapy and the foal's condition is deteriorating.

Antibiotics, Nutrients, and Intestinal Inoculant Administration to Foals

The administration of antibiotics to the newborn foal to help guard against infectious diseases is controversial. A long-acting penicillin injection is commonly used. Proponents contend that it helps protect the foal when it is most vulnerable and exposed to a variety of infectious organisms in its new environment out of the uterus. Adversaries, including this author, assert that using antibiotics in this manner has a greater potential for harm than benefit. It is unlikely to help the foal, and it increases organisms resistant to that antibiotic. In addition, penicillin is a poor choice because many septicemias in foals are not susceptible to it. The incidence of diarrhea in foals is several times higher in those given antibiotics at birth than those not given them. It is recommended that antibiotics not be given to healthy foals to try to prevent disease unless foals are born and raised in filthy environments or have low plasma immunoglobulin levels, in which case cleaning the environment and increasing the foal's plasma immunoglobulin levels, as described later in this chapter, are much more beneficial than is antibiotic administration. Proper hygiene, colostrum intake, and good management cannot be replaced by giving antibiotics.

The only supplemental nutrients whose administration to the newborn foal appears to have a potential for being beneficial are vitamins A and E, and selenium in areas deficient in it (Fig. 2-4). Vitamins A and E, are not transferred across the placenta. Therefore, regardless of the mare's intake or body content of these vitamins, the foal is deficient in both at birth. Selenium is transferred across the placenta, depending on the mare's selenium status. Thus, in selenium-deficient areas, without supplementation the foal at birth will be deficient in selenium, as well as in vitamins A and E. All three of these nutrients are secreted into the milk and are particularly high in the colostrum if the mare has adequate intake, or for vitamin A only, if the mare has adequate body stores available. If not, the foal's deficiency will persist. The foal is quite susceptible to and commonly affected by vitamins A and E and selenium deficiencies. The effects of these deficiencies are described in Chapters 2 and 3. One effect of a deficiency of any one of these three nutrients is increased susceptibility to infectious diseases, particularly of the respiratory and intestinal tracts, resulting in pneumonia, septicemia, or diarrhea.

Because of these factors, it is frequently recommended that within 6 to 24 hours of birth all foals be given an intramuscular or subcutaneous injection of 250, to 500, IU of vitamin A, 50 to 200 IU of vitamin E, and in areas where selenium deficiency is known to occur (Fig. 2-4), selenium at the manufacturer's recommended dosage. Vitamin D is present in many vitamin A preparations at a nonharmful level, and, therefore, may be given along with the vitamin A. However, if the brood mares are on a good feeding program, as described in Chapter 13, and the foal receives the amount of colostrum necessary for adequate immunity, as discussed later in this chapter, giving newborn foals vitamins is unlikely to be of benefit. Although it is unlikely that their administration in the amounts given above is harmful, in one study diarrhea in 1- to 14-day-old foals was higher in those given vitamins than in those not given vitamins. Differences other than vitamin administration may have been responsible. However, there was no indication of any benefit from the administration of the vitamins, and the administration of some nutrients to newborn foals may be harmful. This was dramatically illustrated by the death of many foals following the oral administration of an iron-containing intestinal inoculant.

In 1982 and 1983, a previously unrecognized form of acute liver failure occurred in many newborn foals in many locations in the United States. The disease was characterized by lethargy and jaundice at 2 to 3 days of age, followed by diarrhea, bleeding from the nose and in the urine, increased excitability, often blindness, and incoordination with death at 4 to 6 days of age. The disease was found to be caused by the oral administration of a digestive inoculant made and recommended for foals. This inoculant contained several viable bacterial cultures and fermentation products, vitamins A, D_3, E, and B_{12}, and iron, which later was found to be the toxic principal in the inoculant. The dose of iron that will cause acute toxicosis in newborn foals is much lower than the amount toxic to other species or to the foal after the first several days of life. A vitamin E or selenium deficiency also appears to increase the foal's susceptibility to iron toxicosis, as it does in baby pigs.

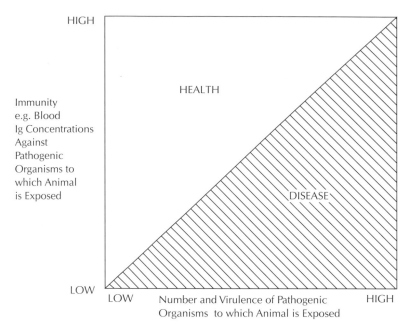

HIGH

Immunity
e.g. Blood
Ig Concentrations
Against
Pathogenic
Organisms to
which Animal
is Exposed

HEALTH

DISEASE

LOW

LOW   HIGH
Number and Virulence of Pathogenic
Organisms to which Animal is Exposed

Fig. 14–1. Effects of immunity and exposure to infectious organisms on disease occurrence and severity.

Foal Immunity Attainment, Determination, and Enhancement

Two things are necessary to minimize the risk of infectious disease in the foal: (1) minimize exposure to disease-producing organisms, and (2) maximize the foal's immunity or resistance to these organisms. As indicated in Figure 14–1, an infectious disease does not occur even if immunity is low if the animal is exposed to few disease-producing organisms, or conversely, if immunity is high even if the animal is exposed to many highly virulent disease-producing organisms. In contrast, an infectious disease does occur when immunity is low with respect to the number and virulence of organisms to which the animal is exposed. Providing as clean an environment as possible for foaling and the first few weeks of life, as described earlier in this chapter, in the sections on "Preparation for Foaling" and proper umbilical care, are the first steps to minimizing the foal's exposure to infectious organisms. The next step is after foaling, when the mare is standing and before the foal nurses: wash the mare's udder with a mild disinfectant solution and rinse and dry it off. At this time, make sure that the teats are open and that colostrum or first milk secreted is present. Take a sample to determine its immunoglobulin (Ig) or antibody concentration.

Antibodies or Ig necessary for resistance to infectious organisms and diseases caused by them can be produced by the equine fetus. However, at birth, the foal is virtually devoid of circulating Ig. This is because: (1) normally, while in the uterus, the fetus is not exposed to any infectious organisms that would stimulate Ig production, and (2) maternal Ig cannot cross the placenta and thus be transferred to the foal during pregnancy. Following birth, the foal will begin producing Ig against nonoverwhelming numbers of infectious organisms to which it is exposed, but it takes several weeks to produce an amount of Ig sufficient to be protective. Thus, during the first few weeks of life, the foal has little immunity or resistance against disease-producing organisms except for the Ig against them that it receives in the colostrum. Colostrum contains Ig against organisms or their toxins to which the mare has been exposed either by vaccination or in her environment. However, their concentration in the colostrum and the foal's ability to absorb them decreases rapidly to near zero in the first day following foaling. Thus, a failure to obtain sufficient Ig for prevention of infectious diseases may occur in any one of three ways: (1) low colostral Ig concentration, (2) failure of the foal to ingest a sufficient amount of colostrum, and (3) failure of the foal to absorb sufficient amount of ingested Ig because colostrum intake is delayed too long after birth.

The higher the colostral Ig concentration, and the more of it and the sooner following birth the foal obtains it, the more Ig absorbed and the higher the foal's plasma Ig concentration and, therefore, resistance to infectious diseases. A failure to obtain or absorb sufficient colostral Ig is the most important factor predisposing the foal to acquiring an infectious disease; even on well-managed farms, unless corrected, generally this occurs in 10 to 20% of all foals.

Mare's Colostrum

Colostrum is produced during the last month of gestation, with most of the Ig it contains secreted during the last 2 weeks. Colostrum is produced only once during each pregnancy. The mare's colostrum contains three major types of immunoglobulin: IgG, IgM, and IgA, which normally at foaling are present at concentrations of approximately 4000 to 10,000, 500 to 1500, and 50 to 200 mg/dl, respectively. IgG and IgM, but not IgA, are absorbed by the foal. However, the concentration of IgG and IgM in the mare's colostrum decreases as they are removed from the udder since what remains in the udder is diluted by milk, which is what the mare is now secreting—not colostrum. By 6 hours following first removal of colostrum from the udder, its IgG concentration is about one half of the concentration present at foaling; by 8 to 10 hours it is 20 to 40%; and by 12 to 18 hours, 5 to 25% of that present initially. Colostral IgG concentration is below that necessary to ensure adequate passive immunity for the foal by 8 to 16 hours after foaling in most mares. Colostrum also contains proteins that enhance the efficacy of absorption of Ig and that aid in defense against microorganisms.

In contrast to the decrease in IgG and IgM concentrations, the IgA concentration in mammary secretions increases after foaling. Although ingested IgA is not absorbed into the circulation, it and other nonabsorbable colostral and milk components are quite beneficial in providing local protection for the gastrointestinal tract against infection-induced diarrheal diseases. The foal's resistance to infectious diarrhea is probably more dependent on the quantity and quality of milk IgA than on colostral IgG; whereas resistance to other infective diseases, such as septicemia and pneumonia is dependent on the amount of colostral IgG absorbed.

While Ig is not usually concentrated in the colostrum until induced by hormonal changes occurring just prior to foaling (Fig. 13-3), in some mares this may occur earlier and the mares may begin to leak colostrum before foaling. As a result, the colostrum high in IgG and IgM is lost, and their concentration progressively decreases in subsequently remaining or secreted colostrum so that reduced amounts are available for that mare's foal. This is a major cause of a failure of adequate passive antibody transfer to the foal. The cause of colostrum loss before foaling (colostrum or milk streaming or leakage) is not known. It is not related to previous occurrences in that mare, bearing twins, or to placental infection, insufficiency, or premature separation. It may be more common in older multiparous mares.

Colostral Ig levels decrease not only as colostrum is produced but also as the duration of gestation increases or decreases above or below 338 to 350 days. Inducing foaling, regardless of gestation length, may also result in lower colostral Ig levels. Colostral IgG levels are also lower in older mares, with the decrease beginning after 10 years of age. As a result, the prevalence of failure of adequate passive antibody transfer to foals may be higher in foals born to mares 15 years of age or older than in those born to younger mares.

The colostral Ig concentration before, but not after, the foal nurses is the most important factor determining, and directly related to, the serum IgG concentration of the 24- to 72-hour-old foal that has nursed that mare. This amount, in turn, is inversely related to the incidence and severity of infectious diseases in foals. Thus, the higher the prenursed colostrum IgG concentration, the higher the foal's serum IgG concentration, and the lower the risk an infectious disease will occur in that foal. The prenursed colostrum Ig concentration, therefore, is a good indication of the foal's resistance to infectious diseases during its first several weeks of life.

Although a thick, yellow, good-appearing colostrum doesn't guarantee that its Ig concentration is high, a thin, watery or milky-appearing secretion almost always indicates that its Ig concentrations is low and inadequate. Colostrum's specific gravity, which can be quickly and easily measured using a modified hydrometer, does give a good indication of its Ig concentration (Table 14-5). Because a fluid's volume increases and, therefore, its specific gravity decreases, with increasing temperature, colostrum should be allowed to cool from body to room temperature before its specific gravity is measured, or 0.05 should be added to the specific gravity measured at body temperature. Distilled, not tap, water should be used in the hydrometer, and ensure that no air is trapped by the hydrometer or it will give erroneously low values.

Kits are also available commercially for measuring colostrum Ig concentration. The methods best suited for on-farm determination of colostrum Ig concentration are measuring its specific gravity and kits that use the latex agglutination test (Table 14-6). The latex agglutination test is designed to indicate low, medium, and high colostrum Ig concentrations (<2500, 2500 to 5000, and >5000 mg/dl, respectively). Its results have been reported to be more subjective, and for a large number of samples, it is more expensive to use, than those obtained using the modified hydrometer (Equine Colostrometer).

Colostrum available to the newborn foal should contain more than 3000 mg IgG/dl as indicated by a specific gravity of greater than 1.060 (Table 14-5). In one study, only 1 of 169 foals that were born to and left from birth with mares having a colostrum with a specific gravity of 1.060 or greater had a failure of adequate antibody transfer as indicated by a serum IgG concentration of less than 400 mg/dl at 24 hours of age. However, colostral specific gravity is less than 1.060 in about 20 to 25% of mares. Thus, all mares' colostral Ig concentration should be measured before the foal nurses and, if it is too low (below a specific gravity of 1.060 or concentration of 3000 mg/dl), the foal should be given supplemental colostrum that is sufficiently high in Ig, preferably one that contains a specific gravity of 1.090 or greater or over 7000 mg Ig/dl.

Measuring the mare's plasma Ig concentration before

TABLE 14–5
Specific Gravity and Immunoglobulin G (IgG) Concentration Relationship in Mare's Colostrum and Her Foal's Serum IgG Concentration

Colostrum Specific Gravity[a]	Colostrum IgG (mg/dl)		Foal's Serum IgG (mg/dl) at 24 hrs of age	
	Mean	Range	Mean	Range
1.020–1.040	Milk, not colostrum			
≤1.045	<1000	0–1500	150	0–370
1.050–1.055	2200	1100–2900	380	200–500
1.060–1.065	4200	3000–5700	880	500–1300
1.070–1.075	5600	4000–7300	1300	600–1850
1.080–1.085	6400	4650–8500	1400	600–1850
1.090–1.095	7800	7000–8400	1300	850–1500
>1.10	>9100		1600	1400–2000

[a] Measured at room temperature using a modified hydrometer (Equine Clostrometer, Lane Manufacturing, Denver, CO 80222). If measured at body temperature, add 0.05 to the specific gravity measured.

TABLE 14–6
Immunoglobulin Concentration Measurement Tests[a]

Test	Commercial Name	Source	Comments
Latex agglutination[b]	Aglutinate Foal Immunity Test & Equine Colostrum Test	McCullough Cartwright, Barrington, IL 60010, Animal Health, Kansas City, MO 64108 & Cambridge Life Sciences, Cambridge, England	Can use blood, plasma or serum, takes 10 min to run but indicates only if the concentration is above or below a specific value for which the test is made (usually either 400 or 800 mg/dl)
	FoalChek	Miles Labs, Elkhart, IN 46514 & Haver Mobay Corp, Shawnee, KS 66201	
	IgG Screen	Hamilton Thorn, Danvers MA 01923	
Dipstick ELISA[b]	EquiStick	Animal Biotech Corp, Newport Beach, CA	
Membrane Filter ELISA[b]	CITA Semi-Quant Equine IgG Test Kit	INDEXX, Portland, ME: or Worrstadt, Germany	Can use blood, plasma or serum, takes 10 min, indicates if concentration is <200, 200 to 400, 400 to 800, or >800 mg/dl
Glutaraldehyde coagulation[b]	None. Add 0.05 ml 10% glutaraldehyde to 0.5 ml serum. If a solid gel forms that doesn't move when tilted in ≤10 min IgG >800, & in ≤60 min IgG >400 mg/dl		Most accurate test at 400 to 800 mg/dl, cheapest, requires serum, severe hemolysis may result in overestimation & takes <10 to 60 min to conduct.
Coagglutination	D-Tech Foal IgG Test	Pitman-Moore, Northbrook, IL 60062	More complex, difficult to do & interpret, & less accurate than those above.
Zinc sulfate turbidity or precipitation	Equi-Z	VMRD Inc, Pullman, WA 99163	Influenced by time, temperature, hemolysis, carbon dioxide in its reagents, and is less accurate below 400 mg/dl.
Radial Immunodiffusion	RID	VMRD Inc, Pullman, WA 99163 Miles Labs, Elkhart, IN 46514	Most accurate, but requires 48 hrs and isn't suitable for on-the-farm use
Sodium sulfite precipitation			In contrast to bovine serum, it does not give reliable results with equine serum

[a] Colostrum (but not blood, plasma, or serum) immunoglobulin concentration can also be estimated accurately by measuring its specific gravity using a modified hydrometer (Table 14–5). Although total plasma or serum protein concentration can be rapidly and easily measured using a refractometer, they do not correspond to the foal's plasma IgG concentration and, therefore, cannot be used for this purpose.

[b] These four tests provide adequate and equally accurate results in detecting concentrations below 400 mg/dl. The glutaraldehyde coagulation test is the most accurate in detecting concentrations between 400 in 800 mg/dl, but requires serum and takes longer to run if the immunoglobulin concentration is below 800 mg/dl.

foaling has no predictive value as to the level of Ig present in her colostrum or in her foal's plasma after nursing and, therefore, is of no benefit.

Assessing Foal's Passive Immunity

Immunoglobulins, whether passively acquired from the colostrum or given intravenously, or actively produced by the foal, are broken down by the foal at a half-life of 3 weeks. As a result, passively obtained colostral Ig levels begin to decrease immediately following their absorption by the foal so that by several weeks to several months of age their concentrations are below protective levels (different for different organisms, and sooner the lower the amount of Ig absorbed). However, during this period, Ig against organisms to which the foal is exposed are being actively produced by the foal, off-setting the decrease in passively acquired colostral Ig and thus maintaining the foal's plasma Ig level and protection against these organisms. The serum IgG level in normal foals reaches a low point at 1 to 2 months of age, which after the period from birth to nursing is the next most susceptible period for the foal to infectious diseases. This comes earlier if inadequate colostral Ig has been absorbed. Normal adult levels of Ig,

and thus, protection against infectious diseases, are not obtained until the foal is about 5 to 6 months of age. However, by 1 month of age other aspects of the foal's immune system have increased to that equivalent to the adult.

Just as colostral IgG and IgM levels begin to decrease within 4 to 6 hours following foaling, so also does the foal's ability to absorb them. Thus, regardless of the colostral Ig concentration, the foal may not obtain sufficient Ig because of a failure either to ingest a sufficient amount of colostrum or to absorb a sufficient amount of ingested Ig.

Most normal, active light breed foals nurse 3 to 5 quarts or liters during their first 12 hours of life. To determine if the foal has ingested and absorbed sufficient Ig for adequate immunity and resistance to infectious diseases so that additional amounts of Ig may be given if needed, the foal's serum IgG concentration must be measured. This should be done when the foal is 6 to 10 hours of age (not before 3 to 4 hours after nursing or later than 10 hours of age). This allows time for the normal foal to nurse and ingested Ig to be absorbed, but is soon enough so that if the foal's serum IgG concentration is low, it can be corrected by giving colostrum high in IgG orally while intestinal Ig absorptive ability is still high. Waiting longer to determine the foal's plasma IgG concentration is not only unnecessary, it increases the time to past that when it can be corrected by giving colostrum if it is too low. After 12 to 16 hours of age, intestinal Ig absorption has decreased to the extent that correction of a low plasma Ig concentration requires the intravenous administration of Ig.

Foals' survival rates are directly correlated with their plasma IgG concentrations, increasing with increasing IgG levels. However, the prevalence of infectious diseases, their severity, and foal mortality are substantially increased or decreased depending on the cleanliness of the foal's environment and management of and, therefore, the foal's exposure to, infectious organisms. This was demonstrated in foals on a commercial breeding farm with excellent management that included prenatal vaccination of pregnant mares that were year-round residents of the farm, minimization of newborn foal stress, steam cleaning stalls with immediate after-foaling and then every 24-hour changing of bedding, supervised foaling, twice-a-day soaking of the umbilical cord for 5 days, ensuring all foals obtained colostrum high in Ig prior to 5 hours of age, maintenance of consistent mare and dam-foal groups, avoidance of overcrowding, and minimal use of foaling barns and indoor and paddock confinement. This type of optimum management minimizes infectious challenge to the foals and maximizes their passively obtained and actively produced immunity and health. Because of this, there was no difference during the first 21 or 90 days of life in disease incidence or severity, health or survival (which was 100 and 99.2%, respectively, with one foal euthanized because of poor health), between those with serum IgG concentrations above or below either 400 or 800 mg/dl. Thus, good farm management and excellent conditions eliminate the need to determine the foal's serum IgG concentration and to treat those that are low. However, this would not be the case with poorer management or conditions.

The risk of an infectious disease occurring and its severity if it does occur are greater the lower the foal's plasma IgG concentration is below 400 mg/dl. Most ill foals have serum IgG concentrations below this level. Approximately 25% of foals with serum IgG concentrations below 400 and 75% of foals with concentrations below 200 mg/dl may be expected to contract an infectious disease if they are exposed to sufficient organisms. Foals with low plasma IgG concentrations are particularly susceptible to septicemic and respiratory diseases.

Although a plasma IgG concentration above 800 mg/dl is preferred, there appears to be little additional benefit from raising it above 400 mg/dl for foals cared for by good management in a relatively clean environment with no maternal or foaling risk factors. However, with poorer management, a dirty environment, increased stress, weakness, prematurity, or other risk factors, increasing it to 800 mg/dl is indicated.

There is a multitude of tests available for measuring serum, plasma, or whole blood IgG concentration as given in Table 14-6. Some may also be used for measuring colostral IgG concentration.

Treatment of Inadequate Passive Immunity

If the mare's colostral IgG concentration is less than 1000 mg/dl or its specific gravity is less than 1.050 (Table 14-5), its foal, or any foal that is not expected to nurse prior to 6 hours of age, or that is less than 16 hours of age and whose plasma IgG concentration is less than 200 mg/dl, should be given at least 24 oz (7000 ml, or about 15 ml/kg body wt) of colostrum containing greater than 7000 mg/dl IgG or a specific gravity of 1.090 or greater (Table 14-3). A minimum of one-half this amount is adequate if the foal's dam's colostrum IgG concentration is 1000 to 3000 mg/dl or its specific gravity is 1.050 to 1.060 and the foal is nursing her. Supplemental colostrum should be given to the foal as soon as its dam's colostrum Ig content is found to be inadequate; ideally before it nurses its dam. The colostrum may be given by allowing the foal to suckle it from a nursing bottle if the foal is able to suck and swallow with vigor and without difficulty. The bottle should be held no higher than the foal's withers to decrease the risk of aspiration. The colostrum may instead be given by stomach tube. A maximum of 1 pint/100 lbs of foal (8 to 10 ml/kg body wt) may be given at one time to most full-term foals, and if more is needed, this amount may be given again 1 hour later.

A frozen colostrum bank should be maintained as a source of colostrum for foals not receiving colostrum sufficiently high in IgG concentration from their own dam. Colostrum for this bank may be collected every 2 hours from mares whose foals die during delivery, until that mare's colostral IgG concentration falls below 7000 mg/dl or its specific gravity falls below 1.090. For most mares, this will be the colostrum secreted up to 6 hours, and for some up to 12 hours, after foaling. One-half pint (250 ml) of colostrum per mare may also be taken from mares who don't lose their foals and whose colostral IgG concentration is above these levels. It is best if it is taken after their foal nurses. Most multiparous light breed mares produce 2 to 5 quarts or liters of colostrum containing an IgG concentration sufficient to ensure adequate passive immunity for a foal (3000 mg/dl). Thus, taking one-half pint (250 ml) of colostrum still leaves plenty of colostrum for that mare's foal.

Colostrum collected in a clean plastic container and frozen at 0 to 5°F (-15 to -18°C) can be stored for up to 1 year. Lower temperatures (below -13°F, or -25°C) reportedly are required to keep it longer. Frozen colostrum may be thawed in a hot water bath or in a microwave oven with minimal loss of Ig.

If colostrum isn't available, plasma or serum can be given orally; however, 6 to 9 or liters are necessary because plasma and serum are lower in Ig concentration, and their Ig is not absorbed as well as it is from colostrum. Commercially available reconstituted lyophilized hyperimmune equine serum (Coli Endotox, Grand Labs, Larchwood, IA) may also be given orally. A sufficient quantity of it should be given to provide the foal that hasn't received any colostrum 0.5 g/lb (1 g/kg) body weight of Ig. Four to 6 hours after it is given, the foal's plasma IgG concentration should be measured. Foals receiving some colostrum may need less, and sick or weak foals may need more.

Bovine instead of equine colostrum may be given. Foals, like lambs and pigs, tolerate bovine colostrum well and are able to absorb bovine IgG as well as and IgM better than, that from their own species. Bovine colostrum also provides other species and, therefore, probably foals, protection from infectious diseases. However, bovine IgG, but not IgM, is broken down more rapidly by the foal than is equine IgG. The half-life of bovine IgG is 9 days versus 26 days for equine IgG. In addition, bovine colostrum may not contain Ig protective against organisms common to horses but not cattle. Thus, although bovine colostrum is beneficial for the foal, it is not as good as equine colostrum, and, therefore, it should be given only when equine colostrum is not available.

Foal's plasma IgG concentration previously found to be low, regardless of treatment, should be remeasured at 18 to 30 hours of age. Since foals greater than 12 to 16 hours of age can no longer absorb any significant amount of Ig from the intestinal tract, if it is necessary to increase their plasma Ig concentration, Ig must be given intravenously. This is accomplished by giving plasma or serum that has been obtained by taking blood from another horse or by giving a commercially available preparation. Twelve to 24 hours later, this foal's plasma IgG concentration should be redetermined. If the concentration is still below 400 mg/dl, more should be given. Some foals will need to be given 2 to 4 liters over several days. Although, as described previously, this may be unnecessary for normal, healthy, nonstressed foals under excellent management and conditions that minimize the foal's exposure to infectious organisms, for other foals an immediate transfusion to increase their plasma Ig concentration to above 400 mg/dl (or in foals sick, stressed, or in which exposure to infectious organisms may be high, 800 mg/dl) is probably indicated and is routinely advocated by most researchers and veterinarians.

Signs of Illness in Foals

Although most illnesses result in specific clinical signs and alterations, most begin with fairly similar changes. The first indication in foals is usually a decrease in milk intake. There is little concerted effort to nurse, a decreased sucking reflex, and increased lying down. The mare develops a distended or tight udder and/or dripping milk, which may be recognized by a foal with milk on its face from standing under her and not nursing. A milk-faced foal is always a red warning flag of illness. Decreased nursing generally occurs at least 3 to 6 hours or more before other recognizable effects. Most foals that become sick in the first 48 hours of life appear normal following birth but show signs of illness within the first 12 to 24 hours. The period between 3 and 10 hours of age is when changes in the foal are most likely to occur. Thus, the foal's behavior should be watched closely during this period. They frequently don't develop a fever or become noticeably depressed or lethargic until they are quite ill.

Additional indications of illness that should be watched for include changes in mucous membrane color and moistness, increased rate or labored respiration, increased heart rate, increased capillary refill time (over 2 seconds), congestion of the white of the eyes (bloodshot eyes), indications of pain or discomfort, milk accumulation in the nostrils, swelling of the distal joints, lameness, cool extremities (legs and ears), changes in stool consistency, color or odor, and a rectal temperature either above or below the normal range of 99 to 102°F (37 to 39°C). However, many sick foals, including those with an infectious disease don't have an increased body temperature. At rest without excitement or exertion the heart rate (mean and range in beats per minute) normally is 70 (30 to 90) at 1 to 5 minutes after birth, 130 (60 to 200) at 6 to 60 minutes, 95 (70 to 130) at 1 to 48 hours, and 60 at 3 months following birth; compared to 28 to 42 in the adult. Respiratory rate normally is 60 to 90 breaths per minute at 1 to 5 minutes, and 30 to 40 at 1 to 2 hours after birth, versus 8 to 15 in the adult.

Without disturbing the foal, its breathing should be watched from a short distance away, preferably when it is laying on its side. Some foals with pneumonia may show profound abnormal respiratory effort while lying on their side, but will breathe fairly normal when lying on their sternum (setting up) or standing. Some abdominal effort at the end of expiration can be normal, but any marked effort is abnormal. Erratic breathing during deep sleep may be normal. A rippling of the rib cage during expiration may be a subtle, early sign of increased respiratory effort and disease. Flaring nostrils, exaggerated rib retractions, grunting during expiration, and a general increased breathing effort are all definite signs of respiratory distress. These are most often due to pneumonia, but may be due to congenital heart defects or air in the thoracic cavity due to an external wound or a perforated lung, such as from a fractured rib from picking up the foal with an arm under its chest behind, instead of in front of, the front legs.

Any alteration in the foal's normal behavior or any delay in its normal activities following birth from those given in Table 14–2, or any physical change in the foal should be immediately and thoroughly investigated by a veterinarian. Any delay in necessary therapy may result in rapid deterioration and even sudden death. A young foal's condition can change rapidly, much more rapidly than it does in older horses. For instance, a young foal in the incubational stages of septicemia may appear alert with near normal physical parameters yet develop septic shock and die within hours. Time is not an available luxury for the sick foal!

In addition to illness, young previously normal foals may suddenly be reluctant to walk or stand, be severely lame and have one or more distended joints or edema and swelling around the joints. Because these signs may occur suddenly without signs of illness, it is often initially thought that the foal has been stepped on or kicked. Instead, it is often due to joint-ill (septic arthritis). Joint-ill unless treated early and adequately results in death, or impaired future performance ability. Any young foal that suddenly becomes lame, or has swelling and/or pain at or near a joint, should be examined, and if indicated, treated as soon as possible.

Foal Pneumonia

Pneumonia is the major cause of death of foals. From a few to the majority of the foals born some years on some farms are affected, and up to 80% of affected foals in some outbreaks may die. Most cases occur in 1- to 8-month-old foals although younger foals may be affected. Even upon recovery from pneumonia, lung lesions may persist decreasing the horse's future athletic performance ability. This effect may be prevented in most cases by early diagnosis and adequate therapy.

Most cases of pneumonia are thought to occur from inhalation of aerosolized or dust-born organisms, but may occur secondary to septicemia, especially during the first few weeks of life. The incidence, severity and risk of pneumonia, particularly for young foals, increase with poor immunity, poor sanitation, overcrowding, parasitism, poor nutrition, poor ventilation, hot weather, extreme fluctuations in environmental temperature, particularly when humidity is high. In cold climates, both chilling and overprotection from the cold, for instance with blankets or reduced stable ventilation, are detrimental. Procedures for preventing pneumonia include a clean environment, good stable ventilation, a good vaccination program, and a good internal-parasite control program, all of which are described in Chapter 9, and a good brood mare feeding program as described in Chapter 13. Strict separation of brood mares, foals, and yearlings from the rest of the horses has been reported to dramatically decrease the incidence of respiratory disease.

Foals with pneumonia may have a normal appearance with or without coughing and a nasal discharge, or they may experience high fever, profuse nasal discharge, respiratory distress, cyanosis, and sudden death. Coughing is not common, but it is an important clinical sign that occurs more often in the morning or following exertion. If a nasal discharge occurs, it will be from both nostrils, and clear initially but becoming yellowish. Alterations in respiratory rate and character are present in most foals with pneumonia. Some may appear fairly normal at rest but have decreased exercise tolerance, may have an anxious expression, and may develop signs of respiratory distress, cyanosis, and disorientation if stressed or forced to exercise. Fever is common but not invariably present. Behavior and appetite are highly variable. Foals showing any of these abnormalities should receive veterinary care as soon as possible.

Foal Diarrhea

Diarrhea (scours), or an increase in fecal water content, is common in foals during the first few months of life. The percent of foals affected on a farm and in an area, the age affected, and the severity of the disease can differ substantially with different causes and between individuals. The incidence is substantially higher with decreasing basic cleanliness at foaling, and in foals born to mares recently brought to that farm. The occurrence, risk, and severity of diarrhea in foals is lessened by basic cleanliness and procedures to maximize the foal's immunity.

In the majority of cases diarrhea is mild, and the foal doesn't show any other signs of illness. These are generally due to excess milk consumption and/or foal heat diarrhea. However, if the stools are quite watery, contain any blood or are voluminous, or if the foal shows any other signs of illness (decreased appetite, fever, depression, dehydra-

TABLE 14–7
Diarrhea in Foals: Causes and Their Effects

Type	Cause	Most Common Age Affected	Common Stool Characteristics	Common Effects on the Foal
Nutritional	Excess milk or secondary to intestinal inflammation	1–14 d	yellow to green, soft to watery, little ↑ in volume	None—unless other causes of diarrhea occur secondarily
Foal heat	Change in intestine or its organisms	5–12 d	yellow to green, soft to watery, little ↑ in volume	None—unless other causes of diarrhea occur secondarily
Parasitic	Threadworms (Strongyloides westeri)	2–4 wk	variable	
	Strongyles	1–4 mo	diarrhea or constipation ⎫	fever, depression, ↓ nursing, colic
	Ascarids	3–6 mo	diarrhea or constipation ⎭	"summer colds," poor growth, colic
Bacterial	E. coli toxin	2–14 d	watery & voluminous	septicemia, dehydration
	Salmonella	2–14 d	watery, ± bloody, voluminous	sudden death, colic, fever, depression
	Clostridium	2–7 d	bloody, voluminous	sudden death, colic, fever, depression
	Rhodococcus equi	1–4 mo	variable	± pneumonia
	Actinobacillus equuli	2–7 d	variable	secondary to septicemia
Viral	Rotavirus	2 d–2 mo	watery, 4–7 d duration	depression, ↓ appetite, mild colic
	Coronavirus	2 d–2 mo	watery, 4–7 d duration	none to same as Rotavirus
	Adenovirus	2 d–2 mo	watery	primarily in Arabians with CID
Sand	Irritation	2 mo on	chronic progressive	poor growth and condition
Gastric ulcers		<3 mo	moderate diarrhea	colic, teeth grinding, slobber, regurgitation
		>3 mo	chronic loose stools	chronic recurrent colic, ↓ food intake & growth
Combined immunodeficiency disease (CID)	Inherited in Arabians	1–3 mo	May be diarrheic	Pneumonia and death usually by 2 to 5 months of age.

Abbreviations used: ↑ = increase, ↓ = decrease, ± may or may not occur, > = greater than, and < = less than.

tion, etc.), the cause may be bacterial or viral (Table 14–7). If this is the case, the foal should be considered contagious with immediate precautions taken to minimize spread of the disease to other horses. If isolation in a separate barn isn't possible, the mare and foal should be kept either in their own stall, or moved to a stall at the end of the barn with empty stalls or space in-between. Their stall should be the last fed and last cleaned. A foot bath with an effective disinfectant for viral and bacterial pathogens, such as phenolic compounds, should be placed at the stall and always used with a boot brush on leaving the stall. Plastic disposable booties and ideally gloves should be used in the stalls. Hands should be washed with a disinfectant soap immediately upon leaving the stall. Having a pair of coveralls or disposable paper surgical gown for use only in that stall may also be of benefit and necessary. Upon termination of cases found or thought to be infectious, the stall should be cleaned and disinfected thoroughly as described previously in the section of this chapter on "Preparation for Foaling."

Treatment of the diarrheic foal is needed: 1) if diarrhea persists more than 3 days, 2) if diarrhea is sufficiently severe to cause dehydration or decreased appetite, or 3) if the rectal temperature increases above 102°F (39°C). If any of these occur, veterinary assistance should be obtained. Antibacterial drugs should not be given unless veterinary prescribed. Their administration may prevent diagnosis of the cause of the diarrhea, and may themselves cause diarrhea. Diarrhea even in previously healthy foals usually begins 2 to 5 days after administration of an antibiotic is begun. Both orally administered and injected antibiotics may induce diarrhea in foals.

Most properly fed mares produce a high amount of milk almost immediately following foaling with little increase in production during the first 45 to 60 days, at which time production gradually begins to decrease. As the normal foal grows and gets past the first few weeks of age, it can utilize all of the milk produced, whereas at a younger age excess milk intake may cause mild diarrhea. Excess milk intake also occurs if the foal is unable to nurse for several hours and the mare is not milked out before the foal is allowed to nurse. Even without excess milk intake most foals develop soft to watery stools between 4 and 14 days of age. This is frequently when their dam's first heat (estrus) occurs following foaling, and therefore is referred to as foal heat diarrhea or scours. The cause isn't known, but it occurs even in foals of this age not nursing their dams, maintained parasite free, and receiving a synthetic mare's milk replacer. Thus, it probably occurs as a result of normal changes in the intestinal tract or intestinal organisms. Generally the only symptoms are soft to watery stools which, with or without treatment, return to normal after 2 to 3 days, unless a secondary infection-induced diarrhea occurs. Treatment is needed only if diarrhea persists more than 3 days or is sufficiently severe to cause dehydration and decreased appetite, or if a secondary infectious disease occurs resulting in an increased rectal temperature.

Although intestinal parasites must always be considered, they rarely cause diarrhea in neonatal foals. However, threadworms (Strongyloides westeri), large strongyles, and ascarids may all cause diarrhea in foals. The largest number of threadworm larvae are excreted in the mare's milk 2 to 3 weeks following foaling and, therefore, are ingested by the foal at that age. One to 2 weeks after these larvae have been ingested, their eggs are passed in the foal's feces and can be found in fecal flotations. The larvae can also be identified in the mare's milk. Treatment is to deworm the foal; prevention is to deworm the mare the first day after foaling with an effective dewormer (e.g., ivermectin, Table 9–1).

Large strongyles don't induce diarrhea until the foal is consuming enough contaminated pasture forage to ingest a sufficient quantity of infective larvae. Once this happens, diarrhea can occur within a few days. Fever, inappetence, depression, diarrhea or constipation, and colic of several days' duration may occur. Although this may occur in foals as young as 2 to 3 weeks of age, it more commonly occurs in foals over several months of age. Ascarids (Parascaris equorum) can also cause diarrhea if present in massive amounts. But their heaviest infestation, with resultant diarrhea, occurs in 3- to 6-month-old, not neonatal, foals.

Gastric ulcers are also a cause of diarrhea in foals. Gastric ulcers commonly occur in horses of all ages beginning as young as 2 days old. The greatest problem, however, is in foals 1 to 4 months of age. The incidence and severity of gastric ulcer lesions are greater in foals with clinical disorders (diarrhea being the most common disorder present in affected foals), and in adult horses in training and used for athletic performance. These and other studies suggest that stress is a major risk factor for the development of gastric ulcers.

It has been suggested that high protein, high alfalfa or high grain diets may result in a higher incidence of ulcers, but there appears to be little convincing supportive data for the role of alfalfa or protein. However, it has been shown that gastric acid secretion is probably greater when grain is fed than when only hay is fed, and that having free access to hay results in less gastric acidity than when feed is withheld for 24 hours. Horses turned out to pasture and thus graze the majority of the time also have been noted to have less gastric ulcers than horses kept in a stall. Thus, both fasting and high-grain diets predispose to gastric ulcers in horses, and frequent consumption of high forage diets may help prevent them. Gastric acidity and thus the risk of gastric ulcers, also increases from birth up to at least 8 weeks of age, and with the absence of solid food intake. Because of this, it has been speculated that gastric ulcers in foals are more likely to occur when their acid secreting ability has increased, but before they begin eating sufficient solid food to buffer it. If this is true, encouraging the foal to begin eating solid feed at as young an age as possible by feeding a good creep feed, as described in Chapter 15, may be helpful in preventing gastric ulcers in foals.

No symptoms occur, and gastric ulcers heal without treatment in the majority of foals. When symptoms do occur, current or previously occurring diarrhea followed by low-grade abdominal pain or colic, are the most common. Poor appetite, slow growth, poor body condition, a "pot-belly" appearance, and colic, along with chronic loose stools, may occur in older foals and adult horses with gastric ulcers. The severity of colic varies from mild to severe and is characterized by chronic recurrent episodes. In suckling foals, excessive salivation, teeth grinding, and froth around the lips may occasionally occur and, when they do, are quite indicative of the presence of either gastric or duodenal ulcers. Affected foals may occasionally have gastric distention, milk regurgitation, fever, and a preference to lie on their back for prolonged periods. Ulcers may serve as a port of entry to the body for bacteria and toxins, resulting in septicemia and botulism, or shaker foal syndrome.

Gastric ulcers may occasionally perforate the stomach wall. When this occurs it generally results in acute abdominal pain, fever, shock, and death within less than 4 days, although some may live several weeks. Clinically there is a sudden onset of profound depression characterized by a wide-based stance with the head hanging. A very rapid heart rate and respiratory rate, toxic appearing mucous membranes, and marked abdominal distention occur.

Obstruction due to constriction from healing ulcers in the stomach near the entrance to the intestine or in the intestine may occur, most commonly at 3 to 5 months of age. Their presence is suggested by stomach distention and reflux. In some cases, large quantities of saliva and milk run out the nose when the suckling foal lowers its head. Surgery is frequently necessary to alleviate the obstruction.

Hernias in Foals

Four types of hernias occur in foals: umbilical, inguinal or scrotal, diaphragmatic, and traumatic abdominal. Umbilical hernias cause a soft fluctuant swelling at the naval; an infected umbilicus causes a much firmer swelling. Umbilical hernias are present at birth or appear during the first week of life. They rarely cause problems other than their unsightly appearance, although intestinal strangulation may occur, primarily in older foals, if the hernia is sufficiently large. An umbilical hernia will usually correct itself within a few days to a year of age if the hernial ring is less than 1-inch (about 3 cm) in diameter. However, if it is larger than 1-inch, the hernia should be corrected surgically, as intestinal obstruction is more likely and it is less likely to close on its own.

Scrotal or inguinal hernias are characterized by a soft fluctuant swelling on one or both sides of the scrotum due to protrusion of the intestine through the inguinal canal. Most will correct themselves without treatment during the first month of life. They may be corrected surgically although this is rarely necessary in foals, but is in adults. Scrotal or inguinal hernias in adults occur particularly in stallions, but also in geldings, and inguinal hernias have been reported in mares. Abdominal contents enter the hernia resulting in mild to severe abdominal pain, and with scrotal hernias scrotal enlargement. Strenuous physical exertion, e.g., breeding or athletic activity, frequently, but not always precede their occurrence. They are usually diagnosed by rectal palpation, although ultrasonography when available is quite helpful and alleviates the risk of rectal palpation induced trauma. Few horses with hernial bowel incarceration for longer than 8 hours survive, which emphasizes the importance of early diagnosis and treatment.

Diaphragmatic hernias can occur in any age horse and may be congenital or acquired. Most congenital diaphrag-matic hernias don't cause any symptoms. Acquired diaphragmatic hernias are caused by violent exertion, external trauma, or increased abdominal pressure, such as in the foal during delivery. With either congenital or acquired diaphragmatic hernia, abdominal contents may pass through the hernia causing severe colic—or with large hernias, impaired respiratory function—which decreases exercise tolerance and may occur with or without difficult respiration being evident.

Leg Abnormalities in Foals

Two of the most common leg abnormalities of neonatal foals are flexure deformities, often referred to as contracted flexor tendons, and angular leg deformities (deviations toward or away from the midline). Either flexure or angular leg deformities may be present at birth, develop within the first few days of life, or develop during rapid growth following birth. Both are considered to be developmental orthopedic diseases, which are discussed in Chapter 16. In contrast to contracted flexor tendons, which occur most commonly in the front legs, foals may be born with weak or elongated-appearing flexor tendons, which occur most commonly in the hindlegs. The incidence of both weak flexor tendons and angular leg deformities are increased in premature foals.

Weak Flexor Tendons (Dropped Fetlocks)

With weak flexor tendons the fetlocks drop, the pasterns slope excessively, and the foal, when standing, may rock back on its heels, causing the toes to elevate. In severe cases, the foal may walk on the bulbs of the heels, pasterns, or fetlocks, resulting in skin abrasions or abscess formation as well as stress to the limbs.

Most cases of weak flexor tendons improve without treatment within 1 to 2 weeks as the foal gains strength. Exercise is beneficial and should be encouraged. Bandages cause tendons to relax and stretch and are, therefore, harmful except for light protective bandages over any abrasions that may be present. Before treatment, radiographs should be taken to rule out the possibility of congenital abnormalities, or a tearing of the flexor tendons from their attachment to the bone or phalanges.

Corrective trimming involves rasping the quarters and heels to provide a flat, weight-bearing surface and to help eliminate the "rocking" effect. If the heels are allowed to grow long, they grow out in an "underslung" fashion; instead of providing support to the fetlock, the horse will be forced to walk on the bulbs even more and the condition will worsen.

In many instances, weekly rasping of the quarters and heels, exercise, and time will correct the condition. More severe or unresponsive cases may benefit from a shoe with a several-inch (4- to 6-cm) heel extension. This prevents the "rocking" effect and forces the foal to walk on the normal weight-bearing surface of the foot. A simple, lightweight shoe can be made of plywood. Since the hoof walls of the young foal are quite thin and soft, it is difficult to nail a shoe on in the ordinary manner without either tearing the hoof wall or nailing into sensitive tissue. An alternative method is to drill holes in the hoof wall and wire the shoe on or to use glue on shoes (e.g., Dallmer Shoes, Advanced Equine Production, Versailles, KY). Following shoeing, exercise should be continued in a supervised manner. The posterior extension of the plywood shoe repositions the toe on the ground, and consequently the angle of the fetlock will change dramatically.

Knee Swelling

Swelling of any joint may occur as a result of trauma or septic-arthritis-induced inflammation. However, when swelling of the knee is present at birth and there is no pain or inflammatory increase in warmth, it may be due to rupture of the extensor tendon or their failure to unite. Both front legs are usually involved. The swellings are soft, fluid filled, not inflamed, not painful, and on the front outside aspect of the knee. It is important that they be differentiated from inflamed painful knee swellings due to septic arthritis. Many foals with ruptured extensor tendons are somewhat "over at the knees" or have a mild to moderate flexor tendon contraction. The majority suffer no ill effects and will regain normal use of their legs without treatment. Surgery is unnecessary, and bandaging and local medication are of little benefit.

Curbed Hocks

With curbed hocks, when the back of the hock is viewed from the side, instead of there being a straight line from the point of the hock to the fetlock �, there is a bowed or curby appearance ⌠. This is caused by compression of the front portion of small bones in the hock (central and/or third tarsal bones). It may be observed in some foals at birth or within 1 to 2 days afterward, while in others it is not observed until nearer to a month of age. It may occur as a result of collapse of these bones due to premature birth or hypothyroidism (see section on "Iodine Deficiency and Excess Effects" in Chapter 2). In older foals it may occur as a result of septic arthritis.

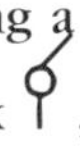

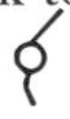

If the angulation is not severe, stall confinement may be sufficient to allow it to correct itself. However, if the angulation is marked, pressure on the front edge of the affected bones is increased and bone deterioration with possible fracture may occur. Casting may be beneficial for some of these cases.

MARE CARE AFTER FOALING

Following foaling, observe the mare and foaling area frequently to ensure that the placenta is expelled. This normally occurs within 1 to 2 hours following foaling. To assist in maternal bonding and thus decrease the risk of maternal rejection of and aggression toward the foal, the placenta should not be removed from the foaling stall for at least 2 hours after foaling. It is normally passed by the mare 15 to 90 minutes following foaling. The expelled placenta should be examined closely to ensure that none is retained. There are two portions to the placenta: the larger, thicker red to reddish tan, blood-vessel-containing water sac (chorioallantois or allantochorion) that attaches to the uterus, and the thinner, white glistening amniotic or foal sac that

surrounded the foal. The water sac normally looks like a pair of pants, with one big leg from the pregnant horn of the uterus and one small leg from the nonpregnant horn, and the umbilical vessels usually going from the crotch of the pants to the foal sac. The placenta should weigh about 10% of the foal's birth weight. If all of the placenta has not been passed or the placenta is abnormal, the mare should be examined and treated as soon as possible.

If premature placental separation occurred at foaling, generally the fetus will die of suffocation and the water sac will show a number of indications that it separated prematurely. The cervical star (an irregular grayish thickening and vascular area devoid of small fingerlike projections or villi where the placenta was near the cervix and through which the fetus generally passes) is not ruptured, but there will generally be a tear across the body of the water sac. The water sac is usually red and edematous. Much of the pregnant horn will be brownish tan and slightly dry. As with any cause of fetal suffocation (e.g., placental separation, dysfunction, thickening or inflammation, or compression of the umbilical cord prior to delivery), the fetus will also be greenish yellow, stained from the passage of fetal stools or meconium prior to birth.

If the placenta thickness, size, or weight is excessive (more than 11% of the foal's birth weight), this may indicate excess uterine fluid or infection of the placenta. Placental infection is also indicated by the placenta being bloody and a red to yellow to leathery brown. Placental infection generally indicates some degree of uterine infection and frequently septicemia in the foal, both of which should be treated as soon as possible and before symptoms occur in the mare or the foal.

If abortion, stillbirth or perinatal death occur, or if the foal is weak or unthrifty at birth, the placenta, along with the fetus or foal should be critically evaluated by a veterinarian and diagnostic laboratory. About one half of these cases are associated with an infectious or noninfectious condition involving the placenta. Placental physical and laboratory findings may help indicate the best treatment of the mare or the newborn foal, and be necessary to determine the cause for these effects, and thus to minimize their occurrence in other mares on that farm.

If the placenta or any part of it is retained by the mare for more than 4 hours after foaling, veterinary assistance in removing it and treating the mare is indicated. There is little reason to wait longer and many reasons not to. Although membranes being retained for up to 8 hours is not usually critical, those retained 12 hours or longer predispose the mare to uterine infection, infertility, and whole body infections and toxemia that can result in death and varying degrees of founder, ranging from painful feet to sloughing of the hooves.

In contrast to many other species, mammary gland infection or mastitis is rare in mares. It may occur, however, causing a painful udder that is warmer than normal to the touch and secretions that are abnormal. Veterinary treatment, including supportive therapy, antibiotics, hydrotherapy, and frequent milking, is needed.

MARE INJURIES IN FOALING

The violent, expulsive effort of the mare during foaling may result in her injury. The most common foaling-induced injuries include cervical, uterine, vulvar, or perineal bruising; hematomas or tears; internal hemorrhage; and uterine, intestinal or rectal prolapse.

Mares, especially maidens, are apt to bruise even during normal foaling and to be sore in the perineal areas as a result. This can lead to impaction colic since the mare may be reluctant to defecate due to the pain of doing so. To reduce the risk of impaction, a cup (8 oz, or 240 ml) of mineral oil may be added to the grain for several days following foaling. If the mare had difficulty in foaling and bruising occurred, having 2 to 4 quarts (or liters) of mineral oil given by stomach tube may be beneficial, as well as adding mineral oil to each grain feeding for 10 to 14 days until she heals.

Colic beginning from 1 day to several weeks following foaling may also occur as a result of injuries to the intestine, bladder, or uterus during foaling.

Foaling-induced hematomas may occur, generally just inside the vulvar lips, and they disappear within a few days. If they don't disappear, it may be necessary to have them drained. Most hematomas are not critical, but if large and severe, they may require earlier treatment and may induce straining, predisposing to vaginal and uterine prolapse.

Tears may occur at the top of the vulva. Most cause few or no problems; however, those of 1 inch (2.5 cm) or more may require surgical repair to retain the normal size and shape of the vulva.

Perineal tears may involve only the vaginal or vulvar mucosa (referred to as a first-degree perineal laceration), go deeper into the vaginal wall (second degree), or penetrate from the vagina into the rectum (third degree). Often a third-degree perineal laceration extends through the anal sphincter, resulting in a rectovaginal opening. Surgical correction of a third-degree perineal laceration is necessary and is usually done about 6 weeks after foaling to allow inflammation and swelling to subside.

Intestines may prolapse through a complete vaginal tear. Prompt replacement of the intestines back into the abdominal cavity is necessary for survival. If the intestine is strangulated for several hours, injured, or torn, chances of survival are poor.

Uterine tears and rupture rarely may occur. Although there is generally a corresponding tear in the placenta that should be detected upon its examination, a uterine tear may occur without a corresponding tear in the placenta. Uterine tears often go unnoticed, particularly if there is no tear in the placenta, until infection in the abdominal cavity and subsequent illness are present. Surgical closure of the tear, abdominal lavage and drainage, and extensive supportive care are necessary and may or may not save the affected mare.

Even without a tear, small uterine vessels and rarely a larger artery may rupture during foaling, resulting in internal hemorrhage. If a larger artery is ruptured, the mare can lose enough blood within 20 minutes to a few hours to cause death. Rupture of a uterine artery has been reported to be a major cause of death of older mares at foaling. Affected mares will generally show signs of colic (e.g., rolling and sweating). If large amounts of blood escape into the abdominal cavity, the mare's mucous membranes become pale, and death may occur during delivery or within 1 hour after. However, signs of pain may continue for hours or days after foaling, with anemia and icterus developing. Edema may occur in the perineum on the affected side. There is no way to prevent or treat the rupture of a large artery during foaling.

Intense and continued straining during foaling may infrequently result in uterine or rectal prolapse. With either, saving the mare requires replacement of the prolapse as soon as possible and no longer than a few hours after it has occurred, along with supportive and antibiotic therapy. Death from shock, hemorrhage, and/or rupture may occur. Other effects include uterine infection and founder. Mares that survive a uterine prolapse are generally unable to produce another foal.

Fracture of the mare's pelvis and/or femur may rarely occur during foaling. It is most commonly caused by the mare doing the splits while the foal is in the birth canal. Affected mares are unable to get up and the ends of the fractured bone rubbing together may be heard.

SUPPLEMENTAL READING RECOMMENDATIONS

Management of the Pregnant Mare and Newborn Foal (1984) by Drs. RK Shideler and JL Voss, two veterinarians who have devoted most of their professional careers of over 30 years each to clinical practice and research, and for which they are noted experts on the topics covered, which include: immunization and parasite control in pregnant mares and foals; pregnancy diagnosis and monitoring; early embryonic loss; fertilization and embryonic development, growth and migration; hormones in gestation; twinning; abortions in mares; foaling; maternal transfer of immunity; post-foaling complications in mares and foals; inducing parturition; and diseases of neonatal foals. This 43-page booklet is available from the Animal Reproductive and Biotechnology Laboratory, Colorado State University, Fort Collins, CO 80523.

Imprint Training of the Newborn Foal (1991) by Dr. RM Miller, a veterinarian with over 30 years of equine practice experience who more than any other individual has made those who own and care for and about horses aware of the benefits of and procedures for imprint training. All associated with foals should be familiar with the information in this 144-page book. Published in 1991 and available from Western Horseman Publications, P.O. Box 7980, Colorado Springs, CO 80933-7980. Two video films by Dr. Miller also available from Millers, P.O. Box 883, Rutherford, NJ 07070 are: (1) "Imprint Training the Foal," Catalog #6676-2, a 60-min video, and (2) "Influencing the Horse's Mind," Catalog #6755-2, a 40-min video.

Chapter 15

GROWING HORSE FEEDING AND CARE

Feeding Growing Horses 264
    Example Calculations of Amount to Feed Weanlings 266
        Example 1 266
        Example 2 267
    Feeding Growing Horses on Pasture 267
    Feeding Nursing Foals 267
Weaning 270

Growth Promotants for Horses 271
Exercise for Growing Horses 271
Vaccination and Internal-Parasite Control for Growing Horses . 272
Orphan and Early-Weaned Foal Feeding and Care 272
    Nurse Mares 273
    Mare's Milk Replacers 274
    Orphan Foal Feeding Procedures 275
    Orphan Foal Feeding Effects 276

FEEDING GROWING HORSES

In feeding the young horse during nursing to maturity, ensure that trace-mineralized salt and all the good-quality water the horse can consume are always readily available. As shown in Table 15-1, protein, calcium, phosphorus, zinc, and copper needs for rapid growth are frequently greater than those present in cereal grains and most forages, and digestible energy (DE) needs are greater than what is provided by forages. Even if an ample amount of feed is available, inadequate amounts of dietary energy will be consumed if the feed is too low in either digestible energy or protein. Growth rate isn't affected by more dietary protein than needed, but it is reduced by inadequate protein intake, and also by inadequate dietary energy intake. A slower growth rate decreases the need for and masks other nutrient deficiencies. If growth rate is slowed sufficiently, mature body size will be reduced. However, at a faster or normal growth rate as shown in Table 15-2, if a deficiency of any of these four minerals (calcium, phosphorus, zinc, or copper) isn't prevented, developmental orthopedic diseases may occur, as discussed in Chapter 16. Even without a mineral deficiency, excessive dietary energy and protein intake results in a rapid growth rate, increasing the risk of developmental orthopedic diseases, and the susceptibility to "bucked shins," or stress fractures of the cannon bone when put into training and racing competition as a 2-year-old.

If the grain mix fed doesn't contain the zinc or copper concentrations given in Table 15-1, it is recommended that the only salt available be high in these minerals and also selenium, unless you are in an area known to be high in selenium (Fig. 2-4). Trace-mineralized salt high in copper (2500 ppm), zinc (7500 ppm), and selenium (25 ppm) is currently available. However, trace-mineralized salt does not contain any calcium or phosphorus, and even if these are added to salt, or are present in any mineral available for free-choice consumption, this should not be relied upon to provide the proper intake of these minerals. Only if the proper amount of calcium and phosphorus are in the grain mix or forage is the growing horse likely to consume the proper amount of these minerals.

To provide sufficient dietary energy for rapid growth, and often for maximum mature size, grain must be fed. However, to prevent excessive dietary energy and protein intake, the amount of grain mix fed should not exceed the amounts given in Table 15-3. A slower growth rate can be obtained by feeding less than the maximum amounts recommended. In addition to containing sufficient quantities of protein and minerals to make up the difference between that needed and that present in the forage being consumed, the grain mix should also be high in the amino acid lysine. If it isn't, growth rate will be slowed (Table 1-5). The concentrations of these nutrients needed in the grain mix to provide the amount of nutrients needed in the total diet (grain mix plus forage, as given in Table 15-1) are given in Table 4-9. Grain mixes that contain these nutrient levels are available commercially, or may be formulated and prepared as described in Chapter 6. Those given in Table 4-10 may also be used. For a creep feed, rolled oats with or without other cereal grains are often preferred because of their high palatability. Throughout growth, soybean meal, canola meal, or an animal-source protein are preferred as protein supplements because of their high lysine content (Table 4-7). Fat or oil may be added to the grain mix fed growing horses, as described in that section in Chapter 4. Adding 10% fat to the grain mix has been shown to be well accepted and in some studies to increase growth rate and feed efficiency (feed to gain-rate ratio), and decrease feed requirements of both weanlings and yearlings without any detrimental effects.

If less grain mix is fed than the amounts given in Table 15-3, the grain mix will need to be higher in nutrient content than the amounts given in Table 4-9 to provide the nutrients needed in the lower amount fed. Even when a lower amount of grain mix is not fed, a grain mix higher in nutrients than needed may be fed to some horses in order to minimize the number of different grain mixes being used. This is often done where there are a small number of horses in each age or feeding group, or when it simplifies feeding procedures and, therefore, decreases the risk of the wrong grain mix being fed. Although this may increase feed costs, the excess amount of nutrients provided isn't harmful.

The best way to ensure that each horse receives the proper amount of the proper grain mix is to feed each horse individually. However, often this isn't practical or possible for horses on pasture. Young horses should be separated into groups: nursing foals and their dams, wean-

TABLE 15–1
Nutrients Needed for Growth as Compared to Their Content in Feeds[a]

	Digestible Energy Mcal/lb (kg) in Dry Matter	% in Dry Matter			ppm in Dry Matter	
		Crude Protein	Calcium	Phosphorus	Zinc[c]	Copper[c]
Needed by:						
Nursing foal[b]	1.5–1.7 (3.3–3.8)	16	0.9	0.6	60	50
Weanling	1.3 (2.9)	14.5	0.8	0.5	60	25
Yearling	1.25 (2.8)	12.5	0.5	0.3	40	25
Long yearling	1.2 (2.65)	12	0.4	0.25	40	10
Two-year-old	1.15 (2.5)	11	0.35	0.20	15	7
Mature maintenance	0.9 (2.0)	8	0.25	0.20	15	7
Composition of:[d]						
Legume (e.g., alfalfa) hays	1.0–1.1 (2.2–2.4)	15–20	0.8–2.0	0.15–0.3	10–45	4–25
Grasses, growing	0.9–1.1 (2.0–2.4)	10–20	0.3–0.6	0.2–0.4	15–45	2–35
Grasses, mature	0.7–1.0 (1.5–2.2)	6–10	0.3–0.5	0.15–0.3	15–45	2–35
Cereal grains	1.5–1.7 (3.3–3.7)	9–13	0.02–0.1	0.25–0.35	10–50	4–11

[a] In addition to these protein and mineral concentrations, it is recommended that a vitamin mix similar to that given in Table 3–5 be fed in the amounts recommended, or that $1/3$ lb of it be added/100 lbs ($1/3$ kg/100 kg) of grain mix.
[b] Needed in creep feed in addition to milk.
[c] These amounts may be added to the grain mix without regard to that naturally present in normal feeds without risk of a harmful excess. This is often done rather than determining the amount present in the feed and adding just enough copper- and zinc-containing minerals to attain these concentrations, as should be done for calcium and phosphorus.
[d] For more exact values see Appendix Table 6 for the specific type of forage or grain being fed. For the most accurate values, have the feed analyzed as described in Chapter 6.

lings, yearlings, often long yearlings, and two-year-olds. If there are more than about 20 horses in any of these groups, and if it is possible, dividing them into still additional groups according to size and/or aggressiveness may be best. If young horses aren't divided into these groups, older larger horses may injure and drive the younger smaller horses away from the feed. This results in the bigger, more aggressive horses getting too much and the others not enough, both of which may be harmful. In addition, fillies and colts 1 year of age or older must be kept separate, as fillies reach puberty anytime from 20 to 24 months of age and colts anytime from 12 to 20 months of age.

Sufficient forage should be fed to make up the difference between the horses' dietary energy needs, as given in Appendix Tables 4, and that provided by the grain mix. This may be done by allowing the growing horse free access to all of the nonlegume forage it will consume. However, if a legume forage such as alfalfa (lucerne) is being used, the amount fed weanlings should be restricted to that needed to provide the amount of digestible energy required for moderate to rapid growth.

The weanling should not be allowed unlimited access to good-quality legume forage. Doing so, just as feeding excess grain, results in excess dietary energy intake, greatly increasing the risk and incidence of developmental orthopedic diseases (DOD) as described in the section on "Feeding Practices that Cause DOD" in Chapter 16. Unless the feed is so low in energy density that the gastrointestinal tract won't hold a sufficient amount to meet or exceed dietary energy needs of the growing horse, intake of a sufficiently palatable diet will depend upon the energy density of that diet: the higher the diet's energy density, the less of that diet consumed; the lower its energy density, the more of that diet consumed until the desired amount of energy has been reached. However, the amount of energy

desired, or the point at which feed intake stops because adequate energy has been consumed, by weanlings being fed grain or a high-protein, palatable legume forage, is about 20 to 50% higher than the amount of digestible energy needed for a moderate growth rate sufficient to allow the horse to reach its maximum potential size.

A fast growth rate doesn't increase mature size, but it does increase the risk of developmental orthopedic diseases. This risk is reduced after 1 year of age because growth rate, particularly skeletal growth rate, which is best indicated by height rather than weight, has slowed considerably. As shown in Table 15–2, the horse normally reaches 90% or more of its mature height and, therefore, skeletal size, by 12 months of age. For example, 100% of the cannon bone's length and 90% of its circumference are reached by 1 year of age. Bone mineral content and strength also increase during growth. Although bone mineral content doesn't peak until 3 to 4 years of age, most of the increase, like growth, occurs during the first year of life. Yearlings, therefore, in contrast to weanlings, may be given unlimited access to legume as well as nonlegume forages with little risk of causing developmental orthopedic diseases induced by excess dietary energy intake.

In summary, in feeding the growing horse the goal is to achieve a steady growth rate from birth to maturity, avoiding any severe growth depression or spurt by ensuring that all nutrients needed are consumed in the proper amount. This is accomplished by:

1. Feeding a properly formulated grain mix (Table 4–9) limited to the amounts shown in Table 15–3.
2. If a nonlegume forage is used, all of it the horse will consume without waste should be available.
3. If a good-quality legume or legume-grass mix forage is used,

TABLE 15–2
Size of Horses from Birth to Maturity as a Percent of Mature Size[a]

| Age (Months) | Light Horse Breeds[b] | | Pony Breeds[c] Weight | Draft breeds[d] Weight |
	Weight	Height[e]		
Birth	8–11[f]	61–64	7.5–8.5	
1	16.5–19.5[f]	67–70	15–17	
3	30–33	76–79	28–31	
6	44–47	83–86	41–45	34–38
9	55–58	87–90	51–59	
12	63–67	90–92	66–75	52–55
18	78–85	94–96	84–86	69–73
24	87–92	96–98	95	75–80
30	91–96	97–99		
36	94–99	98–100		90
48	98–99	99–100		
60	100	100		

[a] Mature size may be estimated from dam and sire's size. Values will be lower than those given if digestible energy intake is limited or protein intake is inadequate. Although colts tend to be bigger than fillies at birth, with this difference increasing with age, colts are not bigger as a percent of their mature size and they tend to reach their mature size more slowly than fillies. In general, both within the same breed and between different breeds, the heavier the horse's future mature weight, the lower the percentage of this weight at any age and the longer it takes to reach a specific weight. Size from birth to 18 mo of age tends to be higher in foals born in the spring (April–June) than those born in the winter (Jan–March), even though gestational length tends to be shorter the longer the hours of daylight. Size at 18 mo of age tends to be larger for foals from middle-aged (7- to 12-yr-old) dams than those from either younger or older dams. Most prefer that the average daily gain of light horse breeds with a mature weight of 1000 to 1200 lbs (455 to 545 kg) approach the following amounts. However, it should not greatly exceed these amounts.

Age (mo):	0–1	1–2	2–3	3–4	4–5	5–6	6–7	7–8	8–9	9–10	10–11	11–12	12–18	18–24
Lbs/day:	3.4	3.0	2.6	2.3	2.0	1.8	1.6	1.4	1.3	1.2	1.1	1.0	0.8	0.6
Kg/day:	1.5	1.35	1.2	1.05	0.9	0.8	0.7	0.65	0.60	0.55	0.50	0.45	0.35	0.25

[b] Thoroughbreds, Quarter Horses, and Arabians with the following mature sizes:

T.B. males	1200 lbs (545 kg) and 63.8 in (162 cm or 16-0 h)
T.B. mares	1100 lbs (500 kg) and 63.0 in (160 cm or 15-3 h)
Q.H. males	1160 lbs (530 kg) and 60.0 in (152 cm or 15-0 h)
Q.H. mares	1090 lbs (495 kg) and 59.0 in (150 cm or 14-3 h)
Arab males	1025 lbs (465 kg) and 60.0 in (152 cm or 15-0 h)
Arab mares	980 lbs (445 kg) and 58.4 in (148 cm or 14-2 h)

[c] Shetland and Shetland-Welsh cross ponies with a mature weight of 385 to 400 lbs (175–182 kg).
[d] Percherons, which tended to be on the high end, and Belgians, which tended to be on the low end, of the ranges given.
[e] Height at withers, which is less variable and less affected by adverse conditions than weight. It is the birth size parameter that best predicts mature size. Body lengths (e.g., that of the head, which is 36 to 40%, elbow to ground 59 to 60%, hock to ground 39 to 40%, knee to ground 29 to 30%, legs, scapula, humerus, femur, tibia and cannon bones) are a relatively constant percentage of wither's height and are not different between horses of different light horse breeds and frame sizes.
[f] Lower end of these ranges for Arabian, and higher end for Thoroughbred foals.

a. for weanlings, restrict the amount of it fed to 0.5 lbs/100 lbs of anticipated mature body weight (0.5 kg/100 kg) daily until 10 months of age, at which age feed an additional 1 lb (0.45 kg)/day each month until 12 months of age, at which time the amount of forage fed need no longer be restricted. A more exact determination of the amount of forage to feed can be determined as shown in the following examples.

b. for yearlings, all of any type of forage the horse will consume should be fed.

4. Allow unlimited access to water and a trace-mineralized salt high in copper, zinc, and selenium (unless you are in an area known to be high in selenium—see Fig. 2–4) unless adequate quantities of these minerals, as given in Table 15-1, are added to the grain mix fed.

Example Calculations of Amount to Feed Weanlings

Example 1. For a 4-month-old weanling with an anticipated mature weight of 1100 lbs (500 kg), the amount to feed for rapid growth can be determined in the following manner:

a. (4 mo old) × (1.5 lbs of grain mix/day/mo of age from Table 15-3) = 6 lbs grain mix/day maximum.

b. (6 lbs grain/day) × (0.9 dry matter [DM] content) = 5.4 lbs grain DM/day.

c. (5.4 lbs grain DM/day) × (1.6 Mcal/lb grain DM from Table 15-1) = 8.64 Mcal/day provided by the grain mix.

d. 14.4 Mcal/day needed from Appendix Table 4-500) − (8.64 Mcal/day from grain) = 5.76 Mcal/day needed from forage.

e. (5.76 Mcal/day needed) ÷ (1.0 Mcal/lb hay DM from Table 15-1) = 5.76 lb hay DM/day needed.

f. (5.76 lbs hay DM/day) ÷ (0.9 DM content) = 6.4 lbs hay as fed/day.

Thus, you should feed 6 lbs (2.7 kg) of grain mix and 6 to 7 lbs (3 kg) of alfalfa hay daily (as compared to 5.5 lbs (2.5 kg) alfalfa/day estimated using the rule of thumb of

TABLE 15-3
Amount of Feed Recommended for Growing Horses[a]

Horse	Age (mo)	Grain mix % in Total Diet	Lb Grain mix/100 lbs (or kg/100 kg) body wt/day	Lb (kg) grain mix/day/mo of age	
				Ponies[b]	Others[b]
Nursing foals	0–4	100[c]	0.5–0.75	0.25 (0.1)	1.0 (0.45)
Weanlings[a]	4–12	70	1.7–2.0	0.5 (0.25)	1.5 (0.7)
Yearlings	12–18	60	1.3–1.7	For all age horses feed grain only up to a maximum of 0.9 lb/100 lb (0.9 kg/100 kg) of anticipated mature wt/day	
Long yearlings	18–24	50	1.0–1.25		
Two-year-olds	24–36	50	1.0–1.25		

[a] Feeding less grain mix than these amounts may slow growth rate and require feeding a grain mix higher in nutrient content (than that recommended in Table 4–9) to provide the nutrients needed in the lower amount fed. All the forage the growing horse will consume should be available except for weanlings being fed an average- or better-quality legume such as alfalfa (lucerne). For weanlings, in addition to limiting the amount of grain fed, when this amount of grain is fed, the amount of good-quality legume fed should be limited to 0.5 lbs/100 lbs of anticipated mature weight (0.5 kg/100 kg) daily until 10 mo of age, at which age feed an additional 1 lb (0.45 kg)/day, and at 11 mo an additional 2 lb (0.9 kg)/day until 12 months of age, at which time the amount of alfalfa fed should no longer be restricted.
[b] With an anticipated mature weight of 500 lbs or less (225 kg) for ponies and 800 lbs or more (365 kg) for other breeds.
[c] 100% grain mix in the creep feed or solid (nonmilk) diet fed.

0.5 lbs/100 lbs (0.5 kg/100 kg) of anticipated mature weight daily).

Example 2. For a 9-month-old weanling with an anticipated mature weight of 1100 lbs (500 kg), the amount to feed for rapid growth can be determined in the following manner:

a. (9-mo-old) × (1.5 lbs/day/mo of age from Table 15-3) = 13.5 lbs grain-mix/day, but this exceeds the maximum of 0.9 lbs/100 lbs anticipated mature weight daily (Table 15-3), so instead feed (0.9 lbs/100 lbs) × (1100 lbs anticipated mature wt), or about 10 lbs of grain mix/day.
b. (10 lbs grain/d) × (0.9 DM content) = 9.0 lbs grain DM/day.
c. (9 lbs grain DM/d) × (1.6 Mcal/lb grain DM from Table 15-3) = 14.4 Mcal/day provided by grain.
d. (19.3 Mcal/day needed from Appendix Table 4-500) − (14.4 Mcal/day from grain) = 4.9 Mcal/day needed from forage.
e. (4.9 Mcal/d needed) ÷ (1.0 Mcal/lb hay DM from Table 15-1) = 4.9 lb hay DM/day needed.
f. (4.9 lb hay DM/day) ÷ (0.9 DM content) = 5.4 lbs hay as fed/day.

Thus, you should feed 10 lbs of grain mix and 5 to 6 lbs (2.5 kg) of alfalfa hay daily (as compared to 5.5 lbs (2.5 kg) alfalfa/day estimated using the rule of thumb of 0.5 lb/100 lbs (0.5 kg/100 kg) of anticipated mature weight daily).

Feeding Growing Horses on Pasture

Because of the facilities available, or to decrease feeding costs and labor, when adequate pasture forage is available many prefer to keep horses on pasture and to give as little additional feed as necessary. If needed, enough grain mix to allow at least a moderate growth rate (such as given in Appendix Table 4) and to ensure that maximum mature size and skeletal development are not impaired should be fed. For nursing foals, regardless of the forage (pasture or hay) available to them, it is recommended that they be fed the amount of grain mix given in Table 15-3. For weanlings on primarily grass pasture, there should be enough good-quality forage for them to eat all they want. In addition, it is recommended that weanlings be fed daily at least 1 lb (0.45 kg), but not over 1.5 lbs (0.7 kg) of grain mix/mo of age (for pony breeds, ⅓ to ½ lb [0.15 to 0.25 kg]/mo of age) up to a maximum of 0.7 to 0.9 lbs/100 lbs (or kg/100 kg) of anticipated mature body weight. However, yearlings or older on good-quality, palatable, growing grass pasture (e.g., Bermuda grass) or winter wheat pasture in early spring, that provide ample amounts of forage even in selectively grazed areas, do not need to be fed any grain or supplemental feed to attain at least a moderate growth rate and their maximum mature size without any detrimental effects. Wheat harvest is not affected by grazing winter wheat early in the Spring (Feb-April in the Central United States).

The amount of pasture forage needed is 60 to greater than 80 lbs of forage dry matter per 100 lbs body wt (or 60 to over 80 kg/100 kg). In a properly fertilized good grass pasture with adequate moisture, this may be obtained with a stocking rate of about 3 yearlings/acre (7 to 8/ha) during the period of forage growth. With lesser amounts of pasture forage available, or poorly palatable forage without supplementation, growth rate will be reduced.

During the winter, or periods when pasture forage is not growing, even when ample amounts of pasture forage are available, at least 5 lbs (2.3 kg) of grain mix daily for light horse breeds must be fed to yearlings or growth and body condition will be reduced.

Cool season annuals, such as wheat, rye and ryegrass pasture providing ample forage, have also been shown to be adequate for yearlings during forage growth (early spring), with little increase in daily gain attained when they were supplemented with a grain mix. In contrast, some pasture forages such as Kleingrass, are not adequate for yearlings even during forage growth, high nutrient content, and with ample quantities available because of poor palatability. Inadequate amounts of a poorly palatable forage will be consumed.

Feeding Nursing Foals

Milk produced by the well-fed normal mare is sufficient to meet all of the foal's nutritional needs for about the first 2 months of life and all of its mineral needs (calcium, phosphorus, magnesium, potassium, sodium, copper, and zinc) for the first 4 months of life. However, most foals will begin nibbling on the mare's grain mix and forage within a few days of birth due to imitation behavior, not nutritional need. Most mares will allow their own foals to

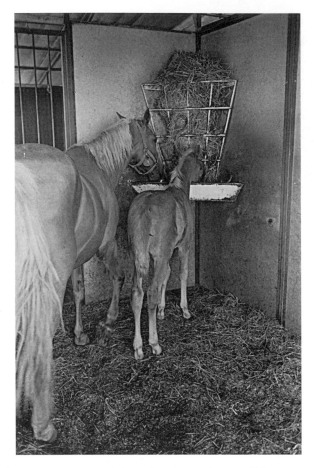

Fig. 15-1. Most foals by a few days of age will begin eating the grain mix and hay fed their dam, which most mares will allow their own foal but not others to do.

eat their grain mix (Fig. 15-1) with them, whereas they will frequently drive other foals away. As the foal grows, it will spend progressively more time consuming solid feed, but even at 5 months of age a foal still with its dam will spend only about 50% of its time feeding as compared to 70% for the mare. The amount of solid feed eaten is usually closely associated with the amount of milk being consumed. The more milk, the less solid feed the foal will eat.

Past 2 months of age, the amount of milk produced by many mares no longer meets all of the foal's nutritional needs. Therefore, beginning when the foal is anywhere from 1 to 2 months of age, a grain mix specifically formulated to meet the nursing foal's needs (Table 4-9) should be fed. Even as young as 3 weeks of age, the foal's efficiency of grain utilization is high, with the foal gaining about 1 lb/4 lb (1 kg/4 kg) of grain consumed. Feed efficiency decreases as the foal gets older and growth rate slows (to 1 lb gain/7 lbs of grain consumed at 4 months of age). Feeding a grain mix creep feed is beneficial not only in ensuring that the nursing foal's nutritional needs are met, but also so that following weaning the foal is accustomed to eating a grain mix separate from what it may eat with the mare.

In foals from 1 to 3 months of age, nursing normal milk-

producing mares, average daily gain (ADG) up to their maximum genetic potential will be the following:

Lbs/day ADG = 2.08 + 0.109 (Mcal DE from nutritionally adequate solid feed consumed daily), or

Kgr/d ADG = 0.95 + 0.05 (Mcal DE from nutritionally adequate solid feed consumed daily).

Thus, if no grain mix is consumed, the nursing foal will gain about 2.08 lbs (0.95 kg/d). From this formula, it can also be determined how much supplemental feed must be fed to attain a faster growth rate. For example, for 2.6 lbs/day gain, 4.77 Mcal DE/day of nutritionally adequate solid feed must be consumed, i.e., [(2.6 lbs/d gain − 2.08) ÷ 0.109 = 4.77 Mcal DE/day]. If the grain mix fed provides 1.6 Mcal/lb, 3 lbs/day would need to be consumed to provide this amount of dietary energy, i.e., 4.77 Mcal DE/day ÷ 1.6 Mcal/lbs of grain mix = 3 lb grain mix/day.

If, during nursing, an adequate amount of nutritionally adequate solid feed is not consumed, then following weaning an adequate diet is consumed, a compensatory growth spurt will occur. This growth spurt greatly increases the risk of the foal incurring and the severity of developmental orthopedic diseases (DOD) (see "Rapid Growth as a Cause of DOD" in Chapter 16). If the foal has been on a good creep-feeding program, this growth spurt, and as a result the risk of DOD, are reduced.

The amount of entirely grain mix creep feed fed should not be restricted until the foals are consuming 4 to 5 lbs (about 2 kg) daily. Prior to this time there should always be feed in the creep feeder. Most foals will eat small amounts frequently. Once the foals are eating 4 to 5 lbs (2 kg) daily, however, the amount of creep feed fed should be limited to that given in Table 15-3 so that growth rate doesn't exceed that given in Table 15-2. If the amount fed isn't limited, some foals may eat excessive amounts, resulting in too rapid growth rate increasing the risk and severity of DOD, as described in Chapter 16.

If the mare is fed in a stall, she can be tied and a separate feeder provided for the foal. Alternatively, a stout board can be placed across one corner of the stall in such a manner that the foal can walk under the board easily to get to a creep feed placed in the corner but the mare cannot. For most light breed horses, a height of 54 inches (137 cm) usually is about right. If the mares and foals are on pasture and the foals are fed in a group, care should be taken that all foals can get to a creep feeder without crowding; if not, dominant or greedy-eating foals may consume more than their share, leaving inadequate amounts for less aggressive or slower-eating foals. If this isn't prevented by having adequate feeding space available, it may be necessary to feed shy, or slow-eating foals separate from aggressive or fast-eating foals. The amount of creep feed needed should be put in the creep feeder in equal amounts at least twice daily after removing any wet or moldy feed that may remain in the feeder.

Creep feeders should be placed close to where the mares are fed, and where there is good drainage, water, salt, shade, or a location attractive to foals, to encourage them to use the feeders. Observations indicate that foals graze only when their mothers do and are more likely to eat, at least initially, and to eat more creep feed, when they see their mothers eating. In addition, they won't use

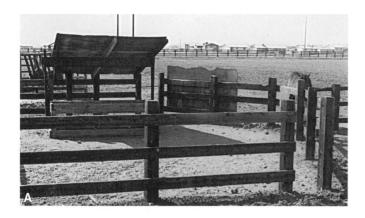

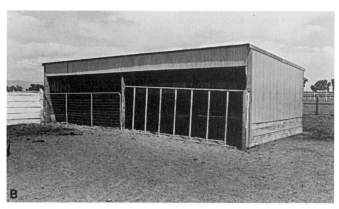

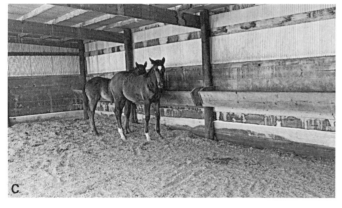

Fig. 15-2(A,B,C). Creep feeders. Figure 15-2 C shows the inside of the creep feeder shown in B. Ensure that the creep feeders are sturdy and safe, and that openings are wide enough and high enough to allow the foal to enter and leave safely while preventing entrance by the mare. Feeders should be large enough to accommodate the necessary number of foals, and covered to keep the feed dry. A feed box containing bars across the top placed close enough together to prevent the mare from inserting her muzzle into the box but far enough apart to allow the foal to eat from the box may also be used as a creep feeder.

a feeder if doing so means being too far away from their dam. As shown in Fig. 15-2, there are numerous ways to make the creep feed available to the foal but not the mare. Foals may have to be shown how to enter and eat from a creep feeder. Often confining several foals inside a feeder for a few minutes, showing them the creep feed, and putting some in their mouths to get them started eating it is adequate so they will act as teachers for the remaining foals.

Although most foals start eating solid feed in the first few days of life, most receiving adequate milk do not drink water, as the milk meets their water needs. In a study of 15 foals with their dams on pasture, the youngest age at which a foal was observed to drink water was 3 weeks, and 8 of the 15 foals were never observed to drink prior to weaning. However, the foal should always have free access to water, particularly after 3 weeks of age. If a nursing foal drinks very much water (for more than 0.5 to 1 min) or often (more than once daily at an environmental temperature of less than 50°F, or 10°C, or more than every 2 to 4 hrs at 50 to 95°F, or 10 to 35°C), the foal probably isn't receiving enough milk. This is also indicated by prolonged or excessive bouts of nursing or by a below-normal weight gain (Table 15-2). During the first month of life, the foal normally nurses for 1 to 2 minutes 3 to 7 times/ hr, and light horse breeds should gain 2 to 3 lbs (0.9 to 1.4 kg) daily. The foal's weight and, therefore, its daily gain can be obtained from a heart girth measurement as described in Chapter 6 under "Obtaining Horse's Weight" or more accurately by weighing the foal. A smaller foal's weight can be obtained as the difference in a person's weight holding and not holding the foal when standing on a scale.

Inadequate milk production by the mare is most commonly due to illness or inadequate nutrition. Following a mild or short-term illness, mares will usually return to adequate milk production. However, they usually won't if the illness is severe or prolonged. If the foal on the mare producing inadequate milk is less than 5 weeks of age, it may be weaned from the mare and all of its milk needs provided as described for "Orphan and Early Weaned Foals" later in this chapter. However, if supplementation for no more than a few weeks is likely to be necessary, it may be preferable to leave the foal with the dam and to give it enough supplemental milk so that it drinks little water and gains the normal amount shown in Table 15-2. Some experimentation may be necessary to determine which method works best to get the foal to accept additional milk. If the foal nurses the mare without obtaining milk, hold a nippled bottle near her udder; the foal may start to nurse from the bottle. Some foals may reject a nipple but drink from a bucket. Some may need to be muzzled or periodically separated from the mare before they will nurse a bottle or drink from a bucket.

The total amount of milk needed by normally nursing foals of light horse breeds has been shown to be about 16 qts (or L)/day (20 to 25% their body weight) for the first 5 weeks of life and about 18 qts (or L)/day thereafter (17 to 20% of their body weight). If the foal is over 5 to 8 weeks of age, milk doesn't need to be given. Instead, the older foal that isn't receiving adequate milk from its dam

TABLE 15–4
Composition of Mare's and Cow's Milk[a]

Time after Parturition	Total Solids (%)	Digestible Energy (kcal/kg)	Protein (%)	Fat (%)	Lactose (%)	Concentration in mg/kg or ppm in Milk as Consumed												
						Calcium	Phosphorus	Magnesium	Potassium	Sodium	Copper	Zinc	Selenium	Sulfur	Manganese	Iron	Cobalt	Molybdenum
Mare:																		
Colostrum	25	1000	19	0.7	5	400	400	100	700	200	0.8	2–3	0.04	100	0.5	1–1.6	0.03	0.09
1–4 weeks	10.7	480	2.7	1.8	6.2	800–1200	500–750	90	700	225	0.3–0.5	2.5	0.01	200	1–1.5	1.3–3	0.05–0.07	0.01–0.02
5–8 weeks	10.5	460	2.2	1.7	6.4	1000	600	60	500	190	0.25	2.0	0.005		0.25	0.5–0.9		
9–21 weeks	10.0	420	1.8	1.4	6.5	800	500	45	400	150	0.20	1.8				0.5		
Cows:																		
Milk	12.5	620	3.2	3.5	4.8	950–1700	700–1600	80–270							0.5			

[a] There appears to be little difference in mare's milk content between different breeds. The amount produced by the normal adequately fed mare is an amount equal to 3 to 4% of her body weight daily for the first 2 to 3 months of lactation, then it gradually decreases. Taurine gradually decreases from about 800 mM/dl in colostrum to about 200 at 3 weeks of lactation on, whereas it is low in cow's colostrum. In contrast, lysine, histidine, alanine and glutamine in the mare's milk increases during the first 8 weeks of lactation, whereas there appears to be no consistent change in the concentration of other amino acids in the mare's milk with the duration of lactation.

may be weaned and fed as a weanling separate from the mare.

Although quite uncommon, a mare may produce adequate quantities of milk but with improper amounts of calcium, phosphorus, or rarely other nutrients. An improper amount of calcium, phosphorus, zinc, copper, or selenium in the milk appears to be unrelated to the mare's diet and cannot be changed by any significant amount by altering her diet. Dietary alterations and nutrient intake affect the quantity of milk produced but have a minimal effect on the nutrient composition of milk. Improper mineral content in the milk may result in DOD (Chapter 18). If a previously normal-appearing nursing foal less than 3 months of age begins developing DOD, either milk with an abnormal nutrient content or excessive dietary energy is being consumed. If an analysis of the mare's milk indicates that it is abnormal, the foal should be weaned. If the mare's milk composition is within the normal ranges given in Table 15-4, the cause is most likely excessive dietary energy intake. This will result in a large well-fed appearing foal with a rapid growth rate that may induce DOD. Excessive dietary energy intake may be caused by either excessive grain (more than 1 lb, or 0.45 kg/day/month of age), excessive milk consumption, or both. To decrease the amount of milk consumed, either reduce the mare's feed intake to decrease her milk production or, if the foal is more than 2 months old, wean the foal.

WEANING

Weaning-induced stress decreases food intake and growth rate, and increases susceptibility to infectious diseases, gastric ulcers, and the risk of self-induced injury. Depending on the degree of stress and sickness, it may take foals several weeks to recover and start doing well—longer if injury occurs. Mares usually have fewer psychological problems at weaning time than do foals; however, some mares will also undergo a high degree of stress. To decrease these risks, procedures should be utilized to minimize weaning stress.

To minimize weaning stress, ensure that the foal prior to weaning is in good health, preferably accustomed to handling, and eating solid feed by feeding a good creep feed. All vaccinations, dewormings, and elective surgery to correct conditions such as umbilical hernias and angular

leg deformities should be completed at least 2 weeks before weaning and should not be done for at least 2 weeks after weaning. Prior to weaning, the foal should be eating 1 lb (0.45 kg) of creep feed/day/month of age, as well as forage. This helps ensure that the nursing foal's nutritional needs are met and, that there is a steady growth rate, and therefore, the risk of problems such as DOD are lessened. In addition, ensure that both the foal's and mare's surroundings following weaning are free of obstructions and protrusions on which the stressed and often fretful animal may injure itself. It is probably best to avoid weaning during periods of adverse weather conditions. Don't change the foal's feed, water, or surroundings; institute any new handling or training procedures; or, unless necessary, conduct any surgical, medical, or diagnostic procedures for at least 1 to 2 weeks after weaning.

Although foals are often weaned at 5 to 7 months of age, earlier weaning offers a number of advantages. With early weaning, less feed is needed for the mare and it allows her longer to prepare for her next foal. Early weaning may allow some mares to return to breeding sooner as some may otherwise have lactation-induced anestrus. Earlier weaning appears to have no detrimental effect on the foal, and most foals grow better when their concern is changed from getting another drink of milk to eating their own grain mix and forage. The best age to wean appears to be as soon as the foal's nutrient needs are no longer provided primarily by the mare's milk and, therefore, must be provided by solid feed intake. For most normal well-fed mares and foals eating the mare's grain-mix, or a grain-mix separate from the mare, this is at about 4 months of age. If creep feeding is not used or there are other reasons, foals can be weaned earlier without any apparent detrimental effects.

Although weaning prior to 2 months of age may initially slow growth rate, if the early weaned foal is fed properly, its growth rate returns to normal within a few weeks and its size, even during the first year of life, is not different from that of foals weaned after 4 months of age. However, the foal's plasma immunoglobulin G concentration and, therefore, immunity is lowest, and its susceptibility to infectious diseases highest, at 1 to 2 months of age and doesn't reach normal adult levels until 5 to 6 months of age. Because of this, and because weaning-induced stress further decreases the foal's immunity, it may be better to wait until the foal's immunity has increased somewhat from that present at 2 months of age before weaning.

There are many methods for weaning foals. Those that are least stressful and most successful are when the foal remains in a safe, familiar place. One method that works well is sometimes referred to as pasture or interval weaning: One or two of the mares with the oldest foals are removed from the herd, leaving their foals with the other mares and foals that the foal has been with. The mares should be removed quickly, quietly, and completely, preferably when the foals are occupied somewhere else, so as to reduce the disturbance to the herd. The mares should be removed to an area completely out of sight and hearing of the herd. After several days, or as additional foals reach the desired weaning age, one or two more mares may be removed until gradually all have been removed. Most foals quickly adjust to the herd of familiar horses, without their mothers, with a minimum of anxiety and stress. However, they should be watched closely to ensure they don't injure themselves, and the pasture fences should be safe and strong.

Putting a companion animal, such as a gentle old mare or gelding, or sometimes even an animal of another species, with the foals before or when the mares are removed may be helpful, particularly if there is only one or a few foals in the group. Contact with people or an older gentle animal appears to decrease weaning stress. Care should be taken, however, that the foal doesn't become overly attached to its weaning companion, or separation from that companion may be nearly as stressful as weaning from its mother. Allowing contact with additional animals beginning the day following weaning may help prevent this. Weaning is complete after 1 week of separation.

It has been found that foals that can see, hear, smell, and touch their mothers through a fence, but not nurse, for 7 days prior to complete separation have lower levels of stress-induced hormones (cortisol) following weaning, and have higher feed intake the first week after weaning, than did foals whose weaning was total, abrupt, and complete. This corroborates behavioral observations in which abruptly weaned foals exhibit more emotional stress (increased vocalizations and activity) than gradually weaned foals. Thus, it appears that gradual weaning is preferable to total and abrupt weaning. Although by the second week following weaning there is no difference in feed intake between foals weaned gradually or abruptly, the major benefit of minimizing weaning stress is reduced risk of injury and disease.

Five to 7 days before weaning, stop feeding the mare grain if possible. For at least 2 weeks following weaning, don't feed her any grain and, if possible, decrease the forage fed to that needed by the nonlactating mare (about 1.5 to 2 lbs/100 lb body wt/day, or 1.5 to 2 kg/100 kg/day). This will decrease her milk production quicker, thus helping to prevent excessive pressure and discomfort. Do not milk out the mare, as this will stimulate increased milk production. Within a week the udder should become soft and flabby, at which time any residue may be milked out.

The newly weaned mare in good condition may be turned out on good pasture and managed as other barren and early pregnant mares. However, if the mare is thin, after lactation has stopped is a good time to feed sufficient forage and grain to increase her body weight and condition to at least moderate and preferably moderately fleshy. This will enhance her reproductive efficiency and rebreeding, and enable her to enter the next pregnancy-lactation cycle with adequate energy stores.

GROWTH PROMOTANTS FOR HORSES

Anabolic steroids and diethylstilbestrol (DES) have occasionally been administered to growing horses to try to increase their feed intake, growth rate, and/or muscle development, but should not be. Their administration can result in premature closure of bone growth plates, thus decreasing mature size. They decrease liver function, and they are of no benefit in increasing growth rate, protein intake or retention, muscling, or athletic or reproductive performance of either the colt or filly in good condition. In stallions, testicular size and sperm production may be decreased with no change in reproductive behavior. In fillies, clitoral enlargement, aggressive stallion-like behavior, and a failure to exhibit heat or to ovulate may occur. For both sexes it may take 2 months to considerably longer for them to return to normal following anabolic steroid or diethylstilbestrol administration.

Growth hormone has also been administered to young horses for many of the same reasons as anabolic steroids, but it is just as ineffective and in many species of animals is known to cause many of the same detrimental effects, including liver and kidney disease, premature sexual development, and early cessation of growth.

Probiotics or live yeast cultures, and enzymes are occasionally added to young horses' diets to enhance feed utilization and/or growth rate and development. As described in Chapter 4, some live yeast cultures may be of benefit for these purposes, at least when the horses are on marginal diets, but like all of these substances, appear to be of little or no benefit when a good diet is fed. Low levels of antibiotics in the feed do appear to increase both the horse's growth rate and feed efficiency by 3 to 12%, just as they do for other species of animals (see Chapter 4). Their use, however, is not recommended, as some are quite harmful and their use in this manner may increase bacterial resistance to that drug. (Feeding zeolite may help).

EXERCISE FOR GROWING HORSES

Sufficient exercise is necessary for normal and strong musculoskeletal development of the horse. Exercise increases the size and strength of muscles, bones, ligaments, and tendons. This is particularly important for young horses, as their bone size, density, and as a result elasticity and strength increase rapidly during the first year of life and then more gradually reaching mature levels at about 3 years of age. However, excessive exercise-induced strain in both growing and mature horses induces bone, tendon, and/or ligament damage as described in Chapter 11. The young horse in which these structures are not fully mature is particularly susceptible. One half of young horses entering race training never race, primarily due to lameness that occurs during training. Nearly 70% of 2-year-olds in training after a fast workout or sprint develop pain on the front of the cannon bones due to bucked shins. The cause is excessive strain due to hard ground with inadequately prepared bones. Like bucked shins, most of these training-induced lamenesses are due to bone, ligament, or tendon damage in the lower leg. This damage and its risk of occurring can be decreased by controlled exercise of weanlings and yearlings or by keeping them and nursing foals on pasture.

Nonstabled foals tend to mature faster than those kept stabled. Stabling weanlings causes a substantial transient slowdown of bone formation. Exercise increases skeletal growth rate, bone mineral content and strength, and increases ligament strength.

Trotting and galloping, as compared to walking, for 15 to 45 minutes 5 days per week from 3 to 24 months of age has been shown to significantly decrease the developmental orthopedic diseases described in Chapter 16. Exercising then resting for 2- to 3-week periods beginning at 1 year of age has been reported to hasten the rate of increase in bone density so that attained at maturity was reached by 2 years of age, whereas those not exercised until 20 months of age did not reach this bone density until 32 months of age. Trotting and some cantering of yearlings during a 6 month period was shown to increase their bone density and strength. Bone density in 2 year olds was also increased with increasing exercise over a 16-week period. These effects do not differ between females, intact males, and geldings.

Ideally, horses from a few days of age until training begins should have free access to pasture or a paddock of a size sufficient to allow them to run. They should also be with similar-age horses to encourage play-induced exercise. If stabling, even with a run, is necessary, the horse from 3 months of age on should be exercised at a trot for 15 to 45 minutes daily. In yearlings, more extensive exercise then rest for alternating 2- to 3-week periods may be beneficial. If exercise is done on a lunge line, be sure to change directions frequently and try to ensure that when cantering, loping, or galloping the horse, uses the correct lead, i.e., that the inside front leg strikes the ground first. This will assist in getting the horse used to using the correct lead, and as a result enhance its athletic ability.

VACCINATION AND INTERNAL-PARASITE CONTROL FOR GROWING HORSES

Foals are born without immunity or resistance to parasites. There are four parasites that require special attention in foals. These are:

1. Intestinal threadworms (Strongyloides westeri), which can be passed to the foal from its mother in her milk.
2. Ascarids or roundworms (Parascaris equorum), which are one of the most damaging and common parasites in the first 6 months of life.
3. Large strongyles or bloodworms (Strongylus spp.).
4. Small strongyles.

These parasites and their life cycles, effects, treatment

and prevention are described in Chapter 9. Ascarids and both large and small strongyle eggs may be ingested and cause damage while the foal is still young and few eggs are being passed in their feces. If parasite infestation is sufficient, the foal may have an apparent general unthriftiness, decreased growth and development, rough hair coat, and coughing. However, even foals not showing any clinical signs may suffer sufficient intestinal damage for feed utilization to be impaired and as a result growth rate and mature size decreased, and sufficient respiratory tract damage to impair the foal's future athletic performance ability.

To prevent intestinal parasites and their effects, mares should be given deworming medication effective against all four of these intestinal parasites (e.g., ivermectin) the first day after foaling. At 6 to 8 weeks of age, the foal should be given an effective deworming medication every 2 months until it is 1 year of age, at which time it should be put on the mature horse internal-parasite control program as described in Chapter 9. But yearlings, as well as weanlings, should be kept separate from mature horses to prevent them from being infected by the older horses.

In addition to control of internal parasites, all foals, brood mares, and growing horses should be on a good vaccination program as given in Table 9–5. This includes the following. Foals receiving colostrum from mares not given tetanus toxoid in the last trimester, or those whose vaccination history is unknown, should be given both tetanus antitoxin (1500 IU) and tetanus toxoid at 1 to 2 days of age. Tetanus antitoxin is unnecessary for foals receiving colostrum from mares known to have been given tetanus toxoid in their last trimester of pregnancy. All foals should be given tetanus toxoid, influenza, rhinopneumonitis (equine herpes virus) and sleeping sickness vaccines at 2 and again at 4 months of age, and all except for sleeping sickness again at 6 months of age. If exposure risk is high, vaccination for influenza and rhinopneumonitis should be continued every 2 to 3 months until maturity. In problem areas or farms, vaccination for strangles (distemper or Streptococcus equi) at 3, 4, and 5 months of age may be helpful (see Chapter 9). Clostridium botulinum type-B toxoid should be given to mares prior to foaling and to the foal at 2, 4 and 8 weeks, and again at 1 year of age on farms or in areas where "shaker foal syndrome" or botulism (as described in chapter 19) in any age horse has occurred. Mares not vaccinated the previous year should be given this vaccine three times, 1 to 3 weeks apart, with the last injection being 2 to 4 weeks prior to foaling. An annual booster vaccination 2 to 4 weeks before foaling is adequate for the mare.

ORPHAN AND EARLY-WEANED FOAL FEEDING AND CARE

A foal sometimes must be raised as an orphan either because its mother has died or because she is unable or unwilling to properly nurse it. If the foal is orphaned at or near birth, the same procedures described in the section on "Neonatal Foal Care" in Chapter 14 are necessary. It may also be necessary to hand-feed the premature or sick foal too weak to stand and nurse.

Nurse Mares

Nurse mares or foster mares, when available, facilitate raising orphan foals and, once the mare has accepted the foal, will decrease the caretaker's time necessary to raise the foal. Generally, a lactating mare will accept another foal, or her foal if she has rejected it, if she is restrained sufficiently so the foal can nurse for a long enough period of time so she becomes familiar with the foal. Care must be taken when this is done to avoid any pain or discomfort to the mare while the foal nurses, otherwise she may associate the discomfort with the foal and the act of suckling. Feeding the mare grain as the foal nurses is helpful in making the occurrence pleasurable and, therefore, in having the mare accept the foal and its nursing.

Mares use smell, sight, and sound to identify their foals. Smell is the primary sense used for close-range identification. Therefore, when trying to get a lactating mare to accept a foal, it is helpful to make the foal smell like the mare by coating it with her placental fluids, milk, sweat, or feces, or by smearing a mentholated ointment in the mare's nostrils and on the foal's head and perianal area.

Initially the mare must be restrained so that she can't prevent the foal from nursing and so that she doesn't injure it. This may be done by tying the mare along the side of the stall, preferably at a feed bunk so she can eat, and placing a bar or pole along her side from the front to the back of the stall. A bar may also be placed behind her if necessary. The nurse mare chute shown in Figure 15–3

has also been reported to work well. When these are used, the foal can remain loose in the stall to nurse freely without the mare's being hobbled or sedated. Although initially she may squeal and try to kick and bite the foal, a healthy hungry foal will not be discouraged from nursing. Tranquilizers should not be given to the mare as most are excreted in the milk, sedating the foal and thus decreasing its attempts to nurse.

The majority of mares accept the foal within 24 hours, and almost all within 12 hours to 3 days, although occasionally it may take as long as 10 days. The responses of both the mare and foal should be observed and restraints gradually removed as acceptance occurs. When both have been loose in the stall for a day without the foal being harmed, they may be turned into a paddock by themselves for an additional couple of days before being placed with other mares and foals.

Draft and draft-cross mares are popular as nurse mares because they produce more milk than smaller mares. However, this may be a disadvantage rather than an advantage if there is only one foal nursing that mare. In one study Thoroughbred foals nursing draft or draft cross mares grew faster than those nursing Thoroughbred mares whether a creep feed was or was not fed. However, 2 of 8 of the draft mare-raised foals developed a developmental orthopedic disease requiring surgery, whereas none of 24 raised on Thoroughbred mares, or of 8 weaned at 5 days of age and

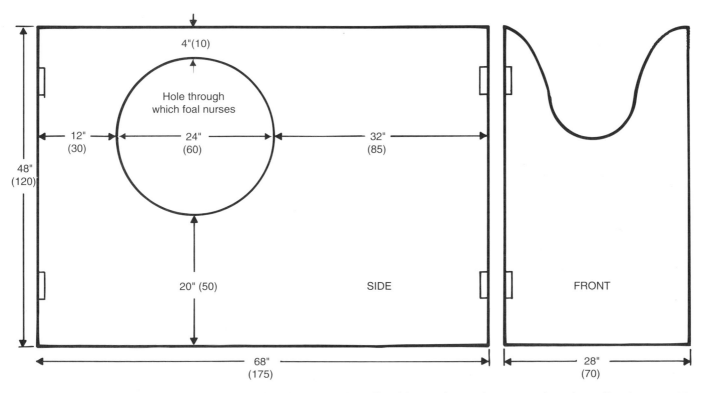

Fig. 15–3. Nurse mare chute. The side is placed in the corner of a stall and fastened 28 inches (70 cm) from the wall with removable pen hinges. The front is fastened to the side with hinges. The chute is swung out to allow the mare to be placed along the side of the stall with her rear in the corner. The chute is then swung closed and the front attached to the wall of the stall using a latch near its top and bottom. At least ¾ inch (2 cm) plywood with strong hinges and latches attached to it with nuts and bolts rather than screws is recommended. The ends of the bolts should be cut off and filed smooth. Dimensions given are in inches (cm) for average-size light horse breed mares.

fed milk replacer, developed any developmental orthopedic diseases.

Nurse mares often aren't available, they are expensive, they make their own foal an orphan unless it has died, and sometimes several days are required to get a nurse mare to accept an orphan foal. Because of these factors, orphan or early-weaned foals are often hand-reared. Many different diets and procedures have been successfully used.

Mare's Milk Replacers

There are numerous replacements for mare's milk that when fed properly have been used successfully, resulting in growth and digestive disturbances no different from that of the foal that remains with its normally lactating mother. These replacements include cow's and goat's milk formulas, nurse goats, foal and calf milk replacers, and acidified milk replacers. In contrast, the enteral formulas intended for people, including some that are occasionally recommended by veterinarians for foals, have all resulted in excessive gas, diarrhea, and colic.

Both cow's and goat's milk are less dilute than mare's milk and contain nearly twice as much fat and one half as much lactose (milk sugar) or carbohydrate but are similar in protein and mineral content (Table 15–5). Because they are lower in lactose and their fat is highly digestible, they can be used for foals. However, unmodified cow's milk may cause diarrhea. Best results seem to be obtained by altering cow's milk to make it more similar to mare's milk. This is done either by using low-fat cow's milk (2% instead of the 3 to 4% in regular milk) or by diluting 2 parts whole milk with 1 part saturated lime water. With either preparation add 4 level teaspoons/quart (20 g/L) or 1 package (2 oz or 57 g)/3 quarts (3 L) of jam and jelly pectin. Jam and jelly pectin is primarily dextrose (glucose), and can be purchased at most grocery stores under many commercial names (Surejel, MCP Pectin, Pen Jel, etc). Saturated lime water is prepared by adding all the lime (calcium oxide) that will dissolve in water, allowing it to stand for several hours, then pouring off the clear saturated lime water.

Dextrose (glucose) is recommended rather than corn syrup or honey, and table sugar (sucrose) should never be used. Corn syrup, honey, and sugar contain disaccharides that are poorly utilized by the foal, and tend to cause diarrhea and colic.

Although goat's milk is similar in nutrient content to cow's milk (Table 15–5), most foals tolerate it and grow well even when it is fed unaltered. This may be because its fat is purported to be more highly emulsified and easier to digest. If digestive disturbances do occur when goat's milk is fed, the same alterations recommended for cow's milk may be helpful. It has been recommended that 1 oz (30 ml) of mineral oil daily be added to goat's milk to prevent firm stools and impactions that reportedly may occur when foals are fed goat's milk alone. In some places, goat's milk can be purchased, but it usually costs several times more than cow's milk. Alternatively, foals have been raised successfully by a nurse goat. Foals may be taught to nurse a lactating goat while on their knees, or with the goat on a platform on a board placed on a couple of bales of hay, and the nurse goat will cooperate fully. The nurse goat may also serve as the foal's companion. Unless the foal is eating some solid feed at an early age to decrease its milk needs, more than one goat may be needed to meet the foal's needs.

There are several good-quality commercial milk replacers specifically formulated for foals (Table 15–5). Foals fed these replacers properly have no more digestive disturbances, or other problems than do foals nursing their mothers; they also grow nearly as rapidly. although growth during the first 1 to 2 months of life may be slightly slower. Stools commonly are soft to watery when milk replacers are fed, although this causes no problems. Intestinal gas accumulation and mild colic may occur during transition to a milk replacer. Constipation and dehydration result if the mare's milk replacer powders are not diluted sufficiently. To prevent this problem, ensure that they are diluted to 10 to 17% total solids or dry matter. This requires 1 to 1.5 lbs of dry milk replacer/gallon of water (110 to

TABLE 15–5
Composition of Milk and Mare's Milk Replacers[a]

Nutrient	Milk			Mare's Milk Replacers		
	Mare[b]	Cow	Goat	Foal-Lac[c]	Mare's Match[d]	NutriFoal[e]
Total solids (DM)—%	10.7	12.5	13.5	20	10	17
Protein—%	25	27	25	20	24	29
Fat—%	17	29	34	14	18	21
Carbohydrate—%	58	38	31	53	46	36
Crude Fiber—%	0	0	0	0.2	0.15	0.2
Calcium—%	11	1.1	1.0	0.9	1.1	1.3
Phosphorus—%	0.7	0.7	0.8	0.75	0.6	0.9
Zinc—ppm	23	40	30	9	40	100
Copper—ppm	4	3	2	6.6	10	30

[a] Values for total solids or dry matter (DM) are for the milk as secreted or the replacers as diluted as recommended by the manufacturer. All other values given are for the amount in the total solids or dry matter (DM).
[b] During first 4 weeks of lactation, excluding colostrum.
[c] Pet-Ag, Inc, Hamshire, IL.
[d] Land-O-Lakes, Fort Dodge, IA.
[e] Reported to provide 691 Kcal or 0.69 Mcal/qt (730 Kcal/L or 0.73 Mcal/L) (KenVet, Ashland, OH).

190 g/L). Some manufacturers' directions for reconstituting milk replacers result in a concentration nearly twice that of mare's milk; these directions should not be used.

Although a mare's milk replacer is preferred, a good-quality calf milk replacer has been used quite successfully to raise foals. Those used should preferably contain all milk protein (e.g., skim milk, buttermilk, whey or casein), rather than soy protein isolate, soy protein concentrate, soy flour, a grain protein or flour, brewers' dried yeast, distillers' dried solubles, fish protein, or meat solubles. This should be indicated on the feed label's list of ingredients and by a crude fiber content of not more than 0.2% (those containing soy protein concentrate and soy flour will contain 0.5% to 1.0% crude fiber). However, specially processed soy protein, such as protein modified soy flour, has been shown to be as good as milk protein for calves, and therefore may be for foals. The milk replacer should contain at least 20% crude protein and 15% fat, although at least 22% protein and 20% fat has been shown to be preferable for calves, and may be for foals. In contrast to milk replacers for calves, those for lambs may not be satisfactory for foals, as most are considerably higher in fat and protein and for lambs are fed less diluted.

Acidified calf milk replacers have also been used to raise foals successfully and are reported to be better than nonacidified calf or mare milk replacers. Acidification enhances nutrient digestibility and keeping quality when reconstituted. They are intended for free-choice feeding. Reconstituted, they are reported to stay fresh for up to 3 days, to be well tolerated even by very young foals, to meet all of the foal's nutrient requirements, and to be higher in most nutrients, to be more palatable, to cause fewer digestive disturbances, and to be less expensive than nonacidified mare's or calf milk replacers. A formula called Acidified Cold Ad Lib Formula (Milk Specialties Co., Dundee, IL) packaged and sold under a variety of names, has been recommended.

Orphan Foal Feeding Procedures

The young foal has a very high dietary energy requirement, needing for its normal rate of growth 50 to 60 kcal DE/lb (110 to 130 kcal/kg) of body weight, which is about 3.5 times that needed by the mature horse for maintenance. Yet, the mare's milk is quite dilute, providing during the first few weeks of lactation about 500 kcal of digestible energy/qt or L (Table 15-4). As a result, a large amount of milk must be consumed: an amount equal to 20 to 25% of the foal's body weight for the first 5 weeks of life and 17 to 20% thereafter. For light horse breeds, and thus foals weighing at birth 90 to 110 lbs (40-50 kg), this amount is 14 qt (or L)/day at birth, increasing by 1 qt/week up to 18 to 20 quarts, and then this amount is fed until weaned. These amounts, which are normally received by the nursing foal, are over twice that recommended in the past for orphan foals. The lower amounts previously recommended seemed to have been based primarily on the amount of milk normally fed to calves, which is inadequate for the foal.

Ideally, the amount of milk needed daily should be fed in equal amounts every 4 hours for the first 1 to 2 weeks of life. However, even in the first week of life, the night feeding may be omitted. From 1 to 2 weeks of age to 3 to 4 weeks of age, feed milk 4 times daily (morning, noon, early evening, and before going to bed works well for many people) and thereafter 3 times daily. If too much milk is fed at one time, it will result in diarrhea and colic. To assist in preventing the occurrence of digestive disturbances, it is best to begin by feeding one half of the amount of milk needed then gradually increasing this over the following 36 to 48 hours. If diarrhea or colic occur, don't feed for 4 to 8 hours, then increase the frequency of feeding so that not so much is given at one time.

Regardless of the feeding procedure or mare's milk replacer used: (1) all diet changes should be gradual, (2) water should always be easily available, (3) milk should be supplemented with solid feed as soon as possible, (4) all feeding equipment should be well cleaned after every feeding, and (5) the following should be closely monitored: foal's attitude, appetite, hydration (based on skin turgor, mucus membrane moistness, and urine volume, appearance, and, if available, specific gravity, which should be less than 1.015), fecal output and consistency, and growth rate. The foal should be bright, alert, playful, and always hungry before being fed; if not, the cause should be determined and quickly corrected.

Most hungry foals will readily suck a nursing bottle or drink from a pan or pail. Regardless of the feeding method used, it works best if the foal is hungry (it has been 4 to 6 hours since the foal last received any nourishment), but still strong and vigorous when first fed. If a nursing bottle is used, a nipple for infants is accepted best by most foals until after the first 1 to 2 weeks of life, when a lamb nipple works well. The hole in the nipple should be small enough to prevent milk from streaming freely when the nursing bottle is inverted. The risk of aspiration is reduced by keeping the foal's nose below the level of its eyes to avoid overextension of the foal's head and neck and to facilitate swallowing.

Feeding by bucket rather than nursing bottle is preferred by most because a bucket is easier to keep clean, and feeding is much easier and faster. Plastic buckets with wide openings rather than deep, narrow, or metal buckets are best. To start the foal drinking from the bucket, let it suck on a milk-wet finger. If the foal does not suck the finger, move the finger against the palate and the tongue to stimulate the foal's sucking response. As the foal sucks on the finger, slowly and gently move it, and the foal's mouth, down into the milk until the foal begins sucking milk from the bucket. After a short while, remove the finger. It may take several attempts, slow, gentle patience and 10 minutes to 2 hours before the foal will learn to drink unassisted from the bucket. Once the foal has learned to drink from the bucket, it, containing milk, should be hung in a convenient and easily accessible location for the foal. It is best to use a light-colored bucket so the foal can see it easily. There is no benefit in warming the milk before feeding. Milk at the foal's environmental temperature is preferred because its temperature remains more constant.

Milk may be left in the bucket for the foal at all times without fear of overeating. The foal will drink small amounts frequently during the day and night, just as the foal nursing the mare does. Excessive milk consumption and gorging don't occur. Because small amounts are ingested frequently, feed-induced digestive disturbances are minimized, although soft stools may occur as they often do when a milk replacer is being fed. The amount of stool excreted is small, however, so dehydration or other problems don't occur. When the foal is drinking well from a bucket, two to three similar-age foals with a similar number of buckets containing milk may be put together in the same stall, paddock, or pasture. This may be helpful in providing them companionship.

When this feeding regimen is used, acidified milk or reconstituted milk replacer is preferred, but not necessary, as it will stay fresh for several days. However, the milk should be changed and replenished twice a day. Each time the milk is changed, the bucket should be thoroughly cleaned. If this is not done, bacteria will rapidly multiply in the warm milk and container, souring the milk and infecting the foal, resulting in decreased consumption and digestive disturbances. Foals may also be allowed continual free access to mare's milk replacer in an automatic nipple feeder sold for calves.

When the foal is several days old, foal milk replacer or milk transition pellets should initially be placed in the foal's mouth several times a day; as much as the foal will eat should always be available. Any pellets remaining should be removed twice a day and fresh pellets placed in the feed bucket. Pellets removed can be fed to older horses or discarded. When the foal is eating 2 to 3 lbs (1 to 1.5 kg) of milk replacer pellets daily, a good-quality grain mix creep feed intended for nursing foals (Table 4–9) may be added to the pellets in increasing amounts as increasing amounts of this mixture are consumed. The bucket containing the solid feed, like that containing milk, should be cleaned and filled with fresh feed twice daily. By about 8 weeks of age, the foal should be eating 4 to 6 lbs (2 to 2.5 kg) of milk replacer pellets or grain mix daily, at which time milk feeding can be stopped, although continuing it for several more weeks may be beneficial. Having milk replacer pellets and a grain mix both available until the foal is 4 months old may result in faster growth than if only the grain mix is fed. After 4 months of age, the foal may be fed as a normal weanling. In addition to milk replacer pellets and grain mix, good-quality hay or pasture forage should be available for the foal to eat all that it wants by at least 1 month of age. Occasionally, a young foal will overeat a good-quality palatable legume forage and develop loose or watery stools, particularly if adequate milk isn't available. This may be corrected by ensuring that adequate milk replacer pellets or grain mix and milk are fed, and limiting forage intake until stools firm up.

Orphan Foal Feeding Effects

Orphan foals allowed all they will consume of a reconstituted milk replacer, milk replacer pellets, a grain mix, water, and forage often grow more slowly for about the first 1 to 2 months of life but not thereafter. The foals should have companionship—if not other foals, then an old gentle gelding or mare, or even a sheep, goat, or burro. In addition to companionship, the animal will teach the foal to eat solid feed as the foal watches the animal eat and imitates it. The older animal should not, however, be able to drink or eat the foal's feed.

There has been concern that orphan-raised foals later may not learn as rapidly and, therefore, be as easy to train as normally raised foals. This does not appear to be the case, however. Although orphan foals initially take more time to walk through a simple maze, they make no more errors and learn the maze just as rapidly as normally raised foals. Their slower exploration of the maze or a novel environment is similar to that observed in early-weaned dogs and cats, but in contrast to these species the orphaned foal's learning ability isn't slowed or impaired. Both orphan and normally raised foals learn faster than the mares. Thus, as with other species of animals, young horses appear to learn faster than older horses, as has also been observed for trainability. There is no correlation between mares and their foals, in dominance hierarchy, weight or age of the mares and their foals' learning ability.

Chapter 16

DEVELOPMENTAL ORTHOPEDIC DISEASES IN HORSES

Effects of Developmental Orthopedic Diseases	277	
Growth Plate Enlargements (Physitis)	277	
Wobblers Syndrome	279	
Angular Leg Deformities	279	
Joint Cartilage Damage	281	
Contracted Flexor Tendons (Leg Flexure Deformities)	282	
Congenital Leg Flexure Deformities	282	
Acquired Leg Flexure Deformities	282	
Causes of Developmental Orthopedic Diseases	283	
Rapid Growth	283	

Trauma to Bone Growth Plates	284
Genetic Predisposition	284
Nutritional Imbalance	285
Dietary Energy Excess	285
Protein Imbalance	285
Calcium and Phosphorus Imbalances	286
Copper and Zinc Imbalances	286
Feeding Practices	286
Nonsurgical Management of Developmental Orthopedic Diseases	287
Supplemental Reading Recommendations	288

Developmental orthopedic diseases (DOD) in horses is currently the favored name for what has been referred to as epiphysitis or the epiphysitis syndrome, and as metabolic bone disease. Both names are less commonly used now than in the past. DOD includes all general growth disturbances resulting from any alteration in normal bone-formation or growth. The disease and its many manifestations are a problem primarily in large, fast-growing, light horse breeds. It most commonly affects those used for athletic activity, including racing, dressage, jumping, roping, or cutting. It may result in (1) enlargements of the bone growth plates (physitis), (2) "wobblers syndrome," (3) angular leg deformities, (4) flexure leg deformities, and (5) joint cartilage damage resulting in a bone cyst or a loose piece of bone or cartilage in the joint (which is referred to as osteochondritis dissecans or OCD). These may result in juvenile arthritis (also referred to as degenerative joint disease or osteochondritis). How closely related these various manifestations of DOD are isn't known. However, most believe they all have a similar set of causes or predisposing risk factors. Often affected horses have a varying severity of more than one of these manifestations of DOD simultaneously, and a number of horses on a farm are affected.

DOD occurs due to a failure of growing cartilage to become properly ossified or converted to bone. This may occur at either, or both, the cartilage in the growth plate for the shaft of the bone or in the cartilage for the bone at the joint. In either case, lack of calcification of the cartilage results in its becoming thickened and enlarged. The increased cartilage thickness inhibits nutrition of underlying cartilage, which may result in its damage. The causes and effects of DOD as described in this chapter are summarized in Figure 16-1.

Developmental orthopedic diseases are quite common. Lesions are reported to be present in 20 to 25% of Thoroughbreds, with about 20 to 25% of these being in the vertebrae and the remainder in the legs. Only 5 to 10% of these lesions, however, are sufficiently severe to result in clinical or radiographic alterations.

Radiographically visible lesions in the hock joints and in the fetlock joints were found in 14.3 and 11.8%, respectively, in 60% of Standardbred trotters born in Norway in 1988. In a Canadian study, radiographic lesions of juvenile arthritis were present in 48%, joint cartilage lesions in 31%, bone cysts in joints in 11%, inflammation of fetlock, sesamoid bones in 22%, and bone growth plate enlargement or physitis in 1.4% of 17-month-old Standardbreds. No DOD lesions were found in only about 25% of these Standardbreds. However, the lesions observed were not sufficiently severe to result in clinical signs, and they appeared to have no long-term detrimental effect on these horses. No decrease in the amount won or racing times were found between horses that as yearlings did, or did not, have nonclinical but radiographically visible osteochondrosis lesions. However, future performance ability will be impaired and lameness will occur in horses sufficiently severely affected.

EFFECTS OF DEVELOPMENTAL ORTHOPEDIC DISEASES

Growth Plate Enlargements (Physitis)

Thickened growth cartilage and callus formation may cause a visible swelling at the growth plate, or physis. This is commonly referred to as either physitis or epiphysitis. The swelling most commonly occurs in the cervical vertebrae and at the distal end of the radius above the knee and at the distal end of the cannon bone above the fetlock, but may also occur in the hock at the distal end of the tibia. Frequently all legs are affected to some degree. The enlarged radial growth plate, which is generally most marked at 12 to 18 months of age, gives the knee a dished-in appearance in front when viewed from the side and is referred to as "open knees" (Figs. 16-2 and 16-3). The growth plate enlargement that occurs at the distal end of the cannon bones, which is generally most evident at 5 to 9 months of age, results in enlarged fetlocks and, if severe, gives the fetlocks an hourglass appearance (Fig. 16-3).

No lameness occurs in some horses with physitis; with others there is a variable degree of lameness which may be mild and intermittent and result in no more than the appearance of a generalized stiffness. Severe cases may

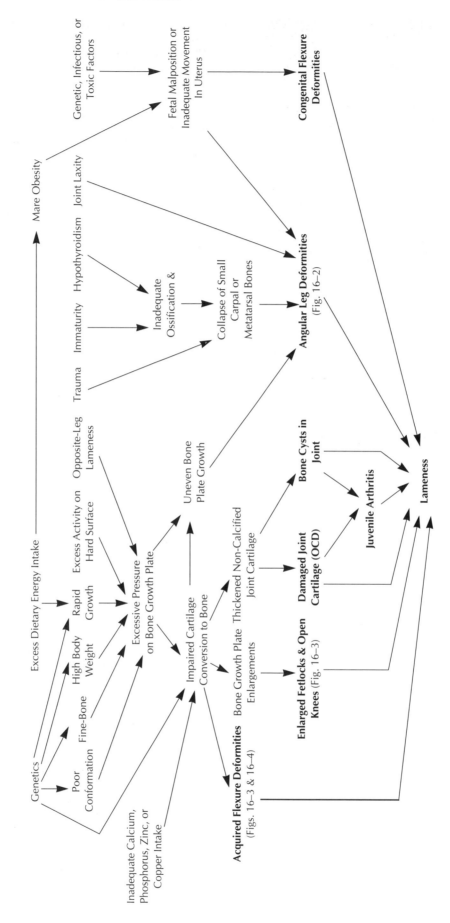

Fig. 16–1. Causes and Effects of Developmental Orthopedic Diseases

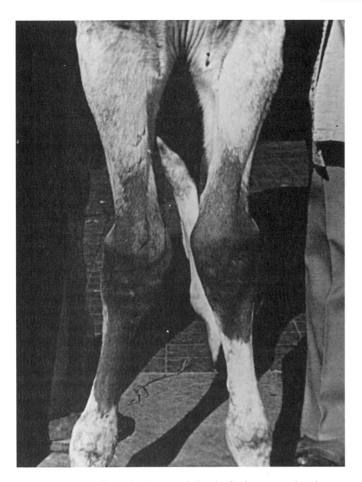

Fig. 16–2. Midline deviation of the foal's knees and enlargement of the distal radial growth plates just above the knees.

have increased warmth and pain in response to deep palpation over the affected regions. Those affected may not play as actively as others in the herd. From one to all similar-age horses in the herd may be affected. Often other manifestations of DOD will be present in affected individuals or others in the herd. The condition is self-limiting, disappearing as growth slows or the growth plates close, unless cystic lesions occur in the bone. Flaring, broadening, asymmetry, sclerosis, and an irregular width of the growth plate or physis may be evident on radiographs. Lesions involving the joint surfaces may be present.

Wobblers Syndrome

Swelling of the growth plates of the vertebrae of the neck causes compression and, if sufficiently severe, damage to the spinal cord. This can be detected radiographically as a narrowing of the vertebral canal. The onset of clinical signs often, but not always, occurs after a traumatic incident, such as being tied up for the first time, being cast, or falling. Clinical signs include an incoordinated gait, a wide-base stance, going down, and spasticity. These signs generally occur on both sides and first and most severely in the back legs. They are most noticeable when the horse is walking slowly or in tight circles, and frequently can be exaggerated by exercising the horse on a slope with the head elevated. Incoordination may be more obvious when the horse is backed. Because of these symptoms, it is commonly referred to as "wobblers syndrome."

Wobblers syndrome may occur as a result of anything that causes spinal cord damage. In 383 cases seen in one university veterinary clinic, 45% were due to EDM (equine degenerative myeloencephalopathy) (discussed in that section in Chapter 2), 31% to a protozoan organism, and 24% to a swelling of the vertebral growth plates. However, spinal cord damage due to a swelling, of the vertebral growth plates is the most common cause of wobblers syndrome in horses less than 4 years old. Less frequent causes of posterior incoordination in the horse include rhinopneumonitis (see Chapter 9), injury, tumors, infarcts, intervertebral disc protrusion, Sudan grass toxicosis (discussed in section on Neurologic-Disease-Inducing Plants in Chapter 18), equine infectious anemia, (swamp fever, see Chapter 9) and a migrating parasite larvae (see Strongyles, Chapter 9).

Growth plate swelling-induced spinal cord compression rarely may be so severe the neck is fixed in a flexed position (Type I), with the onset of signs occurring anytime from birth to several years of age. Compression may instead occur only during neck flexure (Type II), which occurs primarily in nursing and weanling foals. Most often, however, compression is neither relieved nor worsened by neck flexion (Type III), with the onset of signs occuring at 1 to 3 years of age after the horse is put into training, but they may not occur until up to 10 years of age. Compression is often, but not always, continuous by the time it is diagnosed. With all types, an acute onset of signs is often triggered by a traumatic incident.

Dietary management, as described later for all DOD effects, is fairly effective for prevention and for treatment prior to obvious signs. Once signs are obvious, surgery may be indicated. The shorter the duration of clinical signs before surgery and the further forward the compression, the greater the chance of success.

Angular Leg Deformities

Impaired cartilage nutrition due to its thickening slows bone growth. If this occurs unevenly, with one side growing slower than the other, an angular leg deformity occurs. Anything causing more pressure on one side of the growth plates can also cause angular leg deformities. Such factors may include joint laxity, malpositioning in the uterus, poor foot trimming, and excessive trauma due to a large body size for the bone size, excessive physical activity, or lameness in the opposite leg. Excess feed intake during the latter half of pregnancy by previously poorly fed mares was the only common factor recognized on one farm in which angular leg deformities were present in 17 of 30 foals born. It was proposed that the excess feed intake may have resulted in sufficient abdominal fat to compress the uterus, causing fetal malpositioning resulting in congenital angular leg deformities. Impaired or delayed, conversion of bone growth cartilage into bone may result in collapse of the small bones in the knee or hock, or traumatic luxation or fracture of these bones, will also cause

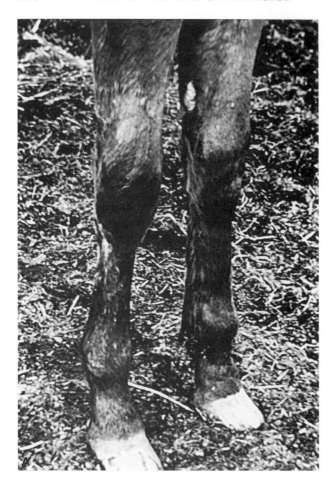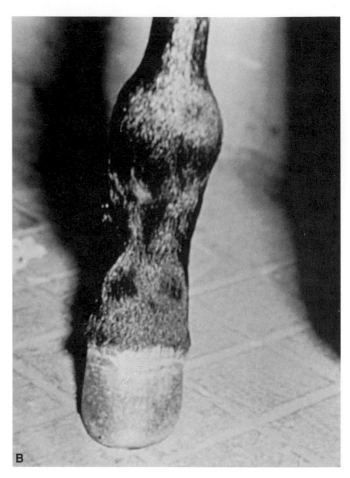

Fig. 16–3(A,B). Distal radial metaphyseal or bone growth plate enlargements giving the knee a dished-in appearance in front, referred to as "open knees," and enlarged fetlocks due to enlargements of cannon bone growth plates. Upright or straight-appearing pasterns due to the occurrence of mild acquired flexure leg deformities are also evident.

angular leg deformity. Angular deformities are most common at the knee, followed by the hock and fetlocks.

Foals may have congenital angular leg deformities present at birth or occurring within the first few days of life, or the deformities may be acquired within several weeks to months of age (Fig. 16-1). Varying degrees of knee joint laxity may be present in newborn foals, particularly those that are premature. The surrounding tissues are not strong enough to support the knee and an angular leg deformity occurs. Unless the deformity is quite mild (less than 5° deviation), it is best to keep the affected foal and its dam confined to a stall and run until muscle tone increases sufficiently to tighten the support and bring about correction. Hoof trimming and balancing should also be done. Squaring or rounding of the toe may help force a more normal break over the foot. However, if the deformity worsens, if substantial improvement has not occurred by 2 weeks of age, or if the deviation exceeds 12° to 15°, thorough investigation as to the cause, and treatment accordingly, should be instituted. Delaying treatment greatly decreases the chances for recovery and future athletic performance ability.

Conversion of growth cartilage to bone in the small bones of the knee and hock normally occurs during the

last few weeks of pregnancy and continues during the first month of life. In some foals this may not be sufficiently complete at birth as a result of normal variation, immaturity, or inadequate thyroid function. Hypothyroidism delays bone formation. This may result not only in the collapse of these bones, but also in bone cysts, contracted flexor tendons, extensor tendon rupture, mandibular prognathism (overbite or parrot mouth) and/or scoliosis (abnormal curvature of the back). As described in Chapter 2, hypothyroidism in the foal may be caused by either inadequate or excessive iodine intake by the mare during pregnancy or lactation.

Radiographs of at least one knee and one hock should be taken of foals that appear immature at birth. If normal ossification of the small bones isn't complete, the foal and the dam should be kept confined until ossification is complete. Radiographs to determine this should be taken every few weeks. Exercise prior to complete ossification may result in collapse of these bones or abnormal ossification with subsequent development of juvenile arthritis. Stall confinement for a maximum of 2 months may be the only management necessary.

Collapse of the small bones of the knee will result in angular deformity of the knee, whereas collapse of the small bones of the hock will result in an increased flexion angle, or sickle hocks. These deformities may be present without improvement since birth. Both knee and hock bone collapse, if treated prior to secondary changes, can usually be straightened under general anesthesia and a splint changed every few days, or a tube cast changed every 1 to 2 weeks, until there is radiographic evidence of adequate symmetrical ossification. This usually takes 2 to 4 weeks but may take as long as 2 months. The cast or splint is stopped at the fetlock, because if the foot is included, dropped fetlocks may occur when support is removed. The leg is usually wrapped for several days after the cast or splint is removed to provide some transitional support.

With acquired angular leg deformities, the foal is born with relatively straight legs that after a few weeks to months of life begin to deviate. The cause may be an unrecognized angular leg deformity present at birth (congenital) that becomes more severe, a growth plate injury, or the other causes of other DOD effects as discussed in that section later in this chapter. Poor conformation or improper hoof trimming that result in more weight and as a result pressure on one part of the growth plate than another have also been thought to cause angular leg deformities. However, it is doubtful that poor hoof trimming is a cause, as it has been shown that altered pressures resulting from attaching a wedge to the hoof, which elevated the lateral aspect 12° to 15°, progressively returned to normal within 10 days. In cases that don't respond to more conservative management or that are severe (in excess of 12° to 15° angulation), both conservative management and surgery are necessary for correction.

Joint Cartilage Damage

Joint cartilage damage may occur because inhibited nutrient diffusion through the thickened noncalcified cartilage results in degeneration of its basal layers. Subsequent physical stress may result in the cracking or fissuring at the periphery of the affected joint. Joint swelling, pain, and lameness may occur as a result of these effects. Avulsion of a piece of the damaged cartilage may occur, resulting in what is referred to as OCD or osteochondrosis dissecans. This damaged piece of cartilage may remain attached or become detached and form "joint mice". In either case this loose piece of cartilage or bone may cause erosions of the opposing joint surface, resulting in juvenile arthritis (also referred to as degenerative joint disease and osteoarthrosis). This is the major cause of juvenile arthritis in the horse and leads to chronic lameness.

The sites most commonly affected by OCD include the stiffle, hock, and less commonly the fetlocks and shoulder. Often multiple joints are affected to varying degrees.

Most horses with OCD of the stifle or hock joints are $\frac{1}{2}$ to 2 years of age but may be older or younger. The majority are 1 year of age or less when signs first become apparent, and lesions tend to be more severe the younger the horse. In slightly over one-half of the cases both hocks are affected.

Typically there is joint distention and mild lameness, which are increased following holding the leg for several minutes in a position to flex the joint (flexion test). Lameness may be severe and worsened by training, or not obvious, although affected horses may have an asymmetric or awkward gait that minimizes flexion of the affected joint. Mature horses frequently present with a sudden onset of clinical signs thought to be associated with the development of osteochondral fragments. Young foals that are affected may have difficulty getting up or are lame. Radiographic changes are usually evident.

Hock joint distention, or bog spavin without lameness, in horses from 6 to 18 months, but up to 3 years of age, is the most common manifestation of OCD in the hock. However, lameness may occur, particularly in horses over 2 years of age in training, and may be worsened by flexion for several minutes. It is a common problem in Standardbreds, with twice as many males as females affected. In one study of 114 cases, joint swelling was evident in 62% and lameness in 43% of affected horses, but previously affected horses had similar lifetime race earnings as did nonaffected horses regardless of whether they had been treated surgically or conservatively. Those affected did have significantly fewer race starts, particularly affected females. Surgical removal of OCD fragments preferably via arthroscopic surgery is recommended for those with joint swelling or lameness.

Horses with OCD or bone cysts, of the shoulder are usually younger than 12 to 18 months and have an intermittent foreleg lameness of insidious onset. In a series of 43 cases, in 37 only 1 shoulder, and in 6, both shoulders were affected. The lameness may have a swinging component and stumbling. Flexing and extending the shoulder joint may cause pain. A loss of muscle size over the shoulder and a smaller foot may be evident. Joint swelling generally is not evident. Arthroscopic surgery is often necessary, but difficult, with about one-half achieving athletic soundness.

OCD in the fetlock joints causes thickening over the front aspect of the joint, and joint swelling. Lesions, although not clinical signs, are frequently present in the legs on both sides. No lameness is usually present, although some may have severe joint pain, and lameness may be worsened by flexing the fetlock for several minutes.

Instead of cracking and fissuring at the periphery of the thickened degenerative joint cartilage, resulting in OCD, this may occur at the center of the joint, leaving an entrance for synovial fluid and creating a bone cyst. Sites in which this most commonly occurs in decreasing order of incidence are the stifle, knee, fetlock, pastern, and the hock. Problems due to bone cysts are usually recognized at a later age than those due to OCD and generally occur after the horse is put into training. They can generally be detected on radiographs.

Bone cysts in the hock typically result in an intermittent gait abnormality worsened by exercise and alleviated following rest. However, in some cases acute lameness may occur. Horses from 3 months to 5 years of age, but most commonly from 5 to 24 months old are most commonly affected. The onset of lameness may be associated with some traumatic event, such as the commencement of training. There is a supporting leg lameness with a shortened stride generally noticeable only at a trot. As with OCD of most joints, flexion may worsen the lameness. Swelling and joint effusion generally doesn't, but may, occur as a result of bone cysts.

Bone cysts in the knee, hock, or fetlock joints usually cause no effects until the horse is put into training and these effects are worsened by several minutes of flexion. In contrast, cystic lesions in the pastern and coffin joints generally result in obvious lameness and swelling. Lameness often occurs suddenly when the coffin joint is affected.

Surgery (generally arthroscopically) is usually recommended for removal of fragmented OCD chips, and for debridement of bone cysts. If chips or fragmentation are not evident, and initially for bone cysts without radiographic evidence of juvenile arthritis, surgery may not be necessary. Injections into the affected joints of substances that decrease inflammation and prevent or slow joint degeneration, along with rest may be adequate. Rest is an important aspect of therapy to give the articular cartilage time to repair. Rest for at least 3 months is necessary and should be followed by radiographic and lameness evaluation to determine if continued rest is necessary. A longer period of rest is required in some cases. The younger the horse and the smaller the bone cyst, the better the prognosis. However, if lameness persists, arthritis is present, or the bone cysts are large, surgery should be considered. Surgery has been recommended over nonsurgical treatment of bone cysts of the elbow, hock, and shoulder joints.

Lesions believed to have a high probability of affecting athletic performance, regardless of treatment, include all OCD of the shoulder and elbow; major OCD lesions of the stifle and hip joints; bone cysts of the distal cannon bones and the phalanges, and lesions that have already initiated juvenile or degenerative arthritis. The clinical course is unpredictable for cartilage flap lesions of the stifle and OCD lesions. With proper treatment, athletic performance may not be affected by small OCD lesions at the rear surface of the first phalanx, most fragments within the hock, and small fragments of the front of the fetlock joints.

Contracted Flexor Tendons (Leg Flexure Deformities)

Flexure deformities of the legs are often referred to as contracted flexor tendons. However, the tendons are not contracted; the effective functional length of the muscle-tendon unit is less than necessary to maintain normal leg extension, resulting in a flexure deformity. Flexure deformities may be present at birth or develop within the first few days of life (congenital), or they may be acquired during growth following birth. Most congenital flexure deformities affect both front fetlocks. Less commonly knee flexion may be present. All flexure deformities associated with bone malformation are fixed and generally not treatable. More than one-half of the lethal congenital defects, which are present in about 1% of Thoroughbred foals, are reported to be due to fixed leg flexure deformities.

Congenital Leg Flexure Deformities

Congenital flexure deformities have classically been attributed to malpositioning or a lack of normal fetal movement in the uterus. Obesity during pregnancy has been proposed as a cause. Genetic factors and intrauterine in-sults to the fetus, such as infectious or toxic agents, may also be responsible in some cases. Dietary nutrient intake by the mare is not known to be a factor, although if obesity is a cause, excess dietary energy intake during pregnancy would be responsible.

Most congenital flexure deformities do not involve the bone and are not fixed. Most of these are alleviated shortly after the foal stands if the foal is able to place the bottom of the toe or the sole on the ground. However, if they do not correct within a few days, early and effective therapy is necessary to prevent juvenile arthritis or degenerative joint disease which may limit the horse's future athletic performance ability. The earlier adequate therapy is begun, the greater the chance of success.

Box stall confinement of the mare and foal for several days may be sufficient for spontaneous correction to occur. Oxytetracycline is commonly given during this period. It has been shown to be a safe and effective method of decreasing the young foal's fetlock joint angles. But it may not be safe for foals with existing renal compromise, septicemia, or other extensive medical problems, or if diuretics or methoxyflurane anesthesia is administered.

Leg wraps from the coronary band to the elbow may be beneficial in some cases. If used, the leg should be rewrapped daily and carefully managed to prevent formation of pressure sores. Correction of nonfixed congenital flexure deformities should occur within 1 week. If it does not, or if the foal cannot stand, or stands on the front surface of the hoof, pastern or fetlocks, splints or casts are generally needed to apply forced extension. Pneumatic splints may work well for this. Forced extension is generally successful if the foal can walk on the sole of the foot so that weight-bearing causes extensor tension, and if pressure sores from the splint or cast can be minimized. If not, they are generally unsuccessful, and surgery may be necessary, although in these cases prognosis for normal limb function is guarded.

Acquired Leg Flexure Deformities

Acquired flexure deformities occur in horses born with straight legs. They may occur gradually over several months or more rapidly over several weeks. They may occur on either one or both sides, although one leg is generally worse than the other. There are two major types: those involving primarily the deep digital flexor tendon, and therefore the coffin joint, and those involving primarily the superficial digital flexor tendon, and, therefore, the front leg fetlock joint.

Acquired flexure deformities involving primarily the coffin joint are characterized by a raised heel and a "club footed" appearance. As a result, the heel tends to grow long and the toe stays worn off. Sole bruises and abscesses in the toe area may occur. In severe cases the front aspect of the hoof wall is past vertical, and knuckling over of the fetlock joint may occur. Flexure involving primarily the coffin joint tends to occur most often in nursing or weanling foals 6 weeks to 6 months of age, whereas flexure involving primarily the fetlock joint or superficial digital flexor tendon tends to occur in older weanlings and in yearlings.

Flexure involving primarily the fetlock joint is characterized by a moving of the pastern and fetlock joint forward and a knuckling at the fetlock joint, with the sole of the foot remaining level so the heel remains on the ground (Fig. 16-4). The leg may at first appear to be upright or straight at the pastern and fetlock (Fig. 16-3). As the horse walks, the fetlock may occasionally knuckle forward. As this condition worsens, the horse may stand with the fetlock in a knuckled-over position. Prolonged abnormal flexion results in a failure of structures (tendons, ligaments, and joint capsules) to elongate normally with growth so that straightening becomes more difficult with time. Thus, the longer a flexure deformity exists, the less likely it can be successfully corrected.

Chronic leg pain, such as that due to OCD, bone cysts, arthritis or degenerative joint disease, chronic joint infec-

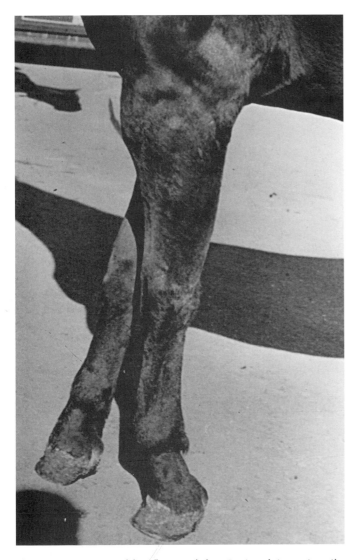

Fig. 16-4. Acquired leg flexure deformity involving primarily the superficial flexor tendon and fetlock joint. The right fetlock is abnormally straight and the left knuckled forward, but the heel remains on the ground, helping to differentiate the deformity from one involving primarily the deep digital flexor tendon and coffin joint.

tions, fractures, or soft tissue damage, causes a shifting of body weight to the nonpainful leg. The pain may result in a contraction of the flexor muscle-tendon unit of either the painful or non-painful leg. A low heel, rapid growth rate, and inadequate exercise have each been thought to predispose to acquired flexure deformities. However, even all three of these factors together did not result in flexure deformities in Quarter Horse weanlings studied from the age of 4 to 10 months.

For acquired flexure deformities involving primarily the coffin joint or deep digital flexor tendon, surgical treatment generally does not detract from future athletic ability. In contrast, few horses in which surgery is done after 5 months of age ever race successfully. For severe or long-standing cases in which the front of the hoof is past vertical, surgery may correct the flexure deformity in some cases, but in others fibrosis and contraction of the joint capsule and associated ligaments don't allow correction of the deformity. In addition, cosmetic appearance and functional ability are often unsatisfactory following surgery. Surgery may also be necessary and beneficial for acquired flexure deformities involving primarily the superficial flexor tendon or fetlock joint. However, results are less predictable than those for primarily coffin joint flexure because of the multiple structures that may be involved.

CAUSES OF DEVELOPMENTAL ORTHOPEDIC DISEASES

The major factors predisposing the growing animal to any of the developmental orthopedic diseases (DOD) are (1) rapid growth; (2) trauma to the bone growth plates or articular cartilages; (3) genetic predisposition; and (4) nutritional imbalances. These four factors are interrelated, and there are many additional factors that affect each one (Fig. 16-1). A combination of two or more of these factors will increase the risk of occurrence and the severity of DOD, although any one of these factors may be responsible. For example, if a growing animal is forced to bear an excessive amount of weight on a leg as a result of pain in the opposite leg, the increased weight bearing may result in DOD in that leg. On the other hand, nutritional excesses or imbalances may result in DOD regardless of the amount of trauma to the bone growth plates or articular cartilages.

Rapid Growth as a Cause of DOD

Rapid growth appears to be the major factor in causing DOD. This has been documented in numerous studies in various species of animals, including horses, dogs, swine, and cattle. The rate of body weight gain is the major factor affecting bone growth plate width. From 4 to 5 times more bone aberrations occurred in light horse weanlings gaining 2.3 lbs (1.05 kg)/day than in those gaining 1.5 lbs (0.67 kg)/day. In one study, growth rates of 5 of 8 Thoroughbred foals that developed compression-induced wobblers syndrome was faster from birth to 3 months of age, but not later in life than that of 44 herd mates whose growth rates were similar to the average for that breed. Two of 8 Thoroughbred foals raised on draft or draft cross mares, who produce more milk than Thoroughbred mares, developed stifle OCD lesions requiring surgery prior to 1 year of age, whereas none of 24 Thoroughbred foals left with their own dam developed any DOD. The foals nursing the draft mares had a 25% faster growth rate up to 6 weeks of age (3.6 versus 2.9 lbs or 1.64 versus 1.30 kg/day gain) but not from 6 to 24 weeks of age (2.2 versus 2.15 lbs or 0.98 versus 1.00 kg/day gain).

A rapid growth rate is promoted by the animal's: (1) genetic capacity; (2) high energy intake; and (3) slow growth early in life followed by a compensatory growth spurt as a result of increased feed intake. In one study, flexure leg deformities occurred in four of six 4-month-old foals whose food intake was restricted sufficiently to slow growth to 0.66 lb (0.3 kg)/day for 4 months and later allowed free access to feed, whereas none of the six foals that were continually fed the same diet free choice developed deformities or any DOD. Not providing adequate amounts of a properly formulated creep feed to the nursing foal, then, following weaning, feeding for rapid growth, is a common cause for a compensatory growth spurt. This should be avoided by feeding foals properly, as described in Chapter 15. The larger the body size and the faster the growth, whether due to genetics or a compensatory growth spurt, and the more dietary energy and protein consumed to permit this rapid growth to occur, the greater the risk of DOD occurring.

Trauma to Bone Growth Plates as a Cause of DOD

Although, as described in Chapter 15, exercise for the growing horse is quite beneficial for optimal musculoskeletal development, excess trauma to areas of bone growth may increase the occurrence and severity of DOD. In some cases, too much exercise can be a major cause. This is common in young foals when they are adapting to exercise in a large paddock or a pasture. After a period of exercise, the foal will move stiffly, lie down excessively, and while standing, tremble, usually at the knee. This indicates that structural damage has occurred resulting in inflammation and pain. The decreasing activity the pain induces may allow recovery. However, if damage accumulates, a stiff stilted gait occurs, with the foal becoming over at the knees, and club-footed with upright pasterns due to contracted flexor tendons.

The problem generally isn't exercise per se, but instead a sudden increase in the amount of exercise, and therefore stress on the growing bone. This is particularly dangerous in inducing DOD. Deprivation of exercise because of confinement of the mare or foal for any reason can result in the bone formed during that period being unable to withstand the stress of normal, and often overexuberent, exercise when it is resumed. A few days is generally of little consequence, but a few weeks can result in a significant amount of unstressed and therefore structurally weaker bone. When exercise is resumed, the now larger foal's normal activity can cause trauma to this weaker bone resulting in DOD. Thus, if exercise during growth is curtailed for more than 2 to 3 weeks, it should be resumed gradually to decrease the risk of DOD. If the return to exercise is accompanied by signs of DOD (most evident as bone growth plate enlargements and lameness), then the amount of exercise should be reduced until these signs subside; then exercise gradually increased.

Trauma to areas of bone growth increase not only with exercise but also with increased weight per unit of area involved. Thus, the greater the weight, the smaller the bone, and the more the horse's conformation increases compression to a particular part of the growth plate or joint cartilage, the more susceptible the animal is to DOD. Decreased weight bearing on one leg for any reason increases the risk of DOD in the opposite leg because of increased weight bearing on it. This situation and the occurrence of DOD lesions has been induced by tying up one foreleg. Trauma is the reason DOD also occur more commonly in horses with short upright pasterns or other conformational defects, and faster-growing, larger, finer-boned horses; DOD occur less frequently in draft horses, presumably because they have larger bones and reach mature size more slowly, and in ponies, because of their smaller body size.

It has been thought that abnormal hoof balance would alter compressive forces on the leg, increasing DOD lesions in areas of increased compression. However, it doesn't appear that abnormal hoof balance has any lasting effect on compressive forces. When a wedge was placed under the outside surface of the foot, although it greatly altered compressive forces and strain on the leg initially, these changes returned to normal within 10 days.

Genetic Predisposition to DOD

There may be both a direct genetic predisposition to the occurrence of DOD and an indirect genetic predisposition to it as a result of a genetic predisposition for a rapid growth rate, a high body weight, fine bones, and/or poor conformation, all of which would increase trauma or pressure on the growth plate (Fig. 16–1). A direct genetic predisposition to DOD has been demonstrated in people, dogs, swine, and horses. A case of eight foals with severe flexure deformities resulting from a dominant gene mutation in the sire has been reported. The incidence of DOD lesions has been reported to be higher in offspring from certain stallions and as a result the Danish Warmblood Registry will not allow stallions with osteochondrosis to be registered. In one study, many of the affected cases related back to two sires. In another study, of 22 foals whose dams and sires both had compression-induced wobblers syndrome, regardless of the foals' diets, 10 had DOD lesions of which 9 were bone growth plate enlargement, 7 acquired flexure leg deformities, and 4 radiographic evidence of compression-induced wobblers syndrome, suggesting a high degree of heritability of these DOD. It was found that the incidence of DOD lesions in the hock in 325 trotting breed horses from 9 different stallions ranged in these 9 different progeny groups from 3 to 30%, indicating a strong genetic influence on its occurrence. The stallions whose progeny had the highest incidence of DOD lesions showed no radiological signs of the disease themselves. It was estimated that the heritability of DOD lesions in the hock joint of trotting horses in Denmark was 0.26, whereas in Standardbred trotters in Norway it was estimated to be 0.52, and in the fetlock joints 0.21. Radiographically visible DOD lesions in the hock and in the fetlock joints of 6- to 21-month-old Standardbred trotters in different progeny groups was found to range from 0 to 69% and 0 to 41% respectively, thus occurring in the majority of some progeny and not at all in others. However, there was no correlation between stallion breeding values for DOD lesions in the hocks and in the fetlocks, indicating there were few common genes coding for lesions in these two locations. Thus, one stallion may be more likely than others to produce offspring with hock lesions, while a different stallion is more likely to produce offspring with fetlock lesions.

Nutritional Imbalance as a Cause of DOD

The excessive or inadequate ingestion of several nutrients may predispose to DOD. Nutrients that may be involved for horses include energy, protein, calcium, phosphorus, zinc, and copper. As described in Chapter 2, a manganese deficiency is known to cause similar DOD in newborn and growing ruminants, swine, and poultry, and has been implicated as a cause of DOD in newborn foals, resulting from a decrease in manganese availability caused by extensive liming of the soil. However, this is the only known case or report of a suspected manganese deficiency in the horse.

Dietary Energy Excess as a Cause of DOD

Excessive dietary energy intake results in rapid growth and is a major factor associated with DOD in most situations. It is sometimes stated that DOD are due entirely to excessive energy intake and not to other nutrient imbalances. However, the amount of nutrients needed in the diet for bone growth depends entirely upon the rate at which growth is occurring. For example, 0.25% phosphorus in the weanling's diet may be adequate for proper bone growth to occur if growth rate is slow, even though 0.5% is necessary for maximal growth rate (Appendix Table 1). If growth rate is rapid, however, a phosphorus deficiency will be manifested. DOD frequently attributed to excessive energy or protein intake may instead be caused by an amount of phosphorus, calcium, zinc, or copper in the diet inadequate to support the rate of growth permitted by the amount of energy and protein consumed. A lesser amount of energy or protein in the diet simply masks the deficiency by slowing the growth rate, or with greater amounts unmasks it by permitting a faster growth rate to occur. Thus, to prevent DOD the diet must provide the nutrients necessary to support the rate of growth occurring. To accomplish this, feed the growing horse as described in Chapter 15. However, even when the horse is fed adequate quantities of all nutrients thought to be necessary for maximum growth rate, DOD may still occur in some rapidly growing horses.

In several species, including the horse, excessive energy intake during growth has been shown to decrease bone density, thickness, and ash content, and result in DOD lesions. In one study, OCD joint lesions were present in all foals that received for 4 months 29% excess digestible energy; they were also present in 4 of 6 receiving 26% excess crude protein; whereas they were present in only 2 of 12 receiving 100% of the recommended amounts of digestible energy, crude protein, calcium, and phosphorus. The number of lesions present were also more numerous and severe in the foals receiving the high-energy diet than in those receiving either the high-protein or the control diet, and also than in those receiving 3.4 times more calcium or 3.9 times more phosphorus than recommended (Appendix Table 1). Thus, excess energy intake can induce DOD lesions within a few months. The incidence and severity of DOD alterations are decreased when dietary energy intake is decreased.

Protein Imbalance as a Cause of DOD

Although DOD occur most commonly in the overfed horse, they may occur in the underfed horse as well. This is thought to occur as a result of inadequate protein in the diet. Since protein constitutes 20% of the bone matrix, as might be expected, inadequate protein intake may interfere with proper bone growth and development. However, because bone matrix is produced at the site of bone formation, unless deprivation is fairly severe, a protein deficiency appears to be an unlikely cause of most cases of DOD. Inadequate protein intake sufficient to interfere with bone growth would be likely to result in poor condition in the horse (Fig. 16-5). However, foals consuming diets containing 9% protein (14.5% needed) had reduced growth of cannon bone diameter without any effect on the rate of height growth. This was interpreted to demonstrate the inhibition of bone remodeling as a result of a protein deficiency, which may contribute to DOD. A diet containing 9% protein is fairly typical of one consisting of mature grass hay or pasture forage, and a cereal grain mix containing little or no protein supplement.

Feeding more protein than the animal needs does not increase growth rate above that achieved when the diet just meets protein requirements. Feeding horses less pro-

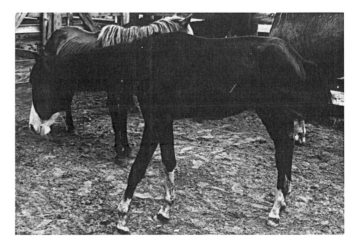

Fig. 16-5. Acquired leg flexure deformity and enlargement of the distal cannon bone growth plates in a horse receiving inadequate quantities of feed. These developmental orthopedic diseases occur more commonly in overfed horses, but may also occur in underfed horses, as shown here. This is thought to be due primarily to a protein deficiency.

tein than needed, however, decreases feed intake and protein digestibility, and as a result decreases their growth rate and skeletal development. Although a sufficient protein deficiency will decrease both weight gain and bone growth in the young horse, if the protein deficiency is mild and energy intake is adequate, only bone growth (not weight gain) may be decreased. Thus, increasing the protein content of a protein-deficient but energy-sufficient diet results in faster bone growth, particularly in its diameter. If the diet does not contain adequate minerals, such as calcium and phosphorus, to support a faster rate of bone growth, alterations in bone growth and DOD may occur. This is the most likely explanation for the implications frequently made but never confirmed that excessive protein intake predisposes to or causes DOD in horses. Although excessive protein intake increases urinary calcium excretion in people and rats, it does not appear to have an adverse effect on calcium or phosphorus utilization or musculoskeletal development of growing horses.

Calcium and Phosphorus Imbalances as a Cause of DOD

Adequate amounts of calcium and phosphorus must be available for bone ossification to occur. Without adequate quantities of calcium or phosphorus, bone growth cartilage becomes thickened, bone density and growth decrease, and DOD occur. The diet must not only contain adequate amounts of calcium and phosphorus, the animal must be able to absorb and utilize these nutrients. As described in Chapter 2, a sufficient excess of either mineral will decrease the absorption of the other. Thus, if the amount of one mineral with respect to the other, or the Ca:P ratio, in the growing horse's diet is outside a range of about 0.8:1 to 3:1, alterations in bone growth resulting in DOD may occur.

Excessive dietary calcium can decrease the intestinal absorption of not only phosphorus but, in a number of species other than horses, zinc, manganese, and iron. However, this isn't known to occur in horses, and although excess calcium has been alluded to as having negative effects on bone development in horses, skeletal calcium contents in horses have been found not to be affected by high calcium intake. In contrast, diets containing 5-times young foals' phosphorus requirement consistently resulted in DOD lesions, but without signs of a calcium deficiency.

Copper and Zinc Imbalances as a Cause of DOD

Copper is involved in stabilizing bone collagen and elastin synthesis. A copper deficiency impairs these functions, resulting in DOD. Ruminants are particularly susceptible and are most commonly affected, but horses also may be affected.

Plasma and liver copper concentrations fell, while diarrhea, a stilted gait, and ultimately, walking on the front of the hoof and DOD lesions occurred, in all foals fed an experimental, low-copper milk replacer. In contrast to copper-deficient ruminants, the growth rate of the copper-deficient foals wasn't reduced, and anemia and decreased hair coloration did not occur. However, it has been shown that, in contrast to what has been theorized, the mare's

milk supplies adequate copper and also zinc for the nursing foal for the first few months of life, and that neither the mare's milk nor the nursing foal's blood concentrations are affected by copper and zinc concentrations in the mare's diet.

A correlation between the occurrence of DOD in horses and reduced amounts of calcium, phosphorus, zinc, and copper, but not with the amount of other nutrients in weanling's diets, has been observed. The incidence of these diseases decreased significantly when these minerals, particularly copper, were increased in the diet.

Because of these studies, even though other studies suggest that lower amounts of dietary copper and zinc may be adequate (as discussed in Chapter 2), and because there is no risk of harm from doing so, it is recommended that copper and zinc be added to the growing horse's diet to the amounts given in Table 15-1.

In contrast to ruminants, excess zinc, sulfur, or molybdenum, at concentrations even up to several times those present naturally in feeds, does not appear to interfere with copper absorption or utilization by horses (see Chapter 2). Excessive zinc intake does, however, decrease calcium absorption, so if dietary calcium is sufficiently low, the excess zinc may cause a calcium deficiency, which in turn may result in DOD. DOD are a consistent manifestation of excessive zinc intake in horses, swine, cattle, and rats. Hock swellings, joint cartilage detachment from underlying bone, radiographic lesions of OCD, stiffness, lameness, and leg flexure deformities may occur in horses as a result of excessive zinc intake.

A zinc excess may be caused by adding excessive zinc to the diet (greater than 200 ppm), grazing pastures contaminated with efflux from nearby smelters, or drinking water containing greater than 15 ppm zinc.

Feeding Practices That Cause DOD

The major feeding practices responsible for the nutritional imbalances causing DOD in horses are: (1) feeding too much grain; and (2) allowing weanlings unlimited access to alfalfa or other legumes, both of which may result in excess dietary energy intake; and (3) feeding a grain mix that is inadequate in possibly copper and zinc, and when a legume forage is being consumed, inadequate in phosphorus, and when a grass forage is being consumed, inadequate in calcium, phosphorus, protein, and lysine. Both grass forages and cereal grains contain less calcium, phosphorus, protein, and lysine (and legumes contain less phosphorus) than is needed by the rapidly growing horse (Table 15-1). Since a grass forage is deficient in all of these nutrients needed for growth, as well as generally digestible energy, growth is slowed and as a result DOD generally don't occur. However, if the diet is not corrected, mature body size may be reduced. The smaller size, but soundness, of many wild horses is an example of this and of growth being reduced in accordance with the nutrients available.

Excessive amounts of grain are most commonly fed when 1) the foal is allowed continual access to a high-digestible-energy-low-fiber creep feed; and 2) a grain mix is fed in amounts greater than those recommended (Fig. 15-3). Although cereal grains contain inadequate amounts of phosphorus for the growing horse, they contain 3 to 20 times more phosphorus than calcium; i.e., cereal grains have a Ca:P ratio of 0.05:1 to 0.3:1. In addition to a low calcium content, cereal grains contain about 1% phytate. The high phytate and low Ca:P ratio decrease calcium absorption. Thus, a major effect of excessive grain intake is a calcium deficiency and with respect to dietary calcium, but not with respect to the growing horses needs, an excess of phosphorus. Cereal grains are also high in digestible energy. They contain 50 to 70% more available energy than most forages. Thus, a diet high in cereal grains is high in energy, which promotes rapid growth, but is inadequate in calcium and also phosphorus, which are necessary for proper bone development. The result may be DOD. Excess energy intake resulting in a rapid growth rate and DOD may also occur as a result of excess intake of a good-quality legume forage by the weanling.

It has been commonly thought that excess dietary energy from cereal grains is more likely to cause DOD than that from forages. This belief is based on the perception that the incidence of DOD are greater in young horses being fed diets high in grain than in those fed diets high in forage. This perception appears to be valid if a primarily grass forage is fed, but not if a good-quality legume, such as alfalfa, is the forage fed. The incidence of DOD is as high in weanlings fed primarily alfalfa as in those fed primarily grain.

The higher incidence of DOD in young horses fed diets high in grain than in those fed diets high in a grass forage therefore doesn't appear to be due to differences in the source or type of dietary energy consumed. Instead, it is because grain and grain mixes are higher in energy and protein density than is grass and, therefore, the intake of these nutrients is generally greater and, as a result, growth is faster when a high-grain diet is fed. In contrast to a grass forage, when weanlings are given free-choice access to diets high in good-quality legumes, their digestible energy and protein intakes, and as a result their growth rate, are not lower than when a high-grain diet is fed. This, and because the source of dietary energy doesn't appear to matter, are the reasons that the incidence of DOD are as high in young horses fed primarily alfalfa as in those fed primarily grain.

This doesn't mean that alfalfa shouldn't be fed during growth; instead, it emphasizes the need to regulate its intake, just as grain intake must be regulated, to prevent excessive dietary energy intake. The weanling should not be allowed unlimited access to either a good-quality legume forage or to a grain mix. Grain intake should be limited to that given in Table 15-3, and legume forage intake limited to that necessary to make up the difference between digestible energy needs (Appendix Table 4) and that provided by the grain mix as described in Chapter 15.

The cause of DOD with excess alfalfa is unlikely to be due to excess protein or calcium intake, as these nutrient excesses do not appear to have an adverse effect on musculoskeletal development of young horses, providing intake of other nutrients is adequate. Instead, it appears, that a high dietary energy intake is most likely responsible, either due to the faster growth rate it induces or to the increased physical activity it produces. Voluntary physical activity of both growing and mature horses is directly related to dietary energy intake. Increased activity may result in greater concussive stress on growing bones, which may contribute to a higher incidence of DOD.

NONSURGICAL MANAGEMENT OF DOD

Feeding the growing horse properly by feeding a diet that provides an adequate amount of all nutrients with enough digestible energy for a steady moderate growth rate, not a rapid growth rate (Appendix Table 4), as described in Chapter 15, will prevent DOD in many horses. However, because of the many non-nutritional factors that cause or predispose to DOD (Fig. 16-1), it may occur in some horses even when they are properly fed. Proper feeding, however, is the first and most important factor in preventing DOD, and the diet of all young horses on a farm where cases occur should be evaluated and altered if necessary. It is one of the few causative factors that is readily controllable; other factors, such as genetics, may not be. In addition, altering the diet can be quite helpful in the management of affected horses.

In horses showing any sign of DOD, it is recommended that growth rate be slowed immediately by decreasing dietary energy and protein intake, and that trauma or pressure on the bone growth plates and joint cartilage be reduced by decreasing physical activity. Dietary energy and protein intake can be reduced by feeding as much good-quality grass or cereal-grain hay as the horse will consume. These are preferred to a legume forage such as alfalfa. Their lower energy and protein content slows growth rate and increases the chances for recovery. Both, however, provide inadequate calcium and phosphorus, which should be corrected by adding the proper amount of these minerals to just enough grain to ensure that the horse consumes them. The additional amount of both calcium and phosphorus needed when these forages are fed is approximately 15, 10, 4, 2, and 0 g/horse daily at 4, 6, 9, 12, and 18 months of age, respectively. The amount of supplemental minerals needed decreases with increasing age because growth slows, and because with increasing size, more feed and therefore minerals in it are consumed. The amount of additional minerals needed may be provided by adding about 4 oz (125 g) at 4 months, 3 oz (85 g) at 6 months, 1 oz (33 g) at 9 months, and 0.5 oz (16 g) at 12 months of age of a mineral containing 12% calcium and 12% phosphorus (proportionally more or less for minerals providing different amounts) e.g., (15 g Ca & P needed) ÷ (12% Ca & P in mineral-used) — 15 g ÷ 0.12 = 125 g of that mineral needed to provide 15 g of Ca & P. It is preferred that a grain containing molasses be used to prevent added minerals from sifting out. If the grain does not contain molasses, it may be necessary to dampen it with water when it is fed and the mineral is added to it. Dampened grain, if not consumed within a few hours, may become moldy and should be discarded.

Exercise is important for normal bone growth. However, once DOD occur, exercise is likely to be detrimental. Exercise will cause greater trauma to the bone growth plates, slow recovery, and may increase the severity of the condition. Because of this, complete (24-hour-a-day) stall confinement is recommended for horses that are sore or in pain and those with angular leg deformities. Many mild angular leg deformities will return to normal with stall confinement. Foot trimming and balancing should also be done. A decrease in exercise by confining the affected foal and its dam to a small paddock, but not stall unless necessary, is recommended for horses with growth plate enlargements and those with acquired leg flexure deformities that are sufficiently mild so that weight can be put on the sole to cause extension and stretching of the flexor muscles and tendons, which helps to correct these. For leg flexure deformities involving primarily the superficial flexor tendon and fetlock joint, it may be helpful to have the toe as long as possible and to elevate the heel; whereas for flexure deformities involving primarily the deep digital flexor tendon and coffin joint, the heel should be lowered, and it may be beneficial to raise the toe. For more severe cases of both types of flexure deformities, it may be beneficial to put a 1- to 2-inch (0.4- to 0.8-cm) extension square on the shoe in front of the toe. The toe extension may force the heel to the ground when the horse is bearing weight on that foot, and delay breakover when the horse is in motion, both of which may stretch the flexor tendon. Glue on shoes may be helpful.

Analgesics and anti-inflammatory drugs should not be used in horses in which angular leg deformity is the major problem. Their use decreases the pain, resulting in increased physical activity, which in turn increases the trauma to the bone growth plates. This may slow recovery or increase the severity of the condition. In the case of bone growth plate enlargements and flexure deformities, however, relief of pain is indicated, so these products may be beneficial.

Bone growth plate enlargements, angular leg deformities, and leg flexure deformities generally show improvement by 4 to 6 weeks of the management described. Even if recovery is not complete after this length of time, gradually over several weeks allow increased exercise and begin feeding 0.5 lbs/100 lbs body weight/day (0.5 kg/100 kg/day) of a grain mix properly formulated to meet the horse's requirements (Table 15–1). If improvement is inadequate or the condition is severe, surgery or other treatments, as described previously in this chapter in the sections on each of the effects of DOD, are indicated.

The benefit of the management described was well illustrated in one study in which it resulted in significant clinical and radiographic improvement in affected Thoroughbred weanlings with the disappearance of spinal cord compression and lesions. If left untreated, fed to allow for rapid growth, and allowed unlimited exercise, the horses would have probably experienced progressive spinal cord compression, rendering them useless as performance animals. However, if the horse is severely affected by spinal cord compression-induced wobblers syndrome and is more than 1 year old before dietary management is started, the management described is not likely to be successful because extensive spinal cord damage will already be present and the time for vertebrae remodeling to occur before rapid growth is over will be inadequate. In this study, when radiographs of the vertebrae were taken monthly, beginning at 1 month of age, and the management described was instituted whenever any narrowing of the vertebral column was noted, no horse developed signs of wobblers syndrome during the 3-year period this was done. Once clinical signs are severe, prognosis, with or without surgery, is poor.

In another study, conservative management, not as rigorous as that recommended, resulted in recovery of 47% of 76 horses 4 to 15 months of age showing signs, primarily gait abnormalities, due to DOD lesions affecting the stifle (62%), hock (14%), shoulder (9%), and other joints (15%), with 54%, 45%, 0%, and 50%, respectively, showing improvement. Those that didn't recover were unable to attain a reasonable level of performance ability. Those not severely lame were allowed to continue or start training, and nonsteroidal anti-inflammatory drug administration was recommended. Only if severe lameness occurred was stall confinement with controlled exercise used.

SUPPLEMENTAL READING RECOMMENDATIONS

Adams' Lameness in Horses (Williams & Wilkins, Baltimore, MD, 1987) by multiple authors, all leading specialists on topics they cover, and edited by Dr. Ted S. Stashak, an equine surgeon and one of the leading authorities of equine lameness. This book initially written in 1962 by Dr. O. R. Adams has long been recognized as the bible on equine lameness. The current updated and much-expanded 4th edition continues this tradition, not only in text but in hundreds of outstanding drawings and pictures. Topics covered include: anatomy; relationship between conformation and lameness; lameness diagnosis; radiology; nutritions role in musculoskeletal disease; diseases of bones; diseases of joints, tendons, and ligaments; lameness; shoeing; gaits; and methods for lameness therapy.

American Association of Equine Practitioners, 39th Annual Convention Proceedings, pages 35 to 89 (December, 1993), contains 10 articles on developmental orthopedic diseases by Drs. C. Wayne McIlwraith, L. R. Bramlage, and G. D. Mundy, specialists in these diseases.

Equine Osteochondrosis in the '90s, edited by Drs. L. B. Jeffcott and G. Dalen contains many articles describing current research results, clinical experiences, and thinking on this topic by many of the world's leading authorities. Cambridge University Press, Cambridge, England (1992).

Chapter 17

FEEDING AND CARE OF HORSES WITH HEALTH PROBLEMS

Inadequate Feed Consumption	. . . .	289
Hoof Defects	. . . .	290
Heaves (Chronic Obstructive Pulmonary Disease)	. . . . . .	291
Diarrhea	. . . .	293
Sand-Induced Diarrhea	. . . .	293
Intestinal Impaction	. . . .	294
Intestinal Calculi (Stones)	. . . .	294
Intestinal Removal or Dysfunction	. . . .	295
Large-Colon Removal or Dysfunction	. . . .	295
Small-Intestinal Removal or Dysfunction	. . . .	295
Rectal/Vaginal Surgery or Lacerations	. . . .	295
Liver Disease	. . . .	295
Kidney Failure	. . . .	296
Urinary Tract Calculi (Bladder Stones)	. . . .	296
Heart Disease	. . . .	297
Potassium Induced Periodic Paralysis	. . . .	297

Most horses, healthy or sick, do not need a special diet. A diet that meets or exceeds nutrient requirements for their particular stage of life and activity, as described in Chapters 10–13 and 15, is quite adequate. Stabled horses do not require the high amount of feed needed by working horses. Most can be well maintained on a diet of primarily hay fed free-choice at an amount equal to 1.5 to 2 lbs/100 lbs (or 1.5 to 2 kg/100 kg) body weight daily. The hay may be any type, but it should be good quality. One to 2 pounds (0.5 to 1 kg) of any cereal grain fed twice daily helps maintain appetite and adaptation to grain. Like all horses, water and salt should be always accessible.

For some specific disease conditions a specialized diet may be beneficial in minimizing the effects of and maximizing recovery from that disease. A specialized diet is one that contains more and/or less of one or more nutrients than diets commonly fed to the normal healthy animal. These differences in the specialized diet's nutrient content may be beneficial for the horse with some diseases because of a decreased ability to tolerate excess nutrients and/or a need for a higher amount of other nutrients.

Nutrients consumed in excess of needs, but below toxic levels, are either not absorbed or are absorbed and excreted by the animal with normal healthy body functions and, as a result, are not harmful. The body's ability to tolerate excess nutrients and to conserve nutrients when there intake is low provides a wide latitude in the types of feeds and diets that may be consumed. In disease, however, these abilities may be decreased. A nutrient excess normally not harmful may become so when there is a decreased ability to metabolize or excrete that nutrient or its metabolites. In contrast, an increased amount of other nutrients may be needed for body defense or repair, or to compensate for a decreased ability to utilize that nutrient or increased loss of that nutrient from the body. For these specific disease conditions, as described in this chapter, diets containing a greater amount of some nutrients and/or a lessor amount of other nutrients may minimize dysfunctions and clinical signs due to that disease and be quite helpful or necessary for recovery from that disease. However, more important than the type of diet fed is that there is adequate feed intake. Some horses with health problems have a decreased ability or desire to eat. A number of procedures may be used to increase these horses' feed intake.

INADEQUATE FEED CONSUMPTION

Inadequate feed consumption due to a decreased ability to eat or desire to eat (anorexia) occurs with many diseases. A decreased ability to consume and utilize food may occur because of facial, oral, pharyngeal, esophophageal, or gastrointestinal damage or dysfunction. Anorexia may be due to alterations in the ability to taste or smell, and to numerous medical problems, including organic disease, inflammation, trauma, and cancer. Pain, fear, and other components of emotional stress also inhibit the desire to eat. Regardless of the cause, it is important to realize that inadequate feed intake is much more than a sign of disease, damage or dysfunction. The absence of food intake, even for a few days, particularly in conjunction with disease or trauma, adversely affects all body systems, making it more difficult for the animal to resist the effects of the disease, to recover, and to respond to therapy.

Nutrient deprivation need not add insult to the injury of disease. Nutritional support is, however, supportive therapy only. For example, without antibiotics, all the food or nutrients possible will not cure the animal with a severe bacterial infection throughout the body. But neither will all the antibiotics possible save the starving animal. Both are necessary. Successful antibiotic therapy depends on a functional host defense system, which in turn depends on adequate host nutrition. Even in healthy horses, infectious organism defense ability and immunity decrease as fast as 5 days without food intake. They are decreased even further in the sick horses and improve with nutritional support. Nutritional support reduces the number of disease-related complications and shortens recovery and healing time.

The horse's intestinal tract is particularly sensitive to even relatively short periods of starvation. Complete food deprivation for more than 3 to 5 days may result in diarrhea, which can be fatal. Therefore, rather than waiting until obvious laboratory or clinical signs of undernutrition have occurred, nutritional support should be provided as early as possible, preferably as soon as the patient's fluid, electrolyte, and acid-base status have stabilized.

If the horse's nutritional needs aren't provided, the effects of these deficiencies will occur as described in Chapters 1, 2, and 3; the major effect is a dietary energy and protein deficiency, which slows or prevents recovery. All of the horse's nutrient needs may be provided by, in order of preference, appetite stimulation, tube feeding, or intravenous feeding. The simplest method for which there are no contraindications should be tried first. If the animal's needs can't be met completely by that method, other feeding methods should be instituted. Frequently a number of feeding methods must be used together to provide sufficient nutrients to meet the horse's needs; any single procedure alone may not be totally effective.

The horse should be encouraged to eat if it is able to do so and there are no reasons that it can't eat, such as sufficient pharyngeal or esophageal damage. The horse should be checked thoroughly, particularly the mouth and pharynx, to determine if there is any physical reason it can't or won't eat. If the mouth is painful or the horse can't swallow, trying to stimulate the appetite is unlikely to be of benefit.

If it is painful for the horse to eat, besides treating the lesions and giving something to decrease pain, feeding green grass or a feed mash (such as can be made by adding water to a complete pelleted feed, alfalfa pellets or meal, or bran) may decrease the pain associated with eating sufficiently so that the horse will consume food voluntarily. Fever and pain, not just oral but anywhere, may depress feed intake, in which case administering drugs that reduce pain and fever may be helpful. Drugs such as aspirin, and butazolidone may be helpful in decreasing body protein breakdown fever and pain and stimulating the horse to eat.

Feed intake is encouraged by feeding small amounts frequently, removing feed that remains uneaten more than 2 hours, and offering a variety of fresh feeds (e.g., leafy alfalfa hay, grains, sweet feeds, bran mashes, and fresh fruit and vegetables). Lush green grass, grazed or freshly cut, is quite palatable for most horses. Initial preferences for novel feeds such as fresh fruit or vegetables may soon diminish, so additional feeds should be constantly sought. The concern for the horse with inadequate feed intake is not so much what it eats, as it is if and how much it eats.

Bran mashes are popular with many for feeding sick horses, but for most horses brans are poorly palatable. Mixing the bran with an equal amount of grain (particularly steam-flaked oats, barley, or sweet feed) may improve palatability, and including alfalfa pellets or meal makes it a more adequate complete diet. One or 2 quarts (liters) of the mixture should be steeped in boiling water. Adding molasses (1 cup) and salt (1–3 tsp) may enhance the mixture's acceptance. The mash should be fed warm but not hot.

Occasionally sick horses, like sick people, may have unusual food preferences, so try different feeds. Some sick horses reject feeds normally quite palatable and consume poor hay or bedding. Feed flavoring agents generally are of no benefit in stimulating feed intake, at least in healthy horses, as described in Chapter 4.

Although some horses may eat when lying down, many won't. Therefore, getting them up, using a sling if necessary, may be quite helpful. Once the horse is standing, it may regain its appetite and eat. If the horse is quite weak, several days of tube or intravenous feeding may be necessary before it will have sufficient strength to stand. If or when the horse is able, and if a grassy area is available, it may graze even if it won't eat otherwise. Even short periods of grazing, of even dried pasture grass, several times daily may greatly improve the horse's nutritional status and attitude. Horses may also eat more if they see and hear other horses eating. Some horses prefer to eat from the ground rather than from a manager, hay rack, or feed bunk, so try different feeding locations.

Many people have the impression that giving B-vitamin injections may stimulate eating. Even if they don't, administering B vitamins is beneficial in providing the horse that is not eating its needs. Valium administered intravenously at a low dosage (10 mg/500-kg, horse) when the horse is quiet with minimal noise and distractions and with feed within easy reach, may stimulate immediate eating but lasts for only 15 to 20 minutes. Repeated doses may be administered several times daily although responses are not consistent. However, it should be used cautiously in horses with hepatic dysfunction, as is generally present in the severely debilitated horse. Excessive tranquilization and incoordination may occur, particularly in horses that are severely depressed or debilitated, when valium is administered.

Anabolic steroids and corticosteroids may increase feed intake after several days but don't have an immediate effect. Anabolic steroids are often used in convalescent horses. Their administration once at their recommended dosage is all that is likely to be helpful or that should be given. Repeated or higher doses may adversely affect the reproductive performance of mares and stallions (see Chapters 12 and 13).

If these procedures do not result in adequate food intake, the horse may need to be fed by stomach tube or intravenously.

HOOF DEFECTS

Hoof damage and defects can occur from a multitude of causes and can be minimized with proper foot care as described in Chapter 9. Nutritional causes of hoof defects include prolonged excess selenium consumption, and a protein deficiency. A protein deficiency results in many detrimental effects in the horse as described in Chapter 1, including slowed hoof growth, which may result in increased hoof splitting and cracking. As described in Chapter 18, horses with prolonged excess selenium consumption may walk stiff-legged, with tenderness followed by pronounced lameness. A ring of abnormal hoof growth may occur. In severe cases, transverse breaks and cracks in the hoof wall may develop. When new hoof growth occurs, these breaks move downward and the old hoof may separate from the new growth. The old hoof may not be completely shed, resulting in ragged long hoofs turned up at the ends.

There are a number of products available for repairing hoof wall defects and quarter cracks, and for reconstructing damaged hoof walls and under-run heels. One of the most common hoof repair substances is a flexible resin that expands with hoof, can withstand the high impact and shear forces produced by the horse's activity, and can be rasped, nailed and trimmed.

Biotin supplementation may be helpful in enhancing the repair of hoof defects and in preventing their recurrence. There is good evidence that biotin supplementation may in some cases be of benefit for horses' hooves. Biotin supplements are widely marketed and used for this purpose. Horses with thin brittle hoof walls, cracks in the weight-bearing border of the coronary horn with crumbling of the lower edges of the walls with thin brittle, tender soles, or open white lines that are prone to infection, may benefit from prolonged biotin supplementation. Horses with these hoof conditions were reported to display marked improvement within 5 months of giving 15 mg of biotin/day to Thoroughbreds and twice this amount to draft horses. Improvement in the hooves was reported in all 55 horses treated in these two reports. But no control horses were monitored in either study. However, biotin supplementation was shown to be of significant benefit in a study in which those giving the supplement and evaluating its effects did not know which horses had or had not been given biotin. In this study of 42 Lipizzaner stallions, 90% had the hoof conditions described above. Twenty-six horses were fed daily for 2.5 years 20 mg d-biotin, and 16, initially with equally poor hooves, were fed a similar appearing substance. By 14 months overall hoof condition was 30% better in biotin supplemented than unsupplemented horses at which time it remained unchanged in both groups throughout the remainder of the study. It took 6 months before signs of improvement occurred, and 19 months for an improvement in white line condition, hoof horn histology and an increase in hoof tensile strength to occur. The greatest increase in hoof tensile strength occurred during the period between 19 and 33 months of biotin supplementation, at the end of which tensile strength averaged 22% greater in the biotin supplemented horses.

It is reported that biotin supplementation is effective only for horses with certain types of hoof defects. Biotin supplementation alone was of benefit for three of three horses with one type of hoof defect, but was of no benefit for any of 21 horses with a different type of defect. However, 95% of these horses improved when protein and calcium were added to diets low in these nutrients. Both defects result in similar-appearing hooves that are brittle, thin, and crumbly at the lower edges. Affected horses may be tender on their feet and, as a result, unwilling to step out, resulting in a shortened choppy stride. They may lose shoes frequently and, when shoes are nailed on, parts of the hoof wall may break away. The front feet are generally more affected than the rear. However, since the two different structural defects of the hooves cannot be differentiated clinically or by laboratory procedures generally available, you should ensure that the diet of the horse with the problems described is adequate in protein and calcium to meet its requirements (as described in Chapter 6), and 1.2 to 1.5 mg of biotin/100 lb (3 mg/100kg) of body weight should be added to the diet daily. Improvement may be evident within 3 to 6 months of biotin supplementation, with continued improvement noted for up to 12 months, at which time biotin supplementation may be discontinued. However, an increase in hoof strength may take 1.5 years to occur and continue to increase with biotin supplementation for up to 3 years. A small amount (0.1 to 0.15 mg/100 lb or 0.2 to 0.3 mg/100 kg of body wt, or 0.05 to 0.1 mg/lb or 0.1 to 0.2 mg/kg of total diet) fed continuously may be beneficial in maintaining good hoof structure and preventing recurrence in some horses. This may be provided by feeding a balanced vitamin supplement, as given in Table 3-5. Excess biotin intake by the horse is not known to be detrimental.

HEAVES (CHRONIC OBSTRUCTIVE PULMONARY DISEASE)

Heaves, chronic obstructive pulmonary disease (COPD), asthma or broken wind in horses is due to a hypersensitivity or allergy most commonly to fungal spores present in hay or bedding but occasionally to summer pasture grass pollen. An association also appears to exist between the development of heaves and previous viral respiratory disease. The amount of fungal spores present directly correlates with dustiness in the stable, hay, and bedding. The allergy results in airway constriction, excess mucus, and inflammatory thickening of the gas exchange membrane in the lungs (alveoli). The disease may begin following an episode of infectious respiratory disease; prevention of these diseases, as described in Chapter 9, is an important aspect in preventing heaves. In people, COPD is most often due to cigarette smoking and is the fifth leading cause of death in the United States.

Some horses may suddenly develop difficult respiration, although generally COPD develops gradually with the first effect being decreased performance ability and exercise tolerance. This may progress to a chronic cough, nasal discharge, and labored breathing, first at exercise and later even at rest. Lung elasticity is reduced so that the muscles for the chest and abdominal lifting must be used to exhale. In chronic cases the increased use of these muscles increases their size, which may result in the development of a "heave line" as shown in Fig. 17-1.

Once the allergy develops, it will remain for the rest of the horse's life. But when horses are removed from contact with the cause, lung function returns to normal, although in chronically affected horses function may be permanently impaired. In addition, repeated exposure to the cause results in more rapid and severe effects. The classic situation starts with the horse beginning to cough a little toward the end of the stabling period following competition or for the winter; the cough disappears when the horse is turned out on pasture, but recurs sooner when stabled the next season. For athletic activity, it is not the cough but the airway constriction and alveoli thickening that limit respiratory gas exchange and, therefore, athletic performance ability. The impairment may occur without a cough occurring. If there is doubt about whether a horse has heaves, an airway or bronchiole dilator may be administered intravenously and any alteration in breathing or performance noted; doing so generally will improve these parameters in affected horses but have no effect in unaffected horses. In contrast to what is sometimes claimed, physical fitness doesn't appear to affect heaves, but regular fast workouts may help remove excess mucus.

In contrast to horses with heaves in which fungal spores

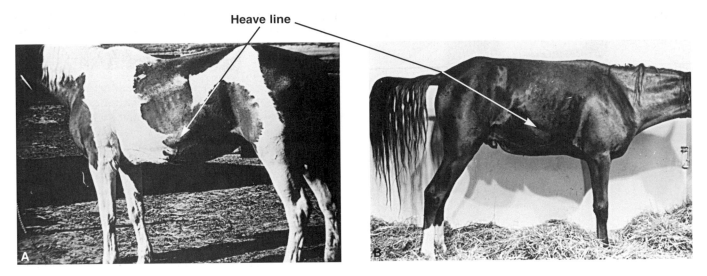

Fig. 17–1(A,B). Heave Line. Note the line formed by the abdominal muscles that runs from the middle of the flank forward and down the rib cage toward the point of the elbow. The heave line develops because of increased use of these muscles for abdominal lifting necessary to push air out of lungs whose elasticity and air exchange ability are reduced because of hypersensitivity or allergy, most commonly to dust and fungal spores in hay, straw bedding, and stable air, which cause chronic obstructive pulmonary disease, or heaves. The bay horse was straining at the time the picture was taken, making its heave line more noticeable. Although the pinto was more severely affected, its heave line isn't as visible.

are the cause and improvement occurs when they are put on pastures away from fungal spores, clinical signs in those in which grass pollen is the cause develop and worsen when they are put on summer pasture with access to grass pollen. In most of these horses, when they are on pasture, clinical signs worsen once yearly when pasture grass pollen develops in the summer and fall, and improve during the winter or when not on pasture. Although most of these cases occur in horses that are on pasture 24 hours a day, less than 12 hours/day of pasture exposure is sufficient to cause the disease.

A change in the affected horse's environment that minimizes their exposure to the cause is vital for both treatment and prevention of the vicious cycle of irritation and further airway destruction. Except for the case in which pasture grass pollen is the cause, affected horses may need to be kept outside and fed pasture forage or hay cubes, pellets, acid-treated hay, haylage, or silage. If loose hay must be used, it should be soaked for at least 5 minutes before being fed. This should be done by putting it in a haynet and immersing it completely in a tank of clean water, or by soaking it well with a hose before placing it inside the stall. Fungal spores released from hay are significantly reduced by soaking the hay for 5 minutes prior to feeding. If the grain is dusty, it shouldn't be fed or should also be soaked prior to being fed. Wet feed not consumed should be replaced frequently, as it may mold. Adding up to 10% fat or oil to the diet, as described in Chapter 4, may also be of benefit in decreasing feed dust, increasing diet caloric density, decreasing diet bulk, and in providing dietary energy in the form which when metabolized produces the least amount of carbon dioxide for respiratory expiration. All feed should be fed close to the ground and not in a deep container, such as a feed trough, so that

particles will tend to fall away from the horse's nose and not be inhaled.

When the horse is stabled, it should be kept in a large well-ventilated stall with the top of an outside door or a window left open. Procedures for ensuring good stable ventilation, as described in Chapter 9, should be followed closely. Straw bedding should not be used, because it greatly increases air contamination (Table 9–7). Instead, wood chips, peat moss, shredded paper, or synthetic bedding material should be used, and the stall should be cleaned daily. Affected, and preferably all, horses should be removed from the stable during and for several hours after stalls are cleaned and bedded and hay is handled.

For these management procedures to be effective, they must be used for all horses sharing an air space with affected horses. For the occasional horse allergic to grass pollen, it must be kept off pasture during late spring, summer, and early fall. Most horses with heaves become symptom-free within 1 to 2 weeks and recover completely in 3 to 4 weeks after their exposure to the cause is minimized, although it takes longer for severe cases. A longer period of time is also required for a reduction in inflammatory secretions and, therefore, improvement in exercise tolerance and performance ability.

Horses in severe respiratory distress may be given corticosteroids, antihistamines, mucolytics, and bronchodilators to help alleviate the distress. However, in a controlled study, medical therapy using combinations of all these drugs did not improve affected horses. This emphasizes the necessity of management changes that minimize the horse's exposure to the cause. Desensitization or immunotherapy is another option to try to prevent recurrence. In one study, it was beneficial in 66 of 99 horses with heaves.

DIARRHEA

Following, if necessary, correction of dehydration, feed should not be withheld from the diarrheic horse unless gastric distention, reflux, or bloating occurs. Feeds, and/or oral fluids either ingested or administered by stomach tube, are necessary in the gastrointestinal tract to maximize its integrity and healing ability. Lack of oral alimentation for more than 2 days, causes a loss of intestinal integrity and function that may contribute to a worsening of or decreased ability to recover from the diarrhea, and may result in disease-producing organisms and their toxins gaining access to the blood, causing septicemia, particularly in the young.

Regardless of the cause of diarrhea, small amounts of high-quality, highly digestible feeds should be fed, frequently. Overly mature and thus poorly digestible hay should be avoided.

If it has been determined that small-intestinal function is adequate, 0.5 to 0.6 lb/100 lbs (0.5 to 0.6 kg/100 kg) body wt/day of grain along with forage always available should be fed. Up to 20% vegetable oil (1 pt/5 lbs, or 20 ml/kg) may be added to the grain fed if additional dietary energy is needed for the maintenance of hydrated body weight. However, if small intestinal function, and as a result, grain utilization is greatly impaired, a primarily forage diet should be fed, as excessive grain intake may worsen the diarrhea. Grain or starch not absorbed in the small intestine pass into the large bowel where excess amounts alter microbial fiber fermentation, decreasing the nutrients derived from forages. Even when small-intestinal function is impaired, this problem can be decreased and at least some grain may be utilized by feeding small amounts frequently so that the intestinal digestive/absorptive capacity is not overwhelmed. Dietary fat, whether absorbed from the small intestine or not, improves energy digestion.

Regardless of the cause of diarrhea, fiber ingestion is beneficial as a source of volatile fatty acids, which, along with the amino acids glutamine and aspartate, are principle sources of energy for the intestine. Fiber may also stimulate intestinal segmental motility (which slows passage of intestinal contents) and add bulk and form to the feces. Because of these benefits, the diarrheic horse should have good-quality forage always readily available. If hydrated body weight is not maintained with forage alone, then grain may be fed in amounts up to 50% of the weight of the feed fed, or a complete pelleted feed containing both grain and forage may be fed with up to 20% vegetable oil added.

If antimicrobial drugs have been administered orally, beginning 2 to 3 days after their administration is stopped, or if there are other reasons to suspect that bacterial fermentation is abnormal, administering by stomach tube cecal or colonic fluid obtained from a horse with normal gastrointestinal function (preferably Salmonella negative), yogurt, or a commercial bacterial inoculant may be beneficial. Many of the organisms in cecal and colonic fluids are temperature sensitive; therefore, only fresh contents are likely to be of benefit, and if they need to be diluted, warm water should be used. Cecal and colonic fluids can sometimes be obtained from slaughter houses or dead horses but should be from those that did not have a digestive disturbance. If equine cecal fluid is unavailable, ruminal fluid instead may be of benefit as their microorganisms appear to be similar.

Sand-Induced Diarrhea

Sand and dirt may be ingested inadvertently with feed or purposely by some horses, particularly foals. Inadvertent consumption with feed is increased in horses on overgrazed and sandy-soil pastures, and when feed is consumed from the ground, particularly if the horses are underfed. The cause for purposeful consumption generally isn't known. It can be, but generally isn't, due to a nutrient deficiency (e.g., phosphorus, sodium or salt, or protein). Purposely eating dirt has been reported to occur as a result of severe intestinal parasitism, but parasitism is not present in most horses with sand-induced diarrhea. An insult to the gastrointestinal tract that alters intestinal motility, impeding the clearing of normal quantities of sand consumed with feed, may be responsible in some cases, and would explain the occurrence of single cases within a herd.

Ingested sand settles to the bottom of primarily the colon and cecum, where it causes damage and irritation-induced diarrhea. Obstructions and impactions may uncommonly occur. Most often there is a chronic diarrhea progressing over several weeks from pasty to semifluid to watery feces with chronic weight loss or poor growth and sometimes poor condition, or an inability to maintain weight compared to herdmates. For horses large enough for rectal palpation, sand may be detected on the sleeve used and may be palpated as a heavy ventral mass. In some, but not all cases, sand can be found in the sediment of a fecal emulsion with water. Although fecal sand excretion has been considered evidence of sand accumulation, a sufficient amount may not be excreted in some affected horses to suggest sand as the cause of the problem. In these cases, radiographic evidence of large amounts of sand in the gastrointestinal tract or sand excretion in response to treatment is necessary for diagnosis, although even with treatment sand excretion may not be consistently detected.

Treatment includes preventing additional sand ingestion and administering soluble-fiber bulk-inducing agents to increase fecal passage of ingested sand. Administering the soluble fiber, psyllium hydrophilic mucilloid (e.g., 3 to 4 oz/foal or 10 oz/adult horse of Metamucil—Searle Pharmaceuticals, or ½ lb or 225 g/adult horse or one-half this amount/foal of Modane—Adria Labs, twice daily) for 2 to 5 weeks in conjunction with a primarily forage diet has been found to be effective. The soluble fiber may be added to sufficient grain mix for its consumption or administered in a water emulsion by stomach tube. Sand-induced diarrhea will generally be resolved within 1 to 3 days of this management. However, treatment should be continued, as recovery may be slow due to sand accumulation, the time necessary for its passage, and chronic bowel inflammation. Infection in the abdominal cavity, but without intestinal rupture, may be present and requires appropriate antibiotic therapy.

Sand or dirt consumption, and thus the risk of sand-induced diarrhea, may be minimized by feeding psyllium daily and ensuring that adequate quantities of a diet consisting of 50 to 100% forage is fed up off the ground, or that the horse's pasture is not overgrazed. Having trace-mineralized salt mixed with equal parts of bone meal available for free-choice consumption may also be helpful in decreasing voluntary sand consumption. In addition, the horses should be kept on a good deworming program as described in Chapter 9, and affected horses should be checked for intestinal parasites and treated accordingly. As with other oral vices or behaviors, as described in Chapter 20, decreasing confinement and providing increased exercise and companionship may be helpful in decreasing purposeful dirt consumption.

INTESTINAL IMPACTION

Normally small intestinal contents are semi-liquid. Intestinal contents become firmer in the large intestine where water is absorbed. If intestinal contents get too dry, they become doughy then firm. If the intestine can't move this mass, or ingested foreign material (e.g., twine, rubber fencing material, etc.), an obstruction occurs resulting in pain from stretching of the intestinal wall by the mass and the intestinal build-up of bacteria-produced gas behind it. This is one of the most common causes of abdominal pain or colic, with colic being the most common medical problem of adult horses. Poor teeth that prevent proper chewing of feed, poor or high fiber feed, inadequate water intake, and ingestion of foreign material are causative factors.

Impaction with ingested feed is one of the most common forms of intestinal-obstruction-induced causes of colic in horses. Sand and intestinal calculi may also be responsible in some cases. Epsom salts (magnesium sulfate), and mineral oil administered by stomach tube are common treatments for feed-induced impactions in horses. Epsom salts has been shown to be an effective laxative in horses. Mineral oil, however, may coat but not penetrate the impacted mass, preventing water from gaining access to and thus disrupting the mass. Gentle manual massage through the intestinal wall of an impacted mass that can be reached by rectal palpation may disrupt the mass so it can be passed. The last, but sometimes necessary, resort is its surgical removal.

To assist in preventing impactions, ensure proper dental care as described in Chapter 9, that fresh palatable water is always readily available and that the horse gets regular exercise and a sufficient quantity of good quality feed. Following successful treatment of impaction, to prevent recurrence, high-fiber, poorly digestible feeds, such as mature forages and straw, should be avoided. Instead, feed low-fiber, highly digestible forages. A growing grass or legume is preferred, as they often produce a soft stool. A low-fiber, complete pelleted or extruded feed (Table 4–11) containing ground alfalfa may also soften the stools. Another alternative is to feed a diet consisting of one-half grain, which for maintenance would be 0.5 to 0.6 lb/100 lbs body wt (or 0.5 to 0.6 kg/100 kg) daily. If necessary to maintain a soft stool, 3 to 4 oz (90 to 120 g) of epsom salts (magnesium sulfate) and regular salt (sodium chloride may be added to the 1100-lb (500-kg) horse's diet daily.

Psyllium added to the diet as described in the previous section on sand-induced diarrhea may also be helpful.

INTESTINAL CALCULI (STONES)

Intestinal calculi or stones (enteroliths) cause impactions and colic and generally must be removed surgically. They form in the large intestine by mineral deposition around a nidus consisting of metal, cloth, or most commonly pebbles, and are composed primarily of magnesium ammonium phosphate (struvite). Their occurrence may be more common in Arabians and Morgans and in western and southern states, particularly California, Florida and Louisiana, although increased occurrences in Indiana and Illinois have also been reported. Their incidence is also high in some herds of zebras. Diets high in wheat bran—and thus high in phosphorus, calcium, magnesium, and protein—and alfalfa hay have been incriminated in their formation although conclusive evidence is lacking. However, several studies have indicated that when wheat bran was removed from the diet, the incidence of intestinal calculi decreased. Alfalfa also promotes alkalinity in the rumen and thus may do the same in the horse's large intestine, which enhances calculi formation. Intestinal calculi have occurred in sufficient size to cause intestinal obstruction in horses as young as 11 months of age, although the mean age of occurrence is 10 years. Thus, intestinal calculi can grow to a size sufficient to cause intestinal obstruction within less than 1 year.

Intestinal calculi cause varying degrees of obstruction and pain depending on the amount of distention and vascular compromise caused. With partial obstruction, the horse will continue to pass scanty amounts of liquid feces, gas, or orally administered mineral oil. The first effect often noticed is a decrease in feed intake, which may become complete. Sometimes the calculus can be palpated rectally, particularly with the horse facing up a slope, allowing the intestinal tract to move back. They vary in location and may be single or multiple stones.

Because the incidence of enteroliths in horses is low and sporadic, and the incidence of recurrence unknown, the need for a diet to prevent their formation isn't known. In species in which magnesium-ammonium-phosphate calculi commonly occur in the urinary tract, such as the dog and cat, feeding a diet low in protein (a source of ammonium), phosphorus and particularly magnesium that results in the maintenance of an acid urine has been shown to prevent their formation and to cause their dissolution. A similar type of diet may be of benefit for preventing formation of the same type of calculi in the intestinal tract of horses, although this hasn't been demonstrated. A diet for the horse low in protein, magnesium and phosphorus may be obtained by feeding a grass forage and grain. Legumes, wheat bran, and, unless needed, protein supplements should be avoided. The horse's water should also be low in magnesium and phosphorus or total solids.

Grass forages and cereal grains tend to be lower in magnesium (0.10 to 0.25% and 0.12 to 0.17%, respectively) than legumes (0.3 to 0.5%). Soybean meal contains about one-half as much magnesium as other oil seed meals (0.3 versus 0.6%). Wheat bran is relatively high in both magnesium and phosphorus (0.6 to 0.7% and 1.2 to 1.3%, respectively).

Feeding apple cider vinegar may also be of benefit, as it may acidify intestinal contents, which increases the solubility of these calculi. Adding ½ cup (110 ml) of apple cider vinegar per feeding of grain has been reported to acidify cecal fluid in ponies. At least twice this amount would be expected to be necessary to have the same effect in mature horses, and anecdotal reports indicate that when this amount is given twice daily, the incidence of intestinal calculi is decreased. Feeding a high-grain diet also acidifies intestinal fluid and thus would be expected to be of benefit. Thus, feeding a diet consisting of one-half grain (0.5 to 0.6 lb/100 lb body wt, or 0.5 to 0.6 kg/100 kg for maintenance), with 1 cup of vinegar added to it twice daily, and grass hay, while avoiding wheat bran and alfalfa, may be beneficial in preventing intestinal calculi formation in horses.

INTESTINAL REMOVAL OR DYSFUNCTION

Surgical removal of devitalized small or large intestine may at times be necessary and is compatible with resumption of a normal life if appropriate diets are fed.

Large-Colon Removal or Dysfunction

Immediately following removal of portions of the large colon, although fasting to allow bowel rest is often recommended, horses usually are able to eat high-quality feeds within 12 to 24 hours of surgery without adverse effects. The diet for the first month following surgery should be relatively high in protein (over 12%) and phosphorus (0.4%), and low in fiber (less than 28%) to compensate for a decrease in their apparent digestibility, which occurs for up to several weeks after surgical removal of the large bowel or inadequate blood flow to the large bowel without resection. A diet of this type can be provided by feeding a good weanling-type diet (Table 4–9). In addition, ensure that water is always easily available, as water losses and, therefore, needs are increased. Vitamin K administration may also be needed because of the loss of its production by cecal and colonic microflora. If the horse's prothrombin, activated partial thromboplastic or blood clotting times are prolonged, vitamin K should be given.

The diet described should be continued for horses with extensive removal of both the left and right colons, as their apparent digestibility of protein, phosphorus, and fiber remains impaired. However, digestive ability and nutritional requirements return to normal in horses with removal of only the left colon or the cecum, and they are able to maintain adequate body condition on even a relatively low protein (6 to 8%) grass hay fed free choice.

Small-Intestinal Removal or Dysfunction

Following small-intestinal removal, the horse should be fasted for 1 to 3 days (1 if horse is in poor condition and up to 3 if in good body condition) to minimize the risk of disrupting suture lines and because of abnormal intestinal motility, although small amounts of a liquid diet may be offered or administered by stomach tube beginning the first day after surgery. The first day of feeding, give no more than one-quarter of that needed for maintenance, with a maximum of 2 lbs (1 kg) of good-quality hay, or a complete pelleted feed, per feeding every 2 to 4 hours. Gradually increase the amount fed over the next 2 to 3 days until estimated needs are met.

If less than one half of the small intestine has been removed or is dysfunctional, nutritional needs are not increased; whereas, they are if the amount is greater than this. Since grain is digested and absorbed primarily in the small intestine, and forage in the large intestine, a primarily forage diet should be fed, whether decreased small-intestinal function is due to its removal or to disease and dysfunction. The forage fed should be of high quality so that it is easily fermentable. Good-quality alfalfa or growing forage is usually best. Feeding small amounts of grain and fat may be beneficial if additional energy for maintenance of body weight and condition is needed. Calcium absorption, which is primarily from the small intestine, may be decreased, although supplementation is unlikely to be needed if a legume forage is being consumed because of legume's high calcium content (Appendix Table 6). Alternatively a complete pelleted feed may be fed. Complete pelleted feeds fed in small amounts frequently maintained body weight and health of ponies with 70% of their lower small intestine removed. Fat-soluble vitamins A, D and E injections may be necessary if removal of the lower part of the small intestine results in sufficiently poor fat absorption.

RECTAL/VAGINAL SURGERY OR LACERATIONS

Decreasing fecal volume, pressure, and straining to defecate may be helpful following rectal or vaginal surgery or laceration repair in order to minimize pressure on the suture line. Defecation and stool volume can be nearly eliminated by tube-feeding a human commercial liquid diet. A lesser decrease in fecal volume, which is generally quite adequate following most rectal or vaginal surgery or lacerations, can be accomplished while still meeting the horse's nutritional requirements by feeding a low-fiber (16 to 20%), high-energy complete pelleted diet (Table 4–11) along with up to 1 pint of vegetable oil/5 lbs of feed (20 ml/kg). This pellet-oil mix provides about 1.7 Mcal/lb (3.7 Mcal/kg), and thus 0.9 lbs/100 lbs (0.9 kg/100 kg)/day will meet the horse's caloric needs for maintenance. Although a complete pelleted feed may be preferable, instead grain with up to the same amount of vegetable oil added may be fed as one-half of the horse's total dry feed intake. For maintenance this would be about 0.6 lbs/100 lbs (0.6 kg/100 kg) body weight/day of both the grain-oil mix and forage. The forage may be a good-quality alfalfa hay or pellets, or green growing grass. Although fecal volume can be reduced by feeding less than needed, this isn't recommended, at least not for more than a few days, as the resulting nutritional deficiencies it causes, if sufficient, will impair wound healing, and ability to resist disease.

LIVER DISEASE

Liver disease may result in central nervous system effects and behavioral alterations. These alterations and effects can be minimized by feeding diets adequate to meet dietary energy and protein needs, but without excess protein, and protein high in certain amino acids (branched chain) and low in others (aromatic).

Without adequate dietary energy intake, body glycogen, fat, and protein are utilized. Peripheral body fat mobilization, particularly in the animal with decreased liver function, may increase fat deposition in the liver, causing a further decrease in liver function. Body, like dietary, protein utilization for energy produces ammonia, which, if there is a decrease in its conversion to urea by the liver, increases plasma ammonia concentration. Sufficient body protein utilization, along with decreased liver production of plasma proteins, may result in decreased blood plasma protein concentration. If this is sufficiently severe, it results in edema (stocking up) or fluid in the abdominal or thoracic cavities, which may be worsened by high salt (sodium) intake and lessened by low salt (sodium) intake. To prevent or alleviate these effects, the diet for the animal with decreased liver function should meet the following criteria:

1. Meet dietary energy needs.
2. Meet, but not greatly exceed, dietary protein needs.
3. Be high in branched chain amino acids and low in aromatic amino acids.
4. Be low in, or at least not contain added, fat or salt.
5. Be high in starch to decrease need for hepatic glucose synthesis.

If the horse with liver disease is not eating adequate feed, it should be tube-fed until it is. A diet for horses that meets the desired criteria for liver disease is one consisting of one-half milo or corn; if a sufficient amount of feed is being consumed to meet energy needs for maintenance, this would be 0.5 to 0.6 lbs/100 lbs (0.5 to 0.6 kg/100 kg) body wt/day. This should be divided into 3 to 6 feedings daily. All the forage the horse will eat should be fed, which should be an amount similar to the amount of grain consumed. A legume forage such as alfalfa may be best because of its high amino acid content if its higher protein content is tolerated. However, if plasma ammonia concentration is increased, as suggested by behavioral or central nervous system disturbances, a lower-protein grass forage should be fed instead. No salt should be added to the diet or be available for consumption. This is particularly important if edema or stocking-up occurs. If liver damage is severe or the course of the disease is for more than a couple of weeks, adding to the diet a vitamin mix, such as that given in Table 3-5, is recommended.

KIDNEY FAILURE

Chronic renal failure occurs most frequently in older horses. Decreased appetite and depression resulting in weight loss are the most commonly noted signs. Increased urination due to an inability to concentrate the urine is also present. This may be detected by an abnormally wet stall and a compensatory increase in water consumption. It can be confirmed by an inability of the horse to increase the urine concentration.

Excessive protein loss in the urine may decrease the blood plasma protein concentrations sufficiently to cause stocking up or edema. Fetid breath and oral ulcers may be present. Anemia and alterations in plasma electrolyte concentrations may also be present. These alterations occur because of a decreased ability of the kidneys to excrete metabolic wastes such as urea from protein, phosphorus, and, in horses, calcium. Insuring adequate dietary energy intake and preventing excess dietary protein intake, so as to prevent both body and dietary protein utilization for energy, decrease urea production. This, and preventing excess phosphorus and calcium intake, prevents or minimizes their accumulation in the horse with kidney failure. However, regardless of diet, unless a cause for chronic renal failure can be identified and alleviated, the prognosis for long-term survival in most cases is poor.

A diet low in protein, phosphorus, and calcium can be provided by feeding a grass forage. If additional dietary energy is needed for maintenance of desired body weight, grain may be fed as up to one-half of total feed intake, which for maintenance would be 0.5 to 0.6 lbs/100 lbs (0.5 to 0.6 kg/100 kg) body weight/day. Any cereal grain may be fed, although corn is higher in energy density and slightly lower in protein, phosphorus, and calcium than other cereal grains (Appendix Table 6). Plasma urea, calcium, and phosphorus concentrations should be monitored. If they are above normal or increase further, additional protein, phosphorus, or calcium restriction is indicated. This can be accomplished by adding up to 20% vegetable oil to the grain feed, which is 1 pt/5 lbs (20 ml/kg). Varying degrees of protein loss in the urine may, however, increase dietary protein needs. To determine if this occurs, the plasma protein and albumin concentrations should be monitored. If they are low or decrease, and the plasma urea nitrogen concentration is not increased, protein intake should be increased by feeding up to 1 lb (0.5 kg)/horse/day of corn gluten, wheat gluten, distillers' grains, casein, or soybean meal. These are lower in calcium and phosphorus per unit of protein than other commonly available protein supplements for the horse (Table 4-7). Legumes should be avoided because they are high in protein and calcium, and bran should be avoided as it is high in protein and phosphorus (Appendix Table 6).

It is recommended that a vitamin supplement, such as that given in Table 3-5, be added to the diet for the horse with kidney failure to compensate for excessive losses of B vitamins in the urine. Water should always be freely available since there is decreased ability to concentrate the urine and thus conserve water, which will result in dehydration and death if sufficient water is not available. It is recommended that no salt be added to the diet, but that it be available for free-choice consumption.

URINARY TRACT CALCULI (BLADDER STONES)

Calculi formation in the urinary tract, although fairly common in many species of animals, is relatively uncommon in horses. When calculi do occur, they are generally in the bladder and in males. Although they presumably form as readily in mares, they are less commonly retained because of mares' much shorter and wider urethra that allows their excretion. Affected horses usually have frequent painful urination, straining when urinating, and bloody urine or bleeding from the urethra after urination. Other clinical signs include colic, stilted gait, and urine scalding of the prepuce or hindquarters.

Dietary and/or medical procedures to dissolve urinary calculi have not been developed in horses as they have in dogs and cats. Thus, bladder stones are routinely removed from horses surgically. Antimicrobial drugs are generally administered following surgery.

Recurrence of bladder stones in horses generally is not, but may be, a problem. Dietary management to decrease the urine concentration of stone forming constituents and to alter urine acidity to make it unfavorable for their formation has been shown to be effective in preventing their recurrence. This management differs with different calculi compositions. In the horse, the calculi are nearly always composed primarily or entirely of calcium carbonate. In recurring cases, this should be confirmed by a quantitative analysis of the calculi.

To prevent recurrence of calcium carbonate calculi, a low-calcium diet should be fed. The diet should ideally just meet but not exceed the horse's calcium, as well as phosphorus, requirements of about 0.2% of both in the diet dry matter, except during growth and lactation (Appendix Table 1). This can be accomplished by feeding a mature grass pasture or hay, or a cereal-grain hay, and grain with no added calcium, and avoiding early growth grass and particularly all legume forages, such as alfalfa and clovers, which are high in calcium.

Increasing salt intake has been used to increase water intake and urine volume and to assist in preventing urinary calculi retention. However, increasing sodium intake increases calcium and phosphorus absorption and retention by horses and, therefore, may not be beneficial in preventing calcium carbonate bladder stones in horses. Feeding urinary acidifiers, such as ammonium sulfate, has also been recommended and used, as calcium carbonate crystals don't occur in a sufficiently acid urine (pH below 6.0). However, urinary acidifiers are fairly unpalatable, and may increase horses urinary calcium excretion, which would enhance the formation of calcium containing bladder stones.

HEART DISEASE

A decrease in cardiac performance impairs the kidneys' ability to excrete sodium and water; if sufficient, this results in sodium and water retention, and, in turn, stocking up and/or fluid in the lungs or abdominal cavity. These effects are prevented or controlled by the following means:

1. Decrease cardiac workload by decreasing exercise or physical activity.
2. Decrease salt (sodium) and water retention by:
   a. restricting salt intake by having no salt added to the diet or available for consumption. All common horse feeds are low in sodium, grass forages generally being lower than legumes (Table 17-1). However, beet molasses is relatively high in sodium (Table 17-1), and many commercially available grain mixes contain added salt and, therefore,

TABLE 17-1
Potassium and Sodium Content of Horse Feeds

Feed	Potassium	Sodium
	(% in feed dry matter)	
Most cereal grains	0.35–0.45	0.01–0.06
Barley	0.50–0.6	0.02–0.03
Hay—immature (grass or alfalfa)	2.2–3.4	0.01–0.15
late maturity (grass or alfalfa)	1.0–1.9	0.01–0.15
cereal grain hay	1.0–1.5	0.01–0.15
Soybean meal	2.2	0.04
Cotton seed meal	1.4–1.5	0.04
Molasses, beet	6	1.5
sugar cane	4	0.2
Requirement	0.4	0.1

should not be fed to horses with decreased cardiac function.
   b. ensuring that palatable water is always readily available.
3. Increase sodium and water excretion if necessary by giving a diuretic. If diuretics or vasodilators such as captopril are given, salt should be always available to allow the horse to compensate for excessive sodium losses that may be induced. If nonpotassium-sparing diuretics are being given, the plasma potassium concentration may need to be monitored. As long as a forage constitutes at least one-half of the diet, potassium intake is generally adequate, as forages are high and grains low in potassium (Table 17-1). However, if the plasma potassium concentration is low, several ounces (60 to 120 g) of potassium chloride should be added to the diet daily. Potassium chloride is available at most grocery stores as sodium-free salt. Since diuretics increase water excretion, they also cause increased excretion of water-soluble vitamins; it may therefore be of benefit to give B vitamins daily or to add a vitamin mix, such as that given in Table 3-5, to the diet.

POTASSIUM INDUCED PERIODIC PARALYSIS

Potassium induced or hyperkalemic periodic paresis (PIPP), or episodic weakness, is an autosomal dominant genetic disease initially found in only the impressive line of Quarter Horses, Paints, and Appaloosas. However, matings of carrier horses to any breed may produce the defect. The same disease also occurs in people. The disease in horses, in contrast to people, is apparently incomplete penetrant, so that the expression of the gene—resulting in clinical signs, frequency, and severity of episodes—is variable.

The disease is characterized by recurrent, intermittent episodes of involuntary muscle quivering or rippling, which may be localized involving one or more muscle groups or generalized resulting in diffuse muscle fasiculations and weakness, which may or may not progress to the horse being unable to stand. These episodes may last for periods of a few minutes to a few hours. During an episode, the horse remains fully conscious and does not appear to be in pain. Generalized sweating, without a fever, and difficult and loud breathing from paralysis of the larynx or pharynx usually occur. Increased fluttery breathing noises may be heard, which may progress to collapse of the larynx or pharynx resulting in difficulty breathing and collapse. Upper airway obstruction may occur in some foals and may be the major problem noted. There may be nervousness, and the third eyelid, or membrane from the inside corner of the eye, may come up over the eye. Death may, but doesn't generally, occur. If it doesn't, spontaneous recovery occurs; the horse appears normal and has no indications of muscle stiffness or weakness.

An attack may be precipitated by a change in diet or weather, or trailering, or anesthesia. The first episode may occur in horses from a month to 15 years of age, but most commonly occur at 2 to 4 years of age. In contrast to what is sometimes stated, it appears that the incidence is similar in both sexes. Affected horses may show no signs throughout their lives, may rarely have attacks, or may have 2 to 3 attacks daily.

The blood plasma potassium concentration is usually increased (hyperkalemic) during and immediately following an episode. Because of this the disease is frequently referred to as hyperkalemic periodic paralysis. However, hyperkalemia may not occur. The plasma potassium concentration may be normal. Even during an episode, the increase in the plasma potassium concentration may be small and is not always present, and the concentration is routinely normal except during an episode. During an episode, an increase in the plasma potassium concentration if it occurs may be only in blood taken from the veins directly draining the affected muscles. But normokalemia has been observed in jugular blood taken from horses during a generalized episode resulting in recumbency induced by giving potassium chloride orally. Mild increases in serum creatinine concentration and creatine kinase activity may be present between episodes.

The disease is due primarily to a defect in muscle membrane permeability to sodium, which results in increased sodium movement into and potassium movement out of the cell. The alterations in these electrolytes across the muscle cell membrane increases the muscles excitability causing the clinical signs, and abnormal muscle electrical activity. No muscle abnormalities are visible.

A DNA blood test to diagnose affected horses and to determine their carrier status is available by sending 5 to 10 ml of blood collected into an EDTA anticoagulant to the Veterinary Genetics Laboratory, University of California, Davis, CA 95616. All foals born to homozygote carriers (genes acquired from both parents having the defect) are affected; 75% of those in which both parents are heterozygotes (so only one of their genes has the defect) are affected; and 50% of those in which only one parent is a heterozygote carrier are affected. Homozygotes are rare, probably because they die in the womb or are so severely affected that they die before diagnosis can be verified. A horse that is positive to the DNA blood test will have PIPP, will pass it on to its offspring, and will have an abnormal muscle electrical activity whether or not it shows signs of the disease. Ideally affected horses should not be used for breeding. An affected horse will pass on the disease as effectively and with similar consequences as any affected horse in its family, regardless of the number of generations they are apart. Thus, in contrast to a common misconception, the disease cannot be "bred-out" with genetic input from nonaffected lines of horses; nor do horses "grow out" of the disease as they get older. Because of these factors, affected horses should not be bred.

Episodes of PIPP must be differentiated from colic, seizures and exertional myopathy or tying-up syndrome. Horses down due to colic will usually have an increased heart rate and congested, muddy-appearing membranes, neither of which are present in horses with PIPP. During an episode of PIPP, the muscles are firm but not hard, as they tend to be with exertional myopathy or tying-up syndrome. PIPP should be suspected in horses with a family history of the disease and showing clinical signs. It can be confirmed by the presence of hyperkalemia during an episode, abnormal electromyographic findings, or induction of an episode by giving potassium.

Provocative testing for PIPP is conducted by giving potassium chloride by stomach tube following a 12-hour fast. Generally, but not always, hyperkalemia and typical clinical signs occur in affected horses 30 to 60 minutes and 2 to 4 hours, respectively, following potassium chloride administration. Treatment should be instituted as soon as clinical signs occur. This test, however, risks injury and heart block induced death of affected horses; therefore, the DNA blood test is preferred.

Diagnosis of PIPP following death is difficult, as the plasma potassium concentration normally rises following death from any cause. The DNA test can be run on splenic tissue but doesn't indicate whether the horse died during an episode of PIPP or from another cause.

Treatment of acute episodes of PIPP is to administer calcium gluconate, or alternatively dextros (glucose), with or without insulin or sodium bicarbonite. Calcium counteracts the effects of hyperkalemia on the muscle membrane. Glucose, insulin and bicarbonate all increase potassium movement into the cells.

The occurrence of episodes of PIPP may be decreased or prevented by decreasing potassium intake, preferably to less than 1% of the dry diet, and by increasing potassium excretion. Exercise and frequent feeding, and avoiding fasting and sudden feed changes are also helpful. As shown in Table 17–1, potassium intake may be decreased by feeding a high-grain mature forage or cereal-grain hay diet, and avoiding immature or growing forages and sweet feeds because of the high potassium content in molasses and the oilseed meals that they often contain. Electrolyte, kelp, and vitamin supplements may also be high in potassium. However, as with all horse diets, grain ideally shouldn't constitute over one-half of total feed intake. There are several complete feeds available commercially that contain less than 1% potassium, and are marketed specifically for horses with PIPP. Even with these low-potassium diets, potassium intake will be substantially greater than that needed (Table 17–1) unless there are excessive potassium losses, such as with sweating or diarrhea. The diet should be changed gradually and kept consistent, as rapid changes in diet, or routine, and fasting and stress may induce an episode of PIPP in affected horses.

Potassium excretion may be increased by increasing the intake of alkalinizing salts. Alkalinizing salts increase acid or hydrogen ion retention, which may in turn increase potassium excretion. The alkalinizer—sodium bicarbonate, or baking soda—has been recommended (1 oz, or 30 g, per horse twice daily). However, increased sodium intake results in increased sodium excretion, which may decrease potassium excretion, off-setting any effect bicarbonate may have on potassium excretion. For this reason, limiting sodium intake by not feeding salt, and adding calcium carbonate (limestone), instead of baking soda, as an alkalinizer to the diet, may be of benefit.

If these procedures don't prevent further episodes, they can generally be prevented by giving diuretics that increase potassium excretion, such as acetazolamide. Acetazolamide may also be helpful in regulating potassium exchange across cell membranes and stimulates insulin release, which increases potassium movement into the cell. It has been shown to be more effective than hydrochlorothiazide. The amount of diuretic given should be as low as necessary to prevent episodes, as their overuse can over time cause a total body potassium deficit. The plasma potassium concentration should be checked periodically when diuretics are being given. Phenytoin, a drug most commonly used in treating epilepsy in people may be used in refractory cases, but is costly and may cause tranquilization.

Chapter 18

PLANT POISONING OF HORSES

Anthony P. Knight*

Salivation-Inducing Plants 301
Colic- and Diarrhea-Inducing Plants 302
  Horse Chestnut and Buckeye (Aesculus spp.) 302
  Field Bindweed (Morning Glory) (Convolvulus arvensis) . . 303
  Oak (Quercus spp.) 303
  Mountain Laurel (Kalmia latifolia) 304
  Pokeweed (Phytolacca americana) 304
  Buttercups (Ranunculus spp.) 306
  Castor Oil Plant (Ricinus communis) 306
  Jimson Weed, Potato, and Tomato (Nightshade or
    Solanaceae) 307
Primary Photodermatitis-Inducing Plants 308
  St. John's Wort or Klamath Weed (Hypericum perforatum) . 309
  Buckwheat (Fagopyrum esculentum) 309
Liver Disease-Inducing Plants 310
  Pyrrolizidine Alkaloid Poisoning 310
    Plant Causes 310
      Senecio species 310
      Hounds tongue (Cynoglossum officinale) 311
      Fiddleneck or Tarweed (Amsinckia intermedia) . . . 312
      Rattlebox or Rattlepod (Crotalaria spp.) 312
    Effects of Pyrrolizidine Alkaloids 312
  Nonpyrrolizidine Alkaloid Liver Poisoning Plants . . . 313
    Indigo (Indigofera spicata) 313
    Alsike Clover & Klein grass (Trifolium hybridum &
      Panicum coloratum) 314
Neurologic Disease-Inducing Plants 314
  Sagebrush (Artemisia spp.) 314
  Locoweeds and Milkvetches (Astragalus & Oxytropis spp.) . 316
    Locoweed Neurologic Poisoning 317
    Milkvetch Neurologic Poisoning 317
  Yellow Star Thistle and Russian Knapweed (Centaurea spp.) . 318
  Horsetail, Marestail, Horserush, or Snake Grass
    (Equisetum spp.) 319
  White Snakeroot and Crofton, Jimmyweed, and Burrow
    Weed (Eupatorium and Haplopappus spp.) 320
  Bracken Fern (Pteridium aquilinum) 320
  Johnson and Sudan Grasses (Sorghum spp.) 321
Lameness- and Muscle Weakness-Inducing Plants 322
  Black Walnut (Juglans nigra) 322
  Coffee Weed or Coffee Senna (Cassia occidentalis) . . . 323
  Plant-Induced Calcinosis 324
    Day-Blomming or Wild Jessamine (Cestrum diurnum) . . 324
  Selenium Excess 324
    Causes of Selenium Excess 325

Two-Grooved Milkvetches (Astragalus spp.) 325
Golden Weed (Haplopappus engelmannii) 326
Woody Aster (Xylorrhiza glabriuscula) 326
Prince's Plume (Stanleya pinnata) 326
White Prairie Aster (Aster falcatus) 326
Broom, Turpentine, Snake or Match Weed (Guterrezia
  sarothrae) 326
Gumweed or Resinweed (Grindelia spp.) 326
Saltbush (Atriplex spp.) 328
Indian Paintbrush (Castilleja spp.) 328
Beard Tongue (Penstemon spp.) 328
Effects of Selenium Excess 328
Diagnosis of Selenium Excess 330
Treatment of Chronic Selenium Excess 330
Anemia-Inducing Plants 330
  Onions (Allium spp.) 330
  Red Maple (Acer rubrum) 331
  Spoiled Sweet Clover (Melilotus spp.) 331
Teratogenic Plants 332
Sudden Death-Inducing Plants 334
  Cyanide-Induced Sudden Death 334
    Plant Causes of Cyanide Poisoning 334
      Serviceberry or Saskatoon Berry (Amelanchier alnifolia) . 334
      Wild Blue Flax (Linum spp.) 335
      Western Chockecherry (Prunus virginiana) 335
      Elderberry (Sambucus spp.) 335
      Sorghum (Johnson & Sudan) Grasses 335
      Arrow, Pod or Goose Grass (Triglochin spp.) . . . 335
    Effects of Cyanogenic Glycosides 336
  Cardiac Glycoside Induced Sudden Death 337
    Plant Causes of Cardiac Glycoside Poisoning 337
      Milkweed (Asclepias spp.) 337
      Foxglove (Digitalis purpurea) 337
      Oleander (Nerium oleander) 338
      Yellow Oleander, Be-Still or Lucky Nut Tree
        (Thevetia spp.) 338
    Effects of Cardiac Glycosides 338
  Larkspur or Poison Weed (Delphinium spp.) 340
  Monkshood (Aconitum spp.) 341
  Poison Hemlock (Conium maculatum) 341
  Water Hemlock (Cicuta spp.) 342
  Yew (Taxus spp.) 343
  Death Camas (Zigadenus spp.) 344
  Avocado (Persea americana) 344
Supplemental Reading Recommendations 344

Plant poisoning of horses and other livestock in the United States has been recognized since these animals were introduced to North America by the early Europeans. As early as 1873, large numbers of horses were reported to have died from a neurologic disease appropriately named locoism, a name derived from the Spanish word meaning

* Written by Anthony P. Knight BVSc, MS, MRCVS, Dipl ACVIM, Professor and Chairman, Department of Clinical Sciences, College of Veterinary Medicine and Biomedical Sciences, Colorado State University, Fort Collins, CO 80523.

crazy. The locoweeds (Astragalus and Oxytropis spp.) responsible for the losses of the horses were, and still are, abundant on many western rangelands. Similarly, in the early 19th century, settlers in the midwestern states experienced severe muscle tremors and deaths in their horses, sheep, and cattle after the animals ate white snakeroot (Eupatorium urticaefolium). People were also affected with similar signs if they drank milk from cows that had been eating white snakeroot.

Although plant poisoning of horses continues to be a problem, the economic impact on the horse industry is not known, as relatively few poisonings are confirmed, and the extent to which the problem occurs has not been investigated. Also, factors such as subclinical poisoning from plants, and the loss of pasture due to the displacement of normal forages by noxious plants, are largely unknown. Indirectly, poisonous plants add to the cost of having horses through the necessity for fencing, herbicides, mowing, and reseeding of pastures where undesirable plants predominate. Typically, horses are at greatest risk when pastures are overgrazed and noxious weeds are able to proliferate. At other times, poisoning can occur when garden prunings are tossed into horse corrals with mistaken good intentions, or when hungry horses are tied adjacent to plants to which they are unaccustomed. Although most plant poisonings occur in horses on pasture during the spring and summer, losses may also occur in horses not on pasture and during the winter if the hay being fed contains toxic plants.

The potential for plant poisoning increases if horses have the opportunity to eat large quantities (green plants in amounts equal to 5 to 10% of their body weight) of a toxic plant over a period of several weeks or months. Rarely is a horse poisoned by a single mouthful of a plant, with the possible exception of the most toxic of plants, such as water hemlock (Cicuta douglasii) and yew (Taxus spp.). Factors such as drought, excessive moisture, fertilization, and soil mineral imbalances can alter the amount of toxin in plants, making them more of a problem in some years than in others. The use of herbicides may also affect plant growth and alter the quantity of toxic substances such as nitrates that will accumulate in the plant.

In describing plant poisoning of horses, it is not the intent to imply that horses are at immediate risk if one or more poisonous plants are present in their pasture. Rather, it is hoped that by recognition of the more common toxic plants the potential for poisoning can be reduced by proper pasture management. To assist in recognition of where poisoning by certain plants should be considered as a cause of health problems in the horse, the most common poisonous plants affecting horses in North America are grouped by the main clinical effects of the plant toxin. These plant toxins may exert their effects on multiple organ systems. The clinical signs they induce therefore vary with the variety and degree of organ involvement. For example, Tansy ragwort (Senecio jacobea) poisoning in horses first recognized effect is most often as a neurologic disease, or occasionally the horse may show severe photodermatitis, yet the underlying problem is one of severe liver disease. Plants that have only been suspected, but not confirmed, of being toxic to horses will not be discussed. Commonly used botanical terms helpful in describing plants, but which may be unfamiliar to those not knowledgeable in botany, like other terms that may be unfamiliar to some, are described in a glossary at the end of the book just preceeding the Appendix Tables.

SALIVATION-INDUCING PLANTS

Excessive salivation or slobbering characterized by frothing or drooling of saliva is generally an indication of traumatic, chemical, or infectious injury to the mouth, or obstruction to the esophagus (choke) that prevents the swallowing of saliva and food. In addition to trauma from sharp points on teeth (as described in Chapter 9), poorly fitting or inappropriately used bits, or infectious diseases such as the virus induced vesicular stomatitis, that causes blister-like lesions of the mouth, as well as a variety of grasses and other plants, may cause trauma to the mucous membranes of the mouth resulting in excessive salivation. Plants with thorns, bristles, stinging hairs, or sharp awns can produce a variety of lesions ranging from reddening of the mucous membranes to deep granulating ulcers on the tongue and gums. Blister-like lesions around the lips, nose, eyes, and anus may also occur in horses bedded on wood shavings containing bitterwood (Quassia simarouba), a tree indigenous to Central and South America, where it is harvested for lumber. Similar blisters occur on the hands and face of people who prune these trees. Affected horses recover completely from the vesicular dermatitis once they are removed from the bitterwood-containing shavings.

Grasses such as foxtail barley (Hordeum jubatum) (Fig. 18-1) bristle grass (Setaria spp.) and wheat or rye awns can become embedded in the mucous membranes of the cheeks, tongue, and gums, causing painful ulcers, excessive salivation, and difficulty in eating. The grass awns are often not visible in the ulcers, as they are covered by a layer of granulation tissue. A wide variety of plants (Table 18-1) have the potential to cause irritation and trauma to the mouth of horses if they are present in hay or are abundant in the pasture. Occasionally these plants can cause trauma to the skin; sometimes potentially serious injury to the eyes may result from bristles of burdock (Arctium spp.) and other plants that become lodged in the tissues around the eyes or cornea.

Eating the following plants may also cause excessive salivation: (1) laurel (Kalmia spp.), (2) azalea (Rhododendron spp.), (3) buttercup (Ranunculus spp.), (4) poison hemlock (Conium maculatum), (5) water hemlock (Cicuta spp.), (6) death camas (Zigadenus spp.), (7) yellow star thistle (Centaurea solstitialis, (8) Russian knapweed (C. repens), or tremetol-containing plants such as (9) white

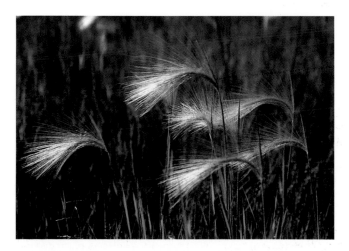

Fig. 18-1. Foxtail Barley (Hordeum jubatum) seed heads

TABLE 18–1

Mechanically Injurious Plants[a]

Common Name	Scientific Name
Burdock bristles	Arctium spp.
Three awn grasses	Aristida spp.
Oat awns	Avena sativa
Sand burrs	Cenchrus spp.
Thistles	Cirsium spp.
Foxtail barley awns	Hordeum jubatum
Barley awns	Hordeum vulgare
Prickly pear cactus, cholla	Opuntia spp.
Rye awns	Secale cereale
Bristle grasses, foxtails	Setaria spp.
Horse nettle	Solanum carolinensis
Buffalo burr	Solanum rostratum
Needle, spear, or porcupine grass	Stipa spp.
Wheat awns	Triticum aestivum
Puncture vine, goat head	Tribulus terrestris
Stinging nettle	Urtica spp.
Cockle burrs	Xanthium spp.

[a] Most commonly cause oral lesions resulting in excess salivation or slobbering, difficulty in eating, and decreased feed intake. Occasionally, some may cause skin trauma; bristles of burdock may cause eye injury.

snakeroot (Eupatorium rugosum), (10) Crofton weed (E. adenophorum), (11) Jimmyweed or rayless goldenrod (Haplopappus spp.), and (12) Burrow weed (H. tenuisectus). However, colic is the major clinical effect of the first three of these plants (Table 18–2). Sudden death is the major clinical effect of the next three plants (numbers 4, 5 and 6) (Table 18–12), and neurologic-disease resulting in an inability to take in or chew feed (numbers 7 and 8) and muscular trembling (numbers 9 to 12) are the major clinical effects of the last six plants (Table 18-7).

Profuse salivation as the only major clinical sign occurs in horses and other livestock eating clover or alfalfa pasture or hay that is infected with the fungus Rhizoctonia leguminicola. The factor responsible has been identified as slaframine, a mycotoxin produced most commonly by this mold on red clover (Trifolium pratense), but may also occur on other common legumes, including alfalfa, white clover, alsike clover, lupines, cow pea, and kudzu. Slaframine is chemically similar to the toxin swainsonine produced by locoweeds (Astragalus and Oxytropis spp.). Under wet or humid conditions, the slaframine producing mold grows on the leaves, producing black or brown spotting. After eating infected legumes for several days, horses begin to salivate excessively, lose weight, and may have excessive tearing or lacrimation, diarrhea, and frequent urination. Pregnant mares may abort if they continue to consume the infected clover. Recovery occurs rapidly once horses are removed from the infected forage. Problem pastures can be grazed if they are mowed, the affected hay is removed, and the regrowth has no brown or black spotting on the leaves.

COLIC- AND DIARRHEA-INDUCING PLANTS

Poisonous plants are but one of many causes of colic and diarrhea in horses. The action of various plant toxins may either have a direct irritant effect on the intestine,

causing increased motility, colic, and diarrhea, or they cause the same effects by acting on the nervous system. Yet other plants may cause severe colic through obstruction or impaction of the small or large intestine, respectively. Fruits of plants such as Cockspur hawthorn (Crataegus crusgalli), mesquite (Prosopis glandulosa), and persimmon (Diospyros virginiana) when eaten by horses can cause obstruction of the small or large intestine. Plants such as halogeton (Halogeton glomeratus), greasewood (Sarcobatus vermiculatus), and shamrock, soursob, or sorrel (Oxalis spp.) contain high amounts of oxalate, which have the potential to cause stomach and intestinal inflammation and diarrhea. Prolonged consumption of low amounts of oxalate from these plants, or other plants containing low amounts of oxalate, may cause a calcium-deficiency as described in Chapter 2.

Plants most frequently associated with either or both colic and diarrhea in horses are listed, along with their toxin and additional effects on the horse, in Table 18–2. Horses eating the fruit, seeds, or leaves of avocado (Persea americana) trees usually die within a few days or less, depending on the amount consumed, as described later in this chapter in the section on "Sudden Death-Inducing Plants." Prior to death, however, colic, diarrhea, and signs of acute congestive heart failure occur. A variety of other common plants also may be incriminated as a cause of colic and diarrhea if horses are deprived of normal forages. Invasive pasture plants such as leafy spurge (Euphorbia esula), wild iris (Iris missouriensis), horsetail or scouring rush (Equisetum arvense), bitter weeds (Helenium spp.), and a variety of mustard plants (Brassica spp.) should be considered as a cause of colic and diarrhea when other causes are not found.

Determining that colic or diarrhea are due to a plant is difficult because generally there are no specific lesions of plant poisoning detectable in the gastrointestinal tract at postmortem examination, and it is difficult to identify plants in the gastrointestinal tract once they have been chewed and acted upon by digestive enzymes. When plants are suspected of causing colic and diarrhea, a careful history and a thorough examination of the horse's pasture and food should be made in an attempt to identify plants given in Table 18–2.

Horse Chestnut and Buckeye

Horse chestnut and buckeye (Aesculus spp.) are common small- to medium-sized shrubs or trees with large palmate leaves, white to red flower spikes born terminally on the branches, and characteristic spiny or smooth fruit capsules containing one to three shiny brown nuts when ripe (Fig. 18–2). A variety of horse chestnut species grow throughout most states but are concentrated in the eastern and southern states. Those reportedly toxic to animals are: Ohio, California, red and yellow buckeyes (A. glabra, californica, pavia and octandra, respectively), and the introduced species horse chestnut (A. hippocastanum). These toxic chestnuts are not related to the edible chestnut (Castanea spp.).

The toxin in buckeyes and chestnuts is aesculin, a glycoside present in the new growth, the leaves, and the nuts.

TABLE 18–2
Colic-[a] or Diarrhea-Inducing Plants

Common Name	Scientific Name	Plant Toxin	Clinical Effects[a]
Foxglove Oleander Yellow oleander Be-Still or lucky nut tree	Digitalis purpurea Nerium oleander Thevetia peruviana Thevetia thevetioides	Cardiac glycosides	Diarrhea, regurgitation, shock, abnormal heart rhythms & death in <24 hrs
Halogeton Greasewood Shamrock, soursob, sorrel	Halogeton glomeratus Sarcobatus vermiculatus Oxalis spp	Oxalates	Diarrhea, rarely kidney disease. Prolonged intake of low amount causes calcium deficiency (Chapter 2).
Horse chestnut, buckeye Corn cockle	Aesculus spp. Agrostemma githago	Aesculin Saponins	Muscle tremors and incoordination
Pokeweed Coffee or senna weed	Phytolacca americana Cassia spp.	Saponins & oxalates Anthraquinone	Diarrhea
Oak, usually Gambels oak or Shinnery oak —	Quercus spp. Q. gambelii Q. harvardii Q. breviloba	Tannins in leaves, bark or acorns, especially when green	Hard, dark feces; later bloody diarrhea. Won't eat, depression. May have oral ulcers & choke signs. Liver & kidney damage.
Field bindweed or morning glory	Convolvulus arvensis	Tropane alkaloids	Slow heart rate & dilated pupils
Laurel Azaleas Fetterbush Mountain pieris Maleberry	Kalmia spp. Rhododendron spp. Leucothoe spp. Pieris spp. Lyonia spp.	Grayanotoxins & arbutin	Salivation, defecation, depression, and incoordination
Privets	Ligustrum vulgare	glycosides	
Buttercup & anemone Hellebore Marsh marigold Clematis	Ranunculus spp. Helleborus spp. Caltha palustris Clematis spp.	Protoanemonin	Salivation & diarrhea
Castor beans Rosary peas Black locust	Ricinus communis Abrus precatorius Robinia pseudoacacia	Lectins	Trembling, incoordination, & diarrhea
Nightshade & potato, Jimson weed (thorn apple) Tomato Jessamine	Solanum spp. Datura stramonium Lycopersicon spp. Cestrum spp.	Hyoscyamine, solamine & hyoscine with atropine effects	Excitement then depression. Diarrhea & weakness.
Avocado (Guatemalan, not Mexican smooth-skin fruit variety)	Persea americana (See section on "Sudden Death" for description)	Unknown toxin in plant. Flesh of ripe fruit not toxic.	Diarrhea, congestive heart failure, edema of abdomen, head & lungs. Death <2 days.
Persimmon Cockspur or hawthorn Mesquite	Diospyros virginiana Cratelequs crusgalli Prosopis glandulosa	Plant & fruit not toxic but fruit may cause impaction	Impaction colic

[a] In addition to the clinical effects given, all plants listed cause colic, except those causing acute oxalate poisoning (halogeton, greasewood, and Oxalis spp.).

Its principal action appears to be on the gastrointestinal tract and nervous system. Colic has been the main problem reported in horses, although muscle tremors, incoordination, and paralysis are possible. There is no specific treatment, but mineral oil given by stomach tube as a laxative, and supportive fluid therapy may be beneficial.

Field Bindweed (Morning Glory)

Field bindweed (Convolvulus arvensis), found throughout North America, is an extremely persistent, invasive, perennial, twining or creeping weed with alternate leaves and white or pink funnel-shaped flowers (Fig. 18–3). The plant reproduces readily from seed and from its extensive root system.

The toxins in bindweed, are present in all parts of the plant. Colic as the result of intestinal paralysis, decreased heart rate, and dilated pupils may result if toxic levels of bindweed are consumed. No specific treatment is known.

Oak

Horses are susceptible to oak poisoning caused by the tannic acid that accumulates in new leaves and acorns that horses will eat when normal forages are scarce. Although all 60 species of oak that grow in North America are potentially toxic, most livestock poisoning is attributed to Gambels oak (Quercus gambelii), Shinnery oak (Q. havardii), and Q. breviloba. Oaks range from shrubs to large trees. All have alternate, simple, toothed or lobed, dark green

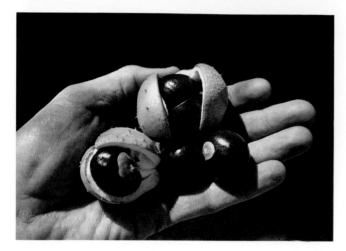

Fig. 18–2. Fruits of horse chestnut or buckeye (Aesculus spp.)

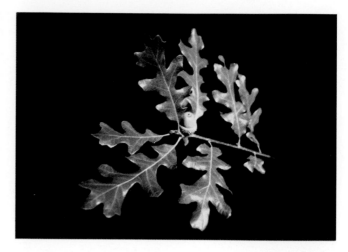

Fig. 18–4. Gambels oak (Quercus gambelii) showing typical leaves and acorn

glossy leaves that become red in the fall (Fig. 18-4). The plants are monoecious, with the staminate flowers occurring in long catkins and the pistillate flowers occurring singly or in small clusters. The fruit, an acorn, is a nut partially enveloped by an involucre of scales (Fig. 18-4).

Tannins found in the leaves, bark, and acorns of most oak species are presumed to be the toxin causing poisoning in animals. Tannins are potent precipitators of cellular protein (astringents), which when ingested cause severe damage to the intestinal tract and kidney. Oaks at any stage of growth are poisonous, but are particularly toxic when the leaf and flower buds are just opening in the spring. As the leaves mature, they become less toxic. Ripe acorns are also less toxic than green acorns. Cattle, sheep, horses, and pigs are susceptible to oak poisoning. Ruminants frequently browse on oak without apparent problems, provided they have ample access to normal forages.

Clinical signs of oak poisoning vary according to the quantity of oak leaves, bark, or acorns consumed. Initially animals stop eating, become depressed, and develop colic. The feces are hard and dark, but a bloody diarrhea often

occurs later in the course of poisoning. Some horses may appear to have choked with ingested food, and saliva passes out the nose. Mouth ulcers may also be present. Severe gastrointestinal, liver and kidney damage and a low blood calcium and phosphorus concentrations are usually present. Horses may die within a 24-hour period after eating large quantities of acorns, or may live for 5 to 7 days after the onset of clinical signs.

Affected animals should be removed from oak pasture and given supportive care in the form of fresh water and hay. Mineral oil, intravenous fluids and drugs to control pain are particularly indicated for colicky horses.

Mountain Laurel

Laurels (Kalmia latifolia) are common branching shrubs or small trees with glossy, green, alternate lanceolate leaves. The characteristic white to pink flowers are produced in showy clusters (Fig. 18-5). Laurels are common to the eastern and southern United States.

The principal toxins in laurels are present in all parts of the plant. Similar toxins are also present in azaleas (Rhododendron spp.) (Fig. 18-6), fetterbush (Leucothoe spp.) (Fig. 18-7), mountain pieris (Pieris spp.) (Fig. 18-8), and maleberry (Lyonia spp.) (Fig. 18-9). The principal effects of the toxin when these plants are ingested are gastrointestinal irritation and disruption of the heart's normal electrical activity.

Although all animals are susceptible to laurel and rhododendron poisoning, horses and donkeys are only occasionally poisoned. Affected animals may show excessive, green frothy salivation, colic, frequent defecation, depression, weakness, and incoordination. If a sufficient quantity of laurel has been eaten, an inability to stand, coma, and death occur. There is no specific treatment. Mineral oil and intravenous fluids may be helpful.

Pokeweed

Pokeweed (Phytolacca americana) is a perennial branching herb 3 to 10 ft (1 to 3 m) tall, with a large taproot,

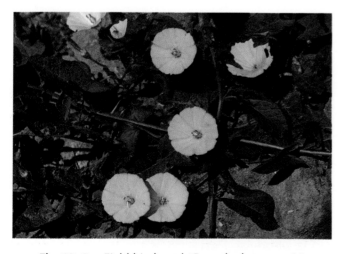

Fig. 18–3. Field bindweed (Convolvulus arvensis)

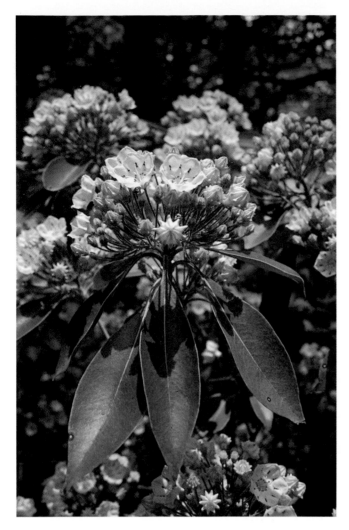

Fig. 18–5. Mountain laurel (Kalmia latifolia)

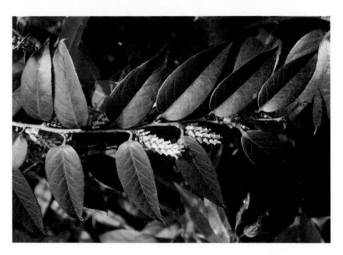

Fig. 18–7. Fetterbush (Leucothoe spp.)

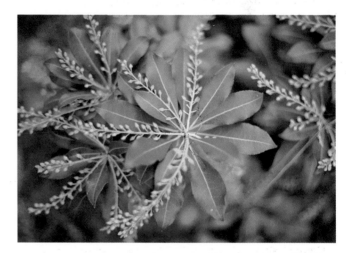

Fig. 18–8. Mountain pieris (Pieris spp.) (Courtesy of Drs. John and Emily Smith, Baldwin, GA)

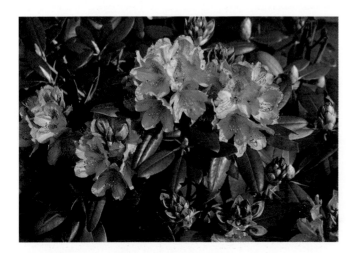

Fig. 18–6. Azaleas (Rhododendron catawbiense)

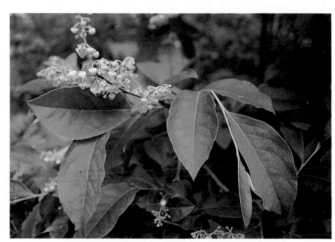

Fig. 18–9. Maleberry (Lyonia spp.)

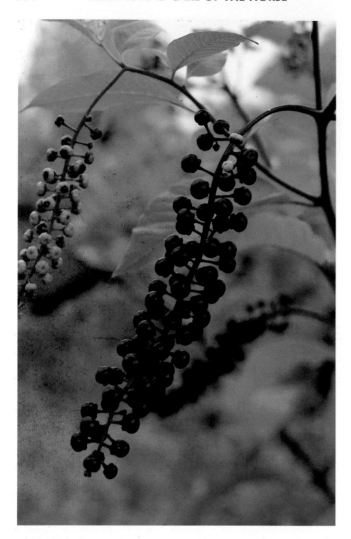

Fig. 18–10. Pokeweed berries (Phytolacca americana) (Courtesy of Drs. John and Emily Smith, Baldwin, GA)

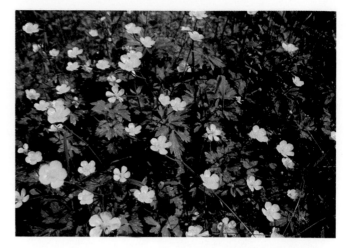

Fig. 18–11. Buttercup (Ranunculus spp.)

protoanemonins include hellebore (Helleborus spp.), marsh marigold (Caltha palustris), clematis (Clematis spp.) and anemone (Ranunculus spp.)

Ingestion of plants containing protoanemonins results in excessive salivation, mild colic, and diarrhea varying in severity depending on the amount the horse has eaten.

Castor Oil Plant

Castor oil plants (Ricinus communis) are common perennial plants of tropical areas, growing 6 to 13 ft (2 to 4 m) high, with a single, hollow branching stem. The stem is often purplish in color with a waxy coating. Leaves are large, alternate, usually 8 lobed, each with a main vein that radiates from the off-centered attachment of the petiole (Fig. 18-12). Yellowish flowers are produced in racemes at the end of the main stem and form fruits covered with soft spines that dry into sharp spines surrounding three characteristic seeds. Poisoning occurs from eating either the plants or grain contaminated with castor beans (Fig. 18-13).

green or purple stems, and large, alternate, petioled and ovate leaves. The flowers are small, white in color, and petalless. The distinctive fruits are shiny purple berries (Fig. 18-10). Pokeweed grows mostly in the eastern and southern United States. All parts of the plant, especially the roots, contain saponins and oxalates. Pokeweed mitogens may also cause mild to severe colic and diarrhea depending on the amount consumed. Fatalities are rare.

Buttercups

Buttercups (Ranunculus spp.) are perennial herbaceous plants with fibrous roots, erect hairless stems, and leaves deeply divided into three lobes. The upper leaves are smaller. The flowers vary from few to many, and have five bright yellow petals and five green sepals (Fig. 18-11). Buttercups are commonly found in wet areas throughout North America.

Some, but not all, species of buttercups contain ranunculin which forms the toxic blistering agent protoanemonin when the plant is chewed or crushed. When dried, buttercups lose their toxicity. Other plants that contain

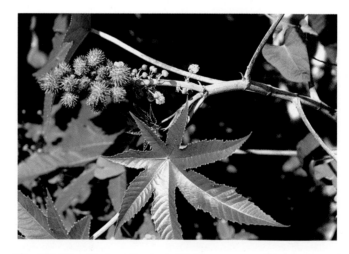

Fig. 18–12. Castor oil plant (Ricinus communis) leaves and spiny fruit capsules

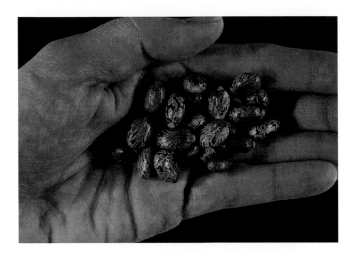

Fig. 18–13. Castor beans (Ricinus communis)

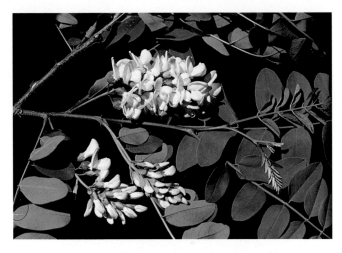

Fig. 18–15. Black locust (Robinia pseudoacacia) flowers, compound leaves, and thorns on branches

All parts of the plant and especially the seeds contain ricin, a highly toxic lectin that inhibits protein synthesis. Similar toxic lectins are found in rosary peas (Abrus precatorius) (Fig. 18-14) and black locust (Robinia pseudoacacia) (Fig. 18-15). Lectins are proteins that have the capability of binding to cells; they can cause agglutination of cells and acute hypersensitivity reactions. Horses are poisoned by eating seeds (castor beans) in an amount as small as that equal to 0.01% of their body weight. This amount could be provided by only 1 to 2% castor beans in the horse's grain. However, castor oil extracted from the seeds is not toxic, as the ricin is insoluble in the oil. The oil is, however, a potent intestinal purgative or cathartic.

Early signs of castor bean poisoning in horses include trembling, sweating, and incoordination which appear several days after the animal has eaten grain contaminated with castor beans. Colic, diarrhea, and a rapid weak pulse develop as the poisoning progresses. Horses that develop clinical signs seldom survive.

Jimson Weed, Potato, and Tomato

In the large family of nightshade (Solanaceae) plants, horses have been poisoned by various genera that include nightshades (Solanum spp.), jimson weed or thorn apple (Datura stramonium) (Fig. 18-16), tomato (Lycopersicon spp.), potato (Solanum tuberosum), and jessamine (Cestrum spp.).

A variety of toxins are found in Solanaceae plants, especially in the green parts of the plant and the unripe fruits. These toxins inhibit the animal's parasympathetic nervous system. They also have a direct irritant effect on the digestive system. Horses are most often poisoned by the feeding of grain contaminated with jimson weed seeds (Fig. 18-17) green or rotting potatoes, or potato or tomato plants. Compared to other livestock, horses may be more susceptible to of solanine toxins.

Initially there may be excitement, but depression follows with decreased heart and respiratory rate, muscle

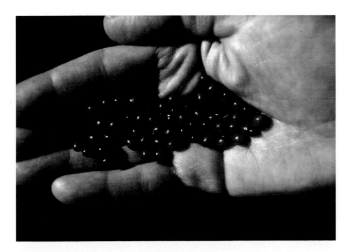

Fig. 18–14. Rosary peas (Abrus precatorius) with characteristic black patch on the scarlet seeds

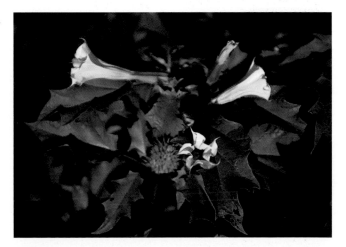

Fig. 18–16. Jimson weed or thorn apple (Datura stramonium) showing characteristic trumpet-shaped flower and spiny fruit (thorn apple)

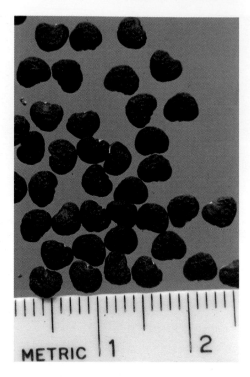

Fig. 18–17. Jimson weed or thorn apple seeds (Datura stramonium)

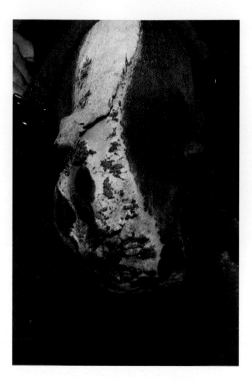

Fig. 18–18. Photosensitization in a horse showing severe dermatitis affecting the nonpigmented skin only

weakness, dilated pupils, colic, and watery diarrhea that may be bloody. When large amounts of solanine are ingested, death results from cardiac arrest. Therapy is symptomatic as no specific treatment exists.

PRIMARY PHOTODERMATITIS-INDUCING PLANTS

The common cause of plant-induced dermatitis or skin inflammation is photosensitization, which can be induced by the consumption of plants given in Table 18-3. These plants induce photodermatitis as a result of the accumulation of photodynamic compounds in the skin, which when exposed to ultraviolet rays from sunlight fluoresce, releas-

TABLE 18–3
Photodermatitis-Inducing Plants

Common Name	Scientific Name	Toxin	Effect[a]
St. John's wort or klamath weed	Hypericum perforatum	Hypericin	Primary photodermatitis
Buckwheat	Fagapyrum esculentum	Fagopyrin	Primary photodermatitis
Spring parsley	Cymopterus watsonii	Furocoumarins	Primary photodermatitis in other livestock and poultry
Bishop's weed	Ammi majus		
See Table 18–4		Liver toxins	Secondary photodermatitis

[a] See Figure 18–18 for effects of photodermatitis. All may also cause excessive tearing and abnormal intolerance to light.

ing radiant energy that causes cellular damage. The less pigmented the skin, the more ultraviolet rays are able to reach photosensitive compounds in the skin, and the more susceptible that skin consequently is to photosensitization (Fig. 18-18). Horses with completely pigmented skin are often fully protected even though the photodynamic pigments are present in the skin. In such animals, excess tearing or lacrimation and an abnormal intolerance to light may be the only manifestations of photosensitivity.

Photodermatitis may be primary or secondary. Primary photosensitization develops when horses eat plants containing photosensitive pigments, which are absorbed and accumulate in the skin. Two plants associated with primary photosensitization in horses are buckwheat (Fagopyrum esculentum) and St. John's wort (Hypericum perforatum). Horses are also potentially at risk from plants such as spring parsley (Cymopterus watsonii) and bishop's weed (Ammi majus), which contain photoreactive substances that induce primary photosensitization in other livestock and poultry and, therefore, may in horses.

Secondary, or hepatogenous, photosensitization occurs more commonly in animals than primary photosensitization. Unlike primary photosensitization, liver disease is the underlying cause for secondary photosensitivity. The plant toxins themselves are not photoreactive, but they cause liver damage. Once 80% or more of the liver is affected, it is unable to eliminate phylloerythrin, a normal breakdown by-product of plant chlorophyll, which then accumulates in the blood. Phylloerythrin fluoresces when exposed to ultraviolet light, causing the cellular damage resulting in photosensitization. The prognosis for animals with secondary photosensitization is always far poorer

TABLE 18–4
Hepatotoxic Plants

Common Name	Scientific Name	Toxin
See Table 18–5	Senecio spp.	Pyrrolizidine alkaloids[a]
Fiddleneck, tarweed	Amsinckia spp.	Pyrrolizidine alkaloids[a]
Rattlepod, rattlebox	Crotolaria spp.	Pyrrolizidine alkaloids[a]
Hound's tongue	Cynoglossum officinale	Pyrrolizidine alkaloids[a]
Salvation Jane[b]	Echium lycopsis[b]	Pyrrolizidine alkaloids[a]
Heliotrope, stickseed	Heliotropium spp.[b]	Pyrrolizidine alkaloids[a]
	Trichodesma spp.[b]	Pyrrolizidine alkaloids[a]
Creeping indigo[c]	Indigofera spicata[c]	Indospicine[c]
Birdsville indigo[b,c]	Indigofera dominii[b,c]	Indospicine[c]
Alsike clover pasture[d]	Trifolium hybridum	Probably a mycotoxin
Kleingrass pasture[d]	Panicum coloratum	Probably a mycotoxin

[a] In addition to signs of liver failure, often first noted by abnormal behavior followed by weight loss, icterus, bloody urine, anemia, and photosensitization (Fig. 18–18), the pyrrolizidine alkaloids also cause cancer, birth defects, and abortion with effects often not occurring for months after its ingestion.
[b] Currently not found in North America, but could be introduced and become a problem. Salvation Jane has been introduced into California; if it escapes, it may become a problematic toxic plant in North America.
[c] Several weeks of eating indigo may also result in incoordination, depression, corneal opacity, difficulty breathing, and abortion.
[d] Horses on contaminated pastures (not hay) during warm, humid weather characteristically develop acute photosensitization of thin haired and white-skinned areas (Fig. 18–18) especially around the lips, nose, and feet, which has been referred to as "dew poisoning."

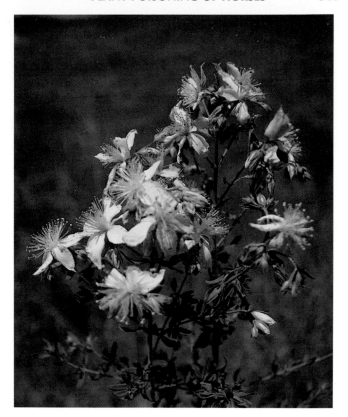

Fig. 18–19. St. John's wort or Klamath weed (Hypericum perforatum)

than that for primary photosensitization because the underlying liver disease is frequently irreversible and eventually fatal in most affected animals. The plants that are most frequently associated with secondary photosensitization in horses in North America are discussed in the next section on "Liver Disease-Inducing Plants," and are listed in Table 18–4. Those most commonly responsible for causing primary photosensitization in horses, buckwheat and St. John's wort, are described here.

Treatment of the dermatitis due to photosensitization, whether it is primary or secondary, is to keep the animal completely out of the sun, preferably stalled. Sunlight through a glass window isn't harmful, as ultraviolet rays are filtered out by the glass. Gentle daily cleaning of the skin with a mild organic iodide solution will aid recovery. Antibiotic therapy may be necessary if there is secondary bacterial infection of the skin.

St. John's Wort or Klamath Weed

St. John's wort (Hypericum perforatum) grows throughout North America. It is an erect perennial herb that grows up to 3 ft (1 m) tall with woody lower stems. The branches are opposite and sterile. Usually both stems and branches are two-edged or winged. The leaves are opposite, sessile, linear-oblong, ¾ inch (2 cm) long, and spotted with tiny dots which are translucent when held against the light. The flowering part of the plant has a cyme arrangement with numerous flowers ½ to ¾ inches (1 to 2 cm) in diameter with five bright yellow petals, five green sepals, many stamens in clusters of three to five and an ovary with three widely spreading styles (Fig. 18–19). The petals have fim-

briate margins and may have black glandular dots on the margins. These dots contain the toxin, hypericin.

Hypericin is a photodynamic pigment that remains chemically intact through digestion and is readily absorbed into the blood. It has no effect on the liver or other organs unless it is exposed to ultraviolet rays. This occurs especially in nonpigmented skin, causing primary photosensitization. Its presence in the glandular dots on the leaves suggests that all Hypericum spp. plants with similar glands are potentially capable of causing primary photosensitization. The young plants are as toxic as the mature plants and more palatable to livestock; they are thus more likely to cause poisoning in grazing animals. However, the toxin is not destroyed by drying and, therefore, hay containing it may also cause poisoning.

Buckwheat

Buckwheat (Fagopyrum esculentum) is a glabrous, herbaceous annual plant with erect stems, alternate with hastate or cordate leaves. The stipules are united as a sheath (ochrea) around the stem at the nodes. The greenish white flowers occur as terminal or axial panicles, and have eight stamens and 3-parted styles, which form 3-angled brown-colored seeds from which buckwheat flour is made (Fig. 18–20). Commonly grown as a cover crop to be plowed under for soil enrichment, it has escaped in many areas to become a weed of waste places.

Both the green and dried plant contain the pigment fago-

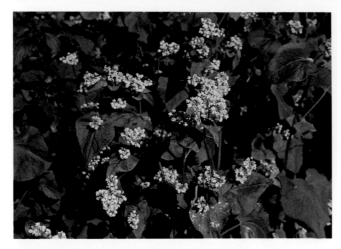

Fig. 18–20. Buckwheat (Fagopyrum esculentum) showing the typical heart-shaped leaves and white flowers

TABLE 18–5
Toxic *Senecio* Species Plants in North America

Common Names	Scientific Name
Tansy ragwort, stinking willie	S. jacobaea
Lamb's tongue groundsel	S. integerrimus
Woolly or threadleaf groundsel	S. douglasii
Ridell's ragwort	S. riddellii
Groundsel	S. plattensis
Broom groundsel	S. spartioides
Butterweed	S. glabellus
Common groundsel	S. vulgaris

pyrin, which, when ingested in sufficient quantities and then exposed to sunlight, is capable of producing primary photosensitization in all domestic livestock.

LIVER DISEASE-INDUCING PLANTS

Surprisingly, few plant toxins cause liver disease, probably because the liver has tremendous capabilities for detoxifying many compounds that are absorbed from the gastrointestinal tract. Furthermore, the liver has a great reserve capacity and will continue to function at near optimal levels until approximately 80% of it is destroyed. Only then will clinical signs of liver failure such as weight loss, depression and abnormal behavior, icterus, bloody urine, anemia, and photosensitization be observed. Photosensitization occurs because of the damaged liver's inability to eliminate the body's normal breakdown products of plant chlorophyll, which then accumulate in the blood. When these photosensitive substances are exposed to sunlight, they fluoresce, causing the skin damage responsible for secondary or hepatogenous photosensitization (Fig. 18–18). As described in the previous section, photosensitization may also be caused by the ingestion of plants, such as buckwheat (Fagopyrum esculentum) or St. John's wort (Hypericum perforatum), that contain photosensitive pigments but do not cause liver damage. Because signs of secondary or hepatogenous photosensitization, or other clinical signs of liver disease, appear only when a majority of the liver's functions are destroyed, horses showing clinical signs as a result of any plant-induced liver disease have a guarded to poor prognosis.

The most important plant toxins responsible for causing secondary photosensitization, as well as other manifestations of liver damage, are pyrrolizidine alkaloids.

Pyrrolizidine Alkaloid Poisoning

Plants Causing Pyrrolizidine Alkaloid Liver Damage

Pyrrolizidine alkaloids (PA), the major plant toxins harmful to the liver are present in a variety of plants listed in

Table 18-4. The most common in North America are the many different species of Senecio.

Senecio spp. There are some 1200 different species of Senecio that are distributed throughout the world, with about 70 species occurring in North America. Approximately 25 of these are known to be poisonous, but all species of Senecio should be considered toxic unless known otherwise. Those most commonly responsible for causing poisoning in horses in North America are listed in Table 18-5. The Senecio species have a wide overlapping geographical range in which they grow, but are selective in their habitats, some preferring high altitude, subalpine, moist conditions, while others prefer dry, rocky, sandy soils at lower elevations.

Identification of individual Senecio species is difficult. However, recognition of a plant as a member of the genus Senecio can be based on the presence of a single layer of touching, but not overlapping, greenish bracts surrounding the flower head (Fig. 18–21). Senecio species have alternate leaves that are generally lanceolate to ovate, dentate, and often irregularly and deeply pinnately divided. Some species are densely covered with white hairs. The composite heads are flattened terminal clusters with showy yellow ray and disk flowers. Seeds have a dense ring of white hairs (pappus) at one end to aid in wind distribution.

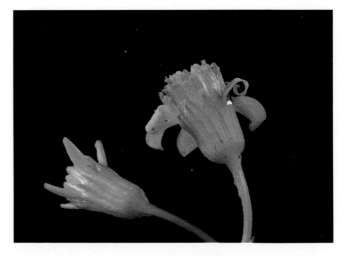

Fig. 18–21. Senecio flower showing the characteristic single layer of green bracts surrounding the yellow petals

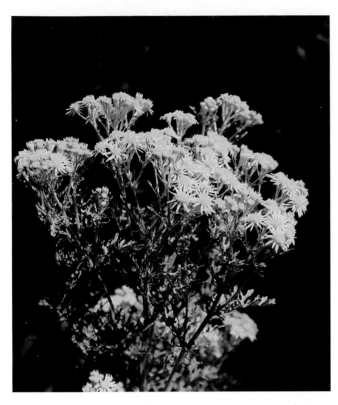

Fig. 18–22. Tansy ragwort or stinking willie (Senecio jacobaea)

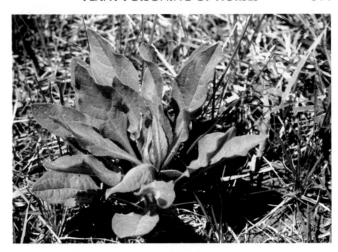

Fig. 18–23. First-year growth or rosette stage of Hounds tongue (Cynoglossum officinale)

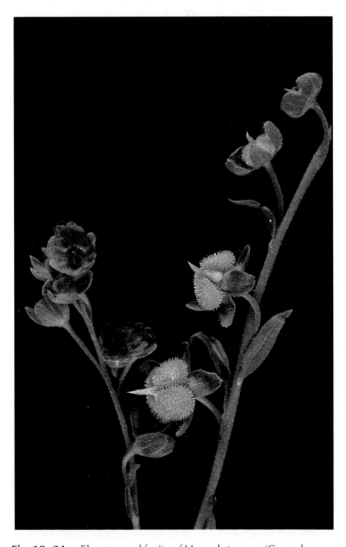

Fig. 18–24. Flowers and fruits of Hounds tongue (Cynoglossum officinale)

The PA concentration and thus toxicity of Senecio species vary considerably with the stage of growth, the mature plant being the most toxic. Ridell's ragwort (S. ridellii), when near maturity, contains exceptionally high concentrations of PA (10 to 18% dry weight). Acute poisoning and death in 1 to 2 days has been associated with a few days' consumption of Senecio plants high in PA concentration in amounts of green plant equal to 1 to 5% of the animal's body weight. Chronic poisoning, however, is more common in horses and cattle, and is usually associated with ingestion of smaller amounts of Senecio over a period of 3 weeks or longer.

Horses eating green tansy ragwort or stinking willie (S. jacobaea) (Fig. 18-22) in amounts in excess of that equal to 1 to 2% of their body weight develop clinical signs 20 days to 5 months later. This equates to a minimum 20-day cumulative or total dose equal to 2% of the animal's body weight of plant dry matter.

Hound's tongue (Cynoglossum officinale) is a PA-containing common biennial weed of cultivated and waste areas that grows up to 3 ft (1 m) tall with alternate tongue-shaped, hairy basal leaves up to 20 inches (0.5 m) long (Fig. 18-23). The upper leaves are lanceolate and sessile. The flowers are small, regular, reddish purple, and produced on terminal racemes. The fruits separate into four brown nutlets at maturity, which are covered with hooked barbs that readily attach to animal hair, aiding in their dispersal (Fig. 18-24). Hound's tongue contains the pyrrolizidine alkaloids heliosupine and echinatine, with the greatest concentration (2.1% dry weight) in the preflowering

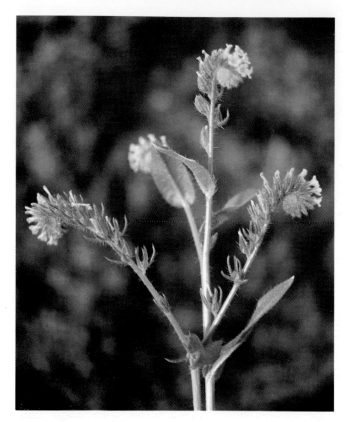

Fig. 18–25. Fiddleneck (Amsinckia intermedia) showing its characteristic fiddleneck and flowers on one side of the inflorescence

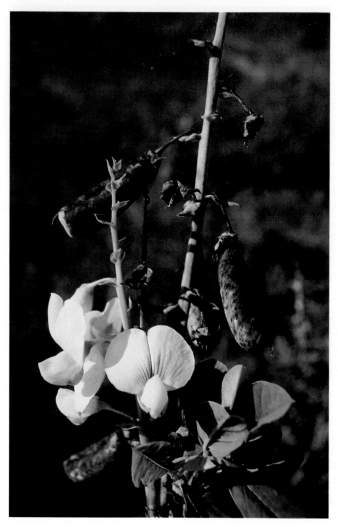

Fig. 18–26. Rattlebox or rattlepod (Crotalaria spectabilis) showing the pea-like flowers and dark seed pods

rosette stage. Although reduced in quantity, the alkaloids remain present in the dried plant.

Fiddleneck or Tarweed (Amsinckia intermedia) is an erect, sparsely branched annual weed that grows up to 3 ft (1 m) tall and is covered with numerous, fine white hairs. Leaves are hairy, lanceolate, and alternate. The perfect five-parted, small, orange to yellow flowers are born terminally on a characteristic fiddleneck-shaped raceme, with the flowers all inserted on one side of the axis (Fig. 18–25). Mature fruits separate into two to four black-ridged nutlets.

Horses, cattle, and pigs have been poisoned by eating fiddleneck plants, especially the seeds. The symptoms and lesions in all species of animals consist of liver damage and fibrosis characteristic of pyrrolizidine alkaloid poisoning. Amsinckia species have also been reported to accumulate levels of nitrate potentially toxic to ruminants but probably not horses (see section on "Nitrate Poisoning" in Chapter 19).

Rattlebox or Rattlepod (Crotalaria spp.) are erect, herbaceous, variably hairy plants that may be annuals or perennials. The leaves are simple, alternate, lanceolate to obovate, with a finely haired undersurface. The flowers are yellow, with the leguminous calyx longer than the corolla (Fig. 18–26). The fruit is a leguminous pod, inflated, hairless, becoming black with maturity, and containing 10 to 20 glossy, black, heart-shaped seeds, which often detach and rattle within the pod. Several species of Crotalaria have

been associated with livestock poisoning, including C. sagittalis, C. spectabilis, and C. retusa.

Crotalaria species contain pyrrolizidine alkaloids, the most notable of which is monocrotaline. It is present in greatest quantity in the seeds, lesser amounts being present in the leaves and stems. All livestock, including domestic fowl, are susceptible to poisoning. Although acute deaths will occur from eating large quantities of the Crotalaria seeds or plant, more often, as with other pyrrolizidine alkaloid-containing plants, clinical signs typical of this toxin develop from a few days to up to 6 months later.

Effects of Pyrrolizidine Alkaloids

Variations in the PA content of plants, the quantity eaten, and susceptibility of individual animal species result in wide variations in the severity of PA poisoning in animals. Flowers tend to contain the greatest amount of the alkaloid, although seeds of rattlebox or rattlepod, fiddleneck, and tarweed contain high levels of PA.

Pigs are the most susceptible to the effects of PA, followed by poultry, cattle, horses, goats, and sheep. Sheep can eat approximately 20 times the amount of Senecio it would take to poison a cow on an equivalent bodyweight basis. Horses show about the same susceptibility to pyrrolizidine toxicosis as do cattle. The chronic lethal dose of dried tansy ragwort (S. jacobaea) in cattle is only 0.02 to 0.05 mg/kg body weight fed over several months. This would equate to a 1000 lb (450-kg) horse eating about 5% of its body weight of green tansy ragwort over a period of 1 to 3 months.

Fortunately, herbivores will not readily eat plants containing PA unless they are forced to do so through lack of other feed. However, the dried plants, which have only a minimal reduction in their alkaloid content, are more palatable, making them a particular risk when present in hay. Although acute poisoning and death can occur from a few days' consumption of plants high in PA, chronic poisoning is more common. The effects of PA are cumulative, so symptoms of liver disease and photosensitization may not appear for many months after animals have eaten toxic quantities of PA-containing plants. This makes identification of the suspected poisonous plants difficult, since the plants will often not be present in the pasture or hay when clinical signs become evident in the horse.

Pyrrolidizine alkaloids are readily absorbed from the digestive tract of horses and are converted in the liver to toxic substances that bind to cellular proteins, causing rapid liver cell death. Similar cellular damage may also occur in the kidneys, intestinal tract, and lungs. Pyrrolizidine alkaloids may also induce cancer, birth defects and abortion. Although secretion of PA in mare's milk has not been established, there is potential risk to the suckling foal, as PA has been shown to be present in small quantities in the milk of cows and goats fed tansy ragwort (Senecio jacobaea).

Acute PA poisoning occurs occasionally in horses that ingest large amounts of alkaloid-containing plants over a few days. Affected animals may show only depression, coma, and death as a result of severe liver damage.

Chronic PA poisoning, which is more common, is characterized by irreversible liver disease clinically manifested by one or more of the following clinical signs: weight loss, nervous signs, icterus, anemia, bloody urine, and photosensitization. Nervous signs due to liver damage are often the first clinical indication of PA poisoning, and may include drowsiness, head pressing, blindness, aimless wandering or "walking disease," frequent yawning, and incessant licking of objects. The first sign of PA poisoning in a small percentage of horses is difficulty in breathing in, destruction of red blood cells and a bloody urine. Photosensitization may occur in some horses that have areas of nonpigmented skin (Fig. 18–18). In these horses, severe dermatitis that develops when the horses are exposed to sunlight results from the liver's failure to excrete phyloerythrin, a photoreactive by-product of chlorophyll breakdown. Photosensitization is described earlier in this chapter in the section on primary photodermatitis.

Pyrrolizidine alkaloid poisoning is usually not suspected and, therefore, not detected until severe liver damage has occurred and clinical signs of liver failure are evident. At the present time, the only widely available and reliable means of confirming PA-induced liver failure is detecting specific microscopic alterations in a liver biopsy. The only

other disease to mimic these alterations is aflatoxin poisoning, which occurs when horses eat moldy grains containing aflatoxins, but which, as described in Chapter 19, is uncommon in horses.

Horses showing signs of liver disease should be fed as described in that section of Chapter 17. However, the prognosis is poor for confirmed cases of PA poisoning.

Animals showing signs of photosensitization should be provided shelter from the sun and preferably kept stalled completely out of sunlight. Sunlight through glass will not induce photosensitization as it blocks ultraviolet rays. Gentle daily cleaning of the affected skin with a mild organic iodine antiseptic solution will aid in the healing process. Antibiotics may be indicated in cases where there is severe secondary bacterial infection of the skin.

Nonpyrrolizidine Alkaloid Liver Poisoning Plants

Indigo

Creeping indigo (Indigofera spicata) is a legume that was introduced into southern Florida, where it has become well established. It causes a fatal neurologic disease resulting from liver failure. The disease of horses known in Florida as "grove poisoning," originally thought to be due to chemicals used in the citrus industry, is now known to be due to horses' eating creeping indigo. In Australia, a similar disease of horses and other livestock referred to as "Birdsville disease" is caused by Birdsville indigo (Indigofera dominii).

Creeping indigo is a prostrate plant of tropical and subtropical areas with many branched runners fanning out from a crown of a white tapering taproot that may be up to 3 ft (1 m) in length. The stems are usually pale green with alternate pinnate leaves and alternate ovate leaflets on a short petiole (Fig. 18–27). The pink to dark red flowers are produced on short spikes from the leaf axils. The pointed seed pods are produced in downward-pointing clusters. The plant is a prolific seed producer and tends therefore to be capable of spreading readily.

The liver poison amino acid indospicine is present in various species of Indigofera. The leaves may contain from

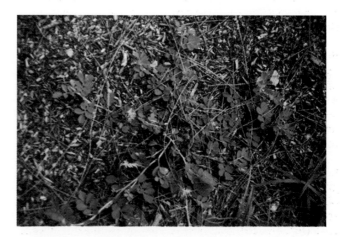

Fig. 18–27. Creeping indigo (Indigofera spicata): young flowering plant showing prostrate form (Courtesy of Dr. Julia F. Morton, University of Miami, Coral Gables, FL)

TABLE 18–6
Protein, Sulfur-Containing Amino Acid, and Arginine Content of Horse Feeds

Feed	% Protein in Air Dry Feed	% Cysteine + Methionine in Air Dry Feed	% Cysteine + Methionine in the Protein[a]	Arginine % in Air Dry Feed	Arginine % in the Protein[a]
Alfalfa	17	0.52	3.1	0.73	4.3
Corn	9	0.18	2.0	0.45	5.0
Cottonseed meal	41	1.5	3.7	4.25	10.4
Fish meal	61–66	2.7–3.2	4.5–4.8	4–4.5	6.5–6.8
Grain, small	11–13	0.3–0.45	3.0–3.5	0.5–0.8	4.6–6.6
Peanut meal	47	1.0	2.1	5.9	12.5
Rapeseed meal	41	1.5	3.7	1.9	4.7
Soybean meal	46	1.3	2.8	3.2	7.0
Sunflower seed meal	47	2.2	4.7	3.5	7.5
Wheat bran	16	0.4	2.5	1.0	6.2
Yeast, brewer's	45	1.2	2.7	2.2	4.9

[a] The most important value to consider in selecting a feed high in these amino acids. It is the (% amino acids) ÷ (% protein) in the feed.

0.1 to 0.5% of this toxin in their dry weight, and the seeds as much as 2.0%. Horses apparently find the plant highly palatable and seek it out. The toxin acts as a specific antagonist of the amino acid arginine and, therefore, is an inhibitor of protein synthesis. Horses fed sufficient peanut meal or cottonseed meal, both of which are rich in arginine, are protected from the effects of this toxin. Arginine constitutes 10 to 12% of the protein in these two protein supplements as compared to 4 to 7% in other horse feeds (Table 18–6).

After consuming creeping indigo for several weeks, affected horses develop incoordination, difficulty in turning, and inability to walk in a straight line; they eventually collapse. They become severely depressed, lose weight, and have been reported to develop corneal opacity and respiratory difficulty. Affected pregnant mares may abort. Death results from liver failure. Animals eating meat from horses that have been poisoned by creeping indigo may suffer similar fatal poisoning.

Alsike Clover and Klein grass

Occasionally horses grazing clover, generally alsike clover (Trifolium hybridum), during wet or humid weather, develop a photosensitivity and hepatitis referred to as trifoliosis. A similar condition may also occur in horses or sheep grazing klein grass (Panicum coloratum) pastures during wet or humid weather. The toxin responsible for either trifoliosis or klein grass poisoning has not been identified, but the sporadic nature of the diseases and their occurrence only during wet humid weather suggest that mycotoxins, or plant metabolites produced under humid, high-moisture growth conditions, may be responsible.

Affected horses on clover pasture characteristically develop an acute photosensitization involving thinly haired and white-skinned areas (see Fig. 18–18), especially around the lips, nose, and feet. The condition has been referred to as "dew poisoning" because there is an association between the location of the dermatitis and contact with moisture present on the dew-laden clover pasture. Affected horses may exhibit icterus and other signs of liver disease. In such cases, there may be significant liver enlargement and evidence of liver degeneration. Horses generally recover rapidly from the photosensitivity if they are removed from the toxic pasture. Horses may graze the

pasture again without problem under different growing conditions in subsequent years or after the pasture dries out.

NEUROLOGIC DISEASE-INDUCING PLANTS

Behavioral alterations, blindness, inability to ingest and chew food, incoordination, depression, convulsions, and other physical abnormalities are all indicators of nervous system disorders. The brain, spinal cord, and peripheral nervous systems are susceptible to a variety of infectious, toxic and congenital diseases that are often indistinguishable clinically. A variety of plants that grow throughout North America are known to produce neurologic abnormalities in horses and, therefore, should be considered in the differential diagnosis of nervous system disorders. These plants, along with the major clinical signs they cause in poisoned horses, are listed in Table 18-7.

Sagebrush

The sagebrushes (Artemisia spp.) of the western United States are perennials ranging from the woody-stemmed 3 to 10 ft (1 to 3 m) tall big sagebrush (A. tridentata) to the smaller sand sage (A. filifolia) (Fig. 18-28) and the low-growing fringed sage (A. frigida) (Fig. 18-29). Considerable variation exists in the 200 or more species of sagebrush. Leaves are usually alternate, covered with very fine hairs that give the leaves a silvery green appearance, and when crushed give the characteristic smell of sage. Flowers are usually inconspicuous and born on panicles from the leaf axils.

The toxins in sagebrush are volatile monoterpenoid oils, which vary considerably in quantity depending on growing conditions and season, being highest in the fall and winter months.

Sand sage (A. filifolia), common in the sandy soils along the eastern side of the Rocky Mountains and south into Mexico, has been associated with a syndrome in horses called "sage sickness." Budsage (A. spinescens) has been reported to cause similar problems in California and Nevada. Recently the author encountered a neurologic disease of horses that were wintered on an overgrazed range in Colorado where fringed sage (A. frigida) was the predominant forage available.

TABLE 18–7
Neurotoxic Plants and Their Effects on Horses

Common Name	Scientific Name	Plant Neurotoxin	Food Intake	Sali-vation	Muscle Tremors	Gait	Abnormal Behavior[a]	Depressed or Weak[a]	Excitable	Miscellaneous	Recovery
Sagebrush	Artemisia spp.	Monoterpenoids	Normal	–	–	Forelimb incoordination & falling	+	–	+	Sage smell on breath & feces	1–2 weeks
Locoweed	Oxytropis and Astragalus spp.	Indolizidine alkaloids (IA)	Decreased	–	–	Incoordination, falling, high steps, head bobbing	+ + +	+ +	+ + +	Lymphocyte vacuoles	Partial only
Milkvetch	Astragalus spp.	Nitroglycosides & IA	Decreased	–	–	Incoordination, posterior weakness	–	+	–	Difficult respiration	Partial
Yellow star thistle & Russian knapweed	Centaurea solstitialis C. or Acroptilon repens	Sesquiterpene lactone?	Can't eat	+ +	–	Possible circling & head tossing	+	–	–	Abrupt onset of open mouth, tongue out, inability to prehend or chew feed	No
Horsetail, marestail, horserush, or snake grass	Equisetum spp.	Thiaminase	Normal	–	±	Rear leg incoordination, reluctance to move	–	+	–	Possible blindness, diarrhea, or constipation	
Bracken fern / Sensitive fern	Pteridium aquilinum Onoclea sensiblis	Thiaminase	Decreased	–	–	Rear leg incoordination	–	+ +	–	Serum thiamin low & pyruvate high	Yes, with vitamin B₁ injections
White snakeroot / Crofton weed / Jimmyweed or rayless goldenrod / Burrow weed	Eupatorium rugosae Eupatorium adenophorum Haplopappus heterophyllus Haplopappus tenuisectus	Tremetol	Decreased; difficulty swallowing, & choking appearance	+ +	+ + +	Incoordination	–	+	–	Patchy sweating, heart degeneration	Recovery or death within a few days
Johnson grass / Sudan grass	Sorghum halepense Sorghum sudanense	Cyanogenic glycosides	Normal	–	–	Rear leg incoordination; and sitting or falling when backed	–	±	–	Urinary incontinence; bladder & possibly vulva, rectum & tail paralysis; rarely sudden death	Yes early; later partial

[a] Also caused by liver disease-inducing plants (Table 18–4) and other causes of neurologic diseases given in Table 19–5.

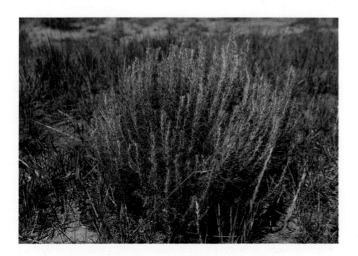

Fig. 18–28. Sand sage (Artemisia filifolia)

Although the actual toxin that causes sage sickness has not been defined, some monoterpenes present in Artemisia species are known to be toxic to the nervous system. Thujone, a monoterpene present in wormwood (A. absinthium), has been associated with a neurologic syndrome in people who chronically consume absinthe, the alcoholic beverage produced from wormwood. A similar poisoning is presumed to develop in horses that consume a sufficient quantity of sage.

Horses appear to develop neurologic signs after they are forced to eat sagebrush because other forage is depleted or unavailable either as a result of deep snow cover or pasture overgrazing. After eating sage for several days, horses suddenly exhibit abnormal behavior characterized by incoordination and a tendency to fall down or react abnormally to stimuli that would not normally have elicited such a response. Tying an affected horse to a fence, for

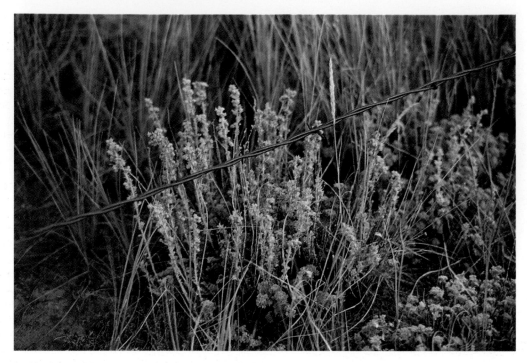

Fig. 18–29. Fringed sage (Artemisia frigida)

example, will cause the animal to pull back violently, eventually throwing itself to the ground in panic. If left undisturbed, the animal will recover and act relatively normal. Incoordination is particularly noticeable in the forequarters, with the hindquarters seemingly normal. Some animals may circle incessantly; others may become excitable and unpredictable. The characteristic smell of sage is often noticeable on the breath and in the feces. Sage-poisoned horses maintain an appetite and have a normal temperature, pulse, and respiration. The clinical signs closely resemble those of a horse that has been poisoned by locoweed. However, unlike "locoed" horses that do not recover, "saged" horses tend to recover in 1 to 2 weeks after they stop eating sage and are fed a nutritious diet. Supportive therapy, including protection from extreme climatic conditions will aid in the recovery. They should not be ridden until fully recovered and evaluated for normal behavior and neurologic function.

Locoweeds and Milkvetches

Several hundred species of locoweed and milkvetch (Astragalus spp.) occur in North America, many of which are known to cause severe poisoning of livestock. This large group of legumes is taxonomically very difficult to identify, even by the experienced botanist. The genus Oxytropis, which like many Astragalus spp. is also commonly called locoweed, is a closely related genus and produces identical locoism in horses, cattle, sheep, and elk. However, not all species of Astragalus are toxic, and some are useful forage plants.

Astragalus spp. are perennial legumes growing to a height of up to 3 ft (1 m), with branching stems from a stout crown and extensive taproot. The leaves are alter-

nate, pinnately compound, with each leaflet being elliptical or oval and minutely hairy. The racemes are usually produced at the ends of the branches and are densely covered with white to purple pea-like flowers, depending on the species. The leguminous seed pods vary considerably in shape and contain many bean-shaped seeds (Fig. 18-30).

Oxytropis species differ from Astragalus in that their hairy leaves and flower stems arise directly from the taproot crown. The leaves are pinnately compound, with each having a single apical elliptical leaflet. The flowers are either white (O. sericea) or purple (O. lambertii) in color and have a characteristic pointed keel (Figs. 18-31 and 18-32).

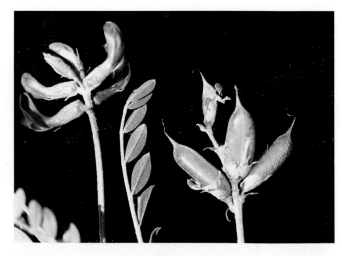

Fig. 18–30. Locoweed (Astragalus spp.) showing the typical flowers, leaves and pea-like seed pods (see also Fig. 18–60)

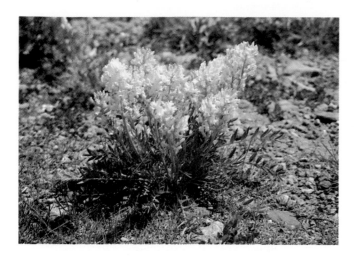

Fig. 18–31. White locoweed (Oxytropis sericea)

Locoism, blind staggers, alkali disease, and a syndrome characterized by respiratory difficulty and incoordination have all been attributed to species of Astragalus and Oxytropis. Three distinct syndromes are now recognized by

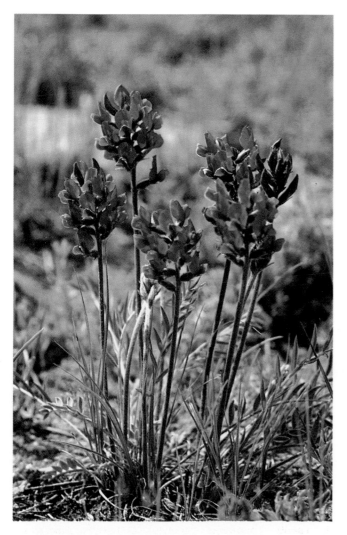

Fig. 18–32. Purple locoweed (Oxytropis lambertii)

virtue of the different toxins that various species of these plants may accumulate. The Astragalus species can be categorized into the locoweeds that contain indolizidine alkaloids (swainsonine), the milkvetches that contain nitroglycosides (miserotoxin) and the milkvetches that, as discussed in the section in this chapter on lameness, accumulate toxic amounts of selenium. Some species may contain more than one of the toxins and consequently may cause a combination of clinical signs in affected animals.

Locoweed Neurologic Poisoning

Locoism results from the cumulative effects of the toxin swainsonine, named after its isolation from various species of Swainsona (Darling pea) in Australia. It has subsequently been demonstrated in Astragalus lentiginosus, A. mollisimus, and A. bisulcatus, amongst others, and Oxytropis lambertii, and O. sericea in North America. Signs of poisoning do not become evident until animals have consumed significant quantities of locoweed over many weeks and the toxic threshold is reached. Some horses develop an addiction for locoweed, seeking it out even when normal forages are present. Young animals are most severely affected, as maturing nerve cells are more vulnerable to the effects of the toxin. The toxin causes a generalized lysosomal storage disease, eventually causing irreversible nerve cell damage similar to the disease mannosidosis in people.

The most noticeable feature of locoism is the change in the normal behavior of affected horses. Incoordination, high stepping gait, head bobbing, marked excitement, and overreaction to various stimuli are typical of locoism. Some horses become totally unpredictable in their response to handling and may fall down when being haltered or ridden. When left alone they become progressively depressed and lose weight due to their impaired ability to take food into the mouth. If removed from the source of the locoweed and fed a nutritious diet, horses will show improvement and appear relatively normal after several months. However, if the horse has been chronically affected by locoism, the animal will recover only partially and will remain a liability to human safety. The prognosis for locoed horses therefore is always poor.

Pregnant mares that consume quantities of wooly loco (A. mollisimus) in early gestation may produce foals with various limb deformities. The teratogenic effects of the Astragalus will be discussed further in the section on teratogenic plants.

There is no proven effective treatment for locoweed poisoning in horses. Further access to the plants should be prevented immediately and in every year thereafter, as horses may retain an addiction to the plants from year to year.

Milkvetch Neurologic Poisoning

Nitroglycosides or nitrotoxins have been demonstrated in some 263 species of milkvetch (Astragalus spp.). These plants are found growing in vast areas of rangelands in the western United States, Canada, and northern Mexico, and have been associated with severe livestock losses. Horses, although not frequently affected, are susceptible to poisoning by these nitrotoxins.

Nitrotoxin-containing Astragalus contains at least two toxic compounds. These toxins, once absorbed from the digestive tract, act primarily on the respiratory and central nervous system, causing initially depression, incoordination, and hindleg weakness. Difficulty in breathing, weight loss, and paralysis of the hindquarters develop as the animal continues to eat milkvetch. Animals appear to recover if they are removed from the source of the plants before neurologic signs become too severe.

Yellow Star Thistle and Russian Knapweed

Horses that eat yellow star thistle (Centaurea solstitialis) or Russian knapweed (C. or Acroptilon repens) for prolonged periods develop an irreversible brain disease called nigropallidal encephalomalacia, because it causes a softening or dissolution (encephalomalacia) of the nigropallidal areas of the brain. This damage destroys the horse's ability to take in and masticate food. The disease occurs only in horses and only in those areas of the western United States, Australia, and Argentina where these plants are abundant. Cattle and sheep appear to be able to eat both yellow star thistle and Russian knapweed without problem.

Yellow star thistle originated in the Mediterranean area. It has become extensively established in California and has spread through the southern states to the Atlantic coast. It is an annual weed, with multiple branching stems growing to 3 ft (1 m) in height. The stems have longitudinal wings or ridges formed by the downward extension of the leaf bases. The basal leaves are markedly lobed, with the stem leaves being linear and covered with fine white hairs. The characteristic, star-like yellow flowers are produced at the ends of the branches and are protected by bracts with long spines (Figs. 18-33 and 18-34). The seeds have a terminal tuft of whitish hairs.

Russian knapweed was introduced from Russia and has become a noxious weed in many Rocky Mountain states. It is a perennial with woody stems up to 3 ft (1 m) tall and invasive, branching underground stems. The name knapweed is derived from the grey hairs, or knap, that cover

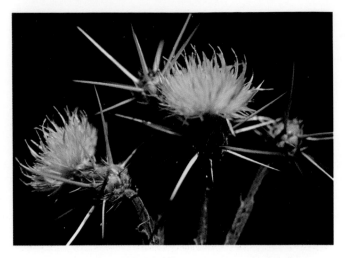

Fig. 18-34. Yellow star thistle (Centaurea solstitialis) showing the long spiny bracts surrounding the yellow flowers

the leaves and stems, giving the plant a grey green appearance. The stems branch terminally and end in a purple thistle-like flower (Fig. 18-35). The bracts are papery white and lack the stiff long spines seen in yellow star thistle. The seed heads tend to remain closed and do not shed the seeds readily.

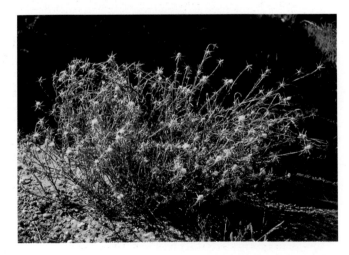

Fig. 18-33. Plant of yellow star thistle (Centaurea solstitialis)

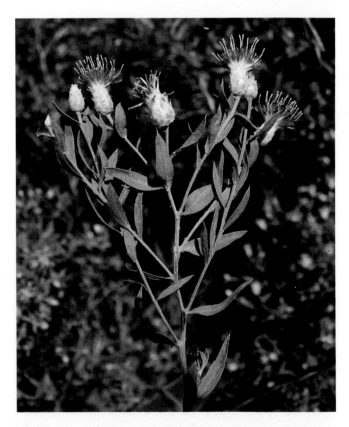

Fig. 18-35. Russian knapweed (Centaurea repens or Acroptilon repens) with spineless papery bracts surrounding the thistle-like flowers

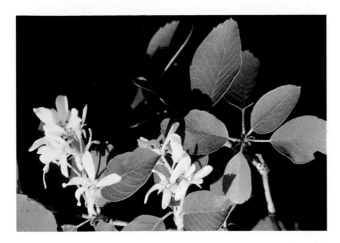

Fig. 18–61. Serviceberry or Saskatoon berry (Amelanchier alnifolia) flowers

bicular in shape and with margins coarsely serrate or dentate (Fig. 18–61). The inflorescence is a raceme with perfect regular flowers (Fig. 18–61). The five petals are white and ¼ to ⅜ inch (6 to 10 mm) long. The ovary has five styles, developing into a purple pome when ripe.

Wild Blue Flax (Linum spp.). This plant is widely distributed throughout North America. It is a herbaceous perennial with tough slender stems and alternate slender leaves. Its bright blue flowers have five petals that drop off by midday (Fig. 18–62). New flowers open each day. The young succulent plants are particularly toxic.

Western Chokecherry (Prunus virginiana). This commonly grows in thickets, especially along waterways, mountainsides below about 8000 ft (2500 m) elevation, and occasionally in the drier plains. It grows to about 8 to 12 ft (2.5 to 3.5 m) high as a shrub or small tree with gray bark marked by lenticels running around the stems. The leaves are simple, glossy, and alternate with serrated margins and a few glands on the petiole or base of the blade. The inflorescence is a cylindrical raceme of showy white fragrant flowers appearing in early spring after the leaves have appeared (Fig. 18–63). The fruit changes from a red to a dark purple drupe when ripe. It is the only edible part of the plant, having an astringent but sweet taste when ripe. Other members of the genus known to be toxic include Pin cherry (P. pennsylvanica) and wild black cherry (P. serotina).

Elderberry (Sambucus spp.). This is a woody shrub growing 6 to 10 ft (2 to 3 m) high and forming colonies from underground runners. Generally, elderberry bushes prefer open areas in the rich moist soils surrounding ponds and along ditches and streams. The stems are thick and are filled with a white pith. The leaves are opposite, pinnately compound, and with lanceolate serrated leaflets. It has conspicuous, terminal, round or flat-topped clusters of white five-petaled flowers about 3/16 inch (4 to 6 mm) in diameter (Fig. 18–64). Drooping clusters of dark purple (S. canadensis) or red (S. racemosa), juicy edible berries with several seeds form from July to September.

Sorghum Grasses. Johnson grass (Sorghum halepense) is a coarse, drought-resistant perennial in the south-

ern states and an annual in the northern states. It has scaly root stalks and relatively broad leaves, and grows 6 to 8 ft (1 to 2 m) tall (Fig. 18–39) as described previously in the section on "Neurologic Disease-Inducing Plants." Sudan grass (S. sudanense) and its hybrids are corn-like in appearance (Figs. 18–40, and 18–41) and are often grown as a forage crop. Cyanide-free varieties are available and are useful as a forage crop.

Arrow, Pod or Goose Grass (Triglochin spp.). This plant grows at most elevations throughout North America, preferring wet alkaline soils. It flourishes in marshy ground and irrigated pastures, often growing in native meadows cut for hay. It is a perennial grass-like plant with fleshy, half-rounded, dark green leaves clumped at the base of the plant. Leaves are 5 to 7 inches (12 to 18 cm) long, linear, unjointed, and sheathed at the base. The inflorescence is a pedicled raceme from 1.6 to 5 ft (0.5-1.5 m) in length that appears as an unbranched, unjoined flower spike (Fig. 18–65). The flowers are inconspicuous and numerous, with a greenish, six-parted perianth. The fruits are made up of three- to six-celled capsules that turn a golden brown before splitting.

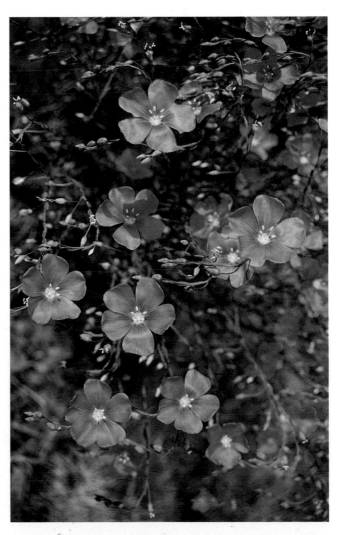

Fig. 18–62. Wild blue flax (Linum spp.)

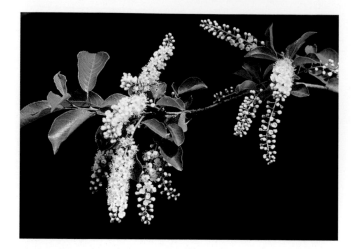

Fig. 18–63. Western chokecherry (Prunus virginiana flowers)

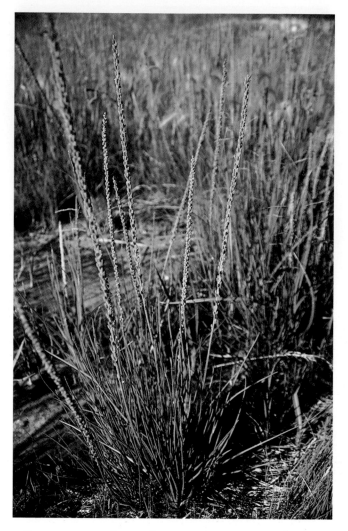

Fig. 18–65. Arrow, pod, or goose grass (Triglochin spp.)

Effects of Cyanogenic Glycosides

Plants rarely contain free hydrogen cyanide (hydrocyanic or prussic acid) but rather have one or more complex cyanogenic glycosides in their leaves and stems. When acted upon by plant enzymes, these glycosides form hydrogen cyanide. This enzymatic conversion occurs when plant cells are damaged or stressed as they are chewed, crushed, droughted, wilted, or frozen. Application of herbicides and nitrate fertilizers may increase the cyanogenic glycoside content of plants. Generally all parts of the plant are toxic, with the young rapidly growing portion of the plant and the seeds being most toxic. Drying of the plant reduces its cyanogenic content.

Ruminants are more likely to be poisoned by plant cyanogenic glycosides than are horses and other simple-stomached animals, because the less acidic rumen (pH 6-7), with its high water and bacterial enzyme content, optimizes the rapid hydrolysis of the glycosides to cyanide. Animals that drink water immediately after eating cyanogenic plants enhance the hydrolysis of the glycosides to

cyanide. Acute cyanide poisoning depends on the rapid ingestion of large quantities of plant material high in glycosides and its conversion to cyanide faster than the animal's ability to detoxify the cyanide.

Cyanide is highly toxic to all animals. It is readily absorbed from the intestinal and respiratory tracts. The cyanide ion binds with iron in hemoglobin, inhibiting its release of oxygen from the blood. This results in the characteristic cherry-red color of venous blood that occurs in acute cyanide poisonings. Normally, small quantities of cyanide are detoxified and excreted in the urine. If there is plenty of other plant material and carbohydrate present in the gastrointestinal tract, formation and absorption of cyanide may be slowed, thus allowing the animal to tolerate a higher dose of cyanide. Plant material containing more than 200 ppm of cyanide (200 mg/kg) in its dry matter is potentially lethal to all animals.

Animals poisoned by cyanide usually die within minutes of consuming a toxic amount. If observed early, poisoned animals show rapid labored breathing, frothing at the mouth, dilated pupils, incoordination, muscle tremors, and convulsions. The mucous membranes are often dark red

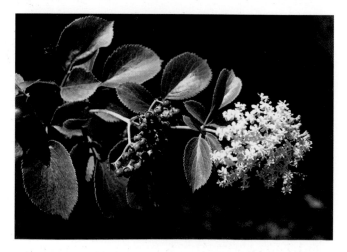

Fig. 18–64. Elderberry (Sambuccus spp.) flowers and fruits

to cyanotic in color because the animal is near death even though the hemoglobin is saturated with oxygen. These acute cyanide poisoning effects are quite different from chronic cyanide poisoning that causes neurologic disease in horses consuming sorghum hays or pasture forages with low levels of cyanide, as discussed previously in the section on Neurologic Disease-Inducing Plants.

Successful treatment of acute cyanide poisoning depends on detoxification of the cyanide radicle to thiocyanate. Traditionally this has been accomplished by intravenously injecting sodium nitrite and sodium thiosulfate.

Cardiac Glycoside-Induced Sudden Death

Plant Causes of Cardiac Glycoside Poisoning

At least 34 plant genera contain cardiac glycosides that are potentially toxic to man and animals, but relatively few have attained notoriety as causes of animal poisoning. The most important cardiac glycoside-containing plants in North America are listed in Table 18-12. These include foxglove (Digitalis spp.), oleander (Nerium oleander), and lily of the valley (Convallaria majalis), which are widely grown as ornamental plants and have escaped to become established in the wild. Dogbane, or Indian hemp, (Apocynum cannabinum) is an indigenous plant containing cardiac glycosides but is rarely a problem to livestock. Milkweeds are common cardiac glycoside-containing plants that are widely distributed throughout much of North America and are toxic green or dried.

Milkweed (Asclepias spp.). The species of milkweeds that have been identified as causes of cardiac glycoside poisoning in sheep, goats, cattle, horses, and domestic fowl are listed in Table 18-13, as are their relative toxicities. Greatest losses have occurred in sheep on western rangelands, but all animals are susceptible to poisoning, especially when other forages are scarce or milkweed is incorporated in their hay.

Milkweed is an erect perennial herb that has either 2.5- to 5-inch (6- to 12-cm) broad-veined leaves or narrow linear leaves seldom more than 1 to 1.5 inches (2 to 4 cm) wide

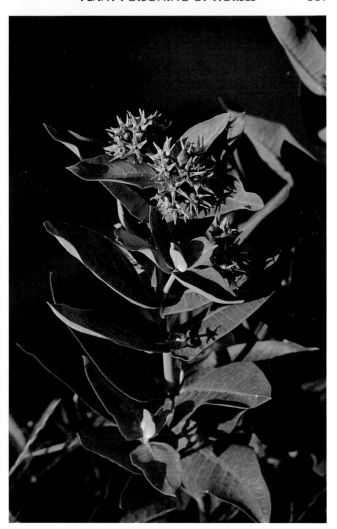

Fig. 18–66. Milkweed flowers (Asclepias speciosa) showing the characteristic horn-like modified petal

TABLE 18–13
Common Toxic Milkweeds

Common Name	Scientific Name	Toxicity[a]
Labriform milkweed	Asclepias labriformis	0.05
Western whorled milkweed	A. subverticillata	0.2
Eastern whorled milkweed	A. verticillata	0.2
Woolypod milkweed	A. eriocarpa	0.25
Milkweed	A. asperula	1–2
Plains or dwarf milkweed	A. pumila	1–2
Swamp milkweed	A. incarnata	1–2
Mexican whorled milkweed	A. mexicana	2
Showy milkweed	A. speciosa	2–5
Broad-leaf milkweed	A. latifolia	1
Narrow-leafed milkweed	A. stenophylla	?
Butterfly weed	A. tuberosa	?
Milkweed	A. hirtella	?
Antelope horn milkweed	A. viridis	?

[a] Amount of green plant as a percent of the animal's body weight that is lethal.

arranged either alternately or in whorls. Most species of milkweed (except butterfly weed, or A. tuberosa) contain a milky sap from which the plant derives its name. The flowers are produced in terminal or axillary umbels consisting of two 5-parted whorls of petals, the inner one being modified into a characteristic horn-like projection (Fig. 18-66). The color of the flowers varies from greenish white to red. The characteristic follicle or pod contains many seeds, each with a tuft of silky white hairs (Fig. 18-67). The narrow-leafed species (Fig. 18-68) generally tend to be the most toxic. They grow in open areas along roadsides, waterways, and disturbed areas, preferring the sandy soils of the plains and foothills. Overgrazing will enhance the encroachment of milkweed.

Foxglove (Digitalis purpurea). Foxglove is a native plant of Europe that was introduced to North America and escaped cultivation to become widespread in the northwest. It prefers disturbed rich soils along roadsides, fences, and unused areas. It is a perennial herb growing 3 to 5 ft (1 to 1.5 m) tall with alternate toothed, hairy basal leaves. The characteristic purple or white tubular pendant flowers

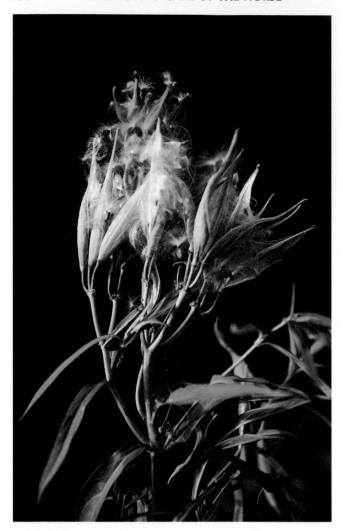

Fig. 18–67. Milkweed pods and seeds (Asclepias incarnata)

triangular, turning yellow to black when ripe. Both species, native to tropical America, are widely cultivated in the southern United States and Hawaii, and are a potential source of cardiac glycoside poisoning to all animals.

Effects of Cardiac Glycosides

Cardiac glycosides are found in all plant parts with their concentrations highest during rapid plant growth. Toxicity varies with the plant and growing conditions; however, all oleanders, foxglove, and milkweed should be considered potentially poisonous, especially the oleanders, foxglove, and narrow-leafed species of milkweeds. Very little of these plants needs to be eaten to invoke the potent effect of these toxins. In cattle and horses, as little as 0.005% body weight, or less than 1 oz for the 1100-lb horse (25 g/500-kg horse) of green oleander leaves, is lethal. About $\frac{1}{2}$ lb of green labriform milkweed is lethal to the 1100-lb (250 g/500 kg) horse. The relative toxicities of the various species of milkweed are given in Table 18–13. Horses, however, rarely eat green oleander or milkweed plants, apparently because of their taste, but do seem to find the dried leaves more palatable. Because the cardiac glycosides

have conspicuous spots on the inside bottom surface of the tube (Fig. 18–69).

Oleander (Nerium oleander). This plant was introduced from the Mediterranean area. It is an evergreen, showy flowering shrub found in southern states from California to Florida. It is also grown as a potted house plant in northern climates. It is a perennial shrub or small tree up to 25 ft (8 m) tall with whorled, simple, narrow leathery leaves. All parts of the plant contain a sticky white sap. The showy white, pink, or red flowers (Fig. 18–70) with five or more petals are produced in the spring and summer. Fruit pods contain many seeds, each with a tuft of brown hairs.

Yellow Oleander, Be-Still or Lucky Nut Tree (Thevetia spp.). Yellow oleander (T. peruviana) is a perennial branched shrub or tree growing 30 ft (9 m) tall with dark green, glossy, alternate linear leaves up to 6 inches (15 cm) long and $\frac{1}{2}$ inch (1 cm) wide containing a milky sap. The yellow to orange, showy, 5-petalled tubular flowers are produced in clusters at the ends of branches (Fig. 18–71). T. thevetioides is similar but tends to be much larger and has larger yellow flowers. Fruits are fleshy and

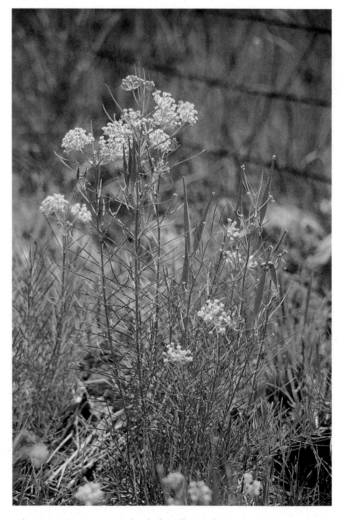

Fig. 18–68. Narrow-leafed milkweed (Asclepias mexicana)

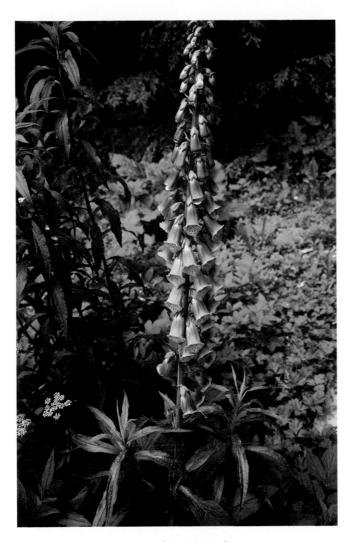

Fig. 18–69. Foxglove (Digitalis purpurea)

vomiting, and diarrhea are also signs commonly encountered in animals poisoned with cardiac glycosides. If observed early in the course of poisoning, animals will exhibit labored breathing which may be rapid, although it is slow in sheep poisoned by milkweed. They also exhibit muscular tremors, incoordination, inability to stand, bloating, and colic prior to death. Horses, once unable to stand, have periods of tetany and chewing movements. The extremities are cold and there is a rapid, irregular and weak pulse due to the decreased heart output. All types of abnormal heart rhythms and heart blocks may occur at various stages of cardiac glycoside poisoning. The duration of symptoms rarely exceeds 24 hours before death occurs. Convulsions prior to death are not common.

There is no specific treatment for counteracting the effects of cardiac glycosides. Affected horses are usually given adsorbents such as activated charcoal by stomach tube with a saline laxative to prevent further toxin absorption. The heart irregularities also may be treated. Poisoned animals should be removed from the source of the plants; given fresh water, good-quality hay, and shade; and kept as quiet as possible to avoid further stress on the heart.

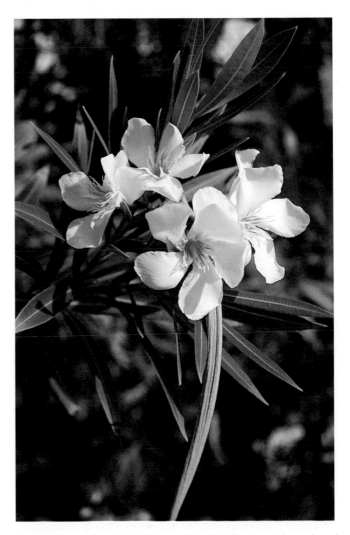

Fig. 18–70. Oleander (Nerium oleander) flower with seed pod

are retained in dried plants, although in reduced quantities, oleander and milkweed pose the greatest threat if present in the horse's hay.

The most important of the cardiac glycosides are digoxin and digotoxin, present in Digitalis spp., oleandroside and nerioside in Nerium oleander, thevetin in yellow oleander (T. peruviana), and cardenolides in milkweed. Acute death from these plants results from their cardiac glycoside ouabain-like toxic effect on the heart. This effect inhibits the cell membrane's sodium-potassium pump, resulting in frequent and irregular depolarization of the cell. This results in disorganized cardiac electrical activity that is manifested as a variety of abnormal heart rhythms and eventually cardiac arrest. The glycosides also act directly on the gastrointestinal tract, causing hemorrhagic enteritis that results in vomiting, colic, and diarrhea. The cardiac glycosides, at least those in milkweed, also act on the respiratory and nervous systems, which may cause difficulty breathing, tremors, seizures, and head pressing.

Animals consuming sufficient cardiac glycoside-containing plants are often found dead 8 to 10 hours later due to the profound effects of the toxins on the heart. Colic,

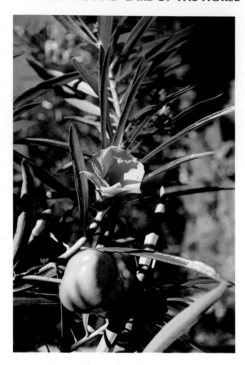

Fig. 18–71. Yellow oleander (Thevetia peruviana) flower and fruit

Animals that have not consumed a lethal dose of the plants recover over several days.

Larkspur or Poison Weed

Larkspur poisoning is of greatest concern for cattle, causing more cattle fatalities in the western United States than any other naturally occurring plant species. Horses are not as susceptible as cattle to the alkaloids in larkspur, and are infrequently poisoned by larkspur. However, consumption of larkspur will cause sudden death of horses, as well as of cattle and other animals.

There are at least 80 species of larkspur or poison weed (Delphinium spp.) in North America, most of which grow in the western United States. They are erect, perennial herbaceous plants with simple or branched hollow stems and alternate, palmate divided leaves. The flowers are perfect and irregular and are carried in terminal racemes. They vary in color from white to red to a dark blue purple. The flower has five sepals, the uppermost one having an obvious spur (Fig. 18–72). The corolla is composed of two sets of two petals each, the two lower ones forming a claw and the upper two extending into the spur.

Larkspur poisoning is related to the quantity of toxic alkaloids in the plant. This varies with the plant species, the stage of growth, the amount ingested, and the duration in which the plant is eaten. Young, rapidly growing plants are the most toxic, the highest concentration of toxic alkaloids being in the leaves and flowers. Delphinium barbeyi is the most toxic of the larkspurs. As little as 0.5% of body weight of green D. barbeyi is lethal to cattle. Sheep can tolerate 3 to 4 times as much larkspur as can cattle, and horses appear to be between cattle and sheep in suscepti-

bility to larkspur poisoning. A horse would therefore be poisoned by eating an amount equal to 1 to 2% of its body weight of green larkspur, depending on the alkaloid content of the plant.

Larkspur alkaloids act primarily at the nerve-muscle junction, causing a curare-like blockade of nerve impulses with resulting muscle weakness and paralysis. Clinical signs of larkspur poisoning are best described for cattle but are similar in affected horses, sheep, and goats. Sudden death is often the first indication of larkspur poisoning. Poisoned cattle initially show uneasiness, increased excitability, and muscle weakness that causes stiffness, staggering, and a base-wide stance. The front legs may be most severely affected, causing the animal to kneel before finally going down. Frequent attempts to stand are uncoordinated and result in rapid exhaustion. Muscle twitching, colic, regurgitation, bloat, and constipation are common. Inhalation of regurgitated rumen contents commonly leads to severe pneumonia and death. Cattle frequently die within 3 to 4 hours of consuming a lethal dose of larkspur.

Early diagnosis of larkspur poisoning through recogni-

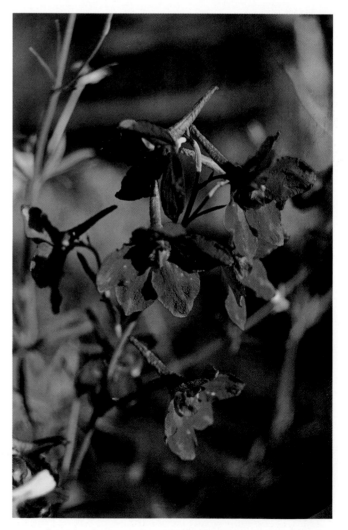

Fig. 18–72. Larkspur or poison weed (Delphinium spp.) showing the characteristic spur protruding from the back of the flower

tion of the clinical signs and observation that horses have eaten larkspur is essential for successful treatment. Stress and excitement of the affected animal should be avoided as it will exacerbate respiratory distress and hasten death.

Monkshood

Monkshood, or aconite, (Aconitum spp.) frequently grows in the same habitat as larkspur, and the alkaloids present in monkshood are similar in effect and toxicity to those of larkspur. The effects and treatment of monkshood poisoning, therefore, are the same as for larkspur poisoning. Monkshood is a perennial herbaceous plant with tall leafy stems. The leaves are alternate, palmate lobed or parted, and similar to those of larkspur. The flowers are usually deep blue purple but occasionally white, and carried on simple racemes or panicles. The flowers have five sepals that are petal-like, the upper sepal being larger and forming a characteristic helmet or hood (Fig. 18–73). There are two to five petals, usually concealed within the hooded sepal.

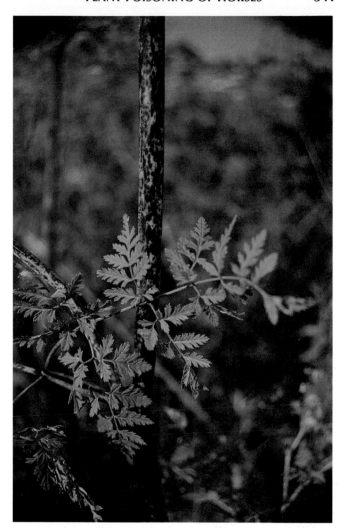

Fig. 18–74. Poison, European, or spotted hemlock (Conium maculatum) showing the purple spots on the stems and the carrot-like leaves

Poison Hemlock

Poison, European, or spotted hemlock (Conium maculatum), although rarely eaten by horses or other livestock, if consumed in even small amounts, will cause sudden death. It is an erect, 3- to 6-ft (1 to 2 m) tall biennial or perennial plant. The branching stems are hollow and hairless, have purple spots especially near the base, and arise from a simple carrot-like tap root (Fig. 18–74). Leaves are alternate, 3 to 4 times pinnately dissected, coarsely toothed, with a fern-like appearance. The terminal inflorescence is a compound, flat-topped, loose umbel with multiple, small, white five-petaled flowers (Fig. 18–75). The fruits are grey brown, ovoid, ridged, and easily separated into two parts. Originally introduced from Europe, poison hemlock is found throughout North America growing along roadsides, ditches, cultivated fields, and waste areas, especially where the ground is moist.

At least five piperidine alkaloids, including coniine, are found in all parts of the plant, but especially in the leaves and stems prior to development of the fruits. Plants grow-

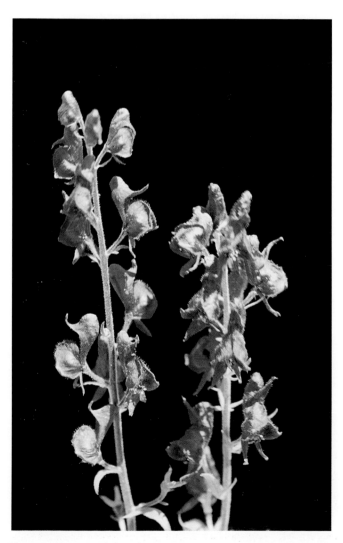

Fig. 18–73. Monkshood or aconite (Aconitum columbianum)

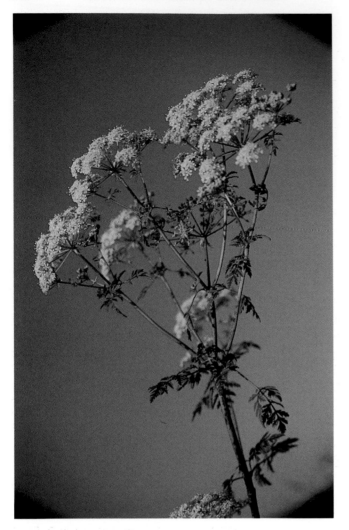

Fig. 18–75. Poison, European, or spotted hemlock flowers (Conium maculatum)

tinguishable from similar deformities caused by the teratogenic effects of Lupinus spp. and Nicotiana spp. Although pregnant mares may exhibit the acute neurologic and gastrointestinal signs of poison hemlock poisoning, the fetus appears to be unaffected.

Treatment is directed at preventing further absorption of the toxin from the gastrointestinal tract and, if possible, providing artificial respiration if respiratory paralysis is imminent.

Water Hemlock

Water hemlock (Cicuta spp.) is extremely toxic, causing violent convulsions and sudden death within hours of consuming even a small amount. It is a stout, erect, hairless perennial growing to a height of 4 to 6 ft (1.2 to 1.8 m) from a close cluster of two to eight thick tuberous roots. At the base of the hollow stem is a series of tightly grouped partitions containing an acrid yellow fluid (Fig. 18-76). The leaves are alternate and 1 to 3 times pinnate; the lanceolate leaflets are 1 to 4 inches (3 to 10 cm) long, with

ing in the warmer southern states appear to be more toxic than those in the northern areas. Poison hemlock is toxic to all animals, including people. People are usually poisoned when they mistakenly eat hemlock for wild parsnips, parsley, or wild carrots. Livestock seldom eat the plant because of its strong pungent odor, but will do so if no other forage is available. Cattle have been fatally poisoned by eating as little as 1 lb (0.45 kg) of the green poison hemlock plant.

Signs of poisoning develop within an hour of eating poison hemlock, and if a sufficient quantity has been consumed, death from respiratory failure occurs in 2 to 3 hours. Salivation, colic, muscle tremors, and incoordination occur initially, followed by difficulty breathing, dilated pupils, weak pulse, cyanosis, coma, respiratory paralysis, and death. Abortions may occur in pregnant animals that survive acute poisoning.

Poison hemlock may cause abnormal fetal development if it is eaten early in gestation by ewes or sows, but not mares. Affected offspring may be born with crooked legs, deformed necks and spines, and cleft palates that are indis-

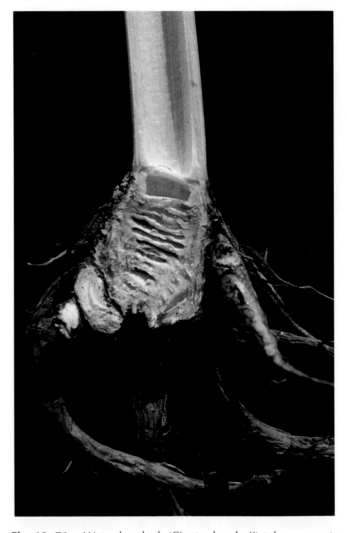

Fig. 18–76. Water hemlock (Cicuta douglasii) tuberous roots and hollow partitioned stems

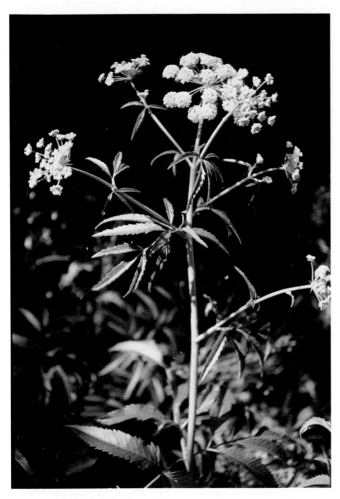

Fig. 18–77. Water hemlock (Cicuta douglasii) umbel inflorescence and leaves

toothed edges. The flowers are white and form a loose compound umbel (Fig. 18–77). The flowers have a stylopodium and evident teeth. The fruits are oval and flattened laterally with prominent ribs. There are many species of Cicuta, but C. maculata found in the eastern half of North America, and C. douglasii in the western half, predominate, preferring wet meadows, riverbanks, irrigation ditches, and water edges, often with their roots underwater.

The toxin in water hemlock is cicutoxin, a highly unsaturated alcohol and one of the most poisonous compounds known. All animals, including people, can be fatally poisoned by eating as little as 0.1 to 0.2 oz/100 lbs (50 to 110 mg/kg) body weight of the plant. The lethal dose of fresh green C. douglasii for an adult horse is about ½ lb (250 g). All parts of the plant, including the fluid found in the hollow stems, are toxic. However, the roots are even more toxic, as the toxin is concentrated in them. The roots are easily pulled up, as the ground is usually wet. Livestock consuming a single root are usually fatally poisoned. The plant remains toxic when dry, although the mature leaves in late summer seem to have minimal toxicity to cattle.

The roots, however, are highly poisonous at all times, with 0.5% body weight of roots, wet weight, being fatal to horses.

Cicutoxin is a potent neurotoxin causing rapid onset of muscle tremors and violent convulsions. Salivation, vigorous chewing movements, and teeth grinding are common. During the convulsions, animals have been known to bite off their tongues. Signs appear within a few hours of eating water hemlock and progress rapidly to convulsive seizures. Poisoned animals have dilated pupils and progress to a state of coma before dying from respiratory paralysis and asphyxia.

There is no specific antidote to cicutoxin. Animals are usually heavily sedated to reduce the severity of the convulsions, and laxatives are often given to remove the plant from the digestive system.

Yew

Horses are highly susceptible to yews (Taxus spp.), whose ingestion results in sudden death following incoordination, nervousness, difficulty breathing, diarrhea, and convulsions. Yews are evergreen shrubs or small trees with glossy, stiff, dark green linear leaves 1.2 to 2.7 inches (3 to 7 cm) long with pointed ends, closely spaced on the branches. Inconspicuous axillary male and female flowers are produced on separate plants, forming showy red to yellow fruits containing a single seed (Fig. 18–78). Several species of yew grow naturally or are grown as ornamental plants in North America; perhaps appropriately Taxus species plants are used extensively for shrubbery around government buildings in Washington D.C. Yews generally prefer humid moist environments. Western yew (Taxus brevifolia) and Canada yew (Taxus canadensis) are two indigenous species. English yew (Taxus baccata) and Japanese yew (Taxus cuspidata) are commonly cultivated species in North America.

Yews contain the potent alkaloid taxine in all parts of the plant, green or dried, except the fleshy aril surrounding the seed. Horses are highly susceptible to the taxine's ef-

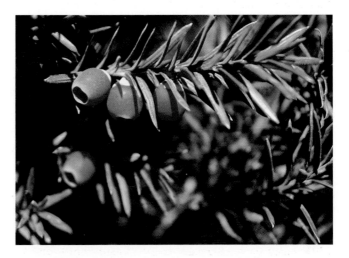

Fig. 18–78. Yew (Taxus spp.) showing the red fruits that resemble a pitted olive

fect on the heart, frequently dying shortly after eating small quantities of the plant (an amount equal to 0.05% of their body weight of green leaves). Livestock are often poisoned when fed trimmings from cultivated yews.

Sudden incoordination, nervousness, difficulty in breathing, slow heart rate, diarrhea, convulsions, and death are characteristic of yew poisoning in all animals. Sudden death may be the only observed sign in horses. There is no effective treatment for acute yew poisoning. A diagnosis of yew poisoning is usually made from the history of sudden death, the absence of postmortem findings, the access to yew, and the finding of yew leaf fragments in the stomach.

Death Camas

Horses that consume 8 to 10 lbs (4 kg) of death camas (Zigadenus spp.) salivate and develop colic and incoordination and die within several days. There are approximately 15 species of death camas, which range from moist mountain valleys to drier sandy hills and plains. They appear in early spring, often growing amongst wild onion. They are herbaceous hairless perennials with grass-like, linear, V-shaped, parallel-veined leaves arising basally from an onion-like bulb 6 to 8 inches (15 to 20 cm) below the soil surface (Fig. 18–79). However, death camas' leaves are not hollow like those of onions, nor do they smell like onions when crushed. The bulb is covered with a membranous black outer coat. The inflorescence, a terminal raceme or panicle, has small, perfect, greenish white to yellow or pink flowers. The six-numbered perianth segments are separated, each with a gland at its base.

Several toxic alkaloids, including zigacine and zigadenine, are found in all parts of the plant, but especially the bulb. Sheep are most frequently poisoned by death camas, but cattle, horses, and pigs may be affected. Poisoning is most likely to occur in early spring when few other plants are available and the succulent shoots are especially enticing.

Sheep show signs of poisoning after eating as little as ½ lb (250 g) of the green plants. Convulsions, coma, and death occur if sheep eat 2 to 3 lbs of green plant per 100 lbs body weight (2 to 3 kg/100 kg). Poisoning may occur in horses after they have eaten about 8 to 10 lbs (4 kg) of the plants. Salivation, colic, muscular weakness, and a staggering gait are reported in horses, with death occurring after several days.

In most cases of death camas poisoning, little can be done to reverse the poisoning. Activated charcoal or kaolin/pectin suspension may be given by stomach tube to decrease further toxin absorption. Supportive therapy and analgesics may be beneficial in managing the signs of colic.

Avocado

Horses, cattle, goats, rabbits, and birds have been poisoned from eating the leaves and other parts of the Guatemalan variety of avocado Persea americana. The Mexican, or smooth-skinned fruit, variety does not appear to be toxic. The flesh of the ripe avocado fruit of neither variety is toxic. Horses are most likely to eat avocado plant parts if they are pastured in avocado orchards and normal forages are depleted.

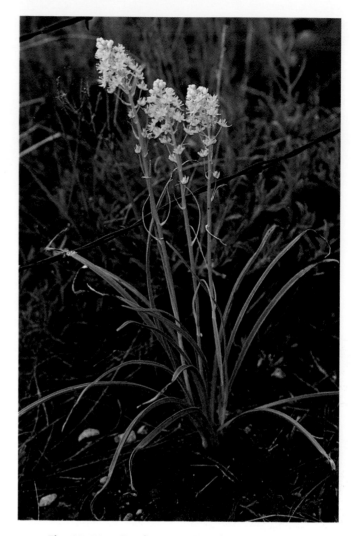

Fig. 18–79. Death camas (Zigadenus venenosus)

Horses, after eating the fruit, seeds, or leaves of avocado trees, develop a variety of clinical signs, including colic, diarrhea, and edema of the ventral abdomen, head, and neck. In severely affected animals there is marked edematous swelling of the head that is painful and causes respiratory difficulty. Fluid may develop in the chest cavity. Goats experimentally poisoned with avocado leaves died within 48 hours of receiving the leaves, and showed heart damage. In addition to the cardiotoxic effects of avocado, lactating mares and goats develop a noninfectious mammary gland inflammation and decreased milk production.

SUPPLEMENTAL READING RECOMMENDATIONS

Poisonous Plants of the United States and Canada by John M. Kingsbury (Prentice-Hall, Inc, Englewood Cliffs, NJ, 1964). Although published in 1964, this text is still the most comprehensive compilation of information on plants in North America documented to cause livestock poisoning. It is particularly valuable when seeking information on early reports of plant poisoning, as it has an extensive bibliography covering plant poisoning reports from the beginning of the 8th century. Botanically, the book covers all groups of toxic plants. The limitation of the book is that it contains relatively few color photographs that would make plant identification easier for those that are not botanists. Since there has been no new edition of the book since 1964, there is much new information on plant toxicology and new toxic plants that are not in the book.

Weeds of the West by Tom D. Whitson. This book, although geographically limited to plants of the Rocky Mountain-Great Plains area of the United States and covering weeds that are not necessarily toxic, has outstanding color photographs of each plant that make identification of them easy. It is written for the benefit of the livestock owner and is a useful book for weed identification important to pasture management. It does not, however, cover the toxicology of the plants other than to mention those that are likely to be a problem to animals. With over 600 color pictures of the common important weeds, this book is well worth possessing. The book is published by the University of Wyoming in cooperation with the Western Society of Weed Science and the Western United States Land Grant Universities Cooperative Extension Services. (Pioneer of Jackson Hole, 132 West Gill Street, Jackson Hole, WY, 83001, 1991.)

Chapter 19

FEED-RELATED POISONINGS OF HORSES

Mycotoxin Poisoning 346
    Diagnosis of Mycotoxin Poisoning 348
       Feed Sampling 350
       Field Mycotoxin Assays 350
    Mycotoxin Destruction in Feeds 351
    Fescue Poisoning in Horses 352
       Cause 352
       Effect 353
       Treatment 354
       Prevention 354
    Equine Ergotism 355
    Grass Staggers in Horses 355
    Moldy Corn Disease in Horses 357
       Cause 357
       Effects 358
       Prevention 359
    Aflatoxin Poisoning in Horses 360

Stachybotryotoxicosis in Horses 360
Ionophore Antibiotic Poisoning in Horses 361
    Diagnosis 361
Forage Poisoning (Botulism) in Horses 361
Lead Poisoning in Horses 363
    Cause 363
    Effects 363
    Treatment and Prevention 364
Blister Beetle Poisoning in Horses 364
    Cause 364
    Effects 365
    Treatment and Prevention 366
Gossypol Poisoning 366
    Cause 366
    Effects 367
    Treatment and Prevention 367
Nitrate Poisoning 368

Poisoning due to substances produced by and present in plants not generally intended as a feed for horses occurs primarily in horses on pasture and was described in the previous chapter. In contrast, toxins ingested in feeds that are intended for the horse occur both in harvested and unharvested feeds and, therefore, in horses both stabled and on pasture. These are described in this chapter. This includes toxins produced by molds (mycotoxins), bacteria (botulism), plants (gossypol and nitrates), insects (blister beetles), or from environmental contamination of plants (lead) or errors in feed preparation (ionophore antibiotics). The largest and most common group of toxins affecting horses is the mycotoxins, of which some are present primarily in harvested feeds (e.g., those causing Moldy Corn disease, aflatoxin poisoning, and stachybotryotoxicosis); others occur more commonly in unharvested feeds (resulting in fescue poisoning and grass staggers); and some occur both in harvested and unharvested feeds (ergotism).

The major clinical symptoms or manifestations of feed-related poisonings are given in Table 19-1, to assist the reader in determining which cause is most likely responsible for a particular case.

Treatment of most feed related poisonings is supportive. Diagnosis of the cause, therefore, is most important in preventing continued and future exposure of that and other animals to the toxin. Frequently no single diagnostic findings occur. A number of criteria must generally be evaluated to arrive at a diagnosis, including: history, clinical and laboratory examination, and, frequently, necropsy (autopsy) alterations and analytical testing or bioassay.

Diagnostic procedures should begin with a thorough review of the history of the herd: how all individuals in it have been affected, their location, new members, their movement, environment and management including the source and type of everything known to be or that may have been ingested (all feeds, supplements, water, plants, chemicals near feeds, etc.). The dates of any changes, such as new pasture or new batches of even the same feed or feeding should be determined. The time from the exposure to something new to the onset of clinical signs can be helpful in determining the cause, and depending on the toxins involved, may be from a few hours to several months. The location of both affected and nonaffected animals may be helpful: e.g., stabled or on pasture downstream, downwind, or near sources of environmental contaminants, such as chemical usage or industrial sites or dumps. Regardless of clinical signs, it is important to rule out nontoxic causes of disease and to avoid focusing too rapidly on poisoning. The absence of effects in others in the herd may be as helpful as are the alterations in affected animals.

Feed samples frequently must be evaluated and should be representative of what the horse has consumed. Toxins may not be present uniformly in a single source of a feed; therefore, a number of samples need to taken from both feed bunks and stored feeds, and equal-size samples from the same source combined for analysis. A complete and systematic necropsy, including microscopic and sometimes analytic examination of affected tissues, animals that have died or are moribund and euthanized by a veterinarian, or if available at a diagnostic laboratory, is frequently necessary. Alterations detectable on necropsy are often critical in diagnosing poisonings.

MYCOTOXIN POISONING

Mycotoxins are poisons sporadically produced by molds. They include many useful antibiotics (such as penicillin, griseofulvin, cephalosporins, and ionophores) which at therapeutic levels are more toxic to bacteria than to animals. Molds are ubiquitous, terrestrial, filamentous one-cell fungi. They are an integral part of the natural decay process of plant materials. Those that produce mycotoxins grow in many feeds; the major feeds affected in the United States are tall fescue pasture and harvested corn, peanuts, and cottonseeds, but they include all cereal grains and for-

TABLE 19-1

Major Clinical Signs, Due to Feed-Related Poisonings of Horses[a]

Causes of Poisoning	Major Clinical Signs
Infected fescue pasture or less often hay cut after seed formation	Prolonged pregnancy & no udder; thick & ± retained placenta; difficult delivery; ± foal weak or dead; no milk produced; ↓ conception & ↓ growth rate
Ergot in grain or seedhead of grasses	Same as fescue poisoning but ergot rarely affects horses
Mycotoxins in ryegrass & Paspalum grasses (e.g., Dallis & Bahia grasses)	Staggers to tetany when moved; without other signs; reversible and not fatal
Moldy corn disease due to fusarium mycotoxins in corn or corn byproduct-containing feeds	Acute onset & rapidly progressive ↓ appetite; uncoordinated; depression, agitation; no fever; sudden death
Aflatoxin in especially cottonseed, corn, & peanuts	Sudden death or ↓ appetite, dehydration, lethargy, & tremors; ± straining; rare in horses
Stachybotrys mycotoxin in sooty-appearing hay or straw. Not reported in North America	Slow progression from lips & oral inflammation to enlarged head, ↓ appetite, & death; less often brain damage signs, lung edema, & death in 1–3 days
Pentachlorophenol (PCP) (in motor oil, wood preservative, & pesticides)	Face, legs, abdomen, and skin irritation, progresses to ulcers & hair loss, especially mane & tail; wt loss & weak; chronic cough, & eye and nose discharge
Ionophores, e.g., monensin, laslocid, or salinomycin in feed usually intended for cattle or poultry	Suspect if following feed change there is feed refusal and ½ to 3 days later loss of appetite, depression, colic, intestinal atony, sweating, incoordination & difficulty breathing; may recover or sudden death without clinical signs
Forage poisoning from botulism toxin in moldy feed. Less often toxin may be produced in an infected wound.	Rapid onset and progression to "shaker foals" & in adult flaccid muscle, loss of tail & tongue tone, difficulty swallowing, reluctance to move & tremors to unable to stand & difficult breathing
Lead-contaminated pasture or hay, rarely paint or herbicide; prolonged consumption	Slow, progressive weakness, incoordination, depression, poor condition, drooping lip, regurgitation, "roaring," difficulty breathing
Blister beetles in alfalfa hay	Shock & sudden death; mild to severe colic, won't eat & depression; frequent voiding and bloody urine, ± splashing water with muzzle; ↑ TPR; congested membranes & ↓ capillary refill time; ± stiff gait, slobbering, & sweating
Arsenic (pesticides on feeds; also paints)	Shock, colic, trembling, hypersalivation; death in <1–3 days
Free gossypol from cottonseeds, possibly with >0.03% in diet for young & >0.1% for adults recommended, but toxicosis not reported in horses	In other species, sudden death or chronic poor condition, difficulty breathing, congestive heart failure, lung edema in young, bloody urine & ↓ performance & ± ↓ fertility in male & female

[a] See Chapter 18 for cause and effects of plant poisonings in horses. Abbreviations used in this table are: TPR = temperature, pulse rate, and respiratory rate; ↑ = increase; ↓ = decrease; > = greater than; < = less than; and ± = may or may not occur.

ages. Their growth and toxin production occur primarily in feeds containing over 12 to 20% moisture, during times of high relative humidity (>70%) when oxygen is available, and generally under alkaline conditions at temperatures of 54 to 117°F (12 to 47°C), although some Fusarium molds produce toxins at temperatures as low as 41°F (5°C). Moisture levels above 13 to 14% are, however, the single most important factor that determines whether mold growth and mycotoxin production occurs. Stress, such as drought or inappropriate application of fertilizers or pesticides, can weaken a plant's natural defenses against molds, and insect and mechanical damage may allow entry of mold spores past a plant's normal physical barrier, allowing increased mold colonization of the plant material.

Under optimum conditions, mycotoxins can be produced within hours and reach a maximum concentration within 1 to 2 weeks. The amount produced varies greatly with different molds and environmental conditions, including the particular type of feed it is in. Mycotoxin poisoning in animals often occurs as an outbreak during a specific season and is often associated with a particular climatic event, such as a wet harvest season preceded by a drought. Because of different growing conditions and cropping systems, mycotoxin production may be regional. Aflatoxins, for example, are most prevalent in corn and peanut meals in Appalachia and southeastern regions of the United States, while Fusarium mycotoxins are most commonly found in corn, and ergot in small grains from

the north central United States and Canada. Although the three genera of molds most commonly responsible for causing mycotoxicosis—Penicillium, Aspergillus, and Fusarium—are all distributed worldwide, Penicillium most commonly causes health problems in temperate areas, Aspergillus in the tropics, and Fusarium in cold climates. However, Fusariume, moniliform, which causes moldy corn poisoning, is also common in the tropics, and aflatoxins can be produced by Aspergillus in temperate and cooler climates. In addition, transport of feeds and their use in commercial feeds may cause a loss of geographic identity. Although feed contamination with most mycotoxins occurs during storage, some mycotoxins (such as ergot alkaloids, slaframine, and some Fusarium spp.-produced mycotoxins) may be produced in the field. Procedures for preventing mold growth and mycotoxin production in stored feeds are described in Chapter 4 (see sections on "Grain Storage" and "Mold Inhibitors").

There are more than 300 chemically different mycotoxins with different sites of action, mechanisms of toxicity, and as a result, effects. Clinical syndromes associated with mycotoxin poisonings in animals range from acute death, debilitation, and interference with reproductive efficiency, to decreased feed efficiency and growth, or poor condition. In general, mycotoxin poisoning is not transmissible from animal to animal but frequently affect more than one animal in a herd, is usually associated with a particular feed and season, and is usually not responsive to treatment of any kind.

The only treatment for mycotoxin poisonings is supportive, including feeding a mycotoxin-free diet that is at least 10 to 20% higher in protein and vitamins than would otherwise be required for that animal. This may assist in overcoming a prior mycotoxin damage-induced decrease in the utilization of these nutrients. In addition to causing detrimental effects in animals, molds and mycotoxins decrease the nutrient content and palatability of feeds. The amount of a number of nutrients ingested also alters mycotoxin effects. A tenfold increase in vitamin E will prevent some of the effects of aflatoxins. A protein, vitamin A, or riboflavin deficiency will increase—and a protein, biotin, beta-carotene, and fat excess will decrease—aflatoxins' detrimental health effects on animals studied. Dietary protein levels have also been shown to have these same effects on the mycotoxin zearalenones effects. In addition, the plasma and tissue concentrations of most B vitamins are decreased during aflatoxicosis. The increased fiber content of alfalfa has been shown to decrease zearalenone and T-2 mycotoxin effects.

Susceptibility to mycotoxins varies tremendously between species, with the young being more susceptible and severely affected than older animals at similar levels of intake of most mycotoxins. Diet concentration of mycotoxin, duration of consumption, and the nutritional and physiologic status of the animal all affect the degree of toxicosis. Three general forms of mycotoxin poisonings occur:

1. Acute primary poisoning occurs when high concentrations are consumed over a short period. This results in specific lesions in target organs, resulting in clinical signs characteristic of that specific poisoning: e.g., moldy corn poisoning.
2. Chronic primary poisoning occurs when moderate to low concentrations are consumed over a prolonged period (several weeks to months). This commonly results in affected animals having a slower growth rate or poorer condition, and a lower reproductive efficiency. Specific lesions in target organs and clinical signs characteristic of that specific mycotoxin poisoning may or may not occur: e.g., fescue poisoning.
3. Secondary poisoning occurs from the continual consumption of low concentrations of a mycotoxin that is carcinogenic or suppresses the immune system and as a result increases the risk or incidence of cancer or infectious diseases.

Feed refusal, reproductive problems, and immune system suppression are the health problems most often attributed, correctly or incorrectly, to mycotoxin consumption in farm animals. However, many other factors may be responsible for these problems. Many factors, including stress, inadequate water intake, and feed palatability for numerous reasons; most diseases of all types, which may be subclinical; as well as moldy feed with or without mycotoxins, may cause feed refusal and must be considered possible causes.

The mycotoxins most commonly implicated in health problems in domestic animals are aflatoxins, fumonisins, and zearalenone, and, to a lesser extent trichothecene, ochratoxins, tremorgenic mycotoxins, and ergot. The clinical effects of these mycotoxins differ both with the amount and rate of their consumption as well as with each individual mycotoxin, depending on which organ systems are affected and to what extent. The major clinical effects, species commonly affected, and feeds these mycotoxins and molds that produce them generally occur in are summarized in Table 19-2.

The only mycotoxin poisonings that commonly affect horses are caused by moldy corn poisoning, due to fumonisins, and the mold, which causes fescue toxicosis. Less commonly, horses may be affected by ergot, aflatoxins, and tremorgenic (tremor producing) mycotoxins that cause grass staggers. Horses may also be affected by the mycotoxins dicoumarol and slaframine, and in the Ukraine, Europe, and South Africa, stachybotryotoxins. Occasionally horses, but more commonly cattle and sheep, in Australia and Europe may also develop lupine poisoning caused by the liver toxins Phomopsis A and B produced by the mold Phomopsis leptostromiformis growing on various species of lupine. In addition, at least 42 species of grasses, the majority of which grow in North America, may contain endophytic molds i.e. molds that grow inside, not on the outside, of the plant. These molds, or their mycotoxins, have the potential to cause disease in horses and other animals consuming them.

Dicoumarol, produced by mold in high-coumarin sweet clover hay, inhibits vitamin K activity decreasing blood coagulation ability, which increases the susceptibility to hemorrhage, (as described in Chapter 3 in the section on "Vitamin K Deficiency"). Slaframine produced by molds in legume pasture forage or hay, particularly red clover, as described in Chapter 18, causes excessive salivation or slobbering diseases in horses, as it does in other herbivores, that stops 2 to 4 days after removal from the contaminated pasture.

Other mycotoxins affecting farm animals include trichothecenes, zearalenone, ochratoxin A, and citrinin. The major effect of trichothecenes is to cause feed refusal, but to do so requires a concentration of at least 1 ppm, and these toxins are rarely found in feeds that animals refuse. They have not been reported to but may cause feed refusal in horses. Zearalenone at concentrations as low as 0.7 to 5.6 ppm is a well-known cause of reproductive problems in swine and much less commonly cattle, but isn't known to affect horses. Under field conditions other mycotoxins have not been found to cause reproductive problems in any species. Most common mycotoxins, particularly aflatoxins and trichothecenes, at concentrations occurring in feeds have been shown to decrease resistance to a variety of infectious diseases in a number of species, but not horses. Usually, reduced disease resistance occurs only after days or weeks of exposure to mycotoxins at levels that cause observable clinical sign and lesions.

Diagnosis of Mycotoxin Poisoning

Mycotoxin poisonings are often difficult to diagnose because of the variation in time from mycotoxin ingestion

TABLE 19–2
Mycotoxin Poisoning: Causes and Clinical Effects

Major Clinical Effects	Mycotoxin and Animals Affected	Feeds Commonly Contaminated	Molds Commonly Responsible
Moldy Corn Disease—neurologic effects, e.g., won't eat, depression, incoordination and sudden death. Less often acute liver failure & icterus.	Fumonisins $FA_{1\&2}$ & FB_{1-4}; affects horses & swine[a]	Corn grain, stalks, hulls or silage	Fusarium monliforme and F. proliferatum
Fescue Poisoning—↓ udder, prolonged pregnancy, thick & retained placenta, difficult delivery of ± weak or dead foals, no milk produced, ↓ conception & ↓ growth.	Probably ergot alkaloids, which affect pregnant & growing horses, cattle, & sheep	Tall fescue grass pasture & less often hay cut after maturity (after seeding out)	Acremonium coenophialum
Grass staggers—mild excitability and muscle tremors to spastic incoordination and tetany followed by recovery.	Tremorgen neurotoxins[b] &	Dallis or Bahia grasses	Claviceps paspali
	lolitrems affect most herbivores, including horses	Perennial ryegrass	Acremonium lolii
Ergot Poisoning—similar to fescue poisoning; grass staggers or dry gangrene of extremities.	Ergot alkaloids affect most species and rarely horses	Grain & grass seeds, especially rye	Claviceps purpurea
Aflatoxin Poisoning—GI disturbances, feed refusal, vomiting, diarrhea, hemorrhage, icterus, anemia, immunity suppression, fatty liver, ↓ weight & growth, oral inflammation, lip & nostril edema.	Aflatoxins (B_1, B_2, G_1, G_2, M_1 and M_2),[c] and	Cottonseed, ground nuts, corn, & less often other grain & hay	Aspergillus flavus & A. parasiticus
	Trichothecenes,[d] and	Especially corn, also hay, barley, oats, wheat, milo, & bean hulls	Fusarium sporotrichioides
	DON.[e] All 3 toxins affect most species & rarely horses.	Corn, wheat, & milo	F. equiseti (roseum)
Estrogen effects—vulval swelling, testes atrophy, vaginal & rectal prolapse, anestrus, nymphomania; ↓ conception, ovulation, implantation, fetal development & neonatal viability.	Zearalenone F-2 & zearalonol affect swine & possibly cattle, but are not known to affect horses	Corn, milo, & wheat	Fusarium graminearum (roseum)
Kidney toxicosis—excess urination & water consumption; ± stomach & intestinal inflammation & liver damage.	Ochratoxin A & citrinin affect most species but not horses	Corn & other cereal grains, beans, peanuts & legumes	Aspergillus ochraceus, Penicillium verrucosum & citrinin toxin by P. citrinum
Slobbering Disease—excess salivation, won't eat, diarrhea, excess urination, stiffness.[f]	Slaframine affects all herbivores, including horses	Legume pasture or hay, especially red clover with black spots or rings on leaves	Rhizoctonia leguminicola
Sweet Clover Poisoning—↓ blood clotting & hemorrhage[g]	Dicoumarol affects all	Moldy sweet clover hay or haylage	Aspergillus spp.
Stachybotryotoxicosis—generally 3 stages occur: 1st: 2–30 days of lip & oral inflammation, runny nose & eyes, ↑ saliva & large head. 2nd: 2–7 weeks of ↓ blood clotting. 3rd: 1–4 days of fever, ± colic, rapid weak pulse & death. **Atypical form**—brain damage signs, lung edema, & death within 1–3 days	Trichothecene satratoxin affects horses, cattle, sheep & swine but currently has not been reported in North America	Dense sooty black spores in hay and straw	Stachybotrys chartarum (atra or alternans)

Abbreviations used in this table are: ↓ = decrease, ↑ = increase, ± = may or may not occur, and GI = gastrointestinal.

[a] Fumonisins also cause lung edema and fluid in the chest cavity in swine but are not known to do so in horses.

[b] Tremorgen neurotoxins also suppress reproduction, lactation, feed intake, and growth of cattle, sheep, poultry, and dogs, but are not known to do so in horses.

[c] Nursing animals may be affected by their mother's ingestion of B_1, the most common and toxic aflatoxin, as well as other aflatoxins and the excretion of their hydroxylated metabolites in the milk.

[d] Includes T-2 mycotoxin and diacetoxyscripphenol (DAS). These may also cause bone marrow suppression, skin inflammation, and a variety of reproductive organ effects, and abortion.

[e] DON (deoxynivalenol or vomitoxin) usually causes only feed refusal and vomiting when present at 1 ppm (1 mg/kg) or greater, and nothing at lower concentrations.

[f] See section on "Salivation-Inducing Plants" in Chapter 18.

[g] See sections on "Vitamin K Deficiency" in Chapter 3 and "Spoiled Sweet Clover" in Chapter 18.

until clinical signs are recognized, and because clinical signs in some cases are not dramatic but instead present as vague or chronic conditions. The only signs in some cases may be poor performance, unthriftiness, or an increased susceptibility to infectious diseases. The effects of low-level feed contamination may not become apparent until days or weeks after the offending feed was consumed; by the time the clinical signs appear, there may be no contaminated feed left to analyze. Attributing clinical signs to the incidental detection of mycotoxin in feed when another cause is responsible is a common error, particularly if any mold is found in the feed. Moldy feed may not contain mycotoxin; conversely, mycotoxins may be present in feed that doesn't appear moldy. Milling and pelleting of feeds can raise feed temperature sufficiently to kill mold, but not destroy mycotoxins. Thus, physical appearance is no definite indicator of the presence or absence of mycotoxins. However, a mycotoxin should be considered as a cause when health problems occur in animals consuming moldy feed.

A diagnosis of mycotoxin poisoning, like any feed-related poisoning, can be made by either reproducing the disease by feeding the suspected feed to other healthy animals, or by identifying from the feed, animal tissues, or body fluids toxins in amounts sufficient to cause a problem. The liver and kidney are most likely to contain mycotoxins in affected animals. The urine of affected horses may also contain aflatoxins. Microscopic evaluation of affected tissue and alternations in blood and tissue constituents can suggest, but not confirm, mycotoxin poisoning. Confirmation requires identification of a mycotoxin at a concentration known to produce disease typical of the clinical signs that occurred in feed representative of that consumed. When feed is moldy, animals may refuse to eat it altogether, or they may eat less of it than normal. Even if the mold is absent, the mycotoxin alone can cause complete or partial feed refusal. In addition, simply determining that a feed representative of that consumed is moldy or contains a mold capable of producing mycotoxins, or finding that small nontoxic amounts of mycotoxins are present, is not sufficient to confirm that mycotoxicosis is responsible for the health problems of concern. However, the true concentration of a mycotoxin in a feed is difficult to estimate accurately by measuring the concentration in a sample taken from the feed because of wide variability of mycotoxins within a feed. In addition, it has been stated that no levels of mycotoxins have been demonstrated to be safe; i.e., any level of mycotoxin carries with it a risk. This may be surprising to those who assume that regulatory guidelines on maximum allowable levels of various mycotoxins in various feeds are based on safety data. Unfortunately, regulatory agencies are required, sometimes by law and by political necessities, to adopt positions not justified scientifically; further, these positions can change for many reasons. Based on such factors, allowable aflatoxin levels in corn have varied from 20 to 300 ppb, and currently are twofold higher for corn for intrastate use than for interstate use, implying that aflatoxin becomes twice as toxic when it crosses a state line. Often a lack of data on safe levels has been responsible for forcing regulatory personnel to adopt subjective positions.

Feed Sampling for Mycotoxin Poisoning Diagnosis

Because of the uneven distribution of mycotoxins in a feed, a number of samples should be taken from representative portions of each feed the animals are consuming. Increases in the size of the sample, number of samples taken, and number of sites sampled all increase the reliability of the results obtained. Most errors in detecting mycotoxins in feeds result from faulty sampling rather than from deficiencies in laboratory analysis.

A sample will be most representative if the feed has recently been mixed or, if not, if small samples are taken from many different locations within the feed, such as from a moving stream of grain being harvested, loaded, etc., or less ideally, probe samples from the perimeter and center of a grain bin at every 6 feet (3 m) of depth. Combine the small samples taken, mix them thoroughly, and analyze a sample of this mixture or submit a composite sample of at least 10 lbs (4.5 kg) for evaluation. In most cases, individual samples of feed from specific problem areas may be useful to detect mycotoxins. These areas might include grain from parts of a bin exposed to water leaks or caked in feeders. Although small amounts of highly contaminated feed may be responsible for an individual case, it is unlikely to be responsible for a herd problem.

Prior to sending a sample to a laboratory for analysis, if the sample is moist, it should be dried to reduce moisture to 12% or less. Drying, as well as chemicals and sunlight, may reduce mold growth and mycotoxin production, but it won't destroy mycotoxins. However, if the feed is to be checked for mold as well as mycotoxins, the sample should not be dried at over 140°F (60°C) to preserve mold viability. A dry feed sample should be placed in a cloth or paper, but not a plastic bag, for transport, as moisture may accumulate if plastic is used. High-moisture feeds should be frozen if not dried, or treated with a mold inhibitor.

Field Mycotoxin Assays

The first and most commonly used means of detecting possible mycotoxins in feed is the "Woods Lamp" or black light. It doesn't, however, detect the presence of mycotoxins. Instead, it detects kojic acid, which is produced by mold that may have but not necessarily has, produced aflatoxins. Thus, under black light or long-wave ultraviolet light (365 nm), a bright greenish-yellow fluorescence indicates only the presence of aflatoxin-producing mold (called "shiners" or "glowers") and not the presence of aflatoxins themselves or the presence of any other mycotoxin. Fluorescence may also occur as a result of substances other than that produced by aflatoxin-producing molds. The use of the "Woods Lamp," therefore, produces many false positives (i.e., suggests a feed contains aflatoxins when it does not). However, it produces few false negatives (i.e., suggests a feed does not contain aflatoxin when it does) and, therefore, serves as a rapid screening test for aflatoxins in finely ground corn and other grains. Feed showing fluorescence under the "Woods Lamp" should be evaluated by additional assay procedures. Feed not showing fluorescence, however, may still contain numerous other mycotoxins.

There are a number of rapid field tests for detecting

TABLE 19–3
Aflatoxin Test Kits

Test Kit	Analysis	Type of Test	Level of Detection (μg/kg or ppb)	Analysis Time[a] (min/sample)	Application	Manufacturer's Telephone and Location
VICAM						
Aflatest[g]	B_1, B_2, G_1, G_2, M_1	Affinity column[b]	1 / 0.1 (M_1)	7	Instrumental, quantitative, fluorometer, HPLC	Somerville, MA 800/338-4381
Neogen Corp.						
AgriScreen[a,c]	B_1, B_2, G_1, M_1	ELISA,[b] microtiter wells	1 / 0.2 (M_1)	12	Visual and instrumental, semiquantitative, quantitative	Lansing, MI 517/372-9200
Intl. Diagnostic						
Afla-20[d]	B_1, B_2, G_1	ELISA,[b] cup	20	4	Visual pass/fail	St. Joseph, MI 616/983-3122
Afla-10			10	4		
IDEXX						
CITE-Probe-aflatoxin	B_1, B_2, G_1, M_1	ELISA,[b] probe	20	4	Visual and instrumental pass/fail	Portland, ME 800/548-6733
Environmental Diagnostic Systems Corp.						
EZ-SCREEN: aflatoxin	B_1, B_2, G_1	ELISA,[b] card	20	7	Visual, pass/fail	Burlington, NC 800/334-1116
BioCode						
Total aflatoxins	B_1, B_2, G_1, G_2,	Affinity column[b]	1	30	Visual (with UV viewer), semiquantitative	York, UK +44-904-430-616
BioCode						
Aflatoxin M_1	M_1	Affinity column[b]	<0.1	30		
Transia						
Aflatoxin test	B_1, B_2, G_1, G_2,	ELISA,[b] microtiter	0	30	Semiquantitative	Lyon, France +33-72-73-03-81
Transia						
Aflatoxin M_1 test	M_1	ELISA,[b] microtiter	0.01	40		
Terra Tek						
Target	B_1, B_2, G_1, G_2,	Selective adsorption[f]	10	10	Pass/fail	Salt Lake City, UT 800/372-2522
Romer Labs, Inc.						
HV Minicolumn	B_1, B_2, G_1, G_2,	Minicolumn	20	10	Pass/fail	Union, MO 800/769-1380

[a] Does not include sample preparation and extraction.
[b] Immunochemical methods: affinity column or ELISA.
[c] Adopted AOAC Official 1st Action for screening for aflatoxin B_1 in cottonseed products and mixed feed; adopted AOAC Interim Official 1st Action for screening for aflatoxin B_1 in corn and peanut butter.
[d] Adopted AOAC Interim Official 1st Action for screening for aflatoxins B_1, B_2, and G_1 in corn, peanut butter, poultry feed, cottonseed, and raw peanuts.
[e] Three-card system available: One sample/card or five sample/card at 20 ppb or one sample/card at 5 ppb.
[f] Modified Holaday–Velasco minicolumn (AOAC method 26,020–26,026).
[g] AOAC approved—Interim Official 1st Action with solution fluorometry or liquid chromatography. FSIS approved.

mycotoxins more reliable than the "Woods Lamp" and that detect nearly all of the clinically relevant mycotoxins affecting horses and other domestic animals. These are shown in Tables 19–3 and 19–4. These tests use one of three types of assay: minicolumn, ELISA, and CSID (chemiselective immobilization and detection). All are rapid, economical, and relatively easy to use. Minicolumn assay, however, is applicable only for aflatoxins and is not as sensitive, repeatable, or selective as ELISA or CSID. But minicolumn and CSID test kits have a longer shelf life than do those for ELISA and can selectively detect a mycotoxin from a mixture of several mycotoxins. Concurrent use of these different assays together in a single test allows for highly reliable detection of various mycotoxins in a wide variety of agricultural commodities. It's been reported that antioxidants, such as ethoxyquin, which are often added to commercially prepared feeds, may interfere with mycotoxin analysis. Therefore, in testing these feeds check with the mycotoxin assay manufacturer to determine if this is a problem with that test. If it is, a diagnostic laboratory test may be necessary. Thin-layer chromatography is currently the standard test used in most laboratories and may require as long as 2 to 4 weeks for the results.

Mycotoxin Destruction in Feeds

There are two approaches for reducing the effect of mold and mycotoxin contamination of feeds: (1) preventing mold growth and mycotoxin production with proper harvesting, storage, and use of mold inhibitors as described in Chapter 4; and (2) destruction or removal of mycotoxins from contaminated feed. Many approaches have been investigated for detoxification of contaminated crops and feeds. Procedures that have been successful include removal of contaminated material by hand and by electronic or pneumatic sorting, extraction with solvents, and various chemical treatments.

TABLE 19–4
Mycotoxin Test Kits

Company	INDEX	Terra Tek	Neogen Corp.	Vicam	Romer Labs, Inc.
Test Name	CITE PROBE Aflatoxin B₁ Test	Target Aflatoxin B₁ Kit	Agri-Screen	Aflatest	Afla-Cup Test
Reagents	None	Toluene, methanol, acetone, salt, & chloroform	Methanol, & water	Column, methanol, & developer	Methanol, water, & developer solution(s)
Detection Limit	20 ppb	10 ppb[a]	5 ppb	1 ppb	10 ppb[a]
Cross Reactivity	—	—	B_2–24%, G_1–51%, G_2–3.6%	—	—
Lab Notes	Transferral between wells requires precise timing	7–10 minute testing time; false positives possible on alfalfa	7–10 minute testing time	Digital readout	None
Storage/Shelf Life	12 months if refrigerated	1 year at room temp.	6–12 months at room temp.	1 year at room temp.	6 months if refrigerated
Cost per Sample	$7.30	$7.00	$4.00–8.00[b]	$6.00–8.00[b]	$6.00–8.00[b]
Other Kits	Aflatoxin M_1	None	DON, zearalenone, T_2 toxin, aflatoxin M_1	Fumonisin, zearalenone, ochratoxin	Zearalenone, DON, trichothecenes, patulin
Special Equipment Needed	Grinder blender	Ultraviolet lamp, grinder, blender	Grinder, blender	Fluorometer, grinder, blender	Grinder, blender
Amount of Sample Required	20 g	50 g	5 g	50 g	50 g
Material Required Not in Kit	Glassware, filter paper	Glassware	None	Glassware, filters	Glassware, filters

[a] Varies according to extraction protocol utilized.
[b] Price varies per number of samples run as a batch.

Heating and most acid or alkali treatments sufficient to destroy the majority of mycotoxin in a feed result in damage to the feed. However, heat treatments used in normal feed processing, such as steam flaking, cooking, roasting, micronizing, and popping, still provide a feasible mechanism for substantially reducing the mycotoxin concentration in feeds. Ammoniation has been shown to be an effective and economically feasible means for reducing the aflatoxin content of feeds without adverse effects. Its efficacy on other mycotoxins is less well known. Solar radiation may be effective but impractical to use in most situations. Adding some clays to mycotoxin-containing feeds has been shown to prevent their effect. Many mycotoxins are adsorbed by compounds such as clay, preventing their adsorption by the animal and enhancing their excretion in the feces. In one study, adding 0.5% sodium bentonite or hydrated sodium calcium aluminosilicate to a diet containing 500 ppb aflatoxin prevented the aflatoxin's inducement of a 30% reduction in feed intake and growth rate of pigs, had a minimal effect on the adsorption of nutrients, and was more effective than five other types of clay tested.

FESCUE POISONING IN HORSES

Fescue poisoning is a commonly occurring problem in mares during the last months of pregnancy and in growing horses grazing mold infected fescue pastures. For other horses, even heavily infected fescue is a good and safe forage. However, during late pregnancy, its ingestion may result in the absence of signs of impending foaling, a prolonged pregnancy, a thickened placenta causing difficult

foaling, the birth of weak or dead foals, decreased or no milk production, retained placenta, and death of the mare or decreased postfoaling conception. In young horses it may decrease their growth rate. Cattle and sheep, as well as horses, are affected by fescue poisoning.

Cause of Fescue Poisoning

Fescue poisoning is caused by the consumption of tall fescue (Festuca arundinaceae) infected with the mold Acremonium coenophialum (formerly referred to as Epichochloele typhina). Poisoning is due to a mycotoxin that produces mold, that causes a decrease in the mares plasma concentrations of the hormones prolactin and progesterone. Tall fescue is usually referred to simply as fescue, although there are other types of fescue that are not infected by this mold. These include chewing fescue (F. rubra var. commutata) used for turf or lawn grass, sheep fescue (F. ovina), meadow fescue (F. elator), and F. pratensis. However, these species of fescue are not grown for forage production because of their lower productivity. Tall fescue is a cool-season, perennial grass that grows in deeply-rooted vigorous clumps. Because optimum growth occurs during cool ambient temperatures and adequate soil moisture, forage-growth surges occur most frequently in spring and fall. Its broad, dark green leaves are ribbed and rough on the upper surface, giving it a coarse texture which reduces its acceptability to horses when it is fully mature, whereas prior to maturity it is well accepted. At maturity it reaches a height of 3 to 4 feet (0.9 to 1.2 m) and seeds out. Two strains of tall fescue, Kentucky 31 and Alta, have been most widely used as a forage crop.

Tall fescue is the most widely grown forage grass, and is the major forage growing on about 35 million acres (14 million ha) in the continental United States, particularly in the transition zone between northern and southern regions in the eastern one-half of the United States. It has been estimated that nearly 700,000 horses are maintained on tall fescue pastures in the United States. Tall fescue is widely grown because of its high productivity, it can be grazed most of the year, and its ability to tolerate wide temperature and moisture extremes, heavy grazing and trampling, and soils varying in texture, moisture, salinity and alkalinity.

The mold causing fescue toxicosis grows inside the plant (i.e. is an endophyte) that moves up the stem and into the seed as the plant grows. The mold is then transmitted via the seed to the next generation of fescue plants. In contrast to most other molds it is not transmitted from plant to plant or from the ground to the plant, but instead is transmitted only in the seed. Because it grows inside, rather than on the outside of the plant its doesn't affect the plant's appearance. As a result, its presence can't be detected by looking at the plant, but can be detected microscopically. Even in infected plants it is not present in their leaf blades or roots, but only in their stems and seeds.

It is estimated that 80% of fescue growing in the United States is infected to varying degrees, usually at levels of 70% or more of the fescue plants in a pasture. It is known that horses grazing fescue pastures are affected at infection levels as low as 25%, and levels below 7% are recommended for fescue toxicosis prevention.

Fescue infection, and as a result the occurrence of fescue poisoning, is greater in warmer humid climates, such as the southeastern and south central United States, particularly in fall pasture regrowth when autumn rains follow a dry summer. Thus, fescue poisoning occurs most commonly during late fall and winter. Although tall fescue is commonly grown and fed to horses in cooler or dryer areas, fescue poisoning is much less common in these areas. Fescue poisoning is most commonly caused by grazing infected fescue pastures, but may also be caused by infected fescue hay. However, the effects of infected hay are minimal if it is cut prior to maturity and, therefore, doesn't contain seeds which contain the highest concentration of the mold and its mycotoxins. Grazing infected fescue pastures that are mature also results in greater effects than consuming either infected hay or grazing immature pastures because horses, like cattle, selectively graze the seedheads if they are present.

Effects of Fescue Poisoning

Gestation in mares consuming infected fescue forage during late pregnancy may be prolonged to more than 13 months, during which time signs of approaching foaling, such as udder development and others (as given in Table 14-1), may not occur and fetal size continues to increase. The placenta is generally edematous with increased collagen, making it thicker and harder for the foal to break through at birth. The thickened, tough placenta, poor re-

laxation of the pelvic ligaments and cervix, and large fetal size lead to difficult delivery, cervical tears, and soft tissue trauma to other components of the mare's reproductive tract. Frequently the foal is in the wrong position for birth, with a 90°-rotation from normal. Premature separation of the placenta may occur resulting in fetal suffocation. Even without premature placental separation foals may be born dead, or weak and fail to breathe, although some may be normal. Affected mares tend to gain less weight during pregnancy, and as a result be in poorer body condition than those not consuming infected fescue. This may be because of reduced intake and digestibility of infected fescue. However, digestibility of infected fescue has been shown not to be reduced at least in growing horses.

In contrast to affected cows and ewes, affected mare's rectal temperature doesn't increase. Following foaling, if premature placental separation did not occur, the placenta is often retained, which in conjunction with dystocia and related trauma, may result in death. If the affected mare lives, she is generally more difficult to get rebred. However, the most consistent effect is decreased or absence of milk production, which in one survey was found to occur in 15% of mares grazing tall fescue pasture as compared to 1.8% in mares on other forages, and to occur in the majority of fescue toxicosis-affected mares. In one study, in 8 mares consuming 94% infected fescue pasture during the last 72 to 181 days of pregnancy, none aborted; of their foals, 4 were stillborn, 2 were weak, 2 were normal at birth, and 3 survived. An abscence of milk production occurred in 7 of the 8 mares, 5 had retained placentas, and only 3 of 7 that were rebred conceived. Identical symptoms occur as a result of ergot ingestion by mares or foals, but as described later in this chapter in the section on ergot, ergot is present in grains or other grasses seedheads but not fescue and rarely affects horses.

It's been reported that 40% of mares grazing infected fescue pastures have decreased reproductive efficiency. Although there are numerous other causes for reproductive problems in mares, as discussed in Chapter 13, it's reported that fescue toxicosis is responsible for the majority of reproductive-related problems in mares grazing heavily infected fescue pastures. Decreased reproduction and milk production has also been reported to occur in cows grazing infected fescue pastures.

Three syndromes may occur in cattle and sheep but haven't been reported in horses grazing infected fescue pastures. These are the following:

1. "Summer Syndrome or Slump," which occurs particularly during hot humid weather and results in: (a) decreased feed intake, gains, and milk production; (b) a rough, dull hair coat; (c) emaciation; (d) listlessness; (e) arched back; (f) a decreased ability to dissipate body heat, or excess body heat production, resulting in an elevated rectal temperature (up to 106°F, or 41°C) and affected animals seeking shade or wet cool areas; (g) increased respiration and heart rates; (h) diarrhea; (i) excessive salivation; and (j) cloudy corneas. These effects are amplified with increasing environmental temperature and humidity.

2. "Fescue Foot," which occurs more commonly dur-

ing late fall and winter and is characterized also by a decreased ability to dissipate body heat as well as symptoms similar to those of ergotism (as described later in this chapter), especially those of dry gangrene of the hind feet.

3. "Fat Necrosis Syndrome," which is characterized by hard fat masses located primarily in the abdominal cavity and which results in symptoms similar to those occurring with "Summer Syndrome," including digestive and parturition problems. Its incidence and severity appear to increase with increasing nitrogen fertilization of infected fescue pastures.

The growth rate and efficiency of feed utilization of horses, like cattle and sheep, grazing infected fescue pasture forage or hay may be decreased. In one study growth rates of both yearling horses and steers were reduced in similar amounts when a high- as compared to a low-endophyte-infected ($\geq$75% or $\leq$25%) fescue pasture with ample forage was grazed. The average daily weight gain was reduced from 1.2 to 0.5 lb/day (0.56 to 0.24 kg/d) for the horses and from 1.5 to 0.5 lb/day (0.69 to 0.23 kg/d) for the steers. Neither species rectal temperatures were increased. The effects of infected fescue forage consumption by growing horses can be prevented by feeding a grain-mix as one-half of the weight of their total diet. This would be the amounts given in Table 15–3.

Treatment of Fescue Poisoning

Removing mares from infected fescue pasture, or not feeding infected fescue hay, is effective in rapidly alleviating fescue toxicosis effects. Even when bromocriptine (which induces all of the effects of fescue toxicosis) is administered to mares up until 320 days of gestation, and until an average of 12 (7 to 17) days before foaling the mares are unaffected. Even mares that are past their expected foaling date because of fescue poisoning will be all right if they are removed from infected pasture and fed a noninfected hay. This was well demonstrated in one report in which 7 of 14 mares on infected fescue pasture had difficult delivery without any prior signs of impending foaling; all 7 foals died, 4 of the mares died, and none of the mares lactated. Within 48 hours of moving the remaining 7 mares to a noninfected pasture, their udder development began, and all delivered live foals within 7 days and lactated without trouble.

Mares not removed from infected fescue should be monitored closely so they can be assisted at foaling. Frequently the placenta must be broken, as it may be too thick and tough to be broken by the mare and foal during delivery. Assistance in delivering the foal is also frequently necessary because of decreased pelvic ligament and cervical relaxation, and because of the foal's larger size due to the increase in the length of gestation. The foal may be dead, or weak at birth and require respiratory assistance. Since most affected mares don't lactate, the newborn foal must be given adequate quantities of good colostrum and fed until the mare recovers sufficiently from the poisoning to produce adequate milk for the foal. This will generally take only about a week after she stops consuming infected fescue forage. If the placenta is retained, the mare must be cared for properly if she is to survive and conceive when rebred. Procedures for providing assistance in delivery and caring for the foaling mare and newborn foal, including providing respiratory assistance, colostrum, and feeding, are described in Chapter 14.

Prevention of Fescue Poisoning

Pastures containing a significant amount of fescue should not provide the major part of the diet for growing horses, or for mares during the last 60 days of their pregnancy, unless it is known not to be infected. If weanlings or yearlings are to be grazed on pastures or fed mature hay containing a significant amount of endophyte-infected fescue, or fescue whose infestation status isn't known, they should be fed a grain-mix as 50% of their total diet (Table 15–3). This will be approximately 1 lb of grain-mix/100 lbs (1 kg/100 kg) body weight daily. Pregnant mares consuming fescue not known to be infestation-free should be closely monitored beginning 6 weeks before their expected foaling date.

If a mare has no udder development by 2 weeks before her due date, she and all other pregnant mares on that pasture should be removed from that pasture and either put on a pasture or fed a hay known to be either noninfected or not fescue. If all the mares can't be fed a nonproblem-causing forage, or removed from a problem-causing pasture, they should be fed alfalfa hay as a substantial portion of their diet (over 10 lbs or 4.5 kg/mare daily) and continue to be monitored closely for fescue-poisoning-induced problems.

Whether a fescue pasture or hay has the potential to cause problems can be determined. To do so collect an equal number of fescue seeds or, (ideally in the fall but anytime from fall to spring) stems from several sites throughout the hay or entire pasture. Collect from at least 5 sample sites/acre or 30 sample sites/pasture. Combine the samples into one composite sample of at least 2 oz per 10 acres or less (60 g/4 ha). The samples should be seedhead, or from the bottom 2 inches (5 cm) of the plant stem above the ground, and be devoid of roots and leaves since the mold is not in them. Put the composite sample into a jar or test tube and fill the container half full of water. Send it to a laboratory able to determine if the Acremonium coenophialum endophyte mold is present. Since the mold is on the inside, not on the outside of the plant, it can't be detected by visual observation. At the laboratory each seed or stem should be stained (e.g., with lactic acid and aniline blue) and examined microscopically to determine the percent of infected fescue plants in the pasture or hay. Infected plants can also be detected by enzyme-linked immunosorbent assay (ELISA) and by tissue-print immunoblot (TPIB). These two methods are comparable in accuracy, and both are more specific than the staining method, but aren't currently available commercially.

If more than 7% of the fescue is infected, to ensure that fescue poisoning doesn't occur, mares must be removed from that pasture or hay during the last 2 weeks, and preferably 2 months, of pregnancy. Feeding grain in amounts up to even one-half of the pregnant mare's energy needs will not decrease the incidence or severity of fescue poisoning if she remains on infected pasture, but may, if the infected forage is hay rather than pasture, since on pasture more seeds which are higher in the mold and its toxins are consumed. Feeding a grain-mix as one-half of the growing horse's diet will prevent any effect of consuming an infected fescue hay, but may not if they are on a heavily infected fescue pasture.

All mature horses, including pregnant mares until the latter stages of pregnancy, may be safely kept on infected fescue pasture, as they are not known to be affected by fescue poisoning. In contrast to previous suggestions, neither increasing nor decreasing nitrogen fertilization or giving pregnant mares selenium have any effect on altering the incidence or effects of fescue poisoning.

Overseeding pastures that have 25% or less infected fescue with legumes, such as red or white clover or alfalfa, so as to maintain at least 20% legumes in the pasture may decrease fescue poisoning, presumably by decreasing the concentration of the mold in the total pasture forage. Overseeding grass pastures with legumes is often also beneficial in increasing both the amount of pasture forage produced and the nutritional value of forage obtained from that pasture, as described in Chapter 5.

Fescue toxicosis can be prevented by killing the fescue in an infected pasture with tillage or a herbicide (e.g., Roundup-Monsanto, or Gramoxone Super) and replanting as described in Chapter 5 with either fescue seed certified to be endophyte-free, or with a different forage. Since the fescue-toxicosis-inducing mold is transmitted only through the seed and, in contrast to most molds, is not in the soil and does not spread from plant to plant, whether a plant is infected depends entirely on whether or not the seed from which it grows contains the live mold. The mold is reported to die in seed stored for more than a year, although 2 years storage has been recommended. Because it is spread only in the seed, its spread is slow and can be prevented by grazing or cutting fescue before it matures and produces seeds. Also, since the seeds contain the highest concentration of the mold, cutting fescue before seeds form decreases the amount present in the hay and thus its detrimental effect; it also results in a more palatable, higher nutritional value hay.

If a mold-free fescue seed is to be planted, ensure that all of the old infected fescue is dead. This can be difficult, particularly in old established sod. It is best to not plant noninfected fescue seed immediately after killing an old infected fescue pasture. If possible, it is best to plant an annual forage or a row crop for at least one growing season prior to planting the noninfected fescue. This reduces the likelihood of the old fescue sod damaging the fescue seedlings; it allows infected seeds that might be present in the soil to age making them less likely to germinate and produce infected plants; and it allows a thorough assessment of the extent to which old plants were destroyed before replanting noninfected seed.

Fescue seed free of infection, which may be referred to as fungus-, mold-, or endophyte-free seed, is available in most areas. There are no known varieties of fescue that are resistant to the mold. However, all of the commercially available seed of some varieties is mold free. For other

varieties, seed bought commercially can be either mold free or mold infected, depending on the source of the seed. Most certified fescue seed now contains a statement on the seed tag as to whether or not it is infected. Only seed that has 5% or less, and preferably zero percent, mold infection should be used to plant an infection-free pasture.

It may be better in some areas, however, not to plant noninfected fescue. Noninfected fescue is less productive and less resistant to insects, flooding, drought, and variations in fertilizer application than is infected fescue. Infected fescue is hardier and will tend to take over noninfected fields. Because noninfected fescue has less vigor, particularly as seedlings, care must be taken to provide favorable conditions during its establishment, including planting at the optimum time, fertilizing and liming according to soil tests, using an adequate seeding rate, and avoiding overgrazing, especially during the first year of growth.

Besides keeping the mare off infected fescue pasture during the last 60 days of pregnancy, or replanting infected fescue pastures, a third alternative that may be beneficial is to feed compounds that counteract infected fescue's effect. The oral administration of domperidone to mares during the last 30 days of pregnancy has been reported to be effective in preventing the effects of fescue poisoning with no negative side effects. Perphenazine, a phenothiazine derivative, fed twice daily at 0.3 to 0.5 mg/kg body wt beginning 1 week before foaling is due has been shown to increase non-pregnant mare's plasma prolactin concentration, back toward normal, induce mammary growth and to initiate milk production. Care must be taken to use a pure perphenazine preparation, because this drug marketed for people, is often combined with the antidepressant drug, amitriptyline. Twice the recommended dosage of perphenazine causes sweating, colic and excessive sensitiveness to activity. Feeding phenothiazine and thiabendazole has been shown to have a preventive effect in cattle, but not horses, grazing infected fescue pastures.

EQUINE ERGOTISM

Ergot is the common name for the mycotoxin-containing hardened covering of the mold Claviceps purpurea and C. paspali. It is unique in that the mycotoxin is produced only during flowering and seed maturation, and not in the mature plant or seed and, therefore, not during their storage. Ergot formation and, therefore, epidemics and cases of ergotism are most likely to occur during damp weather around plant flowering time. Conversely, ergot formation and spread are inhibited by periods of drought.

Ergots are black- to brown-colored, hard, banana-shaped masses from $\frac{1}{4}$ to $\frac{3}{4}$ inch long (0.6 to 2 cm) that project from the plant seedheads. Those produced by C. purpurea are present most often in rye, but also triticale (the cross between rye and wheat) and ryegrass seedheads, but may be present in any of the cereal grains and seedheads of other grasses. Ergots produced by C. paspali are present primarily in Paspalum grass seedheads, such as Dallis and Bahia grasses. C. paspali, in addition to ergot, also produces tremor producing mycotoxins which are probably responsible for causing "Grass or Paspalum staggers" in horses, and not ergotism as described in the following section on this condition.

Ergot produced by C. purpurea is toxic to all animals, including people, and was responsible for the death of thousands of people in the Middle Ages who ate contaminated rye bread, causing what was referred to as St. Anthony's Fire. Although ergot contains many compounds, its alkaloids are its toxic principle. These include the hallucinatory drug LSD, (lysergic acid diamine) which may be responsible for the behavioral effects ergot causes. Ergot alkaloids also cause blood vessel constriction causing dry gangrene of the extremities, and inhibit the reproductive hormone prolactin, which may be responsible for the reproductive effects of ergot poisoning. Thus, in livestock, ergot alkaloids may cause:

1. Behavioral effects—muscle tremors, hyperexcitability, aggression or lethargy, convulsions, incoordination, lameness, difficult respiration, excess salivating, diarrhea, and paralysis of the hind legs.
2. Dry gangrene, swelling, and tissue death or necrosis of the extremities (feet, tail, ears, and skin) due to prolonged artery constriction which resembles "fescue foot" (see previous section on "Effects of Fescue Poisoning"). When ergotism occurs in cattle or sheep in the summer instead of the fall or winter, there tends to be more diarrhea, skin lesions, loss of hair, and increased efforts to dissipate body heat instead of sloughing of extremities.
3. Reproductive effects—abortion, reduced birth weight and viability, and little milk production similar to fescue poisoning.
4. Reduced feed intake and growth.

Cattle and sheep, which appear to be the most sensitive to ergot, may demonstrate any of these clinical effects, whereas swine show primarily the last two effects, but not abortion. Horses are rarely affected by ergotism. Horses fed over 1 lb (500g) of ergot showed only transient symptoms. But horses may show any of these clinical effects, with behavioral changes being most common. Dry gangrene of the legs, difficulty in swallowing, slow respiration, weak pulse, and death of horses ingesting large quantities of ergot-infected ryegrass may occur. No udder development, thickened fetal membranes that required manual rupturing, difficult delivery, poor cervical dilation, and uterine contractions, retained placenta, and uterine rupture has been reported in mares consuming oats containing ryegrass seeds contaminated with Claviceps purpurea and ergot. Their absence of milk production usually did not resolve, although several mares began lactating 10 to 15 days after foaling. Abortions and prolonged gestation also occurred. Embryonic death and anestrus occurred in rebred mares. Affected foals were unable to stand, were icteric, and had no sucking reflex. These effects are similar to those occurring as a result of fescue poisoning. Despite tube-feeding and blood or plasma transfusions, 21 of 33 ergot affected foals died within the first 5 days of life.

GRASS STAGGERS IN HORSES

Staggers, or incoordination, may occur in horses as a result of: (1) moldy corn disease, as discussed in the following section; (2) ergotism, as discussed in the previous section; and as a result of two types of grass staggers: (3) paspalum staggers and (4) perennial ryegrass staggers. Both moldy corn disease and ergotism occur primarily in horses consuming mycotoxin-contaminated grains, generally result in additional clinical signs, and are often fatal. In contrast, grass staggers usually occur when these grasses are grazed, but may occur when they are consumed as hay, straw, or seed cleanings, and are rarely fatal, with affected horses recovering when a noncontaminated diet is consumed.

With both types of grass staggers, behavioral changes usually occur suddenly in horses within 1 to 4 weeks of the continual consumption of a contaminated forage. From 5 to 75% of horses consuming the contaminated feed are generally affected. Clinical signs vary in severity from mild excitability and muscle tremors to spastic incoordination and tetany. Even horses severely affected often appear normal at rest but have a fine tremor of the head or neck, or weave when standing still. When incited to move, affected horses may have a stiff, spastic uncoordinated gait that affects either the forelegs or all legs, exaggerated leg action, muscular spasms, and occasionally tetanic seizures. Those with tetany, when left undisturbed, will recover, generally in less than 20 minutes, stand, and walk off stiffly. Development of abdominal muscle spasms leading to straining may occur. Loss of body weight does not occur.

Clinical signs are predominantly attributable to reversible biochemical, not pathological, changes. As a result, all effects are reversible, and no visible or microscopic lesions occur even in severely affected animals. Treatment is not generally necessary, as the diseases are self-curing when the animals are removed from infected paspalum grasses or perennial ryegrasses. Marked improvement occurs within 2 to 14 days, and complete recovery occurs within a few months or less if a noncontaminated diet is fed.

Paspalum staggers is caused by tremor producing mycotoxins produced by Claviceps paspali primarily in the seedheads of Paspalums spp. grasses—especially Dallis or Bahia grasses. Although this mold may also produce ergot, it is its tremor producing mycotoxins that are thought to cause paspalum staggers in horses. Dallis grass (Paspalum dilatatum) is the most common of the two paspalum grasses responsible for the condition in the United States and, therefore, it is sometimes referred to as Dallis grass staggers instead of paspalum staggers.

Dallis grass is a common pasture grass of the more humid regions of the United States, ranging from southern California to the southeastern states. Under humid conditions it may become infected with C. paspali. This mold invades only the flowering part of the plant and produces a sticky substance referred to as honeydew that is attractive to insects, which aid in the dissemination of the mold. In time, the honeydew dries to form a brown mycotoxin-containing mass that resembles the grass seeds.

Perennial ryegrass staggers is caused by the tremor producing neurotoxins lolitrems, which are produced by, or their production stimulated by, Acremonium lolii. This endophytic mold grows, and the toxin is produced, in the lower outer leaf sheaths, seeds, and seed cleanings of perennial ryegrass (Lolium perenne). Since the toxin is produced in the lower leaf sheaths, the lower to the ground animals graze perennial ryegrass, the more likely they are to be affected. Thus, the disease most frequently occurs in herbivores, including horses, on intensively or overgrazed perennial ryegrass pastures during late summer or fall.

Confirming perennial ryegrass as a cause of the staggering symptoms described is usually based on finding (most commonly in the lower portions of the plant) and identifying the causative mold Acremonium lolii. Diagnosis is also confirmed by the occurrence of clinical signs in mice injected with plant extracts or by assaying for the toxin. Lolitrem concentrations of 5.3 mg/kg for horses and 2 mg/kg for sheep have been found to result in perennial ryegrass staggers.

Paspalum staggers can be prevented by mowing the pasture at or prior to the flowering stage to prevent formation of the toxic mycotoxin-containing mass, which is formed only in the flowering part of the plant. Procedures for preventing perennial ryegrass staggers include: (1) replacement of the pasture with perennial ryegrass free of the causative mold, (2) not overgrazing, (3) removing animals from affected pastures for a few weeks until new growth appears, and (4) supplementing with noncontaminated feed during hazardous periods (late summer to fall in most areas). Replacement of pasture with mold-free perennial ryegrass may be undesirable, as the mold or mycotoxin increases the grass's resistance to insects, and mold-free perennial ryegrass is less productive.

Facial eczema, characterized by lesions on light-colored or exposed areas of the skin around the face, resulting in edema, exudation, blistering, and tissue death sloughing, may occur instead of staggers in sheep, but not horses, grazing ryegrass pastures. Staggers resembling perennial ryegrass staggers may occur in sheep and cattle, but are not reported in horses, grazing annual ryegrass (Lolium rigidum). Annual ryegrass staggers, however, is not due to a mycotoxin poisoning but instead to the neurotoxin corynetoxin. It is produced in annual ryegrass infected with the nematode parasite Anguina agrostis and the bacterium Corynebacterium spp.

Ruminants, but not horses, may also be affected by both "Phalaris Staggers" and "Bermudagrass Staggers" or tremors. Both result in clinical signs similar to those occurring with either type of ryegrass staggers and with paspalum staggers. The cause for Bermudagrass (Cynodon dactylon) staggers or tremors is unknown. Phalaris staggers is caused by hordenine (p-hydroxyphenylathyl-dimethylamine) produced by Phalaris grasses, primarily reed canarygrass (Phalaris arundinacea). It is sometimes referred to as reed canarygrass staggers instead of phalaris staggers.

Hordenine is also produced by sprouting barley, millet, milo and wheat, and is thought to be the hallucination producing compound in peyote cactus. Hordenine has actions similar to epinephrine or adrenalin. It stimulates the heart, constricts blood vessels, and relaxes constricted lung airways. However, there appears to be no evidence that the amount of hordenine in reed canarygrass or sprouted grains has any significant effect on horses. But some racing commissions (e.g., New Jersey and West Virginia) disqualify horses if hordenine is found in their urine, which it may be if they are consuming these feeds.

Hordenine has been associated with decreased feed palatability and poor growth and/or condition in ponies and ruminants grazing reed canarygrass. But chronic phalaris toxicosis or staggers, which may occur in ruminants, is not known to occur in horses. Clinical signs in ruminants may be acute or chronic. Acute poisoning results in a sudden onset of neurologic signs or collapse, abnormal heart rythms, and respiratory distress followed by death or recovery. Chronic poisoning effects, in addition to poor growth and/or condition, include decreased feed intake, loss of control of the tongue or the ability to swallow, excess excitability, incoordination, stiff gait, head nodding, muscle twitching, tetanic seizures, and death. Clinical signs may be delayed for as long as 4 months after ruminants are removed from phalaris pastures. Pretreatment with cobalt pellets apparently prevents clinical signs. Brown pigment may occur in nerve cells in the brain stem and spinal cord of affected ruminants.

MOLDY CORN DISEASE IN HORSES

Moldy corn poisoning in horses and other equine species results in a degenerative softening of the white matter of the brain, i.e. results in leukoencephalomalacia, another name for the disease. It is also referred to as blind staggers (as are locoweed and excess selenium poisonings) which it causes, as well as other neurologic signs. These generally occur for only 4 to 72 hours, but occasionally 1 to 2 weeks, duration, before death. Liver damage may also occur. In addition to moldy corn disease, blind staggers, and equine leukoencephalomalacia, it has also been referred to as leucoencephalitis, encephalomyelitis, cerebrospinal meningitis, fumonisin poisoning, foraging disease, corn stalk disease, epizootic cerebritis and mycotoxic equine encephalomalacia. It affects only horses and other equine species.

It is one of the most common poisonings of domestic horses. Nearly 200 cases were confirmed by veterinary diagnostic laboratories in 11 states in a 2-year period, and outbreaks with many horses affected can occur. The disease occurs worldwide, most often in areas with temperate humid climates following a dry summer and wet fall, such as throughout eastern and midwestern United States. Fusarium, the causative mold appears to increase when hot, dry conditions are present during pollination, and continues to increase when warm temperatures occur during the last 30 days of maturity. Outbreaks of the disease are usually seasonal, occurring from fall through early spring, but cases can occur any time of the year from stored corn containing the mycotoxin. In contrast to most mycotoxicoses, older horses are reportedly more susceptible to moldy corn disease than younger horses.

Cause of Moldy Corn Disease

Moldy corn disease is caused by a fumonisin mycotoxin that injures the lining of blood vessles. The toxin is produced by the molds Fusarium moniliforme, and by F. proliferatum. The presence of fumonisin mycotoxin in a feed, and the occurrence of the disease from the ingestion of that feed, is generally due to the feed becoming contaminated with the causative mold prior to harvesting and not during storage. Although Fusarium molds may grow in a wide range of different feeds and occasionally are isolated from hay and small cereal grains, moldy corn disease has been reported only in horses consuming corn grain or any portion of the corn plant, or feed containing them. The mold can grow at a wide temperature range when the feed moisture content is above 13 to 15%. Infected corn kernels may be recognized by a pink to reddish brown color. Although affected horses are usually associated with shelled or ear corn, the mold may grow in, its mycotoxin be present in, and the disease be due to consumption of, cornstalks and leaves and in commercially prepared mixes and pellets containing any portion of the corn plant. However, corn containing the Fusarium mold may or may not contain the fumonisin mycotoxin and, therefore, be harmful. Fusarium ear rot was found to be present in 50 to 96% of corn fields sampled in Indiana from 1989 through 1992. But fumonisin was present in only 13 to 84% of the samples that contained Fusarium, and there was no relationship between the amount of mold and the amount of the mycotoxin present. Conversely, although non-Fusarium containing corn generally does not contain fumonisins, it may; that is, nonmoldy-appearing corn-product-based feed may cause moldy corn disease. Determining feed that may or has caused moldy corn disease, therefore requires that the fumonisin mycotoxin be found in the feed. In suspected cases all feeds being consumed, not just moldy-appearing corn, should be analyzed as described in the previous section on "Diagnosis of Mycotoxin Poisoning."

Fusarium molds produce a wide variety of fumonisin mycotoxins which have various effects on different species of animals. In horses the mycotoxin appears to damage the lining of the blood vessels in the brain, and in some cases to cause liver damage. Some have suggested that neurologic signs are caused by a low dose of toxin over time, whereas liver damage is a result of a higher dose. However, this has not been found to be the case in some outbreaks. Others have postulated that different toxins cause the liver and the neurologic forms of the disease, with fumonisin B_1 likely responsible for the neurologic form, which is by far the most common form of the disease. Forty-five horses that died from moldy corn disease in one outbreak had been associated with feeds containing over 5 ppm fumonisin with fumonisin B_1 present at levels of 0.6 to 96 ppm and B_2 at 0 to 38 ppm.

Moldy corn responsible for outbreaks of the disease in horses has been fed to numerous nonequine species, including goats, pigs, monkeys, hamsters, rats, mice, guinea pigs, rabbits, and chickens without causing illness or death. However, feeding other horses contaminated feed responsible for outbreaks in horses doesn't always produce the disease either, even after extended exposure.

Clinical Effects of Moldy Corn Disease

The course of the disease depends on the amount and rate of mycotoxin consumption and the individual horse's tolerance to the toxin, which is variable. In most outbreaks, 15 to 25% of horses consuming the contaminated feed are affected, although 100% may be affected and die. The onset of clinical signs is usually 2 to 9 weeks, but may be from less than 1 to 21 weeks, after the onset of continuous consumption of fumonisin-contaminated feed.

Neurologic signs usually appear abruptly and end in death within 4 to 72 hours of their onset, but occasionally the duration may be as long as 4 weeks. However, more subtle signs, such as decreased feed intake and depression, often precede severe neurologic signs by days or weeks.

The clinical signs are characterized by rapidly progressive neurologic alterations. These include intermittent to complete absence of food intake, and mild to profound depression with little response to stimuli, but when affected horses respond they may be quite excitable. Affected horses have a progressive incoordination, may press their heads against something, have delirium, blindness, sweating, circling, or leaning against a wall, but remain standing until shortly before death. Muscle tremors and incoordination lead to an inability to stand. Once down, convulsions may occur prior to coma and death. Outbreaks may individually be characterized by unique predominant clinical signs such as colic, a high incidence of blindness, or although able to eat and drink a refusal to do so resulting in rapid weight loss and dehydration. The temperature of affected horses is generally normal, in contrast to those with sleeping sickness viral encephalopathies. Some horses with moldy corn disease show many, some only a few, and some no clinical signs prior to death. Horses that show neurologic signs generally die, regardless of treatment, although there are instances of horses recovering, but some retain brain damage. In several outbreaks 64 to 100% of horses showing clinical signs died.

Clinical signs associated with the less common moldy corn induced liver disease form, which may occur alone but more often in conjunction with neurologic alterations, include icterus, which is generally severe; swelling of the lips and nose; bloody spots in the mucous membranes; lowered head; reluctance to move; abdominal breathing; cyanosis; and a bloody urine. As with the neurologic form, clinical signs appear acutely and death usually occurs within a few hours to days.

Moldy corn disease should be considered as a cause of an acute onset of rapidly progressive neurologic signs (e.g., incoordination, blindness, absence of feed intake, little response to stimuli, or severe depression to agitation) and death occurring in two or more horses in a group that has been consuming a corn-containing feed for more than 1 week, even if the feed isn't visibly moldy, but particularly if it is, and if the problem occurs from late fall to early spring in areas with a dry summer, wet fall, and humid climate, such as the eastern and midwestern United States. The presence of Fusarium moniliforme or F. proliferatum in affected horses' feed is quite indicative that the problem is due to moldy corn disease but confirmation requires the identification of fumonisins in feed being consumed. Test kits for detecting fumonisins are available (Table 19–4). It has been hypothesized that the fumonisins in contaminated feed may degrade after a variable period, but deaths have occurred in horses consuming fumonisin containing feed stored for over 1 year.

An acute onset of similar neurologic signs with a rapid progression and high mortality affecting more than one horse on a farm may occur as a result of the diseases given in Table 19–5. Other equine neurologic diseases may have similar clinical signs as moldy corn disease but usually occur in a single horse on a farm and generally aren't as rapidly progressive or severe.

TABLE 19–5
Causes of Neurologic Diseases Characterized by an Acute Onset and Rapid Progression
Generally in More Than One Horse in a Group[a]

Disease	History	Season	Common Clinical Signs	Body Temperature
Moldy Corn Disease	Corn, grain or plant ingestion for more than 1 week	Fall to spring	Rapidly progressive incoordination feed refusal, brain damage signs & death; agitation or ↓ responsiveness; ± icterus, nose swelling, & bloody urine	Normal
Rhinopneumonitis (Equine Herpesvirus) (See Chapter 9.)	Exposure to horses with fever, respiratory disease, or late term abortion	All	Hind leg incoordination, urinary incontinence, ↓ tailtone, fecal retention, penile prolapse	↑ before signs occur
Sleeping sickness (See Chapter 9.)	Poor vaccination history	Mosquito season	Incoordination, blindness, head pressing, dementia, can't swallow, seizures, respiratory arrest	High
Rabies (See Chapter 9)	Bitten by rabid animal	All	Facial spasms or paralysis, behavior change, agitation, depression, incoordination, colic	Variable
Botulism	Generally in 1 horse within 4 days after eating often moldy feed, or a wound infection	Spring to fall	Stilted gait, ↓ tail & tongue tone, can't swallow, flaccid muscles	Normal
Theiler's disease (Acute hepatic failure)	Occasionally after therapy with biologic agent of equine origin	Especially fall	Head pressing, circling, seizures, mild colic, incoordination, hemorrhage, icterus, photosensitization, skin damage, usually death or recovery in 5 days	↑ usually
Aflatoxicosis	Especially young eating stored feed, e.g. corn, cottonseeds, or peanuts	Any	Won't eat, lethargy, dehydration, & tremors, ± icterus, straining & incoordination	Normal
Tick paralysis	Tick attached for several days or more. Often a local reaction & pain at attachment site	Spring & summer, but season prolonged with mild, wet weather	Hindleg incoordination; may ascend to complete flaccid immobility & respiratory paralysis within 36 hours; normal sensory function & alertness	Normal
Pyrrolizidine Alkaloid (PA) Liver Damage	Consuming green or dry PA-containing plants (Table 18–4)	All, as plants may be in either hay or pasture	Nervous signs, wt loss, icterus, anemia, bloody urine, sometimes acute depression & death	Normal

Abbreviations used are: ↓ = decrease; ↑ = increase; ± = may occur.
[a] Numerous poisonous plants, listed in Table 18–7 along with their clinical effects in horses, may also cause neurologic disease with rapid progression.

Prevention of Moldy Corn Disease

The following management practices for the prevention of moldy corn disease are recommended, particularly from fall to early spring.

1. Don't feed moldy or suspicious-looking feeds, especially those containing corn or corn byproducts. However, even corn that shows no visual signs of mold can contain mycotoxins.
2. During and following periods of high moisture during harvesting, particularly if there is drought or insect damage to the grain, don't feed corn or corn-byproduct-containing feeds. Use other cereal grains instead.
3. Always feed forages as at least one-half of the horse's total diet.
4. Don't purchase more than several-weeks supply of grain at one time.
5. Buy grain mixes that contain mold inhibitors (described in Chapter 4).
6. Ensure that feed troughs are clean and that all feed fed is consumed between each feeding period.
7. Feed at least twice a day.
8. Check stored feed for high moisture levels (over 13 to 15%). If present, don't use that feed and correct the cause.
9. Watch all horses closely, particularly when feeding. If there is a reluctance for the horses to eat the feed, or if any show any signs of moldy corn disease, examine them thoroughly for other signs and take their rectal temperature. If there is any question, use a different feed and have the suspicious feed

evaluated for both molds (particularly Fusarium moniliforme, Aspergillus spp., and Penicillium spp.) and mycotoxins (particularly fumonisins and aflatoxins).

10. All horses with or without clinical signs should immediately be prevented access to feed suspected of being contaminated. There is no specific therapy or antidote for the causative toxin. By the time clinical signs are apparent, significant irreversible brain damage has generally occurred. As a result, treatment of those showing severe neurologic alterations is rarely successful. For less affected cases, although the prognosis is poor, slow partial recovery over several weeks after the acute illness has been occasionally reported to occur.

AFLATOXIN POISONING IN HORSES

Aflatoxin poisoning, although the most common mycotoxin poisoning affecting most domestic animals, particularly swine, is rarely reported in horses. Aflatoxins are produced primarily by Aspergillus flavus and A. parasiticus most commonly in stored cottonseeds, peanut meal, corn, less commonly other cereal grains, and only rarely hay or straw. Although mainly a grain storage problem, the molds can invade corn and produce aflatoxins prior to harvest if conditions for mold spore transmission and plant infection are optimal. Conditions that promote mold growth and aflatoxin production include insect damage and methods of cultivation, humidity, and drought conditions that cause plant stress. However, not all corn infected by Aspergillus contain aflatoxins. There are four distinct toxic compounds referred to as aflatoxins B_1, B_2, G_1, and G_2, based upon their blue and green fluorescence respectively when examined under ultraviolet light (black or Wood's light). Aflatoxin B_1 is the most common aflatoxin found in animal feeds and associated with the poisoning of animals. Poultry and fish appear to be the most sensitive to the effects of aflatoxin, with pigs and ruminants, followed by horses, being less susceptible to poisoning.

In contrast to species commonly affected by aflatoxin poisoning, the onset and course of the disease in horses are generally relatively short. The onset of clinical signs, other than reduced feed acceptance, which may occur with the first or second feeding, occurs within a few days of exposure to levels as low as 1000 ppb (1 mg/kg) in diet dry matter. However, lower levels of aflatoxin in the diet of young horses may slow their growth and impair their immunity, as it does in other species at dietary levels as low as 100 ppb and possibly 20 ppb. Toxic symptoms have been reported to occur in horses fed aflatoxin at levels as low as 55 ppb.

In horses, as in other species studied, liver damage is the major effect of aflatoxin poisoning, with the young being the most susceptible and severely affected. Complete recovery of affected animals may not occur as the aflatoxin-induced liver damage may not be reversible. Clinical signs of aflatoxin poisoning in horses are those typical of many illnesses, including decreased feed and water intake, lethargy, dehydration, tremors, and terminal prostration. Icterus and abdominal straining producing a bloody diarrhea may occur. Incoordination and convulsions, have been reported in some cases.

All effects of aflatoxin poisoning in horses are similar to those with moldy corn disease. However, moldy corn disease more commonly affects older rather than younger horses, and only liver and/or cerebral lesions are usually present. Factors helpful in the differential diagnosis of these two diseases and other neurologic diseases characterized by an acute onset and rapid progression are given in Table 19–5. Aflatoxin poisoning is confirmed by finding aflatoxins in the animal's liver, kidney, or intestinal contents. Detecting aflatoxins in the feed of horses or other animals (Table 19–3) showing clinical and necropsy signs is strongly suggestive of aflatoxin poisoning.

As in the treatment of any toxicosis, toxin ingestion must be stopped. Increased protein and fat-soluble vitamins have also been recommended to compensate for decreased utilization. Vitamin E and selenium administration may be beneficial.

STACHYBOTRYOTOXICOSIS IN HORSES

Stachybotryotoxicosis in horses has a several weeks to months course that begins with inflammation of the lips and oral mucosa and progresses to head enlargement followed by fever, not eating, and death; or, less commonly, it is characterized by nervous system effects, lung edema, and death in 1 to 3 days after mycotoxin ingestion. Major outbreaks have occurred in Europe, South Africa, and the Ukraine, but currently it has not been reported elsewhere. It is caused by mycotoxins produced by the soil mold, Stachybotrys chartarum, that produces dense, sooty accumulations of black spores primarily in straw or hay. Its mycotoxins cause poisoning in cattle, sheep, swine, poultry, and people, as well as horses.

Clinically the disease manifests in three stages as a prolonged disease, or atypically as a more severe peracute condition. In the first stage fissures develop at the corners of the mouth followed by deeper fissures of the oral mucosa. This is accompanied by excess salivation and nasal discharge. Further swelling under the facial skin and the lymph nodes may occur, producing the impression of an enlarged head. Inflammation around the eyes and excessive tearing may occur. If oral inflammation is sufficiently severe, feed intake is reduced. This stage may be quite mild and short or more severe and present for up to 1 month. If the mycotoxin continues to be ingested, generalized effects typically of 2 to 7 weeks duration occur. During the third stage, fever, not eating, colic, abnormal heart rhythms, and weak pulse followed by an inability to stand and death generally occur within a few days.

Occasionally an acute syndrome, referred to as the "shocking" form resulting in death within 1 to 3 days of the onset of symptoms, may occur. This form generally, but not always, occurs as a result of the ingestion of large amounts of the mycotoxin. In this form, oral lesions don't occur; instead there is nervous irritability and shock. A loss of reflexes, blindness, stupor, reluctance to move, a wide stance, leg crossing, leaning against objects, fever, diarrhea and not eating but drinking excess amounts of water may occur. Lung edema resulting in difficulty breathing and cyanosis are evident.

Treatment is primarily supportive as described previously for moldy corn disease.

IONOPHORE ANTIBIOTIC POISONING IN HORSES

Monensin (Rumensin and Coban-Elanco Prod.), is the most common of the ionophore antibiotics; others are lasalocid (Avatec, Hoffman-LaRoche), salinomycin, and narasin. These antibiotics are mycotoxins produced by Streptomyces spp. molds. They are sometimes added to grain mixes intended for cattle and poultry to increase the efficiency of feed utilization and growth rate, or to treat or prevent their infestation by coccidial organisms. Monensin, which is generally fed to cattle at a level of 5 to 30 g/ton of total feed intake (5.5 to 33 mg/kg) or 200 to 300 mg/head/day, increases by 5 to 15% feed efficiency in cattle consuming a high-grain diet, and growth rate in those consuming a high-forage diet. It also appears to be beneficial in preventing bloat, acute bovine pulmonary edema, and emphysema, and in decreasing face and horn fly pupae in feces, thus helping to control these flies. In poultry the normal or recommended coccidiostat concentration of monensin and lasalocid is about 90 g/ton (100 mg/kg). However, these antibiotics, even at much lower concentrations, are quite toxic to horses that may consume grain mixes containing them.

The amount of monensin that will kill 50% of the animals consuming it (LD_{50}) is 70 to 100 times lower for horses than for chickens, and 10 to 25 times lower for horses than for cattle. The amount that will kill some horses (minimum lethal dose of 1mg/kg body weight) is 50% lower than the LD_{50} and that will cause clinical effects is even lower than this. The relative toxicity difference between species of animals is similar for the other ionophore antibiotics.

For horses, at 30 g monensin/ton of feed the only effect may be a decrease in feed intake and an uneasiness resembling mild colic. At 90 to 110 g/ton, feed intake is decreased by one-half and in one report, 1 of 3 horses died, whereas all horses consuming a feed containing 250 g/ton died within 12 to 24 hours. Supplements may contain up to 1200 g of monensin/ton. Most horses will refuse to eat salinomycin-containing feed after an initial limited intake, and will decrease their intake or be reluctant to eat feeds containing monensin. A reluctance or refusal of healthy horses to eat a grain mix or prepared feed is an important clue that something is wrong with the feed.

Ionophore poisoning is caused by their formation of lipid-soluble complexes with cations such as sodium and potassium destroying their transmembrane concentration gradients so necessary for cell function. The major toxic effects are on highly active organs such as the heart and to a lesser extent the skeletal muscle and kidney. Liver damage may occur as the ionophores are metabolized and excreted by the liver into the feces with none excreted in the urine.

In four stables that inadvertently fed salinomycin containing feed the incidence of horses showing poisoning symptoms ranged from 38 to 100% depending on how hungry the horses were and, therefore, how much they

ate. Monensin or salinomycin poisoning should be suspected when following a feed change there is feed refusal or a reluctance to eat it, and 8 to 24 hours later there is sudden death, particularly following exercise, with no clinical signs, or there is partial to complete refusal to eat and dullness, followed by mild diarrhea, colic, rear leg weakness and incoordination, stiffness, wide stance, and sometimes a reluctance to move. Intermittent profuse sweating, blindness, and head pressing may occur. Straining and excess urination may occur initially, followed by decreased urination and a bloody urine in some horses. Generally the mucous membranes are severely congested, the heart rate is increased and irregular, hyperventilation may occur, and abdominal or gastrointestinal sounds are absent. Eventually the horse will lie down but may rise repeatedly until it is unable to do so. While down, the horse remains alert but may thrash with its legs and have difficult respiration prior to death.

Death may occur within 12 to 24 hours after the onset of clinical signs. However, less severely affected cases may not become incoordinated or unable to stand, and recover in 2 to 3 days, although they may have some exercise intolerance for a period of time and may die of heart damage and scarring weeks to months later. Chronic cases may also occur, resulting in stocking up, dragging of the hind legs, a rough hair coat, loss of condition, and listlessness, but nervousness when handled.

Although not studied in horses, it has been shown in rats that monensin has no effects on reproduction, no teratogenic effects, and does not cause any chronic lesions or tumors when fed continuously to four generations.

Diagnosis of Inophore Toxicosis

Ionophore toxicosis confirmation requires finding the antibiotic by laboratory analysis of the horse's feed or stomach contents. Tissue samples are usually not useful because the small amount of the drug absorbed is rapidly excreted by the liver. It may resemble strongyle induced colic (discussed in Chapter 9), white snakeroot poisoning (see Chapter 18), and selenium/vitamin E deficiency (see Chapter 2).

There is no known specific antidote for ionophore toxicosis. Treatment is to remove the feed containing the antibiotic, and to give drugs and mineral oil to speed the passage of already ingested feed. Large volumes of fluids may need to be administered intravenously and orally if shock is present.

Horses that survive may have an audibly abnormal heart rhythm, and increased heart and respiratory rates. They may stock-up and can die during physical exertion as long as weeks to years after the poisoning, probably as a result of the initial heart damage with subsequent fibrotic repair and scarring. To prevent exertion-induced death, complete stall rest for at least 6 weeks after the horse appears normal is recommended to allow skeletal and heart muscle repair to occur. Then begin exercise gradually. If any abnormality occurs, wait an additional 6 weeks.

FORAGE POISONING (BOTULISM) IN HORSES

Botulism is an uncommon acute disease causing flaccid paralysis. It affects all animals, including people, and is caused by the toxin produced by the bacteria Clostridium botulinum. These bacteria are present primarily in the soil. They produce a number of different toxins that have clinically similar effects on nerve function. Toxin production occurs during bacterial growth and sporulation, which occurs best in neutral or alkaline warm environments with greater than 15% moisture. This environment is most frequently present in decaying plant matter or animal tissue of dead or live animals,—e.g., improperly ensiled haylage or silage, or small animal carcasses present in drinking water or baled into hay and made into pellets or cubes that are ingested. These conditions are also favorable for mold growth, so that incriminated hay or grain may also be visibly moldy. Most cases of botulism in horses occur as a result of contaminated silage or excessively moist hay.

Botulism in foals most commonly occurs as a result of ingestion of spores and their subsequent toxin production in the foals' intestinal tract. This results in the "shaker foal syndrome," which most often is thought to be due to type B botulism toxin. In contrast, in other horses botulism most commonly occurs as a result of the ingestion of feeds contaminated with toxin type B or C produced in the feed before its ingestion, and is commonly known as "forage poisoning." Botulism may also be less commonly caused in horses by the vegetation of spores in wounds producing type B toxin.

Clinical signs generally occur within 1 to 4 days, but may be as long as 14 days, following consumption of contaminated feeds, or 1 to 3 weeks following wound infections. The toxin blocks the neurotransmitter acetylcholine's release, causing a progressive, symmetric, generalized flaccid paralysis. The period from the onset of clinical signs to an inability to stand and death generally takes 1 to 7 days, or recovery an additional 1 to 3 weeks.

Botulism occurs most commonly in foals 2 to 8 weeks, but up to 8 months, of age. Affected foals are often found laying on their side unable to rise or occasionally dead. If observed earlier, they may lie down more than normal, often with their head resting on the ground, and if forced to walk, may have decreased limb flexion and toe scuffing. Difficulty in swallowing is common, with milk spilling from the mouth when nursing is attempted. They may be able to stand for only a short period, develop generalized muscle tremors, and collapse, unable to lift their head, giving rise to the descriptive term for the condition, "shaker foal syndrome." Up to 90% of foals affected may die.

In adult horses the onset of clinical signs may be acute and progress rapidly, or may be slower in onset with a gradual progression over several days. Severely affected cases may die suddenly, often without clinical signs noted. In others, difficulty in swallowing may be the first signs recognized, with spilling of water or feed from the mouth and the presence of feed material in the nostrils. Appetite is usually normal although the horse may be unable to ingest feed or water. Aspiration of food material resulting in pneumonia can result. There may be generalized weakness, depression, muscle tremors, and a reluctance to move; if there is movement, it is with a stiff, stilted gait with short choppy strides and stumbling, but not incoordination. Muscular activity may worsen the clinical signs,

resulting in increased muscle tremors or collapse. There is paralysis and a loss of tail, tongue, and eyelid tone, resulting in little resistance to their being moved. There is difficulty in retracting the tongue, and unresponsive pupils.

A lack of normal intestinal movements may cause decreased abdominal sounds, constipation, and impaction induced colic. Urinary retention and dribbling, and bladder distention may occur. As severe cases progress, collapse due to a flaccid paralysis, difficulty breathing, a rapid heart rate, and death due to an inability to breathe with minimal agonal movements occur.

Botulism should be considered a cause of sudden death or of development within one to a few days of progressive difficulty in swallowing and generalized flaccid muscle weakness in a single horse. Other causes of difficulty in swallowing primarily in mature horses include obstruction or ulceration in the pharynx or esophagus, yellow star thistle poisoning (see Chapter 18), fungal infection of the guttural pouch, tetanus, rabies, lead poisoning, equine protozoal encephalomyelitis, and tick paralysis. Tetanus, however, affects primarily the brain, resulting in muscle rigidity and spasm rather than a flaccid paralysis. Rabies also typically affects the brain. Lead poisoning may also result in a drooping lip, regurgitation, and respiratory noise or "roaring" which develop gradually over weeks to months, whereas effects of botulism develop within a few days or less. Lactation tetany should also be considered as a cause of similar symptoms in lactating mares and potassium induced periodic paralysis considered in genetic lines of horses known to be affected (see Chapter 17). Botulism must also be differentiated from other neurologic diseases characterized as it is by an acute onset and rapid progression. Factors given in Table 19–5 may be helpful for this purpose. In affected foals, selenium deficiency (see Chapter 2), septicemia, and low blood sugar should be considered.

A presumptive diagnosis of botulism can be made upon finding Clostridium botulinum spores in cecal or colonic contents, feed, wounds, or the feces. Spores can be found in the feces of 20 to 30% of affected adults and about 80% of affected foals, whereas they are rarely present in nonaffected horses. A definitive diagnosis requires identification of the toxin. This is usually accomplished by mouse inoculation of gastrointestinal contents, feces, feedstuffs, or liver. Plasma may not contain sufficient toxin to be detected.

Horses with clinical signs of botulism should immediately be confined to a stall and their physical activity minimized. Muscular activity worsens the progressive weakness and increases the likelihood of death. Prognosis is poor for horses that progress to an inability to stand and respiratory distress in less than 2 days. Paralysis and respiratory distress may not develop, and as a result, prognosis is better, in cases in which the other clinical signs develop gradually over several days. Several weeks may be required before recovery is complete.

To prevent botulism only good-quality silage or haylage (as described in Chapter 4) should be fed. Horses should not have access to feeds containing any decayed material. Hay and grain should be kept dry and free of contamination with rodent carcasses. In areas and especially on farms where botulism has occurred, vaccination may be indicated. Because botulism is uncommon, vaccination of either adults or foals may not be indicated otherwise. For horses not previously vaccinated for botulism 3 doses should be given, 1 month apart, with the last dose for pregnant mares given 2 to 4 weeks prior to the expected foaling date. A single booster vaccination should be given annually 2 to 4 weeks before expected foaling. Foals should be vaccinated at 2, 4 and 6 weeks, and again at one year of age. Antibodies obtained from the colostrum do not interfere with the foal's response to the vaccine.

LEAD POISONING IN HORSES

Lead poisoning (plumbism) usually occurs in horses from prolonged consumption of low amounts of lead on contaminated forages. It is one of the most common poisonings occurring in farm animals but is relatively rare in horses. It produces different clinical signs in different species. Affected horses most commonly become progressively weak and depressed, lose condition, regurgitate, and develop a roaring breathing noise, but only slight anemia, which commonly occurs in other species. Lead poisoning should be considered in horses showing signs similar to heaves, depression, weakness, loss of condition, and that have lower lip paralysis, make a roaring breathing noise and/or regurgitate.

Cause of Lead Poisoning

Horses are very sensitive to a low lead dosage over a prolonged period, but are much less sensitive than ruminants to short-term consumption of large doses. This sensitivity difference combined with the horse's more selective eating habits results in a much lower incidence of lead poisoning in horses than in cattle due to common sources of lead such as lead pipes, batteries, some but not all paint, linoleum, some window putty and caulking material, grease, used motor oil, etc. Lead poisoning in horses, particularly adults, is usually associated with forage contaminated by airborne emissions from lead smelters for ores or for reclaiming lead from old batteries and other sources of lead. Airborne and/or water emissions may also occur secondary to other industrial processes that involve lead. Although various lead entrapment devices are used, malfunctions in them do occur and may result in serious environmental contamination. Lead-based herbicide orchard sprays and occasionally flaking or peeling lead containing paint have also caused lead toxicosis in horses.

In areas where low levels of lead contamination in feed over a long period of time have occurred, horses are often the only domestic animal affected, with cattle on the same pasture apparently unaffected. There is a wide variation in horses' susceptibilities to chronic lead consumption. In one study one horse died after consuming a total of 343 mg of lead/kg body weight (as lead acetate), whereas another appeared healthy after ingesting 8.4 times this amount of the same form of lead in a similar diet. Consumption of plants containing 100 ppm (100 mg/kg) may require years to produce poisoning in horses. However, poisoning is hastened by overgrazing because this will increase the risk of soil ingestion, which is much higher in lead than the

plants that are growing on it. Normally there is little uptake of lead from the soil by the plant, so high plant levels will not occur without continued airborne pollution.

Without airborne contamination, most forages contain 3 to 7 ppm (or mg/kg) of lead in its dry matter, which with soil contamination may be increased to 15 to 30 ppm. Concentrations of 260 to 900 ppm and higher have been reported in forages grown near smelters. Less than 30 ppm is considered acceptable, and over 80 ppm has been associated with chronic lead poisoning in horses. An intake of 1.7 to 2.4 mg/kg body weight/day can cause chronic lead poisoning in horses. Experimentally a single dose 1.1 to 1.5 lbs of (500 to 700 g) of lead acetate causes acute poisoning in horses.

Lead on the plant surface is bound so that it will not wash off, and tends to increase with plant maturity so that it remains as a source of lead whether it is grazed or fed as hay or haylage. Alfalfa is less of a hazard than grass because its high calcium content appears to decrease lead absorption by the animal. Increased dietary zinc also decreases lead absorption.

Effects of Lead Poisoning

Absorbed lead binds to red blood cells, with very little free in the plasma. From blood, lead localizes primarily in liver, kidney, and bone as it is formed. A small amount of lead is excreted in bile and the feces. Up to 95% of lead in the body from chronic consumption is gradually incorporated into bone. This is not the case for acute exposure to large amounts of lead, as bone uptake is slow. Lead in bone is not harmful until released during bone turnover. In soft tissues, lead is bound to protein in cell nuclei, which if sufficiently high is visible microscopically as intranuclear inclusions. This accumulation in peripheral nerves impedes nerve impulse conduction, causing the primary clinical problems. Significant but less profound changes may also occur in the kidneys, gastrointestinal tract, and red blood cell producing tissues inhibiting their production.

The major effect of lead poisoning in horses is on peripheral motor nerves, with little loss of feeling or sensory perception. Initially affected horses may appear weak with perhaps slight incoordination and stiffness, and may show some depression and/or loss of body condition. These may be the only signs for many weeks. However, if lead consumption continues, paralysis of the lower lip, rectal sphincter, larynx, pharynx, and esophagus may occur; as a result the lower lip droops, the rectal sphincter is dilated, regurgitation, and "roaring" or breathing difficulty and a roaring breathing noise, particularly during exercise, may occur. Paralysis of the larynx may not be evident until the horse is exercised vigorously for several minutes, which may induce its sudden collapse with accentuated respiratory (particularly inspiratory) sounds or "roaring," and/or difficulty in breathing. Paralysis of the pharynx usually begins with regurgitation of water from the nose when the horse drinks, which may progress to copious amounts of thick greenish ingested material in the nostrils after eating. Aspiration of ingested material resulting in pneumonia with its accompanying marked fever (temperatures of 104 to 106°F, or 40 to 41°C) and difficult respiration are likely effects of this. Terminally there may be severe incoordination, absence of feed intake, weight loss, muscle tremors, and an inability to swallow food.

Additional clinical manifestations of lead poisoning in horses include joint stiffness and lead deposition in bone growth plates, particularly during growth. Young horses are more susceptible to lead poisoning than adults and seem to manifest bone or joint abnormalities more often. Colic and/or diarrhea may occasionally occur. Brain derangements—with teeth grinding, chewing activity, circling, head pushing and bobbing, ear twitching, blindness, excitement, convulsions, and occasionally sudden death—as occur in ruminants, dogs, people, and other species, don't occur in the horse, with the possible exception of consumption of large amounts of lead at a very young age.

Lead readily passes to the fetus and accumulates in its bones, but very little lead is secreted in milk. Mares in advanced pregnancy consuming lead may deliver premature or small weak foals. These foals may never attain normal growth and are quite susceptible to secondary disease complications. Although caudal birth abnormalities have been produced by lead ingestion in laboratory animals, these have not been reported clinically in either women or domestic animals.

A mild anemia with hematocrits 25 to 30% may occur early in some horses with lead toxicosis, even before peripheral nerve dysfunctions are apparent. However, in contrast to other species, anemia, and other effects on the red blood cells are seldom sufficient to be given any clinical significance unless exposure to lead is suspected.

Confirmation of lead poisoning is usually dependent on elevated blood lead concentrations, although concentrations in horses often are not as high as in other species. Blood lead concentration is much more indicative of lead poisoning than is hair lead concentration. Although numerous studies have shown that hair lead concentration directly correlates with excess lead intake in many species, this hasn't been demonstrated in horses. The major source of lead in hair is from external contamination, not from body content. This and numerous other problems with hair analysis make it appear doubtful that hair analysis is of much benefit in the diagnosis of lead poisoning in horses.

Treatment and Prevention of Lead Poisoning

Many of the early effects of lead poisoning are reversible if lead intake is stopped and if prompt adequate chelation therapy to remove body lead is initiated. The severely affected horse is often emaciated and dehydrated because of a loss of appetite and an inability to swallow. Because of this tube-feeding, and fluid and electrolyte therapy are generally necessary for these cases. Affected, as well as unaffected horses should be removed from contaminated pasture. If this isn't possible, alfalfa hay in amounts sufficient to meet their needs should be fed. The high amount of calcium in alfalfa decreases lead absorption.

Lead-contaminated pastures can be reclaimed by cutting and disposing of the forage, tilling or burning the stubble, and adding lime to the soil. Unless continued airborne lead

contamination occurs, these procedures should sufficiently reduce the amount of lead in future forage produced on these pastures, since little lead is taken up by plants from the soil. Avoiding overgrazing is important in minimizing soil and, therefore, lead ingestion. If there is concern about continued airborne lead contamination, it may be best to reseed the pasture with a legume such as alfalfa, and determine its lead content before feeding it. Feed containing over 80 ppm (mg/kg) of lead in its dry matter should not be fed, even though at this level it may require years before poisoning in horses would occur. Lead not in the feed, such as in paint, batteries, oil, etc., does not pose the threat to horses that it does to ruminants because most horses will rarely chew, lick, or eat these items and because horses have greater resistance to acute poisoning.

BLISTER BEETLE POISONING IN HORSES

Blister beetle poisoning occurs primarily from ingesting blister beetles present in alfalfa hay cut after midsummer. Death or recovery occurs within a few days of their ingestion, with clinical signs varying depending on the number of beetles ingested and ranging from a mild fever and loss of appetite, to severe colic due to gastrointestinal and urinary tract irritation, and death due to shock and heart failure.

Cause of Blister Beetle Poisoning

Over 200 species of blister beetles, belonging to the family Meloidae, occur throughout the continental United States. Six Epicauta species are most commonly associated with poisoning in horses, and are shown in Figure 19–1. These species occur from southern Canada and Maine to

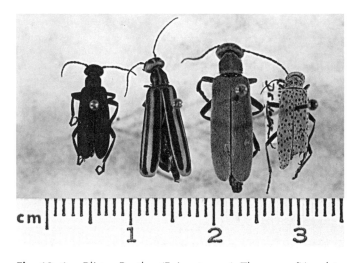

Fig. 19–1. Blister Beetles *(Epicauta spp)*. Those confirmed to cause poisoning in horses have been found only in alfalfa hay and are entirely black or black with yellow orange or gray stripes, or gray or yellowish tan with or without black spots. They vary from 0.3 to 1.3 inches (0.7 to 3.3 cm) in length and have comparatively soft bodies with soft, flexible wing covers. Their distinctive neck, head, and long antennae are helpful in differentiating them from other beetles.

Mexico and Florida, and from the Atlantic coast to Utah, Texas, and New Mexico. Poisoning has occurred in horses from Florida to Arizona and as far north as Illinois. Blister beetle poisoning is the most frequent cause of poisoning of horses in Texas, and is an increasing problem throughout the United States. The peak incidence of poisoning occurs in late summer and early fall.

Cantharidin, thought to be the sole toxic principle in blister beetles, is a highly irritating substance that on any body surface produces inflammation and blisters within a few hours, giving these beetles their common name. Rubbing the eyes after handling the beetles may cause blindness. When the beetle is ingested, cantharidin is absorbed and rapidly excreted in the urine, causing irritation and inflammation of the digestive and urinary tracts. The burning sensation that it causes when excreted in the urine is the basis for the use of blister beetles by people as an aphrodisiac referred to as "Spanish Fly," for which it is of no benefit, unless someone finds a burning sensation upon urinating sexually stimulating.

Cantharidin is toxic to most animals, although horses are most commonly affected and appear to be the most sensitive, while some small animals and birds may be relatively resistant to it. Ruminants, although susceptible to blister beetle poisoning, are more resistant to it than horses. The minimum lethal dose of cantharidin for the horse has not been established but appears to be about 125 beetles for the 1100-lb (500 kg) horse, but considerably fewer may cause severe poisoning.

Blister beetles ingested by horses are generally in hay produced from flowering forages such as alfalfa or clover—most commonly that which is cut, crimped, and swathed all in one operation after midsummer. Crimping crushes the beetles in the hay, whereas when hay is not crimped or swathed, the beetles generally leave the hay after it is cut. The increased use of crimping, which hastens field drying necessary for harvesting, may be one reason for the increased incidence of this poisoning. Cantharidin is quite stable and is toxic in beetles that are alive or in those that have been dead for many years. Thus, storage of contaminated hay doesn't decrease its toxicity.

Blister beetles have only one generation per year, with their adult (toxic) population generally peaking after early summer (June or later in the southern United States and after July in the northern states). Adult beetles mate, and the females lay eggs in the soil. The eggs hatch and the young larvae search out and feed on grasshopper eggs, helping to decrease subsequent grasshopper populations. A few species live in bee nests in the larval stage, where they live on bee eggs and on the food stored in the cells with the eggs. The larvae emerge from the soil or on bees as adult blister beetles the following spring to fall. Thus, the blister beetle population may be increased on years following a high grasshopper population.

Adult blister beetles are primarily pollen feeders but will also feed on blossoms and leaves of plants such as alfalfa. They are rarely present in nonflowering plants such as grasses. Alfalfa hay is the only feed from which blister beetle poisoning in horses has been reported. However, blister beetles have been found in grass hays containing weeds (e.g., silver nightshade and goldenrod) on which the beetles were feeding. The adult beetles congregate in large groups so they are not evenly distributed in a field and, since they are highly mobile, can readily move to other areas. As a result, they may be present in only a few of many bales or in only a portion of a single bale.

Effects of Blister Beetle Poisoning

When decreased feed intake, colic, and depression occur, particularly in more than one horse ingesting alfalfa hay or other feed prepared from alfalfa, blister beetle poisoning should be considered. This suspicion is enhanced if blister beetles are found in the feed. However, the beetles are difficult to find in feed and may be present in only a portion of a single bale. A tentative diagnosis can be made when horses show the effects described (Table 19-1), particularly frequent drinking, nuzzling or splashing water, and frequent voiding of a dilute urine by a dehydrated, depressed, colicky horse. Horses with other gastrointestinal illnesses may also nuzzle and play in water in a similar manner. The best means to differentiate blister beetle poisoning from other causes of acute colic is the presence of low blood calcium and magnesium concentrations.

The severity of clinical signs produced by consumption of blister beetles, like most poisonings, depends on the dosage. Clinical signs vary from a low fever and loss of appetite for a single day (with or without mild colic) to severe pain, shock, and death within a few hours. Clinical signs begin within 2 to 12 hours following blister beetle ingestion and end in death or recovery within 1 to 5 days. The more frequently observed clinical signs include decreased feed intake, varying degrees of colic, depression, frequent voiding of small amounts of dilute urine, and diarrhea or soft stools (which are occasionally but rarely bloody). Sweating, which may be profuse in some cases, may be a response to pain and a reflection of colic severity. Some horses do not have all these signs, and some may show only signs of severe shock, with death occurring within a few hours.

The urine usually appears normal, although in some cases it is blood-tinged or contains blood clots. Very bloody urine may occur in the later stages of the disease. Other less commonly observed signs include thumps (synchronous diaphragmatic flutter as described in Chapter 11), profuse salivating, generally associated with erosion of the gums and oral surfaces; and a stiff, short-strided gait.

Rectal temperature initially is elevated (over 102°F or 39°C) as are heart and respiratory rates (over 60 and 20 per minute, respectively). Occasionally there may be forceful heart contractions that can be noticed through the chest wall. Mucous membranes are invariably dark and congested with a diminished capillary refill time. There is evidence of pain and often retching when a stomach tube is passed.

Blister beetle poisoning can be confirmed by finding cantharidin or blister beetles in stomach contents, or cantharidin in the urine. However, cantharidin is gone from the urine by 3 to 5 days after blister beetles have been ingested, so urine collected early in the disease is necessary for diagnosis. Blister beetles in stomach contents may be identified microscopically; however, parts of other insects (e.g., grasshoppers) frequently are observed in horses stomach contents, so that cantharidin analysis of insect parts found may be necessary for diagnosis confirmation.

Treatment and Prevention of Blister Beetle Poisoning

There is no specific antidote for cantharidin. Early supportive therapy is necessary. The primary goals of therapy are: (1) removal of the toxin source, (2) evacuation of the gastrointestinal tract, (3) hydration and maintenance of normal plasma electrolyte levels, and (4) control of pain.

The continued feeding of the possible offending alfalfa hay or pellets should be stopped. If blister beetle poisoning is confirmed, the offending feed should not be fed to anything. All horses in an affected group, even those not showing signs, are generally given mineral oil by stomach tube, to remove the toxin from, and to help evacuate their gastrointestinal tract.

For severely affected cases, even early and vigorous therapy is rarely successful, whereas for mildly affected cases giving mineral oil alone may be adequate. For cases in between these two extremes, both early and vigorous therapy is necessary and successful. Since initially the severity isn't known, in addition to all horses in the affected group generally being given mineral oil, they should be watched closely and any showing any symptoms should be given additional therapy, such as fluids and analgesics. Recovery or death generally occurs within 1 to 3 days. Complications after recovery usually don't occur. Founder may occasionally occur.

Blister beetle poisoning can be prevented by feeding grass instead of alfalfa hay. However, alfalfa and other legumes cut prior to flowering or prior to midsummer are unlikely to contain blister beetles. Since blister beetles are attracted to flowers, they are rarely present in forages that don't contain flowers or flowering weeds, such as nonflowering plants like grasses, or early-cut legumes. Cutting legumes prior to flowering not only decreases the risk that they contain blister beetles but also results in a higher nutritional value and more palatable hay, as described in Chapter 4. Even legumes in bloom, when harvested prior to midsummer, are unlikely to contain blister beetles, because these beetles have only one generation per year and their population generally doesn't peak until midsummer or later. Not crimping or windrowing hay when it is cut increases the chance that any beetles present in it can get out before it is harvested.

Fields of alfalfa, and other flowering forages, to be cut after early summer when in bloom should be inspected closely before harvesting, particularly near field edges. If any blister beetles are found, the forage in that field shouldn't be cut at that time. After all blooms are gone, blister beetles may no longer be present, although hay harvested after flowering is quite low in feeding value. Forage containing blister beetles may be safely grazed.

No hay from a field or batch found to contain blister beetles or to cause toxicosis should be fed. Spraying infected fields with the insecticide Sevin (a carbamate present in several commercial formulations including Sevin 80SP, Sevimol, and Sevin XLR) at an application rate of 1.5 lb of active ingredient/acre (1.5 kg/hectare) shortly before cutting has been recommended. Hay sprayed with Sevin may be fed to animals with no detrimental effects and no waiting period after spraying. Sevin kills not only blister beetles but also grasshoppers, crickets, cutworms, armyworms, alfalfa caterpillars, and webworms. Whether insecticide killing of blister beetles in a field prevents their inclusion in hay harvested from that field, however, isn't known.

GOSSYPOL POISONING

Gossypol is present in the pigment glands of cottonseeds (Gossypium spp.). Ingestion of a sufficient quantity may cause sudden death or poor condition, difficult respiration and death due to congestive heart failure and lung edema in young animals, and decreased production and fertility in mature animals. All information given on gossypol poisoning is for pigs, cattle, lambs, and rats. Because all results and effects appear to be the same in these four species, the information is probably also valid in horses. Gossypol poisoning in horses has not been reported but would be expected to occur if intake is sufficiently high. The information on gossypol given here is intended to assist in answering questions regarding the effects and feasibility of feeding cottonseed products to horses. For example, Can cottonseed products be fed to horses, and if so, in what amount? What are the effects of feeding cottonseed products to horses? Can certain detrimental effects occurring in horses be due to gossypol? Cottonseed products are occasionally fed to horses, or are not fed because of these concerns.

Susceptibility to gossypol poisoning varies with age and species of animal. Mature ruminants are the most resistant, followed by horses. However, gossypol toxicosis does occur in mature ruminants, and presumably horses, if a sufficient amount is consumed. Swine, dogs, rabbits, rats, poultry, and immature ruminants are all quite susceptible to gossypol poisoning. The younger the animal, the greater its susceptibility.

Cause of Gossypol Poisoning

The pigment glands in cottonseeds, and the leaf, stem, bark, and root of cotton plants, contain a number of pigments, by far the most abundant being gossypol. The amount present varies with growing conditions (being higher the lower the temperature and the higher the moisture during plant growth) and plant variety; it is not present in glandless cotton seeds. However, currently glandless cotton is not widely grown. Unprocessed cottonseeds are more toxic than cottonseed meal because all gossypol in unprocessed seeds is in the free form, which is the form primarily responsible for poisoning. During processing, as much as 65% of the gossypol in the seeds forms complexes with protein, decreasing its availability to the animal. In cottonseed meal, gossypol content and, therefore, toxicity is higher in solvent-extracted meal (which is the only form commonly available currently) than it is in mechanically extracted meal. Storage of cottonseed meal has little effect on its gossypol content. Gossypol is detoxified by cooking during the processing of cottonseed. Gossypol can also be detoxified by treatment of cottonseed meal with a number of salts.

A total diet concentration of free gossypol of 0.010 to 0.015% (100 to 150 mg/kg) is the maximum recommended for young pigs and calves. A concentration of 0.02% (200 mg/kg) slows growth, and in calves causes a rough hair coat and paunchiness. A diet concentration of 0.03% results in death of 50% of piglets and calves within 1 to 3 months. A total dietary concentration of 0.010% free gossypol produced heart lesions in all young lambs after only 30 days of its consumption. Dogs and cats appear to be quite sensitive to gossypol toxicosis, with repeated oral doses as low as 0.001% (10 mg/kg) reported to cause depression, diarrhea, weight loss, loss of appetite, vomiting, a spastic paralysis of the rear legs, lung edema, and death.

In contrast to the low levels harmful to nonruminants and immature ruminants, much of the gossypol ingested by mature ruminants is bound to protein in the rumen which decreases its availability. As a result, mature ruminants can consume diets containing up to 0.20% (2000 mg/kg) free gossypol without apparent adverse effects. However, milk production of high-producing dairy cows is reduced by several weeks consumption of a diet containing as low as 0.225% (2250 mg/kg) free gossypol for several weeks. There is little information available as to the amount of gossypol that is safe for horses. Young horses from 3 to 9 months of age have been fed diets containing 0.030% (300 mg/kg) free gossypol for periods ranging from 56 to 112 days without any detected detrimental effects.

Effects of Gossypol Poisoning

Free, but not bound, gossypol is absorbed from the gastrointestinal tract and transported by the blood to primarily the liver and kidney but also other tissues. It is eliminated primarily in feces after excretion in bile as a gossypol-iron complex, but a small amount is excreted in the urine. None is excreted in the milk.

The toxicity of gossypol is thought to be the result of binding to iron and amino acids, (which occurs with both dietary and body tissue proteins), and its inhibition of oxygen release from red blood cells and of enzymes (particularly those involved with body energy production and transport). Its iron binding results in signs typical of an iron deficiency. Gossypol toxicity can be decreased by increasing protein and iron intake to offset its protein and iron binding effects.

Gossypol poisoning may result in two different clinical syndromes, although lung edema is a major occurrence with both. One syndrome is sudden death without previous signs, although occasionally acute respiratory difficulty may be observed just prior to death. The second is chronic respiratory difficulty. Affected animals may have reduced feed intake and a generalized unthrifty appearance manifested by rough hair coats, poor growth or weight loss, decreased milk production, and a distended abdomen with gastrointestinal stasis and inflammation. There is depression, generalized weakness, diarrhea, and loss of appetite. Affected animals may have short choppy breathing (thumps) and coughing. From the onset of clinical signs to death varies from hours to days. A bloody urine and stools, and hair discoloration may also occur.

Gossypol consumption also decreases fertility in both males and females and may do so without causing other clinical signs. Ingestion of 20 mg of gossypol daily impairs fertility in men. It also decreases the fertility of male rats, monkeys, and hamsters, but not rabbits or mice. It inhibits spermatozoan motility and production. There may be many immature spermatozoa and many with their head and tail separated. Swelling, dissociation, and fragmentation of the spermatozoan acrosome head caps may occur. These effects may be due to gossypol's inhibition of testosterone production or spermatozoan enzymes. In young male rats these effects occurred within 4 weeks of consuming a diet containing 0.0156% free gossypol and were alleviated 3 to 6 weeks after stopping consumption. This amount is below the level that results in other clinical symptoms. In females, gossypol impairs ovum implantation and early pregnancy by a dose-dependent action on early embryo development. Gossypols effect on reproduction in horses isn't known.

Gossypol poisoning should be considered in any animals showing the clinical signs or effects described (including reduced fertility or growth, or sudden death without other signs) if they are consuming any cottonseed products. If necessary, the presence of cottonseed products in the diet can be confirmed by feed microscopy.

Other causes of similar effects that must be differentiated from gossypol poisoning include pneumonia and other causes of lung disease or congestive heart failure. These include monensin poisoning, Cassia (pigweed) poisoning, clostridial diseases, vitamin E/selenium deficiency, and congenital heart defects. Gossypol poisoning must also be differentiated from aflatoxin poisoning and coal tar (pitch) poisoning, both of which uncommonly occur in horses.

Suspicion of gossypol toxicosis is increased by finding dietary free gossypol content in the diet in excess of the amounts given previously, and is confirmed by a high free- or bound-gossypol concentration in the liver or kidney.

Treatment and Prevention of Gossypol Toxicosis

In the treatment of gossypol poisoning, all gossypol intake should be stopped by not feeding any amount of any cottonseed products. Once this is done, supportive therapy is probably adequate, as the effects of gossypol poisoning appear to be reversible.

To prevent gossypol poisoning, the gossypol content of cottonseed products should be known based on analysis or as provided by the supplier, and the products should be fed only in an amount that does not exceed the safe levels given previously. For the young horse, until further information is available, it is safest not to greatly exceed 0.03% (300 mg/kg) free gossypol in the total diet. How much more may be safely fed to mature horses isn't known but the safe level probably exceeds 0.1% (1000 mg/kg). Since the amount of free gossypol in cottonseed products is extremely variable, ranging from 0 to 2% (20,000 mg/kg) in cottonseeds and from 0 to over 0.6% (6000 mg/kg) in cottonseed meal, the amount that can be fed without exceeding these levels must be determined for each cottonseed product as shown in the following example.

Example. Cottonseed meal (CSM) is found to contain 0.5% total and 0.2% free gossypol. Since percent means parts per hundred 0.2% is 0.2 lb/100 lbs, 0.2 g/100 g or 2 g free gossypol/kg CSM. You want to use it as the protein supplement for weanlings. Because, as given above, you don't want more than 300 mg or 0.3 g free gossypol/kg total diet, you could feed 0.15 kg of this CSM/kg total diet (0.3 g gossypol/kg diet ÷ 2 g gossypol/kg CSM), or 15% CSM in the diet (since 0.15 kg/kg = 150 g/1 g = 15 g/100 g = 15%). If the diet consisted of 60% grain mix and 40% forage, the grain mix could contain 25% CSM (15% ÷ 0.60 = 25%). If the CSM is not in the grain mix but instead is added to the grain mix at each feeding, the amount you could feed daily would be 15% times the total amount of feed consumed. The weanling will eat a total amount of feed equal to 3 to 3.5% of its body weight daily if it is available (Appendix Table 1). Therefore, if the weanlings weigh 550 lbs (250 kg), they would eat about 16.5 lbs/day (550 × 0.03) or 7.5 kg day (250 × 0.03). Thus, these weanlings could be safely fed 2.5 lbs CSM/day (16.5 lbs feed/day × 15% = 2.5 lbs) or 1.125 kg CSM/day (7.5 kg feed/day × 15%). If this amount or less provides sufficient protein to meet the horse's requirement (determined as described in Chapter 6), it could be used as the only protein supplement for these weanlings. However, when CSM is the protein supplement used for the growing horse, growth rate and feed efficiency will generally be reduced unless additional lysine is added to the diet (Table 1-5) or enough additional CSM is fed to provide adequate lysine.

Gossypol toxicity of a feed can be reduced by increasing forage intake (particularly alfalfa because of its high protein and calcium content), and by adding iron to the diet. Iron in the form of ferrous sulfate has been shown to be beneficial when added in an amount equal to 1- to 4-times the amount of free gossypol in the diet. Gossypol toxicity has also been shown to be reduced when calcium hydroxide was added to the diet. Iron calcium and protein all appear to decrease free gossypol absorption.

NITRATE POISONING

Nitrate poisoning, although often of concern and occasionally a problem in ruminants, in contrast to what is periodically stated, but without any supportive data, is not known to occur in horses. It is discussed here because of the concerns and questions that arise concerning it in horses, not because it is a problem or even known to occur in the horse.

Nitrate poisoning occurs from the consumption of excessive amounts of nitrate present in plants and rarely water. Nitrate is present in plants after they take it up from the soil and before they convert it to protein. Anything that increases its uptake, or decreases its conversion to protein, increases the plant's nitrate content. Nitrogen fertilization increases nitrate uptake, and anything that decreases the rate of plant growth decreases its conversion to protein. This includes drought, hot weather, early frost, hail damage, or long periods of cloudy weather. After these

periods, a sudden change in growing conditions conducive to plant growth results in plants' taking up nitrate faster than they can convert it to protein. These plants at this time, as well as the stubble remaining after harvesting forage or cereal grains, may contain high levels of nitrate. This occurs in stubble particularly if it begins to grow and thus takes up nitrate, then has its growth stopped by a frost or sudden decrease in temperature before it has converted the nitrate to protein.

Under adverse weather conditions, cornstalks, the stalks of other cereal grains, (but not the seeds or grain itself, and usually not the leaves, because by the time nitrate gets to these locations it has been converted to protein) and stalks of fescue, and particularly Sudan grasses can contain high levels of nitrate. Numerous weeds, and some wild grasses and vegetables, are capable of accumulating large amounts of nitrate. Alfalfa and other legumes, as well as timothy, bromegrass, and soybeans, probably never accumulate enough nitrate to be toxic to either horses or ruminants.

Excessive levels of nitrate in feeds can be prevented by (1) cutting at later stages of maturity, although this will decrease the forage's nutrient value and palatability; (2) ensiling, which may decrease nitrate content 40 to 60%; (3) not cutting for the first few days after a rain; and (4) cutting on the afternoon or evening of a sunny day.

Nitrate may also be present in drinking water. The most common source of nitrates in water is fecally polluted surface or subsurface water, which also have a high bacterial content. High nitrate levels are therefore more common in shallow well water. Nitrate toxicosis is unlikely in ruminants, and even at higher levels in horses, when their drinking water contains less than 400 ppm nitrate (Table 1-3). Nitrate concentrations may be reported in a number of ways and can be converted from one to another based on the following equivalents. 1% nitrate = 0.23% nitrite or nitrate nitrogen; 1% nitrate = 0.74% nitrite; and 1.37% sodium nitrate = 1.63% potassium nitrate. For example: 0.3% nitrate nitrogen (NO_3-N) equals 0.3% ÷ 0.23 or 1.3% nitrate (NO_3); and 0.5% potassium nitrate (KNO_3) equals 0.5% ÷ 1.63 or 0.31% nitrate.

Although a nitrate content above 0.5 to 1% in the total diet dry matter may cause problems in ruminants, horses aren't affected by levels considerably above this. What amount of dietary nitrate is harmful to horses isn't known, but it appears to be above that which may be present in normal horse feeds. No problems occurred when hay containing 1.8 to 2.1% nitrate in its dry matter was fed to either mature or growing horses, or to pregnant or lactating mares.

Although all animals are susceptible to nitrites, ruminants are the most susceptible because ruminal microorganisms reduce ingested nitrates to nitrites. This doesn't occur to any significant extent in nonrumenant animals such as horses. The nitrites formed by ruminal microorganisms from ingested nitrates are absorbed and, in any animal upon contact with red blood cells, convert hemoglobin to methemoglobin, which isn't able to bind oxygen. Thus, if sufficient nitrate is ingested, converted to nitrite, and absorbed so that methemoglobin is produced faster than the body is able to convert it back to hemoglobin, the blood's oxygen-carrying capacity is reduced. This effect can be detected by a drop of blood on white paper turning a chocolate brown color within 1 to 2 minutes after taking it from the animal.

A sufficient decrease in the blood's ability to carry oxygen causes anxiety, increased respiratory rate, and difficulty in breathing. If sufficiently severe, incoordination, muscle twitching, weakness, cyanosis, and death occur. Signs may appear within 0.5 to 4 hours, and death within 12 hours, after ruminants ingest excessive amounts of nitrate.

In non-rumiant animals, such as swine, the major effect of excess nitrate ingestion is irritation of the gastrointestinal tract, which if sufficiently severe, results in colic, vomiting, diarrhea, and frequent urination. Little or no methemoglobin formation, and as a result a lack of oxygen to the tissues, occurs. Although it would seem that this could occur in horses if sufficient nitrate was consumed, neither it nor any other nitrate-induced problems have been confirmed or are known to occur in horses.

Numerous additional health problems, including poor reproduction, decreased growth rate, and a vitamin A deficiency or increased vitamin A requirements, have been attributed, primarily in ruminants, to excess nitrate intake. However, numerous studies have failed to confirm nitrate as a cause of these effects in either ruminants or horses.

Nitrate poisoning is confirmed by finding a high nitrate concentration in an affected animal's serum or eye fluids, or in its diet or drinking water. Nitrate analysis may be done by a field test or sent to a laboratory. Samples sent to a laboratory, or in which analysis is delayed, should be kept cold or frozen to prevent a decrease in their nitrate concentration.

Chapter 20

BEHAVIORAL PROBLEMS IN HORSES

Escape Vices (Pawing, Weaving, Pacing & Stall Kicking) . . .	371	Flight or Fight Vices 376
Oral Vices 372		Aggression (Lunging, Rearing, Striking, Kicking & Biting) . . 376
Wood Chewing 372		Self-Aggression or Mutilation 378
Cribbing and Wind Sucking 373		Maternal Aggression by Mares 248
Tail or Mane Chewing 375		Shying or Bolting 378
Eating Feces or Bedding 375		Balking and Freezing 378
Eating Dirt (See Sand Induced Diarrhea in Chapter 17) . . . 293		Supplemental Reading Recommendations 379

When undesirable and useless behavior becomes a persistent, repetitive bad habit, it is referred to as a stereotypic behavior, or vice. Vices develop most commonly in stabled horses and, therefore, are commonly referred to as stable vices. There are two major types of stable vices: oral vices, that is, those carried out with the mouth and teeth; and escape vices. Both are fairly common in horses kept stabled and uncommon in those kept primarily on pasture with other animals. Another common vice in horses involves flight or fight behaviors. These are appropriate reactions to certain stimuli but become abnormal when the reaction is inappropriate, repetitive, or exaggerated. They include lunging, aggression, bolting or an exaggerated alarm reaction, biting, kicking, and aversion reactions such as shying, balking, and startle reactions. They are considered to be due to a flaw in the horse's temperament, although stabling or feeding management certainly plays a role in some cases.

When you consider the horse's evolutionary development, life, behavior, habits, and needs, it is not surprising that some horses develop vices when stabled. What is surprising is that the incidence and severity of vices aren't much greater. The horse has evolved over millions of years as a free-ranging, primarily grazing, plains dweller whose social unit is a small band with a strict dominance hierarchy or pecking order. By evolution the horse is fearful of confinement, restraint, and being alone because in the wild, these greatly increase the risk of death. Horse management practices of stabling and feeding horses almost completely disregard these normal behavior patterns and well-warranted fears. With common stabling and feeding practices there is frequently insufficient opportunity for the horse to exercise and to engage in species-typical behavior. Instead of spending the majority of their time grazing, their feed is consumed in a few hours and then they have nothing to do, and often no one to do it with. As a result, they become bored, lonely, and frustrated. Frustration, occurring because a horse's needs or desires are unfulfilled, and boredom, or lack of occupation or interest, are the causes of most stable vices. They indicate a psychologic disturbance and stress that a horse tolerates up to a certain level, beyond which a stable vice is likely to occur. The greater and the more rapid the horse's restriction of freedom, isolation, and decrease in exercise and eating duration, the greater the risk of development and the

higher the incidence of stable vices, e.g., when a mature horse that has been on pasture with other horses all its life is suddenly put in a stall by itself. Understanding the occurrence and causes for this horse's frustration and preventing or minimizing them is key to preventing and correcting stable vices.

Horses may also be inadvertently trained to behave badly. For example, the horse paws and someone comes into the stall to see him, or he paws before, or when, he is fed. He associates the behavior, pawing, with the reward, which is relief from boredom and loneliness, or with being fed. Preventing or eliminating this association is then the key to preventing and correcting the undesired behavior. In addition, some stable vices, such as eating wood, dirt or feces, tail or mane chewing, or cribbing, may occur in some horses as a result of imitation and in some may be inherited, or at least the tendency or temperament for them to occur may be inherited.

In one study of over one thousand adult Thoroughbred horses, the incidence in some families as compared to the overall incidence of cribbing was 12.5-fold higher (30% versus 2.4%), of weaving was 10.4-fold higher (26% versus 2.5%) and of stall pacing was 5.2-fold higher (13% versus 2.5%). Imitation of mares by their foals was excluded as the main cause of the vices, although it couldn't be ruled out entirely as a factor in some cases. However, it is doubtful that a vice is inherited; instead, what is inherited is a personality or temperament that makes the horse more or less susceptible to the frustrations that result in stable vices.

Regardless of the cause of a vice, if it continues, it may become repetitive to the point of being a fixation. The repetition may be so continuous that there is fatigue, even exhaustion, and decreased feed intake, performance ability, body condition, and/or weight. Once a fixation occurs, relieving the cause of the frustration—such as providing more feed, exercise, and/or companionship—or punishment may not stop the behavior. Therefore, a vice should be treated and solutions found as quickly as possible; ideally, everything possible should be done to prevent vices from occurring. We can expect the horse to best provide our wants and needs only if we adequately provide the horse's wants and needs, both physically and psychologically. It is unfair to ask or expect anything else. If we don't adequately provide for the horse's physical and psychological needs, stable vices and other behaviors undesirable to us and often harmful to the horse may occur. When they do, it indicates improper care of the horse, just as does poor condition due to inadequate feed or dental problems, overgrown hooves due to inadequate trimming and shoeing, heavy parasitism due to an inadequate worming program, or the occurrence of common preventable infectious diseases due to an inadequate vaccination program. As with all of these problems, they are much easier to prevent than cure, and every effort should be made to do so. If behavior problems do occur and do not respond to conservative treatment, a behavior specialist should be consulted.

The most consistently effective means of stopping a vice is to determine and remove the cause for the vice. If the vice is due to a frustration, everything possible should be done to remove the cause for that frustration. In addition, if the horse by performing the undesirable behavior is receiving something it likes or wants—such as food, a nutrient, chewing, companionship, or decreased boredom—that reward should be prevented, or the association between the vice and the reward prevented. Punishment, even when applied correctly, is rarely as effective in stopping an undesirable behavior as is removing the cause for that behavior. However, when the cause can't be entirely removed, or the vice has become a fixation or habit, punishment is sometimes helpful if properly applied. If not properly applied, punishment is likely to cause more problems than it alleviates.

To be effective, the behavior, not the animal or child, is punished. If the one being punished perceives that it, not the behavior, is being punished, it will become fearful, aggressive, or perhaps sullen and withdrawn, and may or may not stop the undesirable behavior. In contrast to people, however, the animal, like the sufficiently young child, is unable to understand that punishment may be for a prior behavior. Instead, regardless of what is said or done, it associates punishment only with the behavior or situation present at the time it is being punished. An animal, like a sufficiently young child, may act "guilty" when someone arrives and a particular situation is present, such as something broken or a mess. It acts this way not because it knows it's done anything wrong, but instead because it knows from past experiences that when that particular mess is present and someone arrives, it will be punished, which is the situation that existed when it was punished previously. It doesn't associate the punishment with the behavior that caused the problem. For punishment to be effective, it must be given contingent with the undesirable behavior. Even given a few seconds later, it is not as effective because by then the animal is engaging in a different behavior and, therefore, the wrong behavior is punished. Punishment after the undesirable behavior is for revenge and doesn't affect the undesirable behavior; and there is certainly no legitimate excuse for taking revenge on an individual that doesn't realize that it has done anything wrong, anything that it shouldn't or anything that you don't want it to do. This doesn't mean animals can't remember things. Horses, like many animals, have excellent memories, but remembering something in the past is completely different from understanding that the present situation applies to the past.

Punishment to be effective must not only be contingent with the undesirable behavior, it must be swift, sufficiently severe, and consistent. The swifter and more consistent the punishment, the more effective it is. The punishment should not be so severe that it causes fear, submission, or aggression, but sufficiently severe that it causes a satisfactory response. Gradually increasing punishment severity will require a much more severe punishment to prevent that behavior than will punishment sufficiently severe to stop that activity the first time it is applied. But if the punishment causes fear, it is too severe. In addition, the reward the animal gets from the undesirable behavior should be prevented, which is the most effective means of preventing an undesirable behavior with or without punishment. When punishment works, it works quickly and the undesirable behavior ceases within 2 to 10 times. If it doesn't, the punishment is probably not effective and isn't going to be unless the reward the animal gets from the behavior is prevented.

Administration of some drugs (narcotic antagonists) may also be effective in alleviating some vices in horses. Cribbing was prevented, and, stall pacing and weaving and self-mutilation in stallions were greatly decreased for up to several hours after drugs of this type were administered. Although sedation and yawning occurred in the first 30 minutes after their administration, horses were bright, alert, responsive, and could be ridden. However, the vice returns when treatment is stopped, and currently there is no easily administered long-acting form of narcotic antagonist, thus making their use in treating behavioral problems impractical, at least currently. In addition, these drugs are expensive and some may induce colic in horses.

ESCAPE VICES

Escape vices include persistent, repetitive pawing or digging holes; trying to jump out of the stall, run, or paddock; kicking the stall wall; pacing the stall, fence, or paddock; and weaving or just head nodding. Weaving is a rhythmic shifting of the weight from one forefoot to the other while swinging the head. Head nodding may also occur alone without the weight shifting. Although weaving and head nodding are most common in tied horses, they also occur in stabled horses that are not tied. They are also more common in horses with a nervous disposition and in riding horses that are stabled for long periods. Weaving and stall walking can both lead to a considerable loss of body condition and weight. Walking in a stall requires considerable spinal flexion in circling and turning, and can lead to a painful back, adversely affecting performance when ridden. All of the escape behaviors are almost always responses to the horse's frustration of being confined and isolated, and thus inability to obtain food, activity, and/or companionship at will.

Some horses do, of course, habituate to a stall-isolation environment, particularly if unaccustomed to anything else, or if the confinement and isolation aren't too total or continuous. Some young horses that are stalled and develop escape vices may gradually habituate to this environment and stop these activities. Increased daily activity and enforced exercise may help minimize escape vice activities in some cases; however, the mature horse, or any horse that has been doing these activities for months, probably isn't going to habituate and stop these activities unless its environment is changed.

Escape vices can be prevented and stopped prior to fixation by determining the cause for and alleviating the horse's frustration. Ideally the horse should be put on pasture with others. This also is the best means of preventing and, prior to fixation, stopping oral vices. However, if putting the horse on pasture with others isn't possible, provide companionship, increased exercise, increased feeding frequency, and increased feed volume. Sometimes simply having the ability to come and go at will into their stalls will alleviate escape behaviors even if there is only a small run and no other horses are present. A nonaggressive stall companion, such as another horse, pony, goat (without horns), sheep, pig, or dog may be sufficient. Even a small animal such as a chicken or rabbit works well with some horses, although poorly with others. Metal mirrors in the stall, or having a stall in which the horse can see other horses on either side, may help. Increasing feeding frequency and/or feed volume (by feeding less or no grain, and more hay and/or more lower-energy, higher-fiber hay) may be helpful. Hanging a plastic jug or ball from the stall ceiling may help alleviate boredom in some horses if they play with it. For the horse that is pawing or digging, filling the holes with water may stop the pawing, if the cause for the pawing has also been alleviated (i.e., solitary confinement has been decreased). Putting the horse on a wooden floor may help stop both pawing and stall kicking; stall kicking may occur because the horse likes the sound; it may stop when put on a wooden floor because the wood makes enough noise to keep it content.

An additional and by far the most common cause of kicking and pawing, however, is not due to confinement frustration but instead is handler induced. The horse tends to paw or kick at feeding time when it sees or smells food or the feeder in anticipation of being fed. The horse is then fed, thus positively reinforcing that pawing or kicking. It will then begin to paw or kick earlier and earlier to try to receive the reward of being fed. To prevent or eliminate this behavior, the horse should not be fed when it paws or kicks. To break the horse of the habit may require many small meals daily. Initially the horse must not paw or kick for example for only 2 seconds before it is given a half cup of feed, then 5, then 10, then 30 seconds before food is given. Only when the horse will refrain from pawing or kicking for a short time for several feedings should a longer time be tried. The training will go faster if the horse is taught a countercommand such as "stand" for a food reward at the same time.

ORAL VICES

Oral vices include eating wood, dirt, feces, or bedding; tail or mane chewing; cribbing; and wind sucking. Those involving eating or chewing may be referred to as feeding vices and are sometimes thought to have a dietary cause, cure, or prevention, although with some exceptions most cases do not. The oral vices develop almost exclusively in horses that don't have the opportunity to graze. They do, however, occur in both stalled horses as well as those kept in outdoor enclosures. Biting others or themselves is also a vice carried out with the mouth, but is an aggressive vice not restricted primarily to nongrazing horses.

Crib wetting and tongue displacement are additional, less common oral vices. Neither is harmful nor generally warrants treatment. With crib wetting the horse slowly but repeatedly draws its tongue across the edge of some part of the stall or manager. During this the tongue is held still, which differs from licking. It, like repeated licking, may indicate a desire for salt and be alleviated when salt is provided. Tongue displacement includes repeatedly forcing the tongue over the bit or sticking it out the side of the mouth for periods of time. The reason a horse does this isn't known.

Some also consider excessively rapid grain consumption or bolting to be a vice. It is certainly a bad habit and increases the risk of choke. Methods to prevent it are described in the section on "Slowing Feed Consumption" in Chapter 4. Bolting feed may be due to greed, hunger, nervous anxiety, a sore mouth, or mimicry. Another oral vice is excessive water or salt consumption. Both are uncommon and aren't known to be harmful, but they do cause excess urination and, as a result, a wet stall. They can be prevented by first limiting salt intake. If this doesn't alleviate excess water intake, next limit water. However, before doing either, ensure that there isn't a reason for it, such as chronic renal failure, diabetes mellitus, diabetes insipidus, Cushings, or a low blood potassium concentration. With psychogenic water consumption, with or without excessive salt consumption, the urine is quite dilute but its concentration increases with water deprivation and other alterations aren't present.

Wood Chewing

Wood chewing is one of the most common stable vices. Although pastured horses may occasionally chew wood, it is much more common in closely confined horses, but occurs as frequently in those in outdoor enclosures as in those kept in stalls. It is done at any age and by both genders of horse, with no apparent difference among stallions, mares, and geldings. Foals as young as 1 month of age have been observed to mimic their wood-chewing mothers and herdmates.

Although all types of wood may be chewed, the vice appears to be greatest with softer woods, such as pine, aspen, and fir, and also plywood, particleboard and chipboard. Occasionally hardwoods, such as oak and locust, may be chewed, but they appear to be less attractive to the wood chewer. Wood chewing may also increase during cold wet weather. It was thought that this might occur because wood is softer and more aromatic, palatable, and chewable when wet, or because stress or anxiety may be higher in horses during cold wet weather.

Like many behavioral problems in horses, wood chewing may to some extent be a normal behavior that becomes a problem only because it becomes an excessive or repetitious habit. However, any amount of wood chewing may be undesirable because of the damage it causes to facilities. One pony can consume 2 lb (0.9 kg) of wood daily. In boarding facilities constructed of wood, the expense of repairing stalls, fences, and barns destroyed by wood chewers may be second only to the cost of feed. Damage is the major detrimental effect of wood chewing.

Generally, wood chewing doesn't harm the horse. Much of the wood horses chew is dropped, although varying amounts may be ingested by some horses. Occasionally wood splinters may penetrate the tongue, cheek, or gums, causing infections. Wood chewing also increases dental wear. In addition, like many stable vices, wood chewing may become such a fixation or habit with some horses that food and water intake are reduced, resulting in decreased performance ability, condition, and weight. In some cases, wood chewing may lead to cribbing. Even what wood is ingested generally causes no problems. Experimentally ponies have been able to consume a diet containing one-half sawdust with no apparent ill effects. However, sawdust may be quite different from wood splinters, which infrequently may cause stomach and intestinal irritation or obstruction, resulting in impaction colic. The bolus of wood causing an impaction may form in the stomach over a long period of time without any indication of a problem, then when passed caused almost immediate small intestinal obstruction, acute stomach distention, and reflux.

Although horses by nature are primarily grazers, when they have access to brush and trees they may also occasionally browse, eating brush, very small trees, branches, leaves and bark, even when there is no scarcity of grass. Bark eating is often performed by each horse in a group and can lead to many trees being debarked from the ground to as high as the horses can reach. Thus, the horse's propensity for wood chewing may be a vestigial browsing behavior.

The cause of wood chewing in confined horses appears to be a combination of any or all of the following: boredom, insufficient chewing or a desire for more chewing, mimicking others, or a liking for the taste of the wood. Wood chewing increases when there is a decrease in the horse's need to chew its food, such as when it is fed hay instead of being allowed to graze, when loose or cubed hay in its diet is replaced with pelleted feed, or when more grain and less hay is fed. Wood chewing in confined ponies increased from 6 to 30 min/day when they were switched from an entirely hay diet to a high-grain diet. Feeding pellets instead of long-stem hay increased the amount of wood chewed fourfold in one study, whereas there was no difference in wood chewing when hay was fed either loose or cubed. Wood chewing is also increased by decreased frequency of feeding. In one study the amount of wood chewed doubled when feeding frequency was decreased from 6 times to once per day.

A nutritional imbalance is often suspected any time a horse eats, chews, or licks anything abnormal. However, the only nutritional factors that have been associated with increased wood chewing are a protein deficiency and low dietary fiber. Decreased fiber intake, as a result of decreasing forage and increasing grain in the diet, may increase wood chewing both because it decreases the chewing nec-

essary to ingest the diet and because it increases cecal acidity. A salt, other minerals, or vitamin deficiency are not known to have any effect on wood chewing.

Like most stable vices, wood chewing should be prevented or stopped as quickly as possible before it becomes a fixation or habit, to prevent its detrimental effects, and to prevent it from spreading to other horses that might mimic those chewing wood. To prevent, stop, or at least minimize wood chewing, like other stable vices, decrease the horse's confinement and increase the horse's activity and companionship, ideally by putting the horse on pasture with others, if possible. Feed less or no grain or pelleted feeds; feed more hay; and feed as frequently as practical. Ensure that the diet provides adequate protein, and that trace-mineralized salt is always easily available or that 0.5% is added to the diet. If a companion isn't provided, metal mirrors and hanging a plastic jug or ball from the ceiling may be helpful in some cases. If even with these procedures wood chewing occurs, large soft-wood tree trunks may be put in with the horses for them to chew on, thus decreasing property damage. It has also been reported that wood chewing can be inhibited by including sawdust in high-grain diets, however feeding hay instead of grain would be more practical in most situations.

A possibility suggested for the horse that can't be fed more forage, or can't be put on pasture and boredom relieved sufficiently by other means, is the place its feed in a box in which the horse has to push a switch plate with its muzzle to obtain its feed. The device may be set up so the horse has to push the switch from 1 to 20 times to obtain a small amount of feed, thus requiring that it spend more time and energy obtaining its feed and, therefore, making it less likely to chew wood or perform other stable vices.

An electric wire, or covering wood surfaces with metal, creosote, or an unpleasant flavoring, may prevent wood chewing but doesn't provide what the horse wants or alleviate the frustration responsible for causing it to chew wood. As a result, the horse's frustration or unfulfilled need may be expressed in other ways that may be just as undesirable as wood chewing. Compounds put on wood to prevent wood chewing must be reapplied periodically, often stain anything that comes in contact with them, and often have an undesirable appearance.

Cribbing and Wind Sucking

Cribbing or crib biting is a vice in which the horse places its upper incisors on a horizontal solid surface, presses down, arches its neck, and pulls back (Fig. 20-1). As this is done, the horse usually makes a grunting noise and gulps air. This is referred to as wind sucking or aerophagia. Wind sucking, as described in Chapter 13, is also used to refer to the mare that aspirates air (and usually fecal material) into the vagina, particularly when running. Rarely, a horse may crib by placing its upper incisors against its knee or cannon bone. Although both cribbing and wind sucking generally occur together, one may be done without the other. Some cribbers may become wind suckers when measures are taken to try to prevent cribbing; conversely,

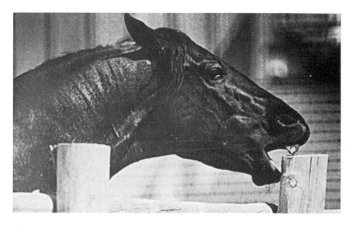

Fig. 20–1. Cribbing or crib biting: a vice in which the horse grasps a horizontal solid surface with its incisors, arches its neck, and pulls back. As it does so, it will probably make a grunting noise and gulp air, called wind sucking or aerophagia. This may occur with or without cribbing. Note the increased size of the throat muscles which, along with wearing of the incisors, may occur as a result of cribbing.

some wind suckers may become cribbers, or do both together.

Wind sucking may occur without the horse grasping anything with its teeth. Individual horses tend to have their own manner of wind sucking. Most horses nod their head and neck several times, jerk their head upward while flexing their neck, and gulp in air. A wind-sucking sound is made by some horses as they swallow the air and by others as they expel some of the air.

Some horses engage in these vices only when alone; some won't do them if they know they are being watched. However, most do them without regard to the presence or absence of other horses or people. Most, but not all, do them only when stabled.

Cribbing is a fairly common behavioral problem, constituting 27% of referrals to one equine behavior clinic. It's reported that nervous hyperactive horses kept in a stall most of the time and exercised and groomed little are most likely to crib or wind suck, whereas these vices are rarely practiced by placid draft horses or ponies. It has also been found that the incidence is as high as 30% in some families of Thoroughbreds as compared to 2.5% in all Thoroughbreds in the study. Imitation of mares by their foals was excluded as the reason for the higher incidence. Thus, inheritance of the vice, or the temperament leading to its occurrence, appears to be an increased risk factor in some cases.

The cause for cribbing and wind sucking isn't known. It is thought to usually start in confined horses due to frustration, boredom, and/or imitation, but once established to commonly persist even when the horse is on pasture. Some believe that cribbing and filling the stomach with air are substitute actions for the natural grazing activity of cropping with the front teeth and filling the stomach with grazed forage. Young idle horses may develop these vices when they are with confirmed cases. These vices have also been observed to increase when a highly palatable high-grain diet is fed. It has been suggested that these

vices may also begin as a response to abdominal discomfort or colic. Conversely, wind sucking is commonly believed to be a cause of colic and passing excess gas because horses can swallow enough air to interfere with stomach and intestinal function.

Cribbing, when continued over a long period, may cause wear and erosion of the upper incisors and pronounced increases in the size of the neck muscles (Fig. 20–1). In severe longstanding cases, tooth wear may progress to such an extent that the incisors no longer meet when the mouth is shut and, therefore, the horse can no longer graze. A few horses may spend so much time cribbing that feed consumption and, as a result, body condition and weight are decreased. However, most horses have no problems as a result of either cribbing or wind sucking; mostly it just annoys those around the horse. Because of this, some have recommended that if the horse is in good condition, ignoring it may be best. However, most people prefer to try to prevent it, and other horses may mimic cribbers and wind suckers. Because of this, cribbers and wind suckers should be kept separate from other horses. But they should be provided with companionship, such as another animal. Solitary confinement will likely worsen the problem or cause others.

Numerous methods have been tried to prevent cribbing and wind sucking. None is universally successful, but some methods may work in some cases. The most common method is fastening a several-inch-wide (5 to 7 cm) leather strap snugly around the throatlatch (Fig. 20–2). When the horse tries to arch its neck to crib or wind suck, pressure from the strap causes pain. To enhance this effect, some cribbing straps have points on the inside or a metal "gullet-piece," which has a recess for the trachea but may put more pressure on the throatlatch when the horse tries to arch its neck (Fig. 20–2B). Some straps have a heart-shaped piece of thick leather that sits between the angles of the jaws with the pointed end protruding back into the pharyngeal area. This may cause additional discomfort when the horse tries to flex its neck to crib or suck wind. Cribbing or wind sucking straps generally decrease or prevent these vices at least initially. However, some horses will resume or continue the vices in spite of the strap and may eventually develop pressure sores from the strap, requiring their removal. Although cribbing straps must be snug to be effective, they shouldn't be so tight that they interfere with breathing, and they may need to be removed or loosened during feeding, although generally they don't need to be.

Another preventive device is a hollow, cylindrical perforated bit, which prevents the horse from making its mouth airtight. A thick rubber or wooden bit that prevents the jaws from closing is sometimes successful but causes acute discomfort and is not recommended. A different approach is to keep the horse in a bare-walled stall without a feed trough, waterer, or anything on which to place its incisors. It's reported that cribbing will stop when this is done. It is likely to recur however, if the horse is returned to the environment in which the vice developed.

Various surgical procedures have also been used to try to prevent cribbing and wind sucking. None is recom-

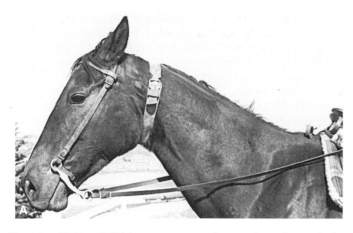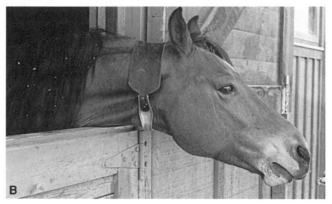

Fig. 20–2(A,B). Cribbing straps: some horses that crib or wind suck will stop doing so when a strap is fastened snugly around their throatlatch. A metal piece at the gullet, as shown in Figure B, with or without points on the inside, may improve the strap's efficacy in preventing these vices in some horses.

mended. The procedures are either ineffective, disfiguring, or associated with secondary complications.

Electric shock collars have also been tried. However, a horse will quickly learn that a shock collar works only when it is on and, for those that are remote controlled, when someone is around to activate it. To prevent the horse's associating a shock with the collar, it should be worn for several days before a shock is administered and the operator should be hidden. To be most effective, initially a shock must be applied immediately and consistently each time the incisors are placed and as the horse begins to arch its neck, preparing to gulp air. It is best to start with quite long treatment sessions, with every occurrence being shocked, followed by a change to short, randomly spaced sessions. The treatment, if effective, will take 4 weeks and, therefore, should not last longer than this. Remote-control shock collars available for training dogs and which depend on a person to activate the shock may be used. The signal for most won't transmit through a wire fence. There are also self-operating collars available with a contact switch under the horse's chin. However, with these there is the risk that the switch may stick and drive the horse into a frenzy by a continuous series of electric shocks.

Punishment or discipline procedures, such as cribbing straps and bits, surgery, and shock collars, however, do nothing to suppress the horse's motivation for cribbing and wind sucking; as a result, when they are used alone other behavioral problems may occur. In addition, even if these disciplinary measures are effective at first, they may lose their efficacy after a time. Thus, it is best to first try to alleviate the cause, and to use cause-alleviation procedures in conjunction with disciplinary efforts only if cause-alleviation procedures by themselves aren't successful. Cause-alleviation procedures include providing a companion animal, decreasing confinement, increasing use and activity, putting metal mirrors in the stall, feeding less or no grain or pellets, and feeding increased hay and/or pasture forage. These may alleviate cribbing and wind sucking without disciplinary procedures in some cases.

Administering narcotic antagonists, as described at the end of the introduction of this chapter, has been shown to be effective in preventing cribbing as well as other vices, but their use, at least currently, isn't practical.

Tail or Mane Chewing

Chewing on the tail, less commonly the mane, and rarely the body hair of other horses, is done primarily by young horses, particularly when they are closely confined in a group and when they are fed a low-forage diet. However, it may also less commonly occur in horses on pasture and in those with free access to hay. The reason horses do it isn't known, but in young horses it may be a part of their play activity and in some cases has been due to a lack of adequate forage. It has been associated with mineral deficiencies but usually occurs in horses receiving a diet providing adequate minerals.

It is primarily a cosmetic problem and not a health problem. However, occasionally sufficient hair may be consumed to cause intestinal obstruction.

Treatment involves decreasing confinement and ideally putting the horse on pasture if possible. Ensure that it's diet is nutritionally adequate, that it consists of 50 to 100% long-stem hay or pasture forage, and that trace-mineralized salt is freely available or 0.5% is added to the diet. Noxious compounds may also be repeatedly and frequently applied to the tail or mane, such as a mineral or plant oil mixed with a spicy compound such as a tobasco or hot pepper sauce.

Eating Feces or Bedding

Ingestion of feces, or coprophagia, is common and fairly normal for young horses, particularly foals up to a couple months of age. It is often thought to be a normal step in the foal's development of feeding and diet selection, and as a way of establishing a normal bacterial population in their intestinal tract. These bacteria allow the foal to switch from milk to a forage diet, because the bacteria are necessary for digestion of forage fiber. Foals usually eat only fresh feces and usually their dam's. As a result, they don't obtain intestinal parasites from this practice because, as described in Chapter 9, these parasites require an incubation period in the feces to become infective.

Mature horses, unlike foals, don't normally eat feces; nor do they eat feed, pasture forage, or bedding contaminated with feces. If feces are placed in areas where they normally graze, they frequently will stop grazing there. However, mature horses will eat feces when on a high-grain diet or on a protein-deficient diet, and will stop when less grain and more forage, or when an adequate protein diet is fed. Mature bored horses confined to a stall with inadequate activity may eat feces, particularly if they have gone from regular exercise to no exercise, or from a regular routine to a neglected routine. These horses may consume from a little to nearly all of their own feces. In addition, most mature horses confined to a stall will occasionally eat their soiled bedding, but with some it may become a habit. Although this may occur in horses that are well fed, imbalanced diets, feeding at the wrong time of day, and heavy intestinal parasitism have all been found to contribute to the increased consumption of soiled bedding.

Treatment for eating either feces or bedding is to alleviate causes or factors associated with it. This includes decreasing confinement and the amount of grain fed, allowing free access to clean hay or pasture forage and salt, feeding on a regular schedule, ensuring there is adequate protein in the diet (as described in Chapter 6), and checking for intestinal parasites and treating accordingly (as described in Chapter 9).

FLIGHT OR FIGHT VICES

The horse has two choices in response to fear—flight or fight. Fear, and thus a flight or fight reaction is a normal response by the horse to new or unfamiliar situations and objects, and to what it perceives as possible danger which may result in it being hurt. The horse shows fear by putting its head and chin up, turning its ears slightly out, flaring its nostrils, sometimes snorting, and showing the white of its eyes. When this occurs the horse's handler should remain calm while letting the horse know the cause for its fear is recognized, and if appropriate, allowing the horse to investigate the cause for its fear so that it realizes it isn't harmful. A horse's last experience with a situation, object or person should, if possible, be a positive, nonfearful and pleasurable experience. A horse tends to remember the last thing that happens in an interaction with much more clarity than previous activities in that situation. If the last thing the horse remembers about a person, object or situation is that it was fearful or unpleasant, it will make the next exposure even worse; whereas if the last thing the horse remembers is that it was not harmful or was pleasant, it will make the next exposure easier. For example, if the last thing a horse remembers about being twitched is jerking a hurting nose out of the twitch, it quite likely will be more difficult to twitch the next time, but it won't be difficult to twitch the next time if the last thing it remembers as the twitch is loosened is getting its nose massaged which felt good. Thus, quitting on a positive note makes the next encounter easier, even if the majority of the time the horse spent with that individual or situation was uncomfortable for it. Thus, this applies not only to a situation,

such as being twitched or ridden, or to an object, such as a flapping piece of plastic, but also to a person, such as you. If you or the situation is remembered as unpleasant, a flight or fight response will occur with increasing repetition and severity each time, and may become a learned behavioral vice.

If the horse is deprived of flight, it must either fight or submit. If it learns from that experience, or remembers from a previous experience, that submission is less harmful or fearful than fighting, or that submission is not harmful or fearful but pleasurable, it submits. This is the basis for most training methods, e.g., imprint training, halter training, tying up a foot, snubbing to or harnessing with an experienced horse, blindfolding the horse so it can't see where to run, round pens and lunge lines. Circling not only prevents flight, thus encouraging submission, but also decreases the horse's ability to buck, rear or run rapidly. A horse that has learned that, at least in its mind, escape is impossible when it is haltered, hobbled, or in its stall, stocks or a corner, is much more cooperative when it is in that situation. However, if it has learned that escape is possible, or that submission is more fearful or harmful than to flee or fight, then flight or fight is what will occur. Again, if this occurs repeatedly, the flight or fight response increases in repetition and severity becoming a learned behavioral vice.

Flight or fight vices include inappropriate, repetitive, and generally exaggerated lunging, aggression, biting, kicking, bolting, or an exaggerated alarm reaction, and aversion reactions such as shying, balking, and startle reactions. These normal responses become a behavior problem when the response is inappropriate or exaggerated, and become a vice when the inappropriate or exaggerated behavior is repetitive. Care must be taken therefore to ensure that they are not a normal response either in purpose or degree, the purpose being a self-preservation instinct in response to fear.

Aggression

Fortunately, few horses are truly mean. However, aggression is one of the most common behavioral problems in horses and includes lunging, biting, kicking, and, less commonly, striking with a forefoot. These aggressive actions may be directed toward people, other horses, or less commonly other animals or themselves, resulting in self-mutilation. The aggression may only occur in certain situations or at certain times, such as at feeding, during heat or estrus, when the feet or face are handled, when in a stall, when being caught at pasture or in a paddock, when the cinch is being tightened, etc. Noting when the aggression occurs or what stimulates it is important in trying to correct it. Maternal aggression toward other horses, animals, people or even the foal may occur as discussed in that section in Chapter 14.

Most aggressive horses are reported to become that way because they have learned that their aggression is tolerated be people, or because they have been abused and react defensively. However, aggression in establishing a dominance hierarchy or "pecking order," and by the mare in protecting her newborn foal, is normal. Nipping behavior by young horses is also normal. Young horses tend to bite at everything they can find simply as normal play and investigative behavior, not as aggression. In the herd, young horses nip each other, pull each other's manes and tails, and rear up at each other. They may think of people as a playmate, particularly when confined and without other playmates. However, their playful nips may hurt and shouldn't be tolerated.

Lunging aggression by a stallion may occur as another stallion and less commonly other animals or people go by it. This occurs most commonly in stabled stallions, particularly when stabled with other stallions. This is a very abnormal environment for the stallion and may initiate aggressive and sexual frustration behaviors that may be alleviated by putting the stallion in a pasture with mares. Lunging aggression may also be done, although less commonly, by horses other than stallions. It is shown most frequently toward people by horses socialized through earlier human contact. It's reported that squirting the horse with a water gun when he lunges may be helpful, although for some a water hose or high-pressure hose from a fire hydrant may seem necessary.

Crowding is another form of lunging aggression in which the horse deliberately crowds or squeezes a person against the stall wall with its body. Punishment in the form of the touch of a whip, a sharp jab, or a pin prick consistently and immediately at the time of crowding may be all that's necessary to stop it. Another procedure is to carry with you into the stall a strong thick stick a bit longer than the width of your body and sharpened at one end. When the horse begins to crowd, place the dull end of the stick against the wall behind you and the sharpened end toward the horse so that as he pushes against it he receives an uncomfortable jab from it, which should be accompanied by a verbal rebuke.

Biting is an occasional aggressive vice of some horses. It is usually in the form of snapping and nipping, often in response to some specific stimulus or situation. Biting attempts are usually very sudden and typically accompanied by laying the ears back, retracting the lips, baring the teeth, and switching the tail. Biting can generally be suppressed by a touch of a whip, a sharp jab, or a pin prick, particularly on the muzzle, given at the same time as the attempted bite. It may be necessary for this to be done consistently by everyone involved until the horse stops biting.

Rearing, or striking with the forefeet with or without rearing, is a dangerous vice of some horses. It may occur when they are first approached, when being haltered or bridled, when being saddled, or at other times. Its occurrence may be quite erratic and unpredictable. Most horses will tense up before doing it. It, like kicking, is difficult and usually virtually impossible to control or stop. Punishment when the horse kicks, rears, or strikes is seldom successful. Kicks frequently aren't delivered with much predictability.

Treatment of most aggressive acts toward people is aimed at rewarding nonaggression, and occasionally also at punishing aggression. The punishment to be of benefit must be swift, consistent, sufficiently severe to stop the aggressive act, and given immediately at the time of the aggression by the person affected. If the aggression is due

to fear, however, punishment may worsen the aggression. With fear, the ears are turned sideways and the tail is either clamped to the rump or stiffened so the hair falls horizontal rather than vertical. In contrast, with non-fear-induced aggression, the horse will lay its ears back and lash its tail. Rewards, such as a small amount of grain, are most effective when given closely following the desired or nonaggressive behavior, although timing is not quite as critical for a reward as it is for punishment.

For example, a horse that kicks or is aggressive when its feet are handled or its head or ears are touched should receive a small amount of grain from a pan following a desired response. Begin by touching as close to the problem area as the horse will allow without an unfavorable response, and reward this response. Gradually touch closer to the problem area, giving a reward for a favorable response. If there is an unfavorable response, either punish it, such as a quick pin prick elsewhere on the body, or preferably withdraw and allow enough time to elapse so that a new training session can begin.

Grain as a behavioral reward may require, or work better when, the horse's feed intake has been reduced so that it is hungry. It's been recommended that especially aggressive horses should receive no other feed or attention (neither animal or people) during such training. The sensory deprivation may heighten the horse's interest in the training sessions and increase the chances that it will exhibit nonaggressive behavior for which it can then be rewarded. The situation should be manipulated however possible to decrease the chances of aggressive behavior and increase the chances of nonaggressive behavior that can be rewarded. The reverse situation—that is, increasing the chances of aggression that is punished—is much less likely to be beneficial.

Quicker, more drastic methods of dealing with aggression are occasionally used but aren't needed for most cases. These include drug-induced immobilization, such as administering succinylcholine, or tranquilizers. Aggression toward other horses may occasionally be treated successfully by administering reposetol progesterone (1 to 2 g,/horse/week) or medroxyprogesterone (65 to 85 mg/horse/day of Ovaban-Schering Corp). Long-term usage in stallions, however, decreases semen quality and libido. Six months may be required to return to normal reproductive capabilities after treatment is stopped, but no permanent changes occur.

Remote control shock collars, such as those available for dogs, may also be used. To ensure that the horse doesn't associate punishment with: (1) the collar, it should be worn for several days before a shock is administered, or (2) with a person, the operator should be hidden. To be effective: (1) the shock must be given at the moment the horse threatens, kicks, or bites another; (2) only one type of unwanted behavior should be punished; and (3) it shouldn't be overused, but use should be consistent. The signal for most shock collars won't transmit through wire fences. In addition, some report that shock collars work only occasionally and often leave the horse more unpredictable, timid, or aggressive. Before punishment, drug or hormonal therapy is used, and ideally, before any vice becomes a fixation or habit, the horse should be referred to a behavioral specialist.

Self-Aggression or Mutilation

Self-directed aggression or mutilation may occur in which the horse bites itself (usually its side or flanks) and is generally accompanied by kicking and squealing. The affected horse may move in a circle, kick, and bite in the air or at its body. Most just nip at themselves, although some may really hurt themselves. The greatest danger is often to anyone or anything in the vicinity, and property damage. Episodes may be precipitated by stressful situations. Colic or pain, peripheral neuritis, central nervous system lesions, rabies, and dermatitis may also cause this behavior. Therefore, these should be ruled out or corrected before other action is taken.

Self-mutilation is thought by some to be likely to be a compulsive disorder, in which case causes would include any factors inducing either conflict or frustration. It may originally develop in a conflict situation, but later in life be displayed again in any situation when arousal is high. It is generally reported to occur most commonly in mature, heavily fed stallions with limited exercise. Stall confinement, limited exercise and social interaction, unstable social hierarchy or dominance order, a high-grain-low-hay diet, and stabling with other stallions are reported to increase the likelihood of it occurring. This is a very abnormal environment for stallions and may initiate aggressive and sexual frustration behaviors, although this hasn't been demonstrated. However, in one report of 31 cases of self-mutilative behavior in horses, only 6 were mature heavily fed stallions with limited exercise, 5 were mature geldings, 3 were yearlings, 2 were foals, and one was a mature mare. The behavior occurred in horses in heavy work, horses kept in pastures with a herd, and horses receiving only pasture or hay forage. In another report of 5 cases all were in mature horses, with 2 in stallions, 2 in geldings, and 1 in a mare. Thus, in contrast to what has been described in the past, there doesn't appear to be a typical type of horse, situation, or management when self-aggression occurs, although it does appear to occur most commonly, but certainly not exclusively, in mature males.

There doesn't appear to be a specific procedure or set of management procedures that successfully alleviates self-aggression. Changing the horse's environment, whatever it may be, seems most likely to be of benefit. Putting stabled horses on pasture with other horses, stallions preferably with mares, is reported to generally alleviate self-aggressive behavior. If this isn't possible, increased activity, decreased confinement, feeding more hay and less or no grain, and a companion, such as a pony, donkey, or goat may be helpful for some cases. In contrast, cases have been reported where self-mutilation stopped only when the horses were brought in from pasture and confined in a stall where they were socially isolated, fed a grain mix, and permitted limited exercise. One horse was found to be most content and free of self-mutilation when cross-tied in a stall away from any other animals; in a larger stall or at pasture, its self-mutilation was life-threatening. In numerous cases all sorts of management changes, even

castration, did not reduce self-mutilation to a safe or acceptable degree. Administration of a beta-endorphin blocker (nalmerfere), or a serotonin reuptake blocker may be helpful, particularly in conjunction with changing the horse's environment.

Self-aggression may be prevented by putting a cradle on the horse's neck so he can't reach his side, but this doesn't change his motivation, and he may continue to lunge at his flank and kick.

Shying or Bolting

With shying or bolting, there is a sudden elevation of either the head, neck, forelegs, or the whole body and generally a sudden movement away from a real or perceived reason for alarm. The alarm may be to almost anything, including visual changes in reflected light, fluttering papers, cloth or even leaves, the sudden movement of a small animal, a person or even their hand, and even stationary objects that they suddenly see. A sharp noise and even possibly an odor may stimulate shying. Shying is of course a normal alarm reaction well developed over millions of years of evolution as an important survival instinct. It becomes a vice not because it may surprise or hurt someone when it happens, but when it is exaggerated, repetitive, and occurs without sufficient cause—a cause that would not alarm most horses.

Shying may be caused by a vision problem or a previous experience. Control methods include a companion horse with a stable temperament, and "blinkers" or "blinders" on the bridle, as are commonly used for driving horses since shying in the shafts can lead to unfortunate consequences. Calm patience, rewarding desirable behavior, and ensuring that undesirable behavior isn't rewarded, are much more likely to be of benefit than punishment.

Balking and Freezing

Balking (jibbing) and freezing (stiff immobility), like shying, are alarm reactions but with the opposite response—an unwillingness or refusal to move instead of a quick alarm movement. The confirmed balker is actively antagonistic toward any effort to get him to move forward. The horse assumes a stubborn stiff state and fights attempts to make him move forward. Instead of balking, some horses may "freeze" in a particular position or posture, most frequently lying down and refuse to rise. They may remain in this state for hours if left alone. Some balking horses may be moved backward or turned and taken out of the situation by doing this. This may gradually eliminate balking in some horses. However, some horses may refuse to move in any direction and no correction is effective. Force, no matter how severe or cruel, often is not effective and is not justified.

Temperament, pain, or overuse may cause balking or lying down. The horse may also sense that it cannot or is afraid to try to perform the task requested and thus balks when asked to do it. Balking or lying down may also occur because the horse has learned that it can successfully avoid work by doing this. To prevent this, the horse should never be allowed to associate these, or any undesirable behavior, with a reward for that behavior, such as avoiding work or getting fed.

When balking or lying down occur, evaluate the situation thoroughly for the cause or a problem before taking action. If the cause is pain, alleviate it. If it's overuse, use the horse less or in a different manner. If it's an inability to perform or a fear of the task requested, ask the horse with authority, and if necessary using a crop or whip, to perform a similar but less difficult or fearful task. Then reward the horse for doing it, such as with a small amount of grain, ensuring that each training session is ended in this manner. Gradually over a number of training sessions work up to the task you want the horse to perform, making sure that it is within the horse's physical and psychological ability.

For the horse that lies down, ensure that there isn't a physical reason for it. The horse that lies down because of a behavioral problem and refuses to get up can be distinguished from the horse that lies down because of illness or weakness and is unable to get up by: (1) the presence of stiff (tonic) rather than flaccid (atonic) immobility; (2) alertness, as indicated by movements of the head, eyes, and ears; (3) a refusal of the horse that appears able to even try to rise in response to stimulation to do so; (4) the horse voluntarily adjusting its legs; (5) normal physiological behaviors, including defecation, respiration, eating and drinking, at least initially; (6) sensitivity to body surface stimulation; and (7) the presence of blink, anal, pedal, and other reflexes. However, reflexes involving changes in body positions—e.g., extension leg movements and righting after laying the horse on its side—are usually slow, and a strong persistence to whichever head posture has been adopted commonly occurs.

The horse may get up on its own at any time or remain lying down for a long period. If the horse does remain lying down for a long period, secondary pathological conditions may occur (such as inadequate blood circulation to some areas, pressure sores, septicemia, and toxemia) to the point the horse may become unable to get up. Even if the condition is only transient, physical injury may occur during transit, or if the horse is in a group of horses, it may be stepped on.

Generally, like the balking horse, force of any type is of little benefit in getting the horse up. However, when both nostrils are held tightly closed, most horses will rapidly scramble to their feet when they run out of air, as this appears to scare of them sufficiently to get up. The horse will also frequently get up if its environment is changed to give the horse more space—e.g., moving the horse from indoors to outdoors. As soon as the horse gets up, but not before, reward it with a small amount of grain.

SUPPLEMENTAL READING RECOMMENDATIONS

Domestic Animal Behavior by Katherine A Houpt, VMD, PhD, who is professor of physiology at New York State Veterinary College, Cornell University, and a leading authority. Dr. Houpt has conducted extensive research and clinical practice, and published widely on animal behavior, particularly that of the horse. Hers is a referenced text covering communication; social structure; biological rhythms; sleep, sexual, maternal, developmental, and ingestive behavior; and behavioral disorders of horses, dogs, cats, pigs, cattle, sheep, and goats. The section on behavioral problems in horses is short, but like all of the book, is quite good without the unproven, often repeated, but frequently incorrect, assumptions made by sometimes excellent veterinarians and horsemen, but without Dr. Houpt's training, experience and expertise in equine behavior. Individuals who read this book will have a much better and accurate understanding of the horse, as well as other animals, and be a better horseman for it. Publisher Iowa State University Press, Ames, IA 50010. 408 pages, Second edition (1991).

The Behavior of the Horse by Dr. Andrew F. Fraser, who is a professor of veterinary surgery at Memorial University of Newfoundland, Canada, and a pioneer in the scientific study of applied animal behavior. This book covers the basics of horse behavior, including normal behavior and one chapter on abnormal behavior. C.A.B. International, Wallingford, Oxfordshire, OXIO 8DE, UK, 288 pages, 1992.

TTouch Horse Video and A-Z Horse Tip Book by Linda Tellington-Jones a well known and respected equine behaviorist who teaches easy and useful methods for gaining the horses cooperation through understanding rather than force. The information shown in the video and 96-page book will help you correct numerous behavioral problems. Her methods are widely used and reported by many to be quite helpful. **TTouch for Horses,** 78-080 Calle Estado, #2B, La Quinta, CA 92253, 1-800-224-5400.

Life Song is by Dr. Bill Schul a clinical psychologist with life-long experience in working with animals and people. In this book he has compiled a multitude of experiences in communications between many different species and people, and the positive result they bring to all involved. I urge you to read this book for a deeper and more rewarding understanding and appreciation of other forms of life. You will enjoy the reading, and even more the wisdom and understanding it will help you have of other creatures with whom we share the earth. Stillpoint Publishing, P.O. Box 640, Walpole, NH 03608, 1-800-847-4014.

GLOSSARY

Abscess: A localized collection of pus in the tissues of the body, often accompanied by swelling and inflammation, and generally caused by bacteria. External rupture or drainage is necessary for healing. Internal rupture is often fatal.

Acid detergent fiber (ADF): See fiber, dietary.

Acidosis: A condition of excess acid or hydrogen ions in the body. The opposite of alkalosis.

Acrodynia: A condition in rats, dogs and pigs due to a deficiency of pyridoxine (vitamin B_6) and marked by swelling and death of tissues of the paws, the tips of ears and nose and of the lips. Not known to occur in horses.

Acute: Occurring over a short period of time; an acute disease is one which develops and progresses to death, or recovery quite rapidly. Opposite of chronic. Often incorrectly used to indicate severity.

Additives (food): A substance purposely incorporated in a feed to provide some desired characteristic, such as color, flavor, enhanced utilization or stability, or resistance to spoilage of any type. See Chapter 4.

Ad lib: Abbreviation for ad libitum, meaning at pleasure, and thus the animal is able to eat or drink at its pleasure, i.e., whenever and however much it chooses.

Aerobic: Aer- or Aero- indicating a relationship to air, so something occurring in the presence of or using air or oxygen. Opposite of anaerobic meaning without air or oxygen.

Agglutination: A phenomenon in which the cells distributed in fluid collect into clumps.

Air dry: In nutrition air dry refers to a feed that has been allowed to dry in the air. As a result, it contains 8 to 12% moisture depending on humidity, but is assumed to be 10%, and thus 90% dry matter.

Air dry basis: Indicates that the value expressed is the amount by weight present in an air dried feed or diet. Nearly all feeds for the horse, with the exception of green pasture forage and ensiled or acid-treated feeds, are air dry, and thus are assumed to contain 90% dry matter. Green growing pasture forage, silage and haylage generally contain about $\frac{2}{3}$ water and $\frac{1}{3}$ dry matter. See dry matter basis for conversion between air dry, as fed and dry matter basis.

Albumin: 1) One of the major proteins in the blood plasma, the other being, globulin. These two proteins normally constitute over 90% of the plasma protein. Both are produced by the liver and a small amount of gamma globulin by the body's immune system. 2) Milk albumin is the coagulated protein fraction from whey.

Alkalosis: A condition of excess base or hydroxyl ions, or inadequate acid or hydrogen ions in the body. The opposite of acidosis.

Allergy: A condition of increased sensitivity to a specific protein (not an amount of protein) so that exposure to that protein causes an excessive response of the body which may be manifested in any one or more of the following effects: a rash, hives, respiratory difficulties, sneezing, nasal discharge, or diarrhea.

Alternate: Botanically it means singly along the stem, one leaf to each node or point of leaf attachment.

Amble: See **gaits.**

Amino acids: Nitrogen-containing hydrocarbon (organic) compounds that are the "building blocks" from which proteins are formed. A protein consists of many amino acids bound together. There are 22 different amino acids. Different types of protein contain different amino acids. Twelve to 14 of these amino acids are produced in the body and do not need to be absorbed from the intestinal tract. These are called nonessential amino acids. The remaining 8 to 10 amino acids must be absorbed from the intestinal tract, and are called essential amino acids. The bacteria in the mature horse's large intestine produce all of the amino acids needed, so it doesn't matter what amount of which amino acids, or type of protein, is present in their diet. However, a high amount of certain amino acids (particularly lysine) are needed in the feed for growth. See Chapter 1.

Amniotic sac (water bag): A translucent membranous sac in the uterus of the pregnant animal that contains fluid and the fetus.

Anaerobic: An- meaning without, and aerobic indicating air or oxygen, thus without oxygen. Opposite of aerobic meaning with air or oxygen.

Anaerobic or lactate threshold: The level of physical activity above which energy can no longer be produced rapidly enough aerobically (using oxygen) necessitating anaerobic (without oxygen) energy production for the physical activity to continue. This is indicated by an increase in the blood's concentration of the end product of anaerobic energy production, lactic acid. This occurs in most horses at a heart rate above 140 to 150 bpm, and at a speed of 2:40 to 5:20 min/mile (5 to 10 m/sec) depending on the horse's physical fitness, weight carried, and difficulty of the terrain covered. See Chapter 11 section on "Plasma Lactate as an Indicator of Fitness."

Anemia: Below normal amount of red blood cells in the blood. Nutritional causes in horses include inadequate or excess vitamin A, and excess selenium or zinc. The most common cause of anemia in horses is excess blood loss due to internal or external parasites. Regardless of the cause, increased intake of nutrients needed for red blood cell production, such as iron, protein and B-vitamins, may be helpful for the most rapid recovery.

Anesthesia: An- indicating absence or without, and -thesia sensation, so anesthesia is a loss of feeling or sensation. This may be in a local area only, or it may be general anesthesia in which there is a complete loss of consciousness.

Anestrus: The seasonal period of time when a female is not experiencing an estrous cycle and is sexually inactive, which for most mares is late fall to early spring.

Anion: A negatively charged particle or ion. See **cation.**

Anhidrosis (dry coat): A decreased ability to sweat. See Chapter 11.

Annual: Yearly. An annual plant being one that lives only one growing season.

Anoplocephala: See **tapeworms** and Chapter 9.

Anorexia: Loss of appetite for food; often used to indicate a decrease in (hypophagia), or absence of (aphagia) food intake; (hypo- meaning below normal, a- an absence of, and -phagia, to eat). Anorexia nervosa, an eating disorder of people, is a specific type of anorexia not known to occur in horses, whereas anorexia is a common sequela to many diseases in all species including horses.

Anterior: In front of, or toward the front or head end of the body. Opposite of posterior.

Anthelmintic: Ant- meaning against, and helminth meaning intestinal worm, thus a dewormer or vermifuge administered to an animal to get rid of intestinal worms.

Antibiotics: Chemical substances produced by fungi or mold that inhibit or destroy bacteria or other micro-organisms, and that are used primarily in the treatment of infectious diseases.

Antibodies: See **immunoglobulins.**

Antigen: A substance that stimulates antibody production, or an allergy.

Antitoxin: Antibodies that counteract a toxin. These are given to an animal to protect it against that particular toxin. An antitoxin does not stimulate the animal to produce its own antitoxins, and therefore it provides protection against that toxin only until it is broken down or eliminated from the body; a period of 1 to 3 weeks. See **vaccine.**

Antioxidant: Anti- meaning against, and oxidation to combine with oxygen, such as in the utilization of carbon containing (organic) compounds for energy converting them to carbon dioxide and water. Thus an antioxidant is a substance which prevents a substance or tissue from being oxidized. See Chapter 4. Common antioxidants used in feeds include tocopherols (vitamin E), citric acid, ascorbates (vitamin C), ethoxyquin, propyl gallate, tertiary butylhydroquinone, butylated hydroxyanisole (BHA) and butylate hydroxytoluene (BHT).

Aril: A fleshy, usually colored covering or attachment to a seed.

Artery: A round, elastic, thick-walled tube that carries blood from the heart to all parts of the body. The blood in an artery is normally well saturated with oxygen it has picked up in its passage through the lungs. This gives it a bright red color, whereas the blood in a vein is dark red because at the capillaries the oxygen has diffused out of the blood into the tissue. Arteries are deeper from the body surface than are veins. The blood in an artery is under high pressure; therefore, if an artery is cut, blood spurts out, whereas the blood in a vein is under very little pressure.

Arthritis: Arthr- referring to an articulation or joint, and -itis inflammation. Thus, arthritis is inflammation of a joint. Common types in horses are:

Serous arthritis—sterile (free from micro-organisms) inflammation of a joint or synovial membrane usually due to trauma resulting in swelling and effusion (escape of fluid into tissues).

Infectious or suppurative arthritis—septic inflammation of the joint from traumatic (exogenous) or blood born (hematogenous or endogenous) invasion of the joint by micro-organisms.

Osteoarthritis—osteo referring to bone, so inflammation of a joint and bone. A chronic condition often developing as a sequel to serous or infectious arthritis.

Ascarids: A large round worm that develops in the intestinal tract of primarily young horses. See Chapter 9.

Ascorbate or Ascorbic Acid: Vitamin C.

As fed or as is basis: Indicates that the value expressed is the amount present in the feed or diet in the form in which it is fed. The amount of nutrients, as given on the feed tag, are on an as fed basis. See dry matter basis for conversion between air dry, as fed, and dry matter basis.

Ash: The mineral or inorganic (non-carbon containing) portion of a substance. See **minerals.**

Assimilation: In nutrition assimilation refers to the processes by which a nutrient or feed is made available to and used by the body: includes prehension, chewing, swallowing, digestion, absorption, distribution and metabolism.

Ataxia: Failure of muscular coordination, resulting in a stumbling, weaving, or drunken-type gait. May be due to weakness, wobblers syndrome, a deficiency of magnesium or vitamins B or E, excess intake of sodium, selenium or vitamin A, or ingestion of neurotoxic plants (Table 18–7), some sudden death-inducing plants (Table 18–12), some feed-related poisons (Table 19–1), and other neurologic-diseases (Table 19–5).

ATP (adenosine triphosphate): A substance produced in the body by attaching 3 phosphate molecules to one molecule of adenosine. Its production requires energy which is derived from the body's utilization of carbohydrates, fats or protein. This energy, which is released when each phosphate molecule is removed from ATP, is the only source of energy that can be used by muscles and other body tissues. ATP, therefore, serves as a means of transferring energy derived from carbohydrates, fats or proteins to body tissues for their activity, such as muscular movement, brain function, etc.

Atrophy: A wasting away or decrease in size of a cell, tissue, organ or part of the body.

Autolysis: Auto- meaning self, and lysis dissolution, so self dissolution or spontaneous disintegration of tissues by the action of their own enzymes, such as occurs after death.

Awn: Bristle usually terminating a plant part.

Axillary: Botanically means located at the junction of the leaf and the stem.

Azotemia: See **uremia.**

Azoturia: Azo- referring to nitrogen containing compounds, and -uria to urine. Thus the excretion of nitrogen-containing compounds in the urine. It is used to refer to a condition in the horse in which, within a few minutes of beginning physical activity, muscle spasms or tetany occur. Affected muscles become hard to the touch, muscle cells die, and muscle proteins, such as myoglobins, are lost and excreted in the urine. See Chapter 11.

B

Balanced diet: A diet which provides the proper amounts and proportions of all the nutrients needed.

Bald: Lacking hair, vegetation or pigmentation, e.g., a bald man, a bald mountain, and a bald eagle or bald-faced horse which have a white head and face, respectively.

"Barn-sour:" A horse that resists being ridden away from the barn; persistently turning the horse all the way around and walking away from the barn is necessary. Once well away from the barn, most barn-sour horses will stop trying to return to it, and gradually become less barn-sour the more they are made to leave the barn.

Barren mare: A mare that has been bred the previous breeding season but failed to either conceive or to carry a foal to term. It is also sometimes used to indicate an older mare that has never conceived or carried a foal to term whether she has been bred or not.

Benign: Not malignant, such as a tumor that will not spread or form new foci in a distant part of the body, i.e., that will not metastasize.

Beta-carotene: A yellow plant pigment that, following ingestion and subsequent absorption, most is converted in the intestinal wall to vitamin A. See Chapter 3.

Biennial: Happening every two years, such as a plant that lives two growing seasons.

Big-head (bran disease): Enlargement of the bones of the skull owing to replacement of their minerals with fibrous connective tissue. The jaw bone and the bones of the face are usually affected to the greatest extent, although all bones in the body are affected. The disease is brought on by excessive secretion of parathyroid hormone (parathormone), which may be caused by a dietary calcium deficiency or phosphorus excess, by parathyroid gland dysfunction, or by tumors (cancer) which may produce a substance that has the same effect as parathyroid hormone. See section on "Calcium Deficiency/Phosphorus Excess" in Chapter 2.

Bilateral: Bi- indicating two, and lateral indicating side. Thus, bilateral means pertaining to both sides or having two sides.

Bishoping: The fraudulent act of making a cup in an aged horse's incisor teeth (Fig. 9–11) by drilling and staining to make the "bishoped" horse appear from age estimation of its teeth to be younger than it actually is.

Bit teeth: See **canine teeth.**

Bleeders (Exercise-induced Pulmonary Hemorrhage): Horses that bleed from the lungs due to strenuous physical exertion. The blood interferes with respiratory gas exchange decreasing physical performance ability. In only a small percentage of affected horses is it sufficiently severe that bleeding from the nose is visible. See Chapter 11.

Blemish: A disfigurement not affecting the normal use of the horse except by its appearance.

Blinders (Blinkers): A solid piece of material attached to the headstall along side of each eye so the horse cannot see to the side without turning its head. They are used to prevent shying at something the horse may see to the side.

Blindness: An inability to see, which may be caused by selenium toxicosis or at night a vitamin A deficiency.

Blinkers: See **blinders.**

Blood counts: Generally refers to the practice of taking a blood sample and measuring the hematocrit (percent of red blood cells) and hemoglobin concentration. The values obtained from the normal-appearing horse at rest are in most instances meaningless (see Chapter 11). If the hematocrit or hemoglobin concentrations are considered to be low, several nutrients such as iron, copper, and B-vitamins needed for red blood cell synthesis are frequently given to the horse and a process called "jugging" may be performed. In most instances, these nutrients are not deficient and giving them or "jugging" the horse is of no benefit.

Blood doping (boosting or packing): Administering red blood cells, which have been separated from the plasma, intravenously. The purpose being to increase the blood's oxygen carrying capacity and thus enhance athletic performance. However, it increases the blood's viscosity which decreases blood flow to the tissues. This is detrimental to athletic performance. Because of this, blood doping has been shown to impair athletic performance in dogs, and would be expected to also be detrimental for horses.

Blood worms: Adult large strongyles. See **strongyles.**

Bloody nose: See **bleeders** and **epistaxis.**

Bloom: When used in reference to an animal, it indicates a glossy hair coat; in reference to a plant it indicates the appearance of flowers.

Blowout: A short (usually 3 to 4 furlongs, or 0.6 to 0.8 km) fast run.

Boil, shoe: See **capped elbow.**

Bone growth plates: See **physis.**

Bone marrow: The soft material that fills the cavities of the bones. Red and white blood cells are produced by the bone marrow.

Body condition score: A score given to an animal based on its overall body appearance ranging from less than very thin (a score of 1), to moderate (a score of 5), to extremely fat (a score of 9). See Table 1–4.

Bolt or bolting: To do something suddenly or rapidly, such as bolting feed or a sudden generally unexpected jump or movement which is also referred to as shying. Sometimes distinguished as shying being to the side, and bolting being straight ahead.

Bots: Bot flies lay eggs on horse's hair. When the horse scratches itself with its teeth or licks itself, the eggs enter the mouth, and hatch. The larvae may invade the tissue of the mouth or be swallowed. Bot worms develop and attach to the wall of the stomach until early spring. They cause inflammation of the stomach, and may cause colic, debilitation, perforations and death. Bot worms are passed in the feces in early spring. See Chapter 9.

Bowed back: When a horse stands with its back pushed or bowed upward. It is indicated by a space between the horse's back and the bottom of the back of the saddle. When horses do this, they are likely to try to buck when you get on.

Bowed tendon: Inflammation of the superficial and/or deep digital flexor tendons and tendon sheaths resulting in swelling behind the cannon bones. See "Tendon and Ligament Injuries" in Chapter 11.

Bract: A small leaf-like structure surrounding or below a flower.

Breeding selection: Selecting matings to increase the probability of offspring having or not having one or more traits. The more traits selected for, the less progress that will be made in any one trait. Major multiple trait selection systems used are:

1. Independent culling levels—in which the breeder sets a minimum acceptable standard for each trait deemed important and only horses at or above *all* minimum standards are bred.
2. Index selection system—in which the breeder places a weight or value on each trait deemed important and calculates an overall score for the total breeding value for each horse. Only those whose overall score is at or above a minimum are bred.

The primary means used for breeding selection for any one or more traits are:

1. Pedigree selection—in which the performance or characteristics of a horse's parents and other relatives are used for breeding selection. This is the most used, because it is the most available, but it is the least indicative breeding selection method. It is useful only when breeding selection must be made before a horse's own performance can be measured.
2. Phenotypic selection—in which the horse's own performance or characteristics are used for breeding selection. The more highly heritable the trait (Table 11-7), the more accurate phenotypic selection is in predicting offspring's traits.
3. Progeny test selection—in which the performance or characteristics of the horse's progeny are used for breeding selection. This is the most accurate method for breeding selection. With enough progeny, a stallion can be ranked quite accurately for the probability of a trait in its offspring even when the heritability of that trait is low (Table 11-7).

Breeding stitch: A stitch inserted surgically into the labial lips to prevent them from separating during breeding where they have been closed by a Caslick's operation.

Breeze: An easy workout.

British Thermal Unit: See **BTU.**

Brittle feet: Dry, cracked hoof walls. See "Hoof Defects" in Chapter 17.

Broken wind: See **heaves.**

Bronchial tubes (bronchi): Tubes, or air passages, formed by the division of the windpipe (trachea) at the point where it reaches the lungs.

Bronchitis: Inflammation of the bronchial tubes.

Bronchiolytic agents: Drugs that help break up mucus in the bronchial tubes.

BTU (British Thermal Unit): The amount of energy needed to raise one pound of water 1°F. Generally used in physical but not biological sciences. 1 BTU = 0.252 kcal or 3.968 BTU/kcal.

Buccal: Pertaining to the cheek or the mouth.

Bucked shins: Inflammation of the tissue or periosteum over the front of the cannon bones, generally due to repeated concussion in the overtrained or overused young horse not yet sufficiently physically fit. See Chapter 11 "Bone Stress Injuries."

Bulbs (buttons): Enlarged nodule at the end of the splint bone, 3 to 4 inches (6 to 9 cm) above the fetlock (Fig. 6-5). Their size varies from no nodule evident to a large prolongation such as in some draft horses.

Bulk limited diet: A diet so low in energy density that the animal is unable to eat enough of it to meet its energy needs because its gastrointestinal tract becomes full first. Thus, the amount consumed is limited by the diet's bulk. In contrast an energy limited diet is one sufficiently high in energy density so the animal is able to eat enough to meet its energy needs. Thus the amount of it consumed is limited by the diets energy density.

Buttons: See **bulbs.**

Buttress foot: New bone growth on the extensor process of the distal phalanx or leg bone causing an enlargement at the coronary band at the center front of the hoof. In early stages there is heat, swelling, lameness and pain to finger pressure. It is due to trauma induced fracture of the extensor process, or excess bone growth in which it is an advanced form of low ringbone. A short and rapid (trappy) gait predisposes to it.

C

Cake: A mass resulting from pressing feeds together. In herbivore nutrition cake generally refers to feed pellets or cubes that are large enough (about thumb size or larger) to be fed on the ground. Usually they are composed of primarily or entirely grains and supplements. They are most often fed to cattle on pasture or on the range, and thus may be referred to as range cake or range cubes.

Calcinosis: A condition in which calcium salts in nodules are deposited in soft tissues such as the muscle, under the skin, tendons, elastic tissues, and nerves. It may be caused by excessive vitamin D or ingestion of plants that contain vitamin D-like toxins. See "Plant-Induced Calcinosis" in Chapter 18.

Calcitonin: A substance (hormone) produced by the thyroid gland in response to an increase in the blood calcium concentration. It inhibits calcium and phosphorus mobilization from the bone and decreases intestinal calcium absorption. In some animals it also increases calcium excretion in the urine. Its function is to prevent or minimize an increase in the blood calcium concentration.

calorie: A unit of energy being the amount of heat required to raise 1 gram of water 1°C. This is known as the small calorie or standard calorie. This unit is not used in nutrition. The smallest unit of energy used in nutrition is the large calorie or kilocalorie. It is equal to 1000 small calories and may be written as 1 calorie, 1 Calorie, 1 kilocalorie, or 1 kcal.

Calyx: An outer series or row of petals.

Camped-out: Standing with the feet too far back, usually because of the horse being too straight at the hock.

Camped-under: Standing with the feet too far foreward, usually because of excessive angulation of the hock. See **sickle-hocked.**

Canine teeth (tusks, tushes, bit teeth, male teeth or fang teeth): Teeth located between the front and middle one-third of the space between the incisors and cheek teeth. They erupt at 4 to 5 years of age. Both upper and lower canine teeth are present in the majority of males and about one-fourth of female horses. They may grow too long and strike the opposite gum making their shortening necessary to prevent this.

Canker: A relatively uncommon chronic proliferation of horn-producing tissues of the foot believed to be due to an infection from unclean stables.

Canter: See **gaits.**

Ca:P ratio (Calcium:phosphorus ratio): The amount of calcium with respect to phosphorus present in the diet or feed with the amount of phosphorus generally being given a value of one. For example, if a diet contained 0.70% calcium and 0.35% phosphorus, the Ca:P ratio of 0.70:0.35 would be converted to 2:1, indicating it contained twice as much Ca as P. This conversion is made by dividing both the amount of calcium and the amount of phosphorus in the diet by the amount of phosphorus.

Capillary: A diffuse network of minute blood vessels between arteries and veins forming a network in body tissues, through which oxygen and other nutrients diffuse in and waste products diffuse out of the tissue.

Capillary refill time: The time it takes for capillary perfusion to return, as indicated by a return of the gums normal color after finger pressure to them is removed. Normally this occurs within less than 3 seconds. If it takes longer, it indicates inadequate capillary perfusion, such as that due to dehydration, shock or heart failure.

Caps: Temporary teeth that after being pushed out by erupting permanent teeth stay attached to the gum. They should be removed, as they interfere with chewing, may lacerate the tongue and cheek, and may interfere with eruption of the permanent teeth. See Chapter 9.

Capped elbow: Inflammation resulting in swelling at the point of the elbow (Fig. 6–5). Usually caused by hitting the elbow often with the front foot when lying down and,

therefore, may be referred to as a shoe boil. It is most common in horses stabled for long periods. The swelling may be extensive but lameness rarely occurs. The elbow may be protected by putting a shoe boot on the front foot.

Capped hock: Inflammation resulting in swelling at the point of the hock (Fig. 6–5). Usually caused by hitting it, often due to kicking a solid object such as the stall; which if done repeatedly is a behavioral problem discussed in Chapter 20.

Carbohydrates: Compounds composed of carbon, hydrogen, and oxygen whose major nutritional function is to supply energy. The most important carbohydrates in the horse's diet are starches, sugars, and the fiber cellulose.

Carcinogen: Any cancer-producing substance.

Caries: The decay of bone or teeth in which it becomes softened, discolored and porous. In teeth it is due to bacterial metabolism of nonfiber carbohydrates to acids which cause tooth enamel, and later dentin, disruption exposing the tooth pulp to destruction.

Carnivores: See **herbivores.**

Carotene: See **beta-carotene.**

Carpitis: Traumatic induced arthritis of the carpal (knee) joint which can progress to degenerative joint disease. Lameness and swelling without radiographic changes are evident early. Predisposed to by calf knees and bench knees, but trauma from kicks and banging a knee on jumps, against stall walls or fences, and in trailers can also cause carpitis.

Carpus or carpal joint: The horse's knee (see Fig. 6–5).

Carrying capacity: The number of animals, or amount of land needed for one animal, that a pasture will provide sufficient forage to meet their needs for one full year.

Casein: A major protein in milk; lactalbumin being another.

Caslick's operation: An episioplasty or surgically suturing the upper portion of the lips of the vulva together to prevent aspiration or wind sucking into the vagina, and as a result, vaginal inflammation and infection which can decrease conception.

Cation: An inorganic (non-carbon containing) atom or molecule, which when free in solution, has a positive electrical charge. Opposite of anion which has a negative electrical charge. For example, when sodium chloride (common salt) dissolves in water the sodium and chloride molecules separate from each other leaving a positively charged sodium atom (cation) and a negatively charged chloride atom (anion). All charged atoms or molecules are called ions: e.g., sodium ion and chloride ion.

Catkins: A scaly, spike-like flowering part of a plant bearing unisexual flowers without petals, as in willows and cottonwoods.

Cecum: A large compartment, or outpouching, of the intestinal tract of some animals, such as horses, rats, and rabbits. Ingested material passes from the mouth down the esophagus to the stomach, small intestine, cecum, large intestine or colon, rectum, and anus. The cecum contains many bacteria that digest much of the cellulose or fiber in feeds that the animal ingests. It serves many of the same functions as the rumen in ruminants such as cattle and sheep. The appendix in humans is the vestige of a cecum (see Fig. 1–1).

Cellulose: A carbohydrate that forms the skeleton of most plants. Animals do not produce the enzymes necessary to digest it, whereas many bacteria do. Animals have these bacteria in their gastrointestinal tracts and are, therefore, able to partially use cellulose as a nutrient because the bacteria digest it for them. The more of these bacteria they have the greater their utilization of cellulose. Ruminants have the greatest, and simple stomached animals such as people, the lowest, ability to use cellulose. The horse is in between, but closer to ruminants, in their ability to use cellulose.

Cereal grains: See **grains.**

Cerebral: Pertaining to the brain.

Cervix (uterine): The neck of the uterus forming the entrance to the vagina.

Chaff: Husks or other seed covering, together with other plant parts, separated from seeds, usually cereal grains, in their harvest such as during combining or threshing. A high-fiber, low-energy feed.

Chelation: A mineral bound to an organic (carbon containing) molecule such as a carbohydrate or protein. If the organic molecule is more readily absorbed than the mineral, chelation will increase the amount of the mineral which can be absorbed. If it is not, it will decrease the mineral's absorption or increase its removal from the body. See section on "Vitamin-Mineral Supplements for Horses" in Chapter 4.

Chemotherapeutic agents: Chemical substances which inhibit or kill bacteria or other micro-organisms, and which are used in the treatment or infectious diseases. Antibiotics are chemotherapeutic agents that are produced by micro-organisms or mold.

Chlorophyll: The green pigment of plants.

Chopped: Reduced in particle size by cutting with knives or other sharp instruments. Sometimes used synonymously with cracked for a cereal grain.

Chronic: Occurring over a long period of time. Opposite of acute.

Cinch-bound: A horse that objects to being cinched-up, also referred to as "cold-backed."

Cirrhosis: A chronic disease of the liver, marked by progressive destruction of liver cells, accompanied by regeneration of the liver with an increase in connective tissue. It can be caused by many infections, toxic and nutritional factors; alcohol being the most common cause in people.

Clinical: Pertaining to or founded on actual observation or treatment, as distinguished from theoretical, experimental or subclinical (e.g., symptoms not sufficiently severe or manifested to be evident).

Club-footed: A deformity causing the horse to walk on the toe. As a result the heel tends to grow long and the toe stay worn off. See "Acquired Flexure Deformities" in Chapter 16.

Cobalamine: Vitamin B_{12}

Coffin bone: The third or distal phalanges, or bone of the foot.

Cold-backed: A horse that objects to being cinched-up, also referred to as "cinch-bound."

Cold-blooded horses: Horses whose major blood line are from the original horses of Europe. In Europe two types of horses were developed; the Celtic pony, which was well-formed, light-weight, sturdy, and rather short-legged; and the Great Horse of the Middle Ages—the large, slow, and powerful heavy horse. This designation has nothing to do with the temperature of the horse's blood. See **hot blooded horses.**

Colic: Clinical signs of abdominal pain resulting from potentially life-threatening diseases of the stomach or intestinal tract of the horse. If the pain is from other organs, such as the urinary tract, liver, reproductive tract or muscles, it is referred to as false colic. Nutritional causes of colic include inadequate fiber intake, low blood magnesium, or excess grain, sodium or vitamin K. Ingestion of blister beetles in alfalfa hay is also a feeding induced cause of colic (see Ch. 19). See chapter 18 for "Colic or Diarrhea Inducing Plants."

Colon: A portion of the large intestine or terminal portion of the digestive tract which extends from the cecum to the rectum. See Fig. 1–1.

Colostrum: The milk secreted by the mare just before foaling, and for about the first day afterwards. It is high in antibodies which protect the newborn against infectious diseases. The amount of antibodies in colostrum decreases rapidly after foaling, as does the foal's ability to absorb them. See section on "Foal Immunity Attainment, Determination and Enhancement" in Chapter 14.

Colt: An immature intact male horse.

Coma: An abnormal state of depressed responsiveness, with absence of response to any stimuli. A state of stupor, or unconsciousness.

Complete feed: A feed that contains all of the nutrients that are needed by the animal, with the exception of water and salt. The term is generally used for commercially prepared diets that contain both forage and grain. See "Grain-Mixes and Complete Feeds" in Chapter 4.

Concentrates: A broad classification of feedstuffs that are high in energy and low in crude fiber (under 18%). Generally considered to be everything in the diet not classified as a forage or roughage, or the part of the diet composed primarily of grains or present in the grain-mix.

Condition score: A score given to an animal based on its overall body appearance ranging from less than very thin (a score for 1), to moderate (a score of 5), to extremely fat (a score of 9). See Table 1–4.

Contagious: Communicable or transmissible from one individual to another.

Contracted tendons: Shortening of the superficial and/or deep digital flexor tendons or check ligaments. See "Flexure Leg Deformities" in Chapter 16.

Convulsions: Spasm or violent, involuntary, uncontrollable contraction, or series of contractions, of the muscles.

COPD: Chronic obstructive pulmonary disease. See **Heaves.**

Coprophagy: Copro- denotes relationship to feces, and -phagy to eat, thus eating feces. This is common in foals and normally decreases with age so that most mature horses try to avoid eating feces and fecally-contaminated feeds.

Cordate: Heart-shaped.

Corn: In regard to feed a cereal grain. In regard to the foot, a contusion of the sole near the hoof wall of its lateral angle. It is usually due to improper shoeing, which may result in a dry, moist or suppurative corn.

Corolla: Collective term for plant or flower petals.

Coronary band (coronet): Located at the hair line along the top of the hoof wall, it is the primary source of nutrients for the hoof wall which grows from it. Injuries to the coronary band usually leave a permanent defect in the growth of the hoof wall. See Fig. 6-5.

Corpus luteum or CL: A glandular mass formed on the ovary by the follicle following ovulation of the ovum or egg. It secretes progesterone which prevents a new follicle from developing. If pregnancy doesn't occur, the CL degenerates and progesterone secretion decreases allowing the development of a new follicle, estrus and ovulation, which in the normally cycling mare occurs 19 to 23 days after the previous ovulation. If pregnancy occurs, the corpus luteum grows and produces sufficient progesterone to maintain pregnancy until the placenta produces enough progesterone (at the 150th to 190th day of pregnancy in the mare) to maintain pregnancy. See Fig. 13-4.

Corticosteroids: Substances that affect the animal in the same manner as hormones produced by the adrenal cortex. Usually used to decrease fever and inflammation, and to give the animal a sense of feeling better or not as ill.

Cow-hocked: A conformational fault in which the points of hocks turn inward instead of straight back.

Cracked: Particle size reduced by combined breaking and crushing. Sometimes used synonymously with chopped for a cereal grain.

Creatinine: A breakdown product of muscle creatine that is excreted in the urine. The amount produced and excreted is directly proportional to the amount of muscle, so the amount excreted daily is fairly constant. The constant quantity of creatinine excreted in the urine can be used to determine the amount of other substances excreted in the urine. The concentrations of all solutes in the urine vary according to the amount of urine excreted, which in turn varies with the amount of water ingested, with kidney function, and with the amount of water lost in sweat and stools. Therefore, comparing the urine concentration of a substance to the urine concentration of creatinine (the substance:creatinine ratio) eliminates the variable of the urine volume and the need for measuring the amount of a substance excreted over a period of time.

Creep feed, or ration: A feed fed to the nursing animal.

Cretinism: Impaired skeletal development leading to coarse heavy extremities and a short body most often due to hypothyroidism, from either inadequate or excessive iodine. This is not known to occur in horses.

Cribbing (crib biting): A vice in which the horse bites or places its upper incisor teeth on some solid object, pulls down, arches its neck and swallows gulps of air which go into the stomach, not the lungs. Not to be confused with wood chewing or wind sucking. See Chapter 20.

Crib biting: See **cribbing.**

Crib wetting: A vice in which the horse slowly and repeatedly draws its tongue across the edge of some part of the stall or manger which holding the tongue still, i.e., not licking. See "Oral Vices" in Chapter 20.

Crimped: A term for grain that is pressed between corrugated rollers to crack the kernels and increase its digestibility. See Fig. 4-12.

Crude fiber: See **fiber, dietary.**

Cryptorchid: An animal past the age when both testicles are normally in the scrotum (10 to 15 months of age for horses) that has one or both testes that are not descended into the scrotum. A cryptorchid horse is referred to by some as a "ridgeling."

Cubes: In equine nutrition the term refers to hay pressed into cubes. These are generally 1 to 2 inches (3 to 5 cm) in size (see Fig. 4-5). Cubes may also refer to range cake or range cubes, which are large pellets or cubes (about thumb size), usually composed primarily or entirely of grains and supplements. Range cubes are useful in feeding grain or supplements to animals on pasture or on the range with no feed bunks available.

Cuboni test: A chemical test for urine estrone content which is high in mares from 120 days of pregnancy to foaling. See Fig. 13-4.

Curb: Inflammation and thickening of the plantar ligaments located behind and below the point of the hock causing a visible swelling. It is caused by trauma from kicking walls, and by violent exertion (which along with sickle hocks and cow hocks) predisposes to this occurrence. It may result in temporary lameness but if periostitis and bone growth occur, lameness may be chronic. Curb may also occur in newborn foals due to hypothyroidism. See section on "Iodine Deficiency and Excesses Effects" in Chapter 2.

Cutaneous: Pertaining to the skin.

Cyanocobalamin: Vitamin B_{12}.

Cyanosis: Blueness of the membrane and skin generally due to insufficient oxygenation of the blood.

Cyathostomes: Small strongyles which are a major internal parasite affecting horses. See Chapter 9.

Cycling: When used in regard to equine reproduction it refers to the mare's estrous cycle; a period of estrus or sexual receptivity followed by diestrous, then estrus again.

Cyme: Flat-topped flower cluster, with the center flowers blooming first.

D

Decubitus: Lying down, such as a decubitus ulcer or pressure sore of the skin that develops because of pressure from prolonged lying down.

Dehy: Meaning dehydrated. In animal nutrition it refers to dehydrated alfalfa pellets. See Fig. 4-6.

Dehydrate: To remove all or enough moisture from a feedstuff to prevent its spoiling during storage.

Dent: The stage when corn kernels are fully mature and develop an indentation.

Dental cup: The recession in the center of an incisor before it has worn down sufficiently to disappear. See Fig. 9-11 and Table 9-6.

Dental star: A darkened spot from the pulp cavity that appears on the occlusal or chewing surface of the incisor teeth in horses over ten years of age. See Fig. 9-11.

Dentate: Tooth-like projections perpendicular to the leaf margin.

Dermatitis: Derm- or dermat- indicating skin, and -itis inflammation, thus inflammation of the skin.

Dermatophytosis: Ringworm infestation. See **ringworm.**

Desmitis: Inflammation of a ligament.

Desmotomy: Desm- referring to ligaments, and -otomy to cutting; thus, the surgical cutting of ligaments.

Deworm: Also referred to as worming. Treating an animal to remove stomach and intestinal parasites; in horses these are primarily ascarids, bots, strongyles, pinworms and occasionally tapeworms. See Chapter 9.

Diarrhea: The presence of an above normal amount of water in the feces. Nutritional causes include inadequate fiber or selenium intake, or excess grain, sodium or selenium intake.

Diaphragm: In anatomy it refers to a thin muscular membrane or wall separating the thoracic cavity, which contains the lungs, heart, and related structures, from the abdominal cavity, which contains such organs as the stomach, intestines, liver, spleen, kidneys, bladder, and, in the female, the uterus.

Dicoumarol: A vitamin K antagonist, found in spoiled sweet clover, which decreases blood coagulation ability. See "Vitamin K Deficiency" in Chapter 3.

Diaphysis: The shaft of a long bone.

Diestrus: Period between times of estrus or sexual receptivity, which for most normally cycling mares is usually 13 to 16 days long. See Fig. 13-4.

Digestible: That part of a feed that the animal is able to digest and absorb. Generally considered to be the portion of the feed that the animal is able to utilize.

Dioecious: Flowers which are unisexual. The staminate (pollen bearing structures) and pistillate (flower with only female reproductive parts) are borne on separate plants.

Dishrag foal: See **hemolytec icterus in foals.**

Distemper: See "Strangles," Chapter 9.

Diterpenoid: A compound with two connected hydrocarbon rings.

Diuretic: A drug that increases the excretion of urine.

Doping: Used to refer to the illicit administration of substances intended to either enhance or impair performance or behavior, or to mask abnormalities.

Dough stage: The period of plant development or growth when the material in the seeds becomes doughy. It follows the milk stage and precedes full maturity.

Dry: When applied to an animal indicates not lactating.

Dry lot: A fenced area devoid of growing edible plants on which horses or other grazing animals are kept. Usually refers to an area smaller than half of a football field and larger than a run (4 to 6 by 6 to 40 yards or meters). May also be referred to as a paddock, although a paddock may instead refer to the area where race horses are saddled and viewed prior to a race.

Dry matter: The part of the feed which is not water. To determine the concentration of a nutrient in the dry matter of a feed, the amount of that nutrient present in the feed is divided by the fraction of the feed which is dry matter. For example, a feed contains 10% moisture and 5% protein. Its dry matter content is 90% (100% − 10%) and it contains 5.55% (5% ÷ 0.90) protein in its dry matter.

Dry matter basis: A method of expressing the concentration of a nutrient to the feed dry matter (DM). In the example given above, the feed contains 5.55% protein on a dry matter basis. If the nutrient content of a feed, its cost, and the like are expressed on a dry matter basis, this value may be converted to the amount present in the feed as fed by multiplying the value times the dry matter content of the feed. The feed given above contains 5.55% protein on a dry matter basis and 90% dry matter; therefore, it contains 5% (5.55% × 0.90) protein on an as fed or as is basis. One should remember to always multiply or divide by the dry matter value, never the moisture content value, of the feed when converting from air dry to a dry matter or to an as fed basis.

% DM = 100% − % moisture content

amount in DM =
(amount in feed as fed) ÷ (% DM ÷ 100)

amount in feed as fed =
(amount in DM) × (% DM ÷ 100)

Whenever any feed comparisons are made (such as nutrient contents or cost of different feeds, or the horse's requirements as compared to its diet) this comparison must be performed with all values expressed on an equal moisture basis. To ensure that this is done, frequently all values are converted to the amount in the feed or diet dry matter.

Duodenum: First portion of the small intestine after the stomach. See Fig. 1-1.

Dyspnea: Difficult or labored breathing. Nutritional causes include a selenium deficiency and vitamin D toxicosis.

Dystocia: Dys- denotes difficult or abnormal, and -tocia birth, thus difficult birth.

E

Early bloom: Period from when plants first begin to bloom until one-tenth are in bloom.

Easy keeper: An animal that requires less feed than others under a similar situation. Opposite of hard keeper.

eCG: See **gonadotropin.**

Eczema: A skin inflammation that results in vesicle formation, a watery discharge, and the development of scales and crusts.

Edema: See **stocking up.**

Electrolysis: The breakdown or decomposition of a substance by an electric current. The electric current may be generated by two unlike metals in water, such as zinc and copper.

Electrolytes: Generally refers to sodium, potassium and chloride. However, electrolytes are any inorganic (non-carbon containing) substances that in a solution dissociate into electrically charged particles called ions. Common examples are table salt, or sodium chloride, that in solution dissociates into sodium ions and chloride ions, and hydrochloric acid that dissociates into hydrogen ions and chloride ions. In contrast, a substance, such as sand, is not an electrolyte because it doesn't dissociate in water into silicone and oxygen. Body salts are electrolytes; the major ones being sodium, potassium, chloride, and bicarbonate.

Elliptic: Tapered at both ends and widest in the middle.

Emphysema: A swelling or inflation due to the presence of air in tissues. It may be under the skin (subcutaneous), gangrenous (due to bacterial gas production) or pulmonary (in the lungs) due to rupture of lung alveoli or air sacs. See **heaves.**

Emaciation: A thin, wasted condition of the body.

-emia: Attached to the end of a word indicating "in the blood."

Enamel spot: A white spot that appears on the occlusal or chewing surface of the incisor teeth for several years after the tooth has worn down sufficiently that the cup is gone. See Fig. 9–11.

Encephalomalacia: Encephalo- indicates the brain, and -malacia indicates softening, thus a softening or dissolution of brain tissue.

Encephalomyelitis: Encephalo- indicates brain, myel- denotes a relationship to the spinal cord, and -itis inflammation; thus an inflammation of the brain and spinal cord which in the horse is referred to as sleeping sickness. See Chapter 9.

Encephalopathy: Encephalo- indicates brain and -opathy denotes disease, thus any disease of the brain.

Endometritis: Endomet- referring to the endometrium, and -itis inflammation; thus inflammation of the endometrium.

Endometrium: The mucous membrane lining the uterus.

Energy, nutritional: Produced by the animal in the utilization of carbohydrates, proteins or fats. These three nutrients may be provided in the diet or mobilized from the body. When they are in a feed, the total amount of energy they provide is referred to as the energy "content" of that feed, and may be expressed as calories, therms, or TDN. The concentration of energy in a feed is referred to as the energy "density" of that feed.

Ensilage: See "Silage," Chapter 4.

Epistaxis: Bleeding from the nose. In the horse this may be caused by trauma, such as from a tube passed through a nostril into the stomach, by blood coagulation disorders, or by blood coughed up from blood vessels in the lungs broken during exertion. See "Bleeders," Chapter 11.

Epiphysis: The end portion of a long bone separated from the shaft of the bone (diaphysis) by the metaphyseal growth plate from which the shaft of the bone grows or develops, whereas the epiphysis or end of the bone develops or grows from the articular (joint) cartilage.

Epiphysitis: Literally it means inflammation of the epiphysis; the end portion of a long bone. It is a misnomer commonly used to indicate an abnormality in the development (dysplasia) of the growth plate for the shaft of a long bone (metaphysis) and no active inflammation is present. Thus, correctly it should be referred to as growth plate or metaphysial dysplasia. The dysplasia results in an enlargement of these growth plates which is most evident just above the knees and fetlocks in young rapidly growing horses. In severe cases pain and a walking-on-eggs type of gait occurs. The condition disappears as the horse ages and its growth plates close (become ossified). This disease syndrome resulting in developmental bone or orthopedic diseases are described in Chapter 16.

Ergot: 1. A fungus (Claviceps spp) which grows under warm, moist conditions affecting and finally replacing the seeds of cereal grain plants, especially rye, oats, and wheat, and the grasses Tobossa, Bahia, Dallis, and Kentucky bluegrass. Ergot is small, hard, and dark brown to black in color, resembling dried mouse feces. It causes constriction of the arteries, and decreasing blood flow to the tissues. If blood flow is decreased sufficiently, the tissue dies and becomes gangrenous. The major tissues affected are the extremities—ears, tail, and limbs. Instead of the gangrenous form other effects may be abortions or nervous system disorders, including excitability, trembling, incoordination, tetany, and death. See "Ergot," Chapter 19. 2. A small mass of horn in the tuft of the hair at the back of the horse's fetlock is called the ergot (Fig. 6–5).

Eruption bumps: Nonpainful bony bumps or protrusions on the bottom of the jaw, or less commonly on the facial bone, at the base of the permanent premolar teeth formed as they push out the temporary premolars. They usually disappear within a few months after the temporary tooth is lost. If they don't, the temporary tooth may have been retained and needs to be extracted.

Estradiol: An estrogen.

Estrogen: A hormone that stimulates the brain to induce sexual receptivity, causes positive feedback on the hypothalamus and anterior pituitary gland resulting in the secretion of lutenizing hormone (LH), and increasing uterine tone, and cervical and vaginal secretions conducive to mating and sperm transport. See Fig. 13–4.

Estrus (heat): The period of sexual receptivity which for most normally cycling mares is 2 to 9 days in length and averages 6 to 7 days, but can vary from 1 to 37 days.

Ether extract: In nutrition it refers to lipids or fatty substances of feeds that are soluble in ether or other fat soluble solvents. The amount is a measure of the crude fat content of the feed.

Euthanasia or euthanatize: Mercifully putting to death an animal suffering from an incurable condition.

Ewe neck: A conformational fault in which the neck curves down excessively just in front of the withers.

Exertion myopathy: See section on it in Chapter 11.

Expanded: As applied to a feed, it refers to an increase in volume as the result of extrusion.

Expectorant: A medicine which aids in the expulsion of mucus or exudate from the lungs, bronchi, and trachea.

Extrusion: In feed processing extrusion is the process of forcing a feed through small openings under high pressure. When the feed comes out of the opening, the sudden release of pressure causes the feed to expand. In contrast, when the feed is forced through openings under low pressure, it remains compacted into a high-density pellet instead of expanding into a low-density extruded feed.

F

Fang teeth: See **canine teeth.**

Far side (off side): Right side of a horse versus the near side which is the left side.

Fartlek: Unstructured alternating periods of slow work and fast work generally below maximum speed but continued until tiring begins. It may be of greatest benefit for endurance and eventing horse training, particularly for events in which there is an intermittent pattern of energy use, such as polo, combined driving and eventing.

Fats: Chemically, fats and oils are triglycerides composed of glycerol with a fatty acid, which is a long chain of carbon atoms, attached to each of glycerol's 3 carbon atoms. Fats are necessary in the diet for the absorption of substances which are soluble only in fats, such as vitamins A, D, E, and K, and as a source of fatty acids needed for body structure. Fats are also used for energy and provide nearly 2½-times more energy than a similar weight of carbohydrate or protein. See "Fat and Oil Supplements for Horses" in Chapter 4.

Fatty acids: A chain of carbon atoms attached to a carboxylic acid (COOH); $CH_3 (CH_2)_n$ COOH, with n indicating from 0 to over 20 carbon atoms. In most dietary fats n is 16 to 20. Bacteria in animal's gastrointestinal tract utilize carbohydrates to form short chain fatty acids in which n is 0 to 2, forming acidic, propionic and butyric acids. These are referred to as volatile fatty acids because of the low temperature at which they volatilize. They are the major source of dietary energy derived from forages and fiber.

Feed efficiency: The number of units of feed required to produce one unit of production (growth or milk); in English units generally the pounds of feed necessary for 1 pound gain in body weight.

Feeders: See self-feeders, timed-feeders, and Fig. 8-1.

Feral: Wild, or existing in a natural, nondomesticated state.

Ferritin: A protein that binds iron for storage in the body, primarily in the liver and spleen. A small amount is present in the blood. Its concentration in the blood is directly proportional to the amount of iron in the body.

Fetlock: The horse's ankle joint. See Fig. 6-5.

Fiber, dietary: A carbohydrate composed of simple sugars bound together by beta bonds. Animals can't break these bonds to digest fiber, but can use the products (primarily volatile fatty acids) produced from fiber by bacteria. These provide most of the energy horses derive from forages and other feeds high in fiber. Fiber consists of insoluble plant structural fibers, cellulose and hemicellulose, and of soluble fibers. Soluble fibers are the parenchymatous portions and secretions of plants, such as sap, resin, gums, pectin and mucilages. Insoluble fiber is the least utilizable carbohydrate in feeds. Crude fiber is an unpredictable underestimate of the insoluble fiber content of a feed, whereas neutral detergent fiber (NDF) is an overestimate. Acid detergent fiber (ADF) underestimates insoluble fiber content, but is the most accurate indication of a feed's poorly utilizable carbohydrate content that is generally available.

Fibrotic myopathy: Replacement of normal skeletal muscle with fibrous connective tissue which may subsequently mineralize. Most commonly affects the hamstring muscles so foot is jerked suddenly downward and backward before being put to the ground. It is treated by cutting or removing a piece of the semitendinous muscle at the level of the stifle.

Filly: An immature female horse.

Fimbriated: Fringed.

Fines: In nutrition fines refer to substances that are small enough and heavy enough to settle to the bottom of a feed.

Fistulous withers: Inflammation of the fluid-filled bursal sac that is located between the nuchal ligament of the neck and the thoracic vertebrae, causing a swelling which may break and drain at the withers.

Flagging: When used in regard to breeding, flagging means movements of the stallion's tail due to the muscular contractions that occur during ejaculation. In many cases, the stallion "flags" without ejaculation occurring which is commonly referred to as "cheating" and is occasionally responsible for stallion infertility.

Flehmen: Curling of the upper lip, which is a common behavior by stallions when teasing mares, and by foals, particularly colts, during the first months of life.

Flexor tendons: The tissue connecting a muscle to a bone which when the muscle contracts, flexes the leg.

Floating the teeth: Filing off sharp points of enamel that develop on the teeth with a file or rasp, which is called a float. These sharp points may lacerate the tongue and cheeks. See Fig. 9-10.

Flowers, disc: A tubular flower in the central part of the floral head as in members of the sunflower family.

Flowers, ray: Single, petal-like symmetrical flowers around the edge of the floral head as in sunflowers.

Flu: See "Influenza," Chapter 9.

Flushing: When used in regard to feeding, it means increasing dietary energy intake prior to some event, most commonly breeding. This has been shown to increase the probability that a thin mare will conceive, and to decrease early embryonic loss in thin mares, but not in mares at or above moderate body condition.

Foal heat: First estrus, or period of sexual receptivity, in the mare following foaling. See Chapter 13.

Fodder: Coarse feeds, such as corn or sorghum stalks, with the grain removed, left standing in the field. When they are harvested they are referred to as stover. See "Straw and Stover" in Chapter 4.

Follicle: In animals, a fluid-filled structure on the ovaries containing the oocyte (egg). In plants, a dry, dehiscent fruit which splits down one side only, e.g., milkweeds.

Follicle stimulating hormone (FSH): A hormone secreted by the anterior pituitary gland that stimulates growth of a follicle and the activity of sperm forming cells. See Fig. 13–4.

Forage: The stems, stalks, leaves and heads of plants, with or without the seeds or grain (grass, legumes or cereal grain plants), consumed by animals by grazing, or by being fed them following harvesting, most commonly as hay, but may be as silage, soilage (green chop), straw, or fodder. Forage is high in fiber (usually defined as greater than 18% crude fiber it it's dry matter). At least 0.5 lbs of forage dry matter/100 lb body weight daily (0.5 kg/100 kg), and preferably no less than one-half of the total weight of the diet dry matter as forage, is needed to prevent diarrhea, colic, founder, and excess non-fiber carbohydrate and dietary energy intake from cereal grains.

Foramen: A natural hole or passage, especially one into or through a bone through which nerves and/or blood vessels pass.

Founder (laminitis): An inflammation of the laminae of the horse's foot. Laminae are interdigitations located between the bone and the hoof wall that contain blood vessels which nourish the hoof. When inflamed, the laminae swell between these two ridged structures causing pressure, pain, and tissue damage. This results in separation of the hoof wall from the laminae. If sufficiently severe, this allows the third phalanx or coffin bone (most distal bone of the foot) to be pushed by the horse's weight downward, so that in extreme cases it may penetrate the sole. The hoof may develop characteristic irregular "founder rings," a long toe that curls up if not trimmed and a dished hoof. Founder may be caused by: (1) consuming excessive amounts of grain (grain founder), (2) consuming large amounts of cold water by the hot inactive horse (water founder), (3) in some horses (particularly pony breeds) consumption of lush green forage (grass founder), (4) infectious conditions such as severe pneumonia, enteritis or uterine infections following foaling (foal founder), or (5) concussion to the feet from running on a hard surface (road founder). There have also been reports of horses foundering after severe "stress" situations, e.g., accidents.

Freezing: When referring to a horse's behavior, it means when the animal becomes stiff and immobile and refuses to move. See "Balking and Freezing" in Chapter 20.

Free-choice or ad libitum: Refers to feed or water being available for the animal to eat or drink as much and as often as it wants. Ad lib or ad libitum means at pleasure and thus at pleasure to eat or drink as it chooses.

Frond: A finely divided leaf, often large, applied to leaves of ferns and some palms.

FSH: See **follicle stimulating hormone.**

Full bloom: When two-thirds or more of the plants are in bloom.

Full-mouthed: A horse that has all of its permanent teeth which occurs at 5 years of age. It is used to indicated a horse that is 5 years of age or older; not a horse that is necessarily 5 years old.

Fungal spores: Small reproductive elements given off by fungi or molds, which, when inhaled by the horse, can cause heaves, bronchitis, and coughing. See "Stable Ventilation," in Chapter 9.

G

Gaits: Natural gaits of the horse are the walk, trot, and run or gallop. The running walk (amble or fox trot), rack (broken amble or singlefoot) and pace (a fast trot) may be either natural or artificial gaits. The canter or lope is a restrained or collected gallop. Walk is a 4-beat gait (a regular sequence of 4 hoof beats at precise intervals occurs): in the following order, near-hind, near-fore, off-hind, and off-fore, with 2 feet always on the ground, and at a speed of 2 to 4 mph (60 to 100 meters/sec or 16 to 27 min/mile). Trot is a 2-beat gait in which opposite fore and hind feet hit the ground together; the usual speed is 7 to 12 mph (200 to 300 meters/sec or 5 to 8 min/mile). Canter or lope is a 3-beat gait in which the hind foot opposite to the forelimb in the lead hits, followed by the other rear foot and the forefoot opposite to it and finally the lead forefoot; the usual speed is 11 to 15 mph (300 to 400 meters/sec or 4 to 5 min/mile). The gallop or run is a 4-beat gait in which the sequence is the same as the canter but with the rear foot hitting before the opposite forefoot instead of them hitting at the same time, the usual speed is 18 to 37 mph (500 to 1000 meters/sec or 1 min:35 sec to 3 min/mile). Backing, like the trot, is a 2-beat gait.

Gallop (run): See **gaits.**

Galvayne's groove: A shallow darkened groove on the outside surface running up and down the center of the third or corner incisor teeth. It is used as a rough estimate of older horses' age. The groove appears from under the gum at 10, is one-half way down the tooth at 15, is full length at 20, is one-half way gone at 25, and is gone at 30 years of age. For other estimates of a horse's age from its teeth, see Table 9–6.

Gangrene: Death of large amounts of body tissue.

Gastrointestinal: Gastro- meaning stomach, and intestinal meaning intestines or guts.

Gastrophilus: See **bots.**

Gavage: Introduction of material into the stomach via a tube.

Gelding: A male castrated horse.

Genetic relationship closeness: Sire or dam 50%, grandsire/dam 25%, great grandsire/dam 12.5%, etc., full-sibling 50%, 3/4 sibling 37.5%, half-sibling 25%, first cousins (by full brothers or out of full sisters) 12.5%. Only first two generations are close enough to be meaningful for breeding selection.

Girth-itch: See **ringworm.**

Glabrous: Botanically indicates smooth, without hairs.

Glowers (shiners): Feed that under black light or the "Woods Lamp" (long-wave ultraviolet light) gives off a bright greenish-yellow fluorescence indicating the presence of aflatoxin-producing mold. The feed may or may not contain aflatoxin. See "Field Mycotoxin Assays" in Chapter 19.

Glucose (dextrose): A simple sugar or monosaccharide that is utilized or metabolized by the animal for energy. It is the major source of energy for the brain.

Gluten: The viscous material remaining when the flour of a cereal grain is washed to remove starch. It is similar in nutrient content to most oilseed meals. See Table 4–7.

Glycogen: A storage form of the monosaccharide or simple sugar glucose present primarily in the muscle and liver.

Glycolysis: The utilization of glucose and glycogen. Without oxygen, lactic acid and small amounts of energy are produced from glucose and glycogen. This is referred to as anaerobic glycolysis. With oxygen available, carbon dioxide, water and 12 to 18 times more energy is produced from glucose and glycogen. This is referred to as aerobic glycolysis.

GnRH: See **gonadotropin releasing hormone.**

Goiter: Enlargement of the thyroid gland, causing a swelling at the throatlatch (Fig. 2–6). It may be caused either by a deficiency or an excess of iodine in the diet, or by the ingestion of large enough quantities over a period of time of substances that interfere with the thyroid function, e.g., kale, white clover, cabbage, rutabaga, and turnip. Thiouracils, thiourea, and methimazole are drugs which may also cause goiter.

Goitrogen: A substance that causes goiter.

Gonadotropin: Equine chorionic gonadotropin (eCG) also referred to as pregnant mare serum gonadotropin (PMSG), is produced by fetal tissue origin endometrial cups from about day 40 to 140 of pregnancy. It apparently stimulates the formation of secondary corpus luteums which are necessary for the production of sufficient progesterone to maintain pregnancy until sufficient placental progestogens are produced. Human chronic gonadotropin (hCG) has luteinizing hormone activity which when administered to the mare with a mature follicle will induce ovulation, generally within 48 hours.

Gonadotropin releasing hormone (GnRH): A hormone released from the hypothalamus upon sufficient daylight stimulation of the pineal gland. It stimulates FSH and LH secretion from the anterior pituitary gland to initiate the estrous cycle.

Goose rump: A conformation fault in which the rump is too flat or curved in as viewed from the side.

Gossypol: A toxic substance present in cottonseeds. See Chapter 19.

Grain: The seed of plants used for food, e.g., corn (maize), milo, oats, wheat, barley, and rye. See Chapter 4.

Grain screenings: Small imperfect grains, weed seeds and other foreign material having feeding value that is separated in cleaning grain by a screen.

Granuloma: A tumor or neoplasm made up of small rounded, fleshy masses.

GRAS: Acronym for Generally Recognized as Safe. A designation of a feed or food additive that has satisfied the Code of U.S. Federal Regulations (21 CFR 573) as being safe for human or animal consumption based on available data and experience of its common usage.

Gravel: In equine medicine gravel refers to a drainage tract at the coronet from an infection which entered through a crack in the white line of the sole (see Fig. 6–5). Referred to as gravel because it was originally and incorrectly thought to be a migrating piece of gravel. It causes lameness until the infection's drainage tract erupts to the outside after which healing may occur.

Graze: To consume standing vegetation.

Grease heel (scratches, mud fever): A bacterial or fungal infection of the skin on the heel and back of the pastern that may occur as a result of the horse's standing in moist, dirty bedding. It can lead to chronic dermatitis that results in scabs, skin cracks and eventually granulation (Fig. 9–12). The affected area can spread to the dorsal aspect of the pastern. It can become very painful and cause lameness. One or most commonly both legs are affected. Conditions that should be considered in differential diagnosis include folliculitis (however it causes papules instead of a diffuse lesion), contact photosensitivity on unpigmented pasterns, dermatophytosis (ringworm), chiggers, chorioptic mange, and allergic contact dermatitis. Treatment is to improve hygiene, remove initiating cause, clip the affected area, wash with a mild soap or chlorhexidine, apply a soothing ointment or zinc oxide. An astringent lotion such as white lotion (zinc sulfate and lead acetate) or calamine lotion, applied several times a day in a soak bandage is indicated in more advanced cases in which exudation has begun. Once exudation stops, apply a steroid/antibiotic cream under a bandage. Chronic cases should be washed twice daily with a povidone-iodine wash followed by a poultice for two days. DMSO, thiabendazole powder and a sulfa cream have been recommended for chronic nonresponsive cases.

Green chop: See **soilage.**

Green horse: An inexperienced or newly trained horse.

Grits: Coarsely ground grain from which the bran and germ have been removed, usually screened to uniform particle size.

Groats: Cereal grain kernels after removal of the hulls, i.e., dehulled cereal grain.

Growth plates, bone: See **physis.**

Gruel: A feed prepared by mixing ground feeds with water.

Guttural pouch: Guttural means pertaining to the throat. In the horse there are two guttural pouches which are large sacs (10 oz or 300 ml) off of each eustachian tube. They are located between the bottom of the cranium (bone under the brain) and the pharynx. The eustachian tubes go from the ear to the pharynx. Domestic animals other than equine species do not have guttural pouches. These pouches may become infected and drain into the pharynx and subsequently the nose. Often only one guttural pouch is infected resulting in drainage from only one nostril, which helps distinguish it from a respiratory disease.

H

Habronema spp.: See stomachworms, Chapter 9.

Habronemiasis: Habronema larval in the skin. See **summer sores.**

Hair analysis: The concentration of numerous substances in the hair have been used to try to determine if there is inadequate or excessive amounts of those substances in the body and, therefore, consumed. Hair analysis for a multitude of nutrients and poisons are readily available, relatively inexpensive, and are commonly promoted for diagnosing nutritional needs or excesses, and poisonings, in many species of animals including horses and people. However, except for excess selenium, and possibly some heavy metal poisonings (mercury, lead, arsenic and cadmium), hair analysis gives no indication of an excess or deficiency of any nutrients.

Hairworms (Trichostrongylus axei): Occur in stomachs of horses grazing or housed with ruminants. See Chapter 9.

Hard keeper: An animal that is nutritionally unthrifty and requires more feed than others under a similar situation. Opposite of easy keeper.

Hastate: A leaf shaped like an arrow head with the basal lobes turned outward.

Hay belly (grass belly): Said of a horse with a distended abdomen which may be due to the presence of excessive amounts of bulky feeds in the intestinal tract.

Haylage: Ensiled grass or leguminous plants that are cut, then not allowed to dry before being packed into a container that prevents the feeds access to air. See Chapter 4.

hCG: See **gonadotropin.**

Head-nodding: A vice in which the horse rhythmitically nods its head either up and down or back and forth. At the same time the horse may shift its weight from one forefoot to the other, which is referred to as weaving. See Chapter 20, "Escape Vices."

Heating feed: A feed in which much of its energy is given off as heat during its digestion, absorption, and utilization. In contrast to popular belief, corn is not a heating feed (see Corn, Chapter 4). The most heat is produced in the utilization of high fiber feeds, such as forages.

Heave line: A ridge of abdominal muscle that has increased in size because of the forced expiration required when heaves is present. In order to push air out of the inelastic lungs, it is necessary to contract the abdomen and push the intestines against the diaphragm. The ridge runs in a straight line from the middle of the flank diagonally forward and down to the rib cage toward the point of the elbow. See Figure 17-1.

Heaves (chronic obstructive pulmonary disease or COPD, pulmonary emphysema or broken wind): A respiratory disturbance resulting from reduced elasticity and rupture of the small sacs (alveoli) in the lungs where gas exchange between the blood and inspired air takes place. Requires forced expiration of air from the lungs. See "Stable Ventilation," Chapter 4 for prevention, and "COPD," Chapter 17, for management of affected horses.

Heels contracted: Contracted heels are pulled together and frog is narrow. The foot may become smaller at the bottom or ground surface than at the top. Results in lameness if not corrected. May be caused by improper shoeing preventing sufficient pressure against the frog when weight is put on it.

Hemagglutination: The agglutination or clumping together of red blood cells.

Hematinics (blood builders): Substances which increase the hemoglobin of red blood cells in the blood. Those most commonly used are iron, sometimes copper, and the B-vitamins particularly vitamin B_{12} or cobalamine. See Chapter 11 "Supplements for Athletic Performance."

Hematocrit: The percent of the blood that is red blood cells. Also referred to as the packed cell volume because the hematocrit is measured by centrifuging the blood and measuring the red blood cells that the centrifugal force has packed into the bottom of the tube.

Hematoma: An enclosed pocket of effused blood, for example, a blood blister, is a small hematoma in the skin.

Hematuria: Hem- indicating blood, and -uria urine, thus blood in the urine. Only nutritionally known cause is vitamin K toxicosis.

Hemoglobin: See **red blood cells.**

Hemolysis: Hem- indicating blood, and lysis dissolution or destruction, thus the breakdown or destruction of red blood cells.

Hemolytic icterus in foals (neonatal isoerythrolysis or "dishrag foals"): Affected foals are normal and healthy at birth. They nurse, and are active for a short period. After 12 to 36 hours they become dull, sluggish, and weak, stop nursing, and may go down. Heart rate and respiratory rate are increased, particularly after exertion. Membranes are pale for the first 24 hours, then become yellowish. Later the urine may become blood tinged. The course of the illness is 1 to 10 days; most foals die at 3 to 4 days of age unless they are given adequate red blood cell transfusions. The cause is the ingestion of colostrum that contains antibodies that destroy the foal's red blood cells. It may be prevented by testing the mare's and stallion's blood for these antibodies and antigens, or by testing the foal's blood for these antibodies. If they are present the foal should be given colostrum that doesn't contain these antigens.

Herbivores: Animals that live from eating or prefer to eat plant materials, in contrast to carnivores who live on or prefer animal tissues. Omnivores are animals that can live on either animal or plant materials. In reality, most animals are nutritionally omnivores, and can utilize both animal and plant materials. However, some require or prefer more plant material, and others, more animal material. Progressing from animals that are more herbivorous to those that are more carnivorous would be cattle, horses, pigs, people, dogs, and cats.

Hernia: The protrusion of a portion of an organ or tissue through an abnormal opening, e.g., the protrusion of abdominal contents through the abdominal wall (abdominal hernia), the inguinal or groin area (inguinal hernia) or the diaphragm (diaphragmatic hernia).

Hives: Small swellings or welts on the skin. They appear suddenly, and are caused by an allergic response to such things as feed, insect bites, drugs, and insecticides. When caused by feed, they may be referred to as protein bumps. See Fig. 1–5.

Hock: The tarsal joint. See Fig. 6–5.

Homeostasis: A tendency to uniformity or stability in the normal body states.

Hoof-bound: A lameness due to chronic contracted hells, which causes pain.

Hops: A flavoring agent mixed with germinated cereal grains in making beer.

Hot blooded horses: Horses that originated from Arabians, Barb, and Turkmene horses. These horses came from northern Africa, along the Mediterranean coast, and the Arabian peninsula. Breeds which have originated at least in part from them include Thoroughbreds, Standardbreds, the American Saddle Horse, the Morgan, the Quarter Horse, and the Tennessee Walker. This designation obviously has nothing to do with the temperature of the horse's blood. See **cold blooded horses.**

Hot feed: To some this means a feed high in energy, such as corn. If the feed provides more energy than the horse can use and the horse feels good, it has a tendency to make the horse high-spirited. Another meaning for hot feed is that which produces a great deal of heat in its utilization, such as forage. This will keep the animal warmer in cold weather, but causes increased sweating and discomfort in warm weather.

Hulls: Outer covering of grain. See "By-Product Feeds for Horses," Chapter 4.

Hyper- : A prefix meaning above normal, e.g., hyperparathyroidism indicates excessive production of hormone by the parathyroid gland.

Hyperesthesia: Excessive sensitiveness to touch, movement and/or sound.

Hyperplasia: The enlargement or overgrowth of a part of the body due to an increase in the number (not size) of its cells.

Hypertrophy: The enlargement or overgrowth of a part of the body due to an increase in size (not numbers) of its cells.

Hypo- : A prefix meaning below normal.

Hypophagia: Hypo- indicating below normal, and phago- relating to eating, and thus a below normal feed intake.

This may be caused by most diseases and inadequate water, feed availability or palatability, a deficiency of phosphorus, sodium, potassium, zinc, vitamin A, D or B_1, or by excess intake of fluoride or vitamin A or D.

I

Icterus (jaundice): Excess bile pigments in the blood, or deposited in the skin and membranes giving them a yellow color. May be caused by liver damage or excessive destruction of red blood cells (hemolysis).

Ileum: Terminal portion of the small intestine. See Fig. 1–1.

Immunity: A condition of security against a disease or poison. The power which an individual may acquire to resist and/or overcome an infectious disease. Immunity is impaired by selenium, vitamin A, energy, or protein deficiency, and by excess iron.

Immunoglobulins (antibodies): Proteins found in body fluids that produce an immunity or resistance to foreign substances such as bacteria or viruses by combining with them and helping to inactivate them.

Incubation: The period between the occurrence of infection and the onset of clinical signs.

Infarct: An area of tissue death due to obstructed circulation to it, e.g., a heart attack is due to a blood clot in an artery to the heart muscle, which if not relieved, results in death of heart muscle supplied by that artery, i.e., a cardiac infarct.

Infectious organisms: Any organisms, such as bacteria, viruses, protozoa, or fungi, that are capable of invading, or entering, the body and causing disease. The resulting infectious disease may or may not be contagious.

Inflorescence: The flowering part of the plant.

Influenza (flu): A highly contagious viral disease. It affects horses of all ages but is most common in horses less than three years old. Following inhalation of the virus, susceptible horses' show clinical signs within 1 to 3 days. It is characterized by fever, depression, often violent coughing, decreased appetite, and usually, a mucoid nasal discharge early in the disease. In the absence of secondary complications, the respiratory lining regenerates and recovery occurs in approximately three weeks. The most common secondary complications are the development of a bacterial pneumonia resulting in a persistent, often productive cough, fever, increase in white blood cells, and a purulent nasal discharge. Occasionally, in young, old, debilitated, or stressed horses, the virus may localize in the muscle, causing inflammation of it (myositis), or in the heart, causing its inflammation (myocarditis). Affected horses should be isolated from other horses, rested and given supportive therapy. See "Influenza" in Chapter 9.

Inguinal: Pertaining to the groin.

Inoculate: See **vaccinate.**

Inorganic: Noncarbon-containing compounds such as minerals.

Intra- : A prefix meaning into or in, e.g. intramuscular, meaning into or in the muscle, or intravenous, meaning into the vein.

Interval training: A method of training using series of 2 to 6 sprints at one-half to full speed for 1 to 8 furlongs (200 to 1600 yds or m) with walking or trotting in between. Its purpose is to allow more intense work for a longer duration than if work were continuous, and to increase aerobic or oxygen-requiring energy production, thus decreasing reliance on anaerobic energy use and therefore glycogen use and lactate production to delay fatigue. See "Fitness Training for Athletic Performance" in Chapter 11.

Involucre: A circle of bracts (small leaf-like structures) under or at the base of a flower.

Ion: An atom or group of atoms having an electrical charge that is positive (cation) or negative (anion).

Ischemia: Isch- indicates to suppress, and -emia blood, thus a suppression or lack of blood or blood circulation to an area, tissue or organ.

Isoantibodies: Antibodies or immunoglobulins produced in the body against the body's own cells or tissues; e.g., anti- red blood cell isoantibodies are antibodies against the animal's own red blood cells which destroy these cells.

-itis: Attached to the end of a word indicating inflamed, e.g., laminitis indicating inflammation of the laminae of the foot.

J

Jaundice: See **icterus.**

Jejunum: Middle portion of the small intestine. See Fig. 1–1.

Jibbing (balking): When a horse becomes stiff and immobile, and refuses to move. See "Balking and Freezing" in Chapter 20.

Joint ill: Joint infection. It may lead to destruction of joint cartilage and permanent impairment of athletic ability. It is caused by an organism gaining access to the body at any location (the umbilicus is a common portal in the newborn), and localizing in the joint.

Joint mouse: A piece of bone or cartilage floating free in the joint. It may have chipped off from trauma or inflammation, i.e., osteochondritis.

Joule: A unit of energy used primarily in England. One joule equals 0.239 calories or 4.1855 kilojoules per kilocalorie.

Jugging: Jugging a horse is a practice in which 500 ml (1 pt), or more, of a sterile solution of amino acids, electrolytes, vitamin B complex, and frequently glucose (dextrose) are given into the jugular vein. Commonly done before an athletic event and doubtful that it is of any benefit.

K

Keratin: The primary component of the dry matter of skin, hair, wool, hoof, and horn. It is a protein high in sulfur containing amino acids.

Ketosis (acetonemia): A condition in which there is excessive production of the ketones or acetones in the body.

These are produced from the incomplete utilization of fat for energy because of inadequate carbohydrate needed for their complete utilization. This may be due to inadequate feed intake or inadequate insulin, i.e., diabetes. It occurs most commonly in ruminants, rarely in horses.

Kibbled: A feed baked then broken into small pieces called kibbles.

Kilocalorie (kcal): See **calorie.**

Kjeldahl: A method of determining the amount of nitrogen in a feed or organic substance.

L

Labile: Unstable, easily destroyed.

Lacrimation: The secretion of tears. Excess lacrimation may be caused by an irritant or a vitamin A deficiency.

Lactate: Lactic acid without its hydrogen ion. Lactic acid is produced when glucose or glycogen are used for energy in the absence of oxygen. Once produced in the exercising muscle it must be removed and transported back to the liver or kidney for its utilization. If it is produced faster than it can be removed and thus accumulates in the muscle, it may inhibit energy production and cause fatigue.

Lactate threshold: See **anaerobic threshold.**

Lactose: Milk sugar. A disaccharide consisting of one molecule of the simple sugars (monosaccharides) glucose and galactose attached together. For utilization these must be split apart, which is accomplished by the lactase enzyme on the surface of the small intestinal cells. Horses only when young have a significant amount of this enzyme and thus can use lactose.

Lameness: Nutritional causes include calcium deficiency or phosphorus excess, and selenium or fluoride excess (see Chapter 2). Feeding related causes include excess grain intake resulting in founder.

Laminitis: See **founder.**

Lanceolate: Lance-shaped.

Larynx: The "voice box" located between the pharynx at the root of the tongue, and the trachea or "wind pipe." It consists of 5 major cartilages (thyroid, cricoid, epiglottis, and two arytenoid or vocal cords) connected by ligaments. It regulates the volume of air in respiration, prevents aspiration of foreign material into the trachea, and is the chief organ for voice.

Late bloom: The period when the majority of blossoms begin to dry and fall off the plant.

Lateral: Toward the side, or farther away from the median plane running from the head to rear through the center of the body. Opposite to medial.

Lathyrism: A neurologic disorder characterized in most species by a spastic paraparesis. In horses its reported to affect the larynx which may result in suffocation during exercise. It is caused by a toxin present in the seeds of some types of peas and vetches. See section on "Beans and Peas" in Chapter 4.

Lectins: A plant protein with carbohydrate binding properties.

Legumes: Plants, such as alfalfa (lucerne), clovers, birdsfoot trefoil, lespedeza, vetches, and peas that obtain nitrogen through bacteria that live in their roots. The plant converts the nitrogen to protein, so that legumes are higher in protein than nonlegumes such as grasses.

Lenticels: Wart-like spots on the bark.

Leukoencephalomalacia: Leuko- means white, encephalo- meaning brain, and -malacia meaning a morbid softening. Thus, a morbid softening of the white matter of the brain. In horses it is caused by a mycotoxin produced by a Fusarium mold, which may be present in moldy corn grain, stalks, hulls, or silage containing feed resulting in moldy corn disease or blind staggers as described in Chapter 19.

Libido: Desire for or the motive for sexual activity.

Ligament: A tough, fibrous band which connects bones or supports viscera.

Lignin: A practically indigestible compound which along with cellulose is a major component of the cell wall of certain high fiber plants.

Lipids: See **fats.**

Lockjaw: See "Tetanus," in Chapter 4.

"Locoed:" An animal (horse, cattle, sheep or wild herbivore) poisoned by the ingestion of locoweeds (Oxythopis spp.), or milkvetches (Astragalus spp.). See section on "Locoweeds and Milkvetches" in Chapter 18.

Lucerne: Alfalfa, a legume forage. See "Types of Hay" in Chapter 4.

Lunge: To train or exercise a horse by having it move around a circle at the end of a lunge line or rope, or a circular track or ring.

Lunge line: A long (e.g. 10 yds or meters) rope fastened to a horse's halter allowing the horse to move in a circle around the person holding the other end of the rope or lunge line.

Lungworms (Dictyocaulus arnfieldis): An internal parasite of horses and donkeys. See Chapter 9.

Luteolytic: Luteo- referring to the corpus luteum, and -lytic to produce lysis or dissolution; thus, luteolytic is something that causes the lysis or dissolution of the corpus luteum. The hormone prostaglandin F_2-alpha and its analogues are commonly used luteolytic substances.

Luteotropic: Luteo- referring to the corpus luteum, and -tropic to turning, changing or development; thus, luteotropic is something that stimulates the formation of the corpus luteum.

Lysine: The amino acid which is most often deficient in the growing horse's diet, the deficiency of which slows growth rate. See "Protein Needs" in Chapter 1.

M

Macro- : Meaning large, e.g., macrominerals meaning minerals needed in large quantities. See **minerals.** Opposite of micro-.

Maiden: 1) a horse that has never won a race, or 2) a mare that has never become pregnant.

Maintenance diet: A diet that is adequate to prevent any loss or gain of weight when the animal is at rest in an environmental temperature in which additional energy is not required to heat or cool the body.

Maize: Corn, see Chapter 4.

Male teeth: See **canine teeth.**

Malignant: Tending to go from bad to worse. Typically it is used to refer to a tumor that is capable of spreading or forming new foci in a distant part of the body, i.e., to metastasize. The opposite of benign.

Malt: The germinated kernels of cereal grains, usually barley, which is mixed with other grains and hops to form mash for making beer.

Mandible (mandibular): Lower jaw bone.

Mash: 1) a mixture of ingredients in small particle size, 2) germinated kernels mixed with other cereal grains, and for beer production hops.

Mating expression or face: An expression that a mare in estrus (heat) may have when near a stallion or gelding. Ears are turned back but not flattened, as if listening, and lips are slack or loose.

Maxilla: The principal bone of the upper jaw.

Meconium: Dark green, brown to black, tarry stools formed prior to birth, which normally begin to be passed within one-half to 6 hours after birth. See Chapter 14.

Medial: Toward the center or closest to the median plane running from head to rear through the center of the body. Opposite to lateral.

Megacalorie (Mcal): One Mcal equals 1000 nutritional calories or kilocalories and 1 therm.

Menhaden: A type of herring from which fish meal is commonly made.

Metabolism: Chemical reactions occurring in the body. Refers to all changes in or utilization of a nutrient that takes place following its absorption from the intestine.

Metabolite: Substance produced by chemical reactions in the body, e.g., urea would be a metabolite of protein because it is produced in the body by chemical reactions that breakdown or utilize protein.

Metacarpal: The front leg fetlock joint, or the cannon bone and splint bones on the front legs (Fig. 6–5).

Metaphysis: Bone growth plate from which the shaft of a long bone (diaphysis) develops or grows.

Metatarsal: The hind leg fetlock joint, or the cannon bone and splint bones of the hind legs (Fig. 6–5).

Methemoglobin: Hemoglobin is the iron-containing compound in red blood cells that binds with oxygen so that oxygen can be transported to the cells. When its iron is converted from the ferrous (+2 valence) to the ferric (+3 valence) state, it is called methemoglobin and can no longer combine with oxygen. This is caused by nitrate toxicosis which rarely, if ever, occurs in horses. See Chapter 19.

Micro- : Meaning small, e.g., microscopic or microminerals. See **minerals.** Opposite of macro-.

Mid-bloom: Period during which one-tenth to two-thirds of plants are in bloom.

Milk stage: The period after a plant blooms when the seeds begin to form and contain a milky like substance which with increased maturity becomes doughy (dough stage) then hard, after which some grain kernels such as corn develop an indentation called the dent stage.

Milk teeth: The deciduous, baby or temporary teeth. See Table 9-6 for description and when they are lost.

Minerals (ash): Noncarbon-containing (inorganic) elements such as salts, calcium, phosphorus, and magnesium. The total amount present is determined by burning the carbon-containing (organic) matter and weighing the residue or ash. This is a relatively meaningless value unless the amounts of the specific substances making up the minerals or ash are known. In nutrition, minerals are classified into two groups according to the amount needed by the animal; macro- meaning large amounts, and micro- meaning small amounts. Macrominerals are sodium chloride (common salt), magnesium, potassium, calcium, phosphorus, and sulfur, and are all needed in the diet in a number of parts per hundred, or percent. Microminerals are iodine, molybdenum, manganese, iron, cobalt, zinc, copper, and selenium, and are all needed in the diet in a number of parts per million (ppm or mg/kg). Microminerals are also referred to as trace minerals. With the exception of iodine, which is a necessary constituent of thyroid hormones, the other trace minerals are necessary primarily as components of enzymes. Enzymes are required for many of the chemical reactions that occur in the body. See Chapter 2.

mM (millimole): A unit of concentration that indicates the number of molecular weights of a substance in milligrams in one liter of water. For example, the molecular weight of sodium is 23, therefore, 23 mg of sodium in 1 L would be 1 mM of sodium.

Monkey mouth (sow mouth or prognathia): A horse with an underbite in which the lower incisors extend out further than the upper incisors. It is less common and opposite to parrot mouth or prognathism in which there is an overbite with the upper incisors extending out further than the lower incisors.

Monoecious: Staminate (pollen bearing structure) and pistillate (female reproductive structure) flowers on the same plant.

Monoterpene: A single ringed hydrocarbon ($C_{10}H_{16}$) compound.

mOsm (milliosmoles): 1/1000 osmoles. See **osmolarity.**

Mud fever: See **grease heel.**

Multiparous: Having had two or more pregnancies which resulted in viable offspring. It may also indicate a species that normally has more than one offspring at a time, such as dogs, cats and swine.

Mycotoxins: Substances produced, particularly under warm, moist conditions, by molds (fungi), which may cause harmful effects to biological systems. Most antibiotics are mycotoxins that are more toxic for bacteria than for animals, and are therefore given to animals to kill infectious bacteria. Many mycotoxins are harmful to the horse and cause a wide variety of symptoms. General symptoms often attributed to mycotoxins are decreased feed consumption, infertility, poor hair coat, decreased performance and growth rate, abortion, diarrhea, liver and kidney damage, nervous system affects (such as tremors, incoordination, and hyperexcitability), hemorrhage, and death. Usually symptoms don't occur until levels of 100 to 300 ppb are present in the diet although this depends on the mycotoxins involved. Except for fatalities, the effects of most of the mycotoxins are reversible once the contaminated feed is removed from the diet. There are 25 to 30 different mycotoxins that may be detrimental to the horse. The best known causes of mycotoxicosis are (1) aflatoxins, ochratoxins, and tremortin A produced by Aspergillus and Penicillium, (2) trichothecene (T-2) produced by Fusarium and Myrothecium, (3) fescue toxicity, which is caused by a mycotoxin produced by Fusarium spp, (4) ergot produced by Claviceps spp., (5) zearalenone (F-2) produced by Fusarium, (6) salframine produced by Rhizoctonia, (7) citrinin and rubratoxin produced by Penicillium, and (8) sweet clover toxicity, caused by the mycotoxin dicoumarin which prevents blood coagulation, resulting in hemorrhage, and is produced by Aspergillus and Penicillium sp. in improperly cured sweet clover hay. A definitive diagnosis of mycotoxicosis is often difficult. Some veterinary diagnostic laboratories are able to analyze for a number of the major mycotoxins. However, portions of a feed may contain high levels of mycotoxins, and in other portions, none may be present. Thus, numerous samples of the suspected feed are necessary. Factors useful in making a presumptive diagnosis include (1) recognition of clinical signs that occur with mycotoxicosis (Table 19-1), (2) failure to isolate infectious agents or the animal to respond to antibiotic therapy, (3) presence of moldy feed, or environmental factors favorable for mold development and mycotoxin production (usually warm, moist conditions), (4) indications are decreased feed palatability, or feed refusal, and (5) test feeding of animals with the suspected feed, remembering that the young are generally the most susceptible and that several weeks may be required before symptoms occur. The best way to avoid mycotoxicosis is to never feed moldy feeds, although not all moldy feeds contain mycotoxins and mycotoxins may be present in feeds that are not visibly moldy. See Chapter 19.

Myeloencephalopathy: Myelo- denotes relationship to spinal cord, encephalo- indicates brain, and -opathy denotes illness; thus, an illness of or involving the brain and spinal cord.

Myopathy: Myo- and my- denote relationship to muscle, and -opathy indicates disease, thus any disease of the muscle or resulting in muscle degeneration, e.g., exertional myopathy indicating muscle degeneration or damage induced by physical exertion. See Chapter 11 for a discussion of this condition.

Myxedema: A puffy, thickened skin due to accumulation of mucinous material under it which produces a swelling of the distal aspect of the legs and sometimes the head. It occurs as a result of an iodine deficiency, rarely in horses, but occasionally in affected foals.

N

National Research Council (NRC): A division of the United States National Academy of Sciences established in 1916 to promote the effective utilization of scientific and technical resources. Periodically, this private organization of scientists publishes bulletins giving the nutrient requirements and allowance of animals. These are considered the best, and when published, the most current information on this topic available. Booklets on numerous species of animals, fish and birds are available for a nominal charge from the National Academic Press, 2101 Constitution Avenue NW, Washington, DC 20418.

Navicular bone: or distal sesamoid bone is a boat-shaped bone situated behind the coffin joint or distal interphalangeal joint (see Fig. 6-5). The deep flexor tendon passes over it to its insertion on the third or distal phalanges (coffin bone).

Navicular disease: One of the most common causes of lameness in mature working horses. Causes an intermittent, often-shifting foreleg lameness which increases with use and usually affects both forefeet to varying degrees with pointing of the more severely affected foot in an attempt to decrease weight on the heels. Landing on toes occurs, shortening the front part of the stride. This causes a rough, shuffling gait and stumbling which tends to wear off the toe, cause sole bruising, contracted, elevated heels, and pain over the center third of the frog. It is predisposed to by trimming the heels too low, repeated concussion and a straight-up conformation causing increased deep flexor tendon pressure on the navicular bone. This causes degeneration and death of fibrocartilage on the flexor surface of the navicular bone and stimulates bone remodeling. Increased vascular activity associated with bone remodeling produces edema, venous hypertension, fibrous adhesions, pain and clinical signs. Initial therapy usually includes rest, anti-inflammatory drugs, and trimming and shoeing to raise the heel and roll the toe. Other treatments include navicular bursa injections, anticoagulants, vasodilators and surgery. Cutting the nerves (posterior digital) to the affected area is a common last resort. Prognosis is poor.

Navel ill: Infection of the umbilicus or navel, which is a major portal for infectious organisms into foals which may cause septicemia, joint infections (joint ill), abdominal cavity infections (peritonitis), internal abscesses, and pneumonia. It can be prevented by proper care of the foal's umbilicus at birth as described in Chapter 14.

Near side: Left side of a horse versus the far or off side which is the right side.

Nebulization: Generally pertains to a treatment in which a substance is converted to a spray so that it can be inhaled; e.g., a vaporizer nebulizes water, and drugs which may be included in the water.

Necrosis: Death of body tissue or cells which are in contact with living tissue.

Necrotic: Dead body tissue or cells in contact with living tissue.

Necropsy: Necro- meaning dead and -opsy to view or examine, thus a necropsy is a postmortem or after-death examination. In people this is referred to as an autopsy, which actually means self-examination rather than post-mortem examination.

Negative nutrient balance: Refers to the state when more of a nutrient is being lost from the body than is being taken in. Opposite of a positive nutrient balance.

Neonatal: Neo- meaning new and natal birth, so the newborn. Usually refers to the first several weeks of life.

Nerving: Term commonly used for the cutting of the posterior digital nerve as a last resort treatment for navicular disease.

Neurologic: Pertaining to the nervous system, e.g., nerves, brain and spinal cord.

Neuropathy: Neuro- indicating nerves or nervous tissue and -opathy any disease, thus nerve disease, specifically a noninflammatory nerve degeneration.

Neutral detergent fiber (NDF): See **fiber, dietary.**

Nits: Eggs laid on the horse's hair by botflies or lice. They are yellow and are about the size of the head of a pin (Fig. 9-3).

NFE (Nitrogen-Free Extract): The portion of a feed consisting principally of soluble carbohydrates, e.g., sugars and starches. The most digestible and utilized carbohydrate fraction of the feed. Used primarily as a source of energy. The percentage of NFE in a feed is determined by subtracting the sum of the percentage of moisture, crude protein, crude fiber, and ash from 100.

Node: Botanically it is the point of leaf attachment to a stem.

Nonprotein Nitrogen (NPN): Nitrogen which comes from other than protein, includes compounds such as urea, ammonia, nuclei acids, etc. If sufficient soluble carbohydrates are ingested, microorganisms in the gastrointestinal tract may use NPN to produce protein. When this occurs in the rumen, the protein is digested and absorbed from the small intestine. However, when it occurs after the small intestine, such as in nonruminant animals like horses, little of this protein is utilized. See Chapter 1.

NRC: See **National Research Council.**

Nutrilites: Bacterial nutrients produced by yeast cultures which when ingested supposedly enhance gastrointestinal bacteria resulting in improved feed utilization.

Nutlet: A small plant nut.

Nuts: In the United Kingdom feed pellets or cubes may be referred to as nuts, a compound nut being a grain mix and forage pellet, often a complete pelleted feed; dehydrated forage pellets are referred to as dried grass nuts in the United Kingdom and as dehy or alfalfa pellets in North America.

Nutrient: Any feed constituent necessary for the support of life. The chief classes of nutrients are carbohydrates, fats, proteins, minerals, vitamins, and water.

Nymphomania: Exaggerated sexual desire in a female.

O

Oatfeed: Oat hulls and oat dust, usual as a pelleted feed, contains in its dry matter about 27% crude fiber, 9% crude protein, and provides 0.87 Mcal DE/lb (1.9/kg).

OBLA: See **onset of blood lactate accumulation.**

Obovate: Botanically indicates an oval leaf with its widest part near the apex and attached to the stem at its narrow end.

Ocrea: United appendages (stipules) surrounding the base of the leaf stock (petiole).

Off feed: Not eating with a normal healthy appetite.

Off side (far side): Right side of a horse versus the near or left side.

Oil: Fats that have a melting point below normal environmental temperature. See Fats, Chapters 1 and 4.

Omnivores: See **herbivores.**

Onset of blood lactate accumulation (OBLA): The speed, exertion, or time at a certain speed or exertion, when the plasma lactate concentration reaches 4 mM/L, above which it increases sharply with small increases in speed or exertion. This occurs in most horses at a heart rate of 170 to 220 bpm and is indicative of endurance or aerobic fitness. See Chapter 11 section on "Plasma Lactate as an Indicator of Fitness."

Open: When used in regard to a breeding female it indicates she is not pregnant.

Open knees: A concave appearance to the front of the knee (carpus) caused by an enlargement of the growth plate just above the knee.

Opposite: Botanically indicates two leaves per point of leaf attachment on the stem.

Ophthalmia: Ophthalm- or ophthalmo- denotes relationship to the eye, and -ia or -itis inflammation; thus inflammation of the eye. Microphthalmia indicating a small eye.

Orbicular: Circular in outline.

Organic: A substance containing carbon.

Organically-complexed: See **chelation.**

Orts: Leftover feed which animals don't eat.

Osmolality: An indication of the number of particles dissolved in a fluid. Water moves across membranes in the body to try to equalize the osmolality, or number of particles in solution, on each side of a membrane. Thus, if the osmolality outside the cells is higher than that inside the cells, water will move out of the cells. This increases the osmolality of the fluid inside the cells, and decreases it outside the cells, i.e., equalizes the osmolality on each side of the cell membrane.

Osselets: Trauma-induced fetlock joint arthritis primarily of the joint capsule causing its thickening and swelling at the front of the joint. Ossification can develop as a chronic change. Often due to overtraining or overuse of the young horse not yet sufficiently physically fit. Acute stage without identifiable bone changes is referred to as "green osselets." Causes an obvious lameness, or if both legs affected a choppy gait, and digital pressure or swelling causes pain.

Treatment includes rest, bandage support and hydrotherapy.

Ossification: Os- indicates bone and -sific to form or become; thus the formation of bone or a bony substance.

Osteoarthritis: Osteo- pertains to bone, arth- pertains to a joint, and -itis indicates inflammation; thus inflammation of the bone and joint.

Osteochondritis: Osteo- referring to bone, chondr- to cartilage, and -itis inflammation. So, osteochondritis is inflammation of the bone and cartilage of a joint. If a piece of cartilage or bone breaks off from the inflamed bone and articular cartilage, it is referred to as osteochondritis dissecans. If the piece is not attached, it is referred to as a joint mouse. See Chapter 16.

Osteopetrosis: Osteo- meaning bone, petro- meaning stone, and -osis disease; thus a bone disease characterized by too much bone due to either excessive bone formation or decreased bone resorption. It may be caused by excessive calcium, vitamin D or vitamin D-like substances in calcinosis inducing plants as described in Chapter 18.

Ovary: The female reproductive gland in which the ova of animals and seeds of plants form. In plants it is the swollen base of the pistil which consists of the ovary, style and stigma.

Ovatel: Egg-shaped in outline. An ovate leaf is egg-shaped and attached to the stem at its wide end.

Overbite: See **prognathism.**

Ovulation fossa: The site on the ovary where rupture of the follicle to release the ovum occurs.

Oxalate: A substance that binds positively charged minerals (cations), such as calcium, decreasing their intestinal absorption. After absorption, oxalates bind calcium in the bloodstream forming a precipitate which is deposited in the kidney, and may thereby cause kidney failure. See "Calcium Deficiency," in Chapter 2.

Oxytocin: A hormone produced by the posterior pituitary gland. Its plasma concentration in the mare remains constant during pregnancy and rises only during the second stage of parturition or foaling.

Oxyuris equi: See "Pinworms" in Chapter 9.

P

Pace: See **gaits.**

Paddock: 1) a small fenced area larger than a run but smaller than a pasture, also referred to as a dry lot if it is without growing edible vegetation. 2) the area where racehorses are saddled and viewed before a race.

Palatability: The desirability of a food for ingestion.

Palmate: Spreading like fingers on the palm of the hand, such as palmate leaf lobes.

Panicle: A compound raceme with the flowers on the terminal branchlets.

Pappus: Bristles at the lip of the single non-splitting fruit of the sunflower family.

Parakeratoses: An abnormality of the skin commonly resulting in dry, flaky crusts.

Parascaris equorum: See **Ascarids,** Chapter 9.

Parathyroid gland: Small glands located on or near the thyroid gland which is in the vicinity of the throatlatch. A decrease in blood calcium concentration stimulates these glands to secrete parathyroid hormone (PTH) that increases intestinal calcium absorption, calcium and phosphorus mobilization from the bone, and phosphorus excretion in the urine. It also decreases urinary calcium excretion. Its function is to prevent or minimize a decrease in the blood calcium concentration.

Parrot mouth: See **prognathism.**

Parturition: The act of giving birth.

Pastern: The area between the fetlock and hoof (Fig. 6-5).

Patella fixation (stifled): Patella (knee cap) catches momentarily or becomes lodged upward in the stifle joint which locks the stifle and hock joint in extension so the leg sticks straight down and back with a flexed pastern. The fixation can usually be relieved by manipulating the leg forward or backing the horse several steps. In horses in which this occurs fixation can be induced by pushing the patella upward and outward. A young horse may outgrow this condition. Surgical correction is possible

Pearled: Dehulled grains reduced into smaller smooth particles by machine brushing or abrasion.

Pecking order: When used in regard to animals it indicates dominance hierarchy or order of dominance. See "Group Socialization, Communication and Feeding" in Chapter 8.

Pedal osteitis: Inflammatory demineralization of the distal phalanx (coffin bone).

Pedicel: Stalk of a single flower.

Pediculosis: Infected with lice (Pediculus) (Fig. 9-7).

Perennial: Lasting for an indefinitely long time, such as a plant that lives more than two growing seasons.

Perianth: Collective term for the flower structures.

Perineal: Pertaining to the perineum the area of the body between the scrotum or vulva and the anus.

Periople: Peri-meaning around, and hople the hoof, so periople is the outer covering of the hoof. It is a smooth, shiny, waxy-like waterproof covering of the hoof wall that minimizes moisture evaporation from the hoof. It is removed by rasping, turpentine, many commercial hoof dressings, and continual standing in dry sand or in urine or wet manure. When the periople is lost, the hoof loses moisture making it when dry, hard, brittle and subject to cracking and splitting.

Peritoneal: Pertaining to the peritoneum, the membrane lining the internal abdominal walls.

Per os: Per oral or administration through the mouth.

Petiole: The leaf stalk.

PGF$_2\alpha$: See **prostaglandin F$_2$-alpha.**

pH: A measurement of acidity and alkalinity. Values may range from 0 to 14. A pH of 7 is neutral, below 2 to 3 is very acid (has a high hydrogen ion concentration or, more exact, activity), and over 10 is quite alkaline or basic (has a low hydrogen ion activity).

Phagocytosis: The engulfing of micro-organisms, other cells and foreign particles by a specialized phagocytic cell. The ingested material is usually digested or destroyed in the phagocyte. Phagocytes are either fixed (e.g., cells of the body's reticuloendothelial system and in lung alveoli) or in the circulation (e.g., the white blood cells, monocytes and polymorphonuclear leukocytes).

Pharynx: The musculomembranous sac located below the nasal passages, and above the mouth at the base of the tongue from which it is separated by the soft palate. It leads into the esophagus ("food tube") and the larynx ("voice box"). When food is swallowed, the soft palate raises, and the epiglottis closes preventing food from entering the larynx and thus the trachea (wind pipe), and allowing the food to enter the esophagus and be swallowed. Because of the horse's soft palate, material cannot be vomited or regurgitated into the mouth.

Photodermatitis: Photo- meaning light, derm- meaning skin, and -itis inflammation, so photodermatitis means sunlight induced skin inflammation. See **photosensitization.**

Photosensitization: A sensitivity to sunlight due to the accumulation of substances in the skin, which when exposed to sunlight fluoresce releasing radiant energy that damages the skin. These substances (photosensitive pigments) are present in buckwheat (Fagopyrum esculentum), St. John's wort (Hypericum perforatum), and possibly spring parsley (Cymopterus watsonii) and Bishop's Weed (Ammi majus), whose ingestion causes primary photosensitization. The causative substances may also be produced in the body because of liver damage and as a result its inability to eliminate normal breakdown products of plant chlorophyll causing a secondary or hepatogenous photosensitization. Any liver disease inducing plant, or toxin, may result in secondary photosensitization. Regardless of the cause, the less pigmented and haired the skin, the more sunlight reaches it and the more severe the effects. See Fig. 18-18.

Photosynthesis: The process by which plants utilize the energy from sunlight to change carbon dioxide, present in air, and water to oxygen and the carbon containing (organic) compounds that make up the plant.

Photoperiod: The relative length of alternating periods of light and dark.

Physiological: Pertaining to the physical and chemical functions of living organisms, as contrasted to mental or psychological functions.

Physis: Bone growth plate. It consists of columns of multiplying (mitotic) cartilage cells (chondrocytes) that become ossified resulting in bone growth. This occurs both at the metaphysis from which the shaft of the bone (diaphysis) grows, and at the articular or joint cartilage from which the end of the bone (epiphysis) grows.

Phytate: A six-carbon ring with a phosphate molecule bonded to each carbon atom. Because of this attachment, its phosphate is poorly available to the animal. The phosphate of phytate binds positively charged minerals (cations), such as calcium, decreasing their absorption. See "Calcium Deficiency" in Chapter 2.

Pica: Depraved or abnormal appetite which results in the consumption of items not normally eaten, such as dirt, wood, hair, feces, etc. May be caused by a sodium chloride (common salt), potassium, phosphorus or protein deficiency. See section on "Feed Selection by the Horse" in Chapter 6.

Pinnate: Resembling a feather. Botanically indicates a compound leaf generally with pairs of leaflets along the main stem bearing the leaves.

Pinworms (Oxyuris equi): Adult pinworms are found mainly in the colon and rectum of the horse (see Chapter 9). They may cause itching and restlessness. Affected horses may rub the tail on any stationary object, and may wear away the hair at the base of the tail and rump.

Pistillate: A flower with only female reproductive structures.

Pituitary gland (hypophysis): A small gland at the base of the brain that produces internal secretions including luteinizing hormone (LH), follicle stimulating hormone (FSH) and oxytocin.

Placenta: The organ in contact with the mother's uterus; it is attached to the fetus by means of the umbilical cord. It is passed after birth and is, therefore, referred to as the "after-birth."

Plasma: See **red blood cells.**

Pleura: The membrane lining the surface of the lungs and thoracic cavity.

Pleuritis: Inflammation of the pleura. Also referred to as pleurisy.

PMSG: See **gonadotropin.**

Poll evil: Inflammation of the fluid filled bursal sac that is located in between the nuchal ligament of the neck and the first (atlas) or second (axis) vertebrae causing a swelling at the poll (Fig. 6–5) which may break and drain.

Polyestrous: Repeated cycles of estrus or sexual receptivity, which in the mare occurs in the spring and summer.

Pomace: Dried fruit or citrus pulp. See Table 4–12 for nutrient content.

Pome: An apple-like fruit.

Popped knee: See **carpitis.**

Posterior: Behind or toward the back or rear-end of the body. Opposite of anterior.

Prebloom: The last one-third of the period of plant growth before blooming.

Prehension: The grasping and conveying of feed to the mouth for its ingestion.

Premix: A mixture of one or more microingredients (those that constitute a very small amount of a feed mix) with a carrier to increase the amount to be mixed into a larger amount, and thus improve the uniformity of distribution of the microingredients into the larger mixture.

Preservatives: A substance added to another substance, such as a feed, to decrease its rate of degradation or the degradation of its contents, such as the nutrients in feeds. It enhances the feed's stability and resistance to spoilage, discoloration, oxidation, mold or bacterial growth, para-

site infestation, etc. See "Feed Additives for Horses" in Chapter 4.

Progesterone: See **corpus luteum.**

Progestogens: Hormones that assist in the maintenance of pregnancy. Progesterone is the primary progestin and is produced by the corpus luteum and the placenta.

Prognathism: A condition in which the upper incisors extend out further than the lower incisors; also referred to as an overbite or parrot mouth. It is more common and the opposite of an underbite (prognathia, monkey mouth or sow mouth) in which the lower incisors protrude out further than the upper incisors.

Prognosis: Prediction of outcome or forecast as to the probable results of a disease or injury.

Prostaglandin F$_2$-alpha (PGF$_2\alpha$): A hormone produced by the uterus which stimulates regression or lysis of the corpus luteum. See Fig. 13–4.

Protein: A nitrogen-containing organic (carbon-containing) compound, made up of many amino acids. It is necessary in the diet, for the body to use in producing all of its tissues. It may also be used by the animal for energy. Crude protein indicates the total amount of protein in a feed; when only protein is stated, crude protein is generally what is meant. Digestible protein indicates only that protein that can be digested, and can therefore be used by the animal. Most protein in natural feeds for the horse is about 75% digestible. Thus if a feed contains 10% crude protein, it would contain about 7.5% digestible protein. If the animal needs 16% crude protein in its diet, it would need 12% digestible protein (16% × 0.75).

Protein bumps: See **hives** and Fig. 1–5.

Protein quality: A term used to describe the amino acid content, balance and useability of a protein. A protein is good, or high-quality, when it contains all of the amino acids in proper proportions needed by an animal, and is poor, or low-quality, when it is deficient in either content or balance of the amino acids needed. It is relatively meaningless for mature horses as it doesn't matter which amino acids make up the protein ingested.

Protein supplements: Feeds high in protein content which are added to diets to increase protein intake. See Chapter 4.

Proud cut: A gelding that shows stallion-like aggressive behavior. Also referred to as a rig or false rig. See section on "Castration" in Chapter 12.

Proximate analysis: A procedure for determining the amount of the following in a feed: (1) moisture, (2) crude protein, (3) crude fat or ether extract, (4) ash or total minerals, (5) crude fiber, and (6) nonfiber carbohydrate or nitrogen free extract (NFE). See Fig. 6–3.

Puberty: The age at which reproductive organs become functional which in both fillies and colts occurs anytime from 10 to 24 months of age, but averages 18. Spermatozoa first appear in colts' ejaculates at an average of 13 months of age. Thus yearlings should not be run with intact horses of the opposite sex, although most fillies will not stand for the stallion, nor will stallions on pasture breed them, until they are 3 or 4 years of age.

Pulmonary: Pulmo indicates relationship to the lungs, so pulmonary means pertaining to the lungs.

Pulmonary emphysema: See **heaves** and "Stable Ventilation" in Chapter 9.

Pulmonary hemorrhage or **bleeding:** See **bleeders.**

Pulses: Beans and peas, which are seeds of leguminous plants.

Pyramidal disease: See **buttress foot.**

Q

Quidding: Slobbering grain often after wallowing it around in the mouth before swallowing. It is usually due to a sore mouth and dental problems. See Chapter 9.

Quittor: A chronic purulent inflammation of the lateral cartilage of the hoof characterized by draining tracts at or just above the coronary band that periodically heal and reopen. It is usually due to a laceration near the coronary band which becomes infected.

R

Rack: See **gaits.**

Raceme: An arrangement of flowers along a stem with one flower per node and the youngest or latest blooming flower towards the apex of the stem.

Rachis: The main stem or axis of a plant bearing flowers or leaves.

Radiographs: Photographs made by using radioactive rays. The radioactive rays are often referred to as x-rays and the radiograph as an x-ray.

Radius: The major bone in the forearm (Fig. 6–5). There are two bones in the forearm, the radius and the ulna. They are united in the horse.

Range cubes (Range cake): Large pellets (usually about thumb size) generally composed primarily of grain and supplements. Their large size allows them to be fed on the ground to cattle on pasture or range where no feed banks are available.

Ration: The feed supplied or available to an animal. Used synonymously with diet, although some consider diet to include water and salt consumed separate from the rest of the animal's ration.

Rectum: The terminal end of the large intestine, or digestive tract, which extends from the colon to the anus. See Fig. 1–1.

Recumbency: The position of lying down.

Red blood cells: The blood consists of a noncellular liquid portion called plasma and the cells suspended in it. The greatest number of cells are red blood cells. These cells contain the iron-containing compound, hemoglobin. Hemoglobin binds oxygen in the lungs and releases it to the cells throughout the body.

Relaxin: A hormone produced by the uterine-placental unit at the same time fetal placental estrogens are produced. It appears to work with progesterone to maintain pregnancy and assist in preventing spontaneous uterine contractions.

Renal: Refers to the kidneys.

Renal Clearance Ratio: The amount of a substance excreted in the urine with respect to the amount of creatinine excreted. The amount of creatinine excreted is fairly constant over time. Thus, comparing the amount of a substance excreted to the amount of creatinine excreted eliminates dilutional effects on that substance's urine concentration and the necessity of doing a quantitative collection of urine over a period of time.

Rhabdomyolysis: Lysis or disruption of muscle fibers following physical exertion. See Table 11–6.

Rhinopneumonitis: A disease caused by equine herpes viruses. It is a common cause of respiratory disease and may also cause abortion and a nervous system disease. The respiratory disease is characterized by fever for 1 to 7 days, mild cough, and a serous, watery nasal discharge. Appetite may be decreased or may remain unaffected. Infrequently, diarrhea and stocking-up may occur. With proper treatment recovery is usually complete within 1 to 2 weeks in uncomplicated cases. It may also cause abortion, most commonly during the eighth to eleventh month of pregnancy, and is characterized by complete and rapid expulsion of the infected fetus and membranes. Less commonly, instead of abortion, infected mares may give birth to a live, but weak, foal, which usually dies of acute pneumonia or pleuritis in the first few days of life. Infections that result in abortion or birth of weak foals usually occur at the same time as an outbreak of respiratory disease in young horses on the farm. Affected mares may never shown any signs of respiratory disease. Rarely there may be infection of the brain, resulting in incoordination frequently associated with urinary incontinence, a decrease in tail tone, and variable anesthesia of the perineal area. In milder cases of brain infection, the horse may recover. Some recovered horses have persistent neurologic deficits; however, when infection of the brain or central nervous system occurs it is usually fatal. See Chapter 9.

Rhizome: An underground, laterally growing stem that sends out shoots above ground and roots below.

Ridgeling: A cryptorchid horse.

Ringbone: New bone growth that occurs near the pastern joint (high ringbone) or coffin joint (low ringbone) and may or may not involve the joint surface (articular or periarticular ringbone, respectively). With periarticular ringbone there may be no lameness, and no heat or pain after the initial stages, whereas with articular ringbone lameness occurs. Ringbone may be caused by trauma, such as a wire cut, or exertion induced strain of tendons and ligaments where they attach to the bone causing inflammation. The strain is increased by overly upright pasterns.

Rig (False rig): A gelding that shows stallion-like aggressive behavior. Also referred to as a proud cut horse. See section on "Castration" in Chapter 12.

Ringworm (Dermatomycosis): A fungal infection of the skin characterized by sharply demarcated, round, gray, dry, scaly areas of hair loss (Fig. 9–8). It occurs most commonly in younger animals.

Road gall (puff): See **wind puff.**

Roaring: A disease caused by a malfunction of the nerve that innervates the internal muscles of the larynx (voice box). It is also referred to as recurrent laryngeal neuropathy and laryngeal hemiplegia. There is an inability to draw the arytenoid cartilage and vocal fold laterally in the normal manner during inspiration. As a result, these structures are vibrated by inspired air producing a whistling or roaring sound during inspiration, and thus the name "roaring" for the disease, or when the sound is a higher-pitched whistle the horse is called a "whistler." The disease decreases maximum oxygen intake ability and, therefore, the horse's athletic performance ability. It is present in varying degrees in most Thoroughbred and Standardbred racehorses at birth or soon after, and its effects increase with age. The degree of impairment can be evaluated by an electrodiagnostic test (as described in Chapter 11 section on "Selecting the Equine Athlete"). It is generally treated by one of three procedures: ventriculectomy, arytenoidectomy (i.e., removing the mucous membrane lining the laryngeal ventricle, or removal of the arytenoid cartilage, respectively), or prosthetic laryngoplasty. The first two have been reported to be poorly effective. Prosthetic laryngoplasty, in which the flapping structures (arytenoid cartilage) is anchored with a suture is sometimes successful. However, a newer procedure using nerve-muscle pedicle grafts to repair the damaged nerve may result in greater success and fewer post-operation complications.

Rolled: In nutrition rolled refers to grain compressed by passing between rollers. See "Grain Processing" in Chapter 4 for its benefit for horses.

Roughage: A non-forage feed, high in fiber (generally over 18% crude fiber) and low in digestible energy, such as cereal grain hulls, straw, corn cobs and stover, beet pulp and fruit pomaces.

Rumen: Often referred to as the first stomach of cud-chewing animals such as cattle, sheep, goats, deer, and antelope. However, it is not a true stomach but a large compartment which, when full, comprises 15 to 20% of the animal's body weight. It is the first compartment ingested foods reach after being swallowed; next is the reticulum, then the omasum, followed by the abomasum, small intestine, cecum, large intestine, rectum, and anus. The abomasum is the true stomach and is similar to that of other animals. The rumen contains many micro-organisms that digest much of the feed that the animal ingests. It serves many of the same functions as the cecum in the horse.

Ruminant: An animal that has a rumen.

Roman nose: An outward hump to the nose when viewed from the side.

S

Saccharides: Soluble carbohydrates, such as starch, sugar and glycogen. The prefixes mono-, di-, tri- and poly- denote the number of these sugar molecules in that substance, e.g., table sugar is the disaccharide composed of the two monosaccharides glucose (dextrose) and fructose; milk sugar is the disaccharide composed of the two monosaccharides glucose and galactose; and starch and glycogen are polysaccharides composed of many molecules of the monosaccharide glucose, with starch being primarily in plants and glycogen primarily in animals.

"Saged:" A horse afflicted with "sage-sickness," a neurologic disease resulting from eating sand sage (Artemisia filifolia), budsage (A. spinescens) or fringed sage (A. frigida). It is characterized by incoordination (particularly in forequarters), abnormal reaction to stimuli, circling, unpredictable behavior, and often the smell of sage on the breath and in the feces. Horses recover in 1 to 2 weeks after not eating sage, whereas symptoms due to locoweed poisoned horses do not recover. See section on "Sagebrush" in Chapter 18.

Saline: Containing the common or table salt, sodium chloride.

Saliva: The clear, alkaline, somewhat viscid liquid secreted into the mouth. It contains a small amount of the enzyme amylase to begin starch digestion, but serves primarily to moisten, soften and lubricate ingested feed. The light breed horse with continuous access to forage secretes about 25 gallons (100 liters) per day. It contains 0.37% protein, and in mmole/L 40 to 50 sodium, 35 to 40 potassium, 40 chloride, 4.6 urea, 3.8 calcium, 1.3 magnesium, 0.3 glucose, and 0.1 phosphorus.

Saponins: Plant glycosides capable of producing a soap-like stable foam with water.

Satiety: The state of having eaten enough to satisfy the appetite.

Sclerosis: A hardening, especially from inflammation.

Scolioses: Abnormal curvature of the back or vertebral column. May occur in foals as a result of hypothyroidism, such as that due to either inadequate or excess iodine intake. See "Iodine" in Chapter 2.

Scours or scouring: Diarrhea most often, but not necessarily, used in reference to young animals.

Scratches: See **grease heel.**

Screened: A feed that has been separated into various sized particles by passing over or through screens.

Section: A part of something. A section of land refers to a square mile which contains 640 acres, 2.59 sq km with 100 hectares/sq km and thus 259 ha/section.

Seedy toe: Separation of the sensitive (dermal) and insensitive (epidermal) laminae of the hoof at the white line at the toe. It may occur as a sequel to chronic laminitis (see **founder**). It can become extreme and cause lameness. Good hoof trimming and keeping the area clean will usually correct or control the condition.

Self feeder: A feed container from which an animal can eat at times other than when feed is first placed in it. This may be because the feeder contains sufficient feed for the animals to eat from free-choice (ad libitum) or whenever and however much it wants, or because the feeder has an automated means of allowing the feed it contains to become available to the animal, such as timed feeders.

Sepal: Outer part of the flower or perianth which is usually green.

Septicemia: Sickness due to the presence of disease producing bacteria and their toxins in the blood. It is the most common cause of illness and death of newborn foals. The bacteria most often gain access via the umbilicus, respiratory tract or gastrointestinal tract. It most often occurs in foals 1 to 4 days of age. Sudden death or lethargy, increased respiratory effort and decreased appetite occur. Even with intensive care the majority of foals with septicemia die.

Serrated: With pointed or sharp forward pointing teeth, such as a serrated leaf.

Serum: The clear portion of any body liquid separated from its more solid elements or cells. Unless otherwise stated, it usually refers to blood serum, which is the noncellular clear liquid which separates from blood after it clots. It differs from blood plasma primarily in that serum doesn't contain fibrinogen which remains in the blood clot.

Sesamoiditis: Inflammation of proximal sesamoid bones. Articular (joint) form is secondary to fetlock joint disease. True or nonarticular form is associated with tearing of suspensory ligament and/or distal sesamoidean ligament attachments due to excessive strain. Occurs most often in racehorses, hunters and jumpers 2 to 5 years old. There is heat, swelling and pain at the posterior surface of the fetlock. Fetlock flexion is painful and worsens lameness. Treatment is to reduce inflammation and immobilize the fetlock. It may result in chronic lameness.

Sessile: Plant without a stalk of any kind.

Settled: When used in regard to reproduction, it means becoming pregnant or conceiving following breeding.

Seven-year hook: An overhang at the back of the upper corner incisor that appears at 7, disappears at 8, reappears at 11, and disappears again by 18 years of age.

Shiners: See **glowers.**

Shock: A condition of acute circulatory failure due to a sudden decrease in heart function, loss of blood, or dilation of peripheral blood vessels. It is characterized by pallor (loss of membrane coloration), decreased temperature of the extremities, a feeble rapid pulse, decreased respiration, restlessness, anxiety, inability to stand or sit up, and sometimes unconsciousness. It may be caused by heart failure (cardiogenic), hemorrhage (external or internal) (hematogenic or hemorrhagic shock), or a loss of nervous control of peripheral blood vessels (neurogenic shock), which may be due to an acute allergic response (anaphylactic shock), head or brain injury, severe pain, or strong emotion (psychic shock). Its treatment requires trying to maintain blood flow to the brain (e.g., by positioning so head is lower than body), warmth, and the rapid administration of large volumes of fluid intravenously.

Shrub: Woody perennial, smaller than a tree, usually with several basal stems.

Shying: A sudden unexpected movement to one side.

Shivering: 1) A reflex trembling in response to fear, excitement or cold which by increasing muscular activity increases body heat production. 2) A nervous or neuromuscular disease characterized by jerking and shaking movements of the legs and tail, especially noticeable when the horse is backed, turned or has to step over an object. Eyelids and ears may also flicker and lips may be drawn backward. Signs usually increase over time. No effective treatment or cause is known.

Shoe boil: See **capped elbow.**

Sickle-hocked: A conformational fault in which there is excessive angulation of the hock (hock isn't straight enough). As a result the horse stands with its rear feet too far forward, or under it which is referred to as camped-under. It predisposes to curb and thus is termed a "curby" conformation (see **curb**). It may also be caused by inadequate conversion of the small bones of the hock growth cartilage to bone resulting in their collapse. See "Angular Leg Deformities" in Chapter 16.

Sidebones: Ossification of the lateral cartilages of the third or distal phalanx (coffin bone) that prevents normal expansion of the foot. Usually occurs as a result of repeated concussion or injury predisposed to by a too straight up conformation. More common in big horses that toe in or toe out. It may or may not cause lameness, but over time may result in contracted heels and abnormal hoof growth.

Silage (ensilage): Fermented forage plants. Corn, sorghum, and small cereal grains are cut and not allowed to dry, or moisture is added to them. The entire plant (stalks, leaves, and grain) is chopped and packed into a facility which protects it from exposure to air. Permits maximum yield of nutrients from a unit of ground. See Chapter 4.

Singlefoot: See **gaits.**

Sleeping sickness (encephalomyelitis, encephalitis, brain fever, or blind staggers): A viral disease transmitted by blood sucking insects, such as mosquitoes, from birds and rodents to horses or people. The bird and rodent are unaffected by the virus, as are animals other than horses and people. The virus is not transmitted from horses or people to other horses or people, i.e., a horse or person cannot get the disease from another horse or person. Symptoms include high fever, incoordination, drowsiness, partial loss of vision, grinding of the teeth, reeling gait, inability to swallow, and, in later stages, paralysis. Once symptoms occur it is usually fatal regardless of treatment. The disease is prevented by vaccinating twice, two to three weeks apart, with annual revaccination several weeks before mosquito season beings. See Chapter 9.

Smooth mouthed: A horse in which all dental cups are gone from the incisors so their occlusal or chewing surface is now smooth. This occurs at about 11 years of age. Thus, a smooth mouthed horse is one that is 11 years **or older.** Some incorrectly believe it means an 11-year-old horse.

Soilage or green chop: Fresh, green forage cut, chopped and fed all in the same day.

Solubles: Liquid containing dissolved substances obtained from processing animal or plant materials. It may contain some fine suspended particles.

Sour: When used in regard to an animal it usually implies a bad attitude, e.g., a barn sour horse which resists being ridden away from the barn.

Sow mouth (monkey mouth or prognathia): A horse with an underbite in which the lower incisors extend further than the upper incisors. It is less common and opposite to parrot mouth or prognathism in which there is an overbite with the upper incisors extending out further than the lower incisors.

Spasm: Sudden, involuntary contractions of a muscle or a group of muscles, attended by pain and interference with function producing involuntarily movement and distortion.

Spavin: A disease of the hock joint of which there are several types:

Blind (occult): Lameness apparently in the hock with no palpable or radiographic signs. May actually be due to changes in the stifle. It is the least common type of spavin.

Blood spavin: A swelling of the saphenous vein crossing a bog spavin.

Bog spavin: Inflammation of the hock joint which causes a chronic swelling primarily at the front-inside aspect of the hock. Lameness usually occurs only with traumatic, or with osteochondritis dissecans-induced bog spavin. Too straight at the hock, and strain such as occurs with quick stops predisposes to it.

Bone, true or jack spavin: Osteoarthritis or degenerative joint disease of the hock of mature horses. Usually there is a gradual onset of lameness that improves with rest, and which the horse warms out of; but results in an inability or refusal (because of pain) to perform normally. There may be a hard enlargement at the inner-front and lower aspect of the hock, and increased lameness following holding the leg up to flex the hock joint for several minutes (spavin test). Often it is associated with excessive concussion from hard work or a traumatic event, and is predisposed to by sickle hocks and by cow hocks. The most common treatment is surgical removal of a portion of the cunean tendon, a procedure referred to as "having the jacks cut." This results in improvement and generally a usable horse if bone changes haven't occurred. Some affected horses may have a persistent mild lameness which they may warm out of. In persistent cases, surgical destruction and ankylosis of the distal intertarsal and tarsal metatarsal joints so they are immobile may result in soundness.

Spermatogenesis: The process by which spermatozoa are produced, which in the horse takes 57 days plus 8 days for transport through the epididymis for a total of 65 days. The time between an event detrimental to spermatogenesis and a decline in semen quality is from 3 days to as long as 65 days, but it will take 65 days after recovery from damage for new unaffected spermatozoa to be ejaculated.

Spirurids: See section on "Stomachworms" in Chapter 7.

Spleen: A glandular organ located near the stomach. It is a flattened oblong shape that varies in size, but in the horse is about 10 by 20 inches (25 by 50 cm) in length. It is dark purple with a soft consistency. It serves as a reservoir for red blood cells, and assists the body in combating infectious organisms.

Splint bones: Small pencil shaped bones (2nd and 4th metacarpal and metatarsal bones) attached by a ligament to each side of the cannon bones (Fig. 6–5). The splint bones taper to a thin stem then enlarge into a variable size nodule at the end referred to as bulbs or buttons, which

in mature light-breed horses are 3 to 4 inches (6 to 9 cm) above the fetlock joints.

Splints: Inflammation of the splint bone (Fig. 6–5) interosseous ligament that binds the splint bone to the cannon bone, or inflammation of the periosteum over the splint bone. Occurs primarily in long yearlings to 4-year-olds in training or use. An elongated swelling occurs several inches (6 to 7 cm) below the knee, most often on the inside surface of the front leg, although trauma such as being kicked can cause it on the outside surface of the leg. Initially there is heat, pain and usually lameness that worsens with exercise on a hard surface. As the inflammation subsides, bone growths often occur. Hard training, poor conformation (such as offset or bench knees, base-narrow, or toe-out conformations), improper hoof trimming and rapid growth predispose to splints. Treatment during the acute phase includes administration of anti-inflammatory agents, cold, pressure support wraps and stall rest, generally with a 10 to 15 minute walk twice daily. During the chronic stage counterirritants are commonly used. If bony exostosis develop, they may be removed surgically.

Sprain: An injury to a ligament from overstress which may result in ligament inflammation (desmitis).

Stallion ring: A ring that is slipped over the stallion's penis to prevent erection and as a result masturbation. Masturbation has been assumed to decrease fertility, and may in some stallions who do so excessively, but in most it does not and may be a normal, not an abnormal behavior (see Chapter 12). Although a stallion ring may aid in preventing masturbation, it may cause damage to the penis, and blood in the semen which makes the semen infertile. Its use is not recommended.

Stall walking: A vice in which a horse continually walks in a circle around its stall. See "Escape Vices" in Chapter 20.

Stamen: Pollen bearing structures of the flower.

Staminate: Having stamens only.

Starch: A carbohydrate composed of many glucose (dextrose) molecules attached together by alpha bonds. These bonds are broken by digestive enzymes releasing the glucose molecules so they can be absorbed and used by the animal. Starch provides the major source of dietary energy derived from cereal grains.

Starch equivalents (SE): An uncommonly used energy term in which the energy provided is compared to that provided by starch. Thus, for example, a feed with a SE of 90% would provide 90% as much energy as starch. Although applicable for ruminants, SE is unsuitable for horses because of their different digestive process.

Steatitis: Steat- indicates fat or adipose tissue, and -itis inflammation, thus inflammation of body fat.

Stiff movement: Nutritional causes include selenium, vitamin E or vitamin B_1 (thiamine) deficiency, or excess selenium, fluoride or vitamin D.

Stifled: See **patella fixation.**

Stillage (slop): What remains following grain fermentation to produce alcohol, and distillation to remove it. It is dried to produce distiller's dried grains and solubles.

Stillborn: Born dead. Nutritional causes for the birth of dead or weak foals or those with bone abnormalities include either an iodine deficiency or excess, and possibly a manganese deficiency. See Table 18-11 for plant poisoning induced causes.

Stipules: Small leaf-like structure just below the leaf's attachment to the stem.

Stocking rate: The number of animals that can be maintained on a unit of ground. Unless specified it generally means for a 1 year period of time.

Stocking up: The accumulation of excess fluid in the tissues (edema) under the skin causing a diffuse swelling of the area. Most commonly occurs in the legs, but may also occur in the prepuce and underline. The most common cause is sudden inactivity, such as putting a horse in a stall, particularly following a period of physical activity. Turning the horse out in a paddock, or exercising a few hours a day, will prevent stocking up. Applying bandages to keep pressure on the legs will also prevent fluid accumulation. Stocking up not associated with inactivity may be due to congestive heart failure, or more commonly, a decrease in the concentration of proteins in the plasma. This may be caused by a decrease in protein synthesis because of liver damage, or excessive losses of proteins from the body such as in blood loss or some forms of diarrhea. High protein diets and alfalfa will not cause or predispose the horse to stocking up. Starvation, however, or a protein deficient diet may, as will a vitamin E deficiency.

Stomachworms (spirurids, Habronema spp. and Draschia): Flies carry stomachworm larvae to the horse where they may cause habronemiasis (summer sores). See Chapter 9.

Stover: Mature, sun-cured stalks of corn or milo which are left standing in the field after the seeds or grain have been removed. If harvested, they are referred to as fodder. See "Straw and Stover" in Chapter 4.

Strangles (distemper): A disease caused by the bacteria Streptococcus equi and characterized by fever, depression, nasal discharge, cough, and swollen lymph glands, particularly those under or behind the jaws. It most commonly occurs in weanlings and yearlings, but may occasionally occur in foals and in older horses. In compromised foals it may cause widespread lymph node abscessation, pneumonia, septicemia, cardiomyopathy and brain abscesses. See Chapter 9.

Straw: Small cereal grain plant residue, stems, or stalks, after removal of the grain or seeds. Used as a feed (see Chapter 4) or a bedding (see Chapter 9).

Stride: The distance between successive imprints of the same foot. In contrast a step is the distance in line of foreward movement between the footprints of two forelimbs or between the two hindlimbs.

Stringhalt: An exaggerated lifting and jerking motion on the forward movement of one or both hocks that is spasmodic and involuntary. Some affected horses show only mild excess hock flexion sporadically during walking, while in severe cases the fetlock may hit the abdomen with each step. Generally signs are exaggerated when turning or backing, during cold weather and after rest, and may disappear for variable periods of time. It must be differentiated from patellar fixation and fibrotic myopathy. In North America only isolated cases occur and the cause is unknown. In Australia and New Zealand outbreaks have occurred in late summer and fall, especially following an abnormally dry summer, in horses grazing pastures where Hypochaeris radicata (catsear, flatweed, or dandelion) constitute 50% of the available forage. Most of these cases recover without treatment when removed from the pasture, although recovery may take 1 to 12 months. Isolated cases are treated by surgically removing the section of the lateral digital flexor tendon that crosses the lateral surface of the hock, after which nearly all cases show varying degrees of improvement.

Strongyles (blood worms): A major internal parasite affecting horses. See Chapter 9.

Stubble: The basal portion of plants remaining above the ground after the top portion has been harvested, either by grazing or by cutting and removing the top portion of the plant.

Style: The stalk attached to the tip of a plant ovary.

Stylopodium: A disk-like expansion of the style of a plant.

Subclinical: Symptoms not sufficiently severe or manifested to be evident.

Subcutaneous: Sub meaning under, and cutaneous pertaining to the skin, thus under the skin.

Sugar: A soluble carbohydrate composed of monosaccharides. See **saccharides.**

Summer sores: Yellow granular type skin lesions that develop during the summer due to stomachworm (Habronema) larvae in the skin. See section on "Stomachworms" in Chapter 9.

Surfactant: A surface-active agent produced in the lungs. It is necessary for preventing collapse of lung alveoli (air sacs) where blood picks up oxygen and releases carbon dioxide.

Supplement: A feed or feed mixture added to a diet to increase the amount of a specific nutrient(s).

Suppurative: Producing or associated with pus, a liquid product of inflammation.

Sweeny: Atrophy (wasting-away) of a muscle. Usually refers to the muscles over the shoulder blade (supraspinatus and infraspinatus muscles) whose atrophy makes the spine of the shoulder blade prominent. Usually due to damage to the suprascapular nerve from harness collar pressure. The horse may be sound with limited use, but often lameness occurs or the horse becomes lame with extensive use. No successful treatment is currently available.

Sweet feed: Refers to a grain mix containing molasses.

Symptomatic: Pertaining to a symptom, e.g., symptomatic therapy would be treatment to lessen symptoms or their effects, as opposed to therapy to correct the cause for the symptoms.

Synchronous Diaphragmatic Flutter (SDF, or

thumps): Contraction of the diaphragm in synchrony with the heart. Clinically, it is manifested by sudden, bilateral, and occasionally unilateral, movements of the horse's flanks, and sometimes hind leg, every time the heart beats. See Chapter 11.

Synergist: Something that in conjunction with something else results in an effect greater than that of either by itself, e.g., drug A and B each alone may be 30% effective, but when used together are 80% effective, and thus they have a synergistic effect.

Synovitis: Synov-referring to the synovial lining of joint capsule, tendon sheath or bursa, and -itis inflammation.

Systemic: Pertaining to or affecting the body as a whole.

T

Tack: The saddle, bridle and other equipment worn by a horse when ridden.

Tapeworms (Anoplocephala): Adult tapeworms are present in horses' intestines where they utilize nutrients and may cause unthriftiness, intermittent colic, diarrhea and anemia. Large clusters can cause obstruction resulting in colic and death. See Chapter 9.

Taproot: The primary carrot-like root of a plant.

TDN: See **total digestible nutrients.**

Teasing: When used in regard to equine reproduction, the term means controlled exposure of the mare to a stallion to increase the signs and thus detection of estrus. It is an important reproductive management procedure for mares not being pasture bred and, therefore, with a stallion. See Chapter 13.

Tearing: See **lacrimation.**

Teart: A condition due to molybdenum toxicosis. See Chapter 2.

Temperature, rectal: Horse's normal rectal temperature is 99 to 101°F (37.3 to 38.3°C). It is increased by excitement, physical exertion and infectious diseases causing a fever, and is decreased by a dilated rectum, shock or other causes of decreased peripheral circulation. The cause for more than a 1°F (0.5°C) variation outside the normal range should be determined and treated if indicated. Monitoring the rectal temperature is one way to monitor the horse's health, and the presence of and response to treatment for an infectious disease or infection. The absence of a fever doesn't, however, mean an infectious disease or infection is not present. A large animal rectal thermometer is beneficial equipment for every horse owner or manager. A clip can be attached to the top end of the thermometer with a string so that after the thermometer is inserted, the clip can be fastened to hair at the base of the tail. This will prevent the thermometer from falling and being broken if the horse has a bowel movement while it is inserted. Before inserting the thermometer, shake it down and cover it with a lubricant such as a petroleum jelly. Two to three minutes in the rectum is sufficient to obtain an accurate rectal temperature.

Tendinitis: Inflammation of a tendon.

Teratogenesis: Terato- denoting relationship to a mons-

ter, and -genesis production or birth, thus the production of a monster due to the development of physical defects in the fetus prior to birth. See Table 18–11 for plant-induced causes.

Tendosynovitis: Tendo- referring to tendon, synov- to the synovial membrane lining the joint capsule, tendon sheath or bursa, and -itis inflammation. So tendosynovitis, or tendovaginitis, is inflammation of both a tendon and the synovial membrane of its sheath.

Teratogenic: Terato- meaning monster and -genic birth, thus tending to produce monsters or offspring with physical defects. See Table 18–11 for plant-induced causes.

Tetanus (lockjaw): A disease caused by the bacterium Clostridium tetani which is widely distributed in soil and manure. After the bacteria enter an injury, such as a cut or puncture wound, they produce a toxin which is absorbed and causes the disease. The disease affects all animals, with the horse being particularly susceptible. Tetanus is characterized by stiffness of any or all muscles. Advanced symptoms include violent spasms, stiff tail and legs, sweating, and fever. Once symptoms occur the disease is usually fatal. Vaccination for all horses is recommended as described in Chapter 9.

Tetany: A condition in an animal in which there are localized, spasmodic muscular contractions, twitching, or cramps. Nutritional causes of muscle tremors, convulsions, tetany or seizures include a vitamin A deficiency, a low blood magnesium concentration, and vitamin D toxicosis.

Therm: An expression of the amount of nutritional energy. One therm equals 1000 nutritional calories or kilocalories (kcal), and 1 megacalorie (Mcal).

Thoroughpin: Strain induced distension of the deep flexor tendon sheath (tarsal sheath) resulting in a soft, fluid filled swelling in the hollow on the outside surface of the hock. The swelling can be pushed freely from the outside to the inside surface of the hock by palpation. Usually no pain, heat or lameness are evident. In contrast with a bog spavin the swelling is lower and is primarily on the front-inside aspect of the hock.

Threadworms: (Strongyloids westeri): An intestinal parasite of horses. See Chapter 9.

Thrifty: In nutrition it means an animal with a healthy appearance.

Thrush: A bacterial infection of the frog and its sulci characterized by the presence of a black necrotic material with a very offensive odor. The infection may penetrate the horny tissue and involve the sensitive structures, resulting in lameness. The major cause is standing in dirty, wet stalls. Prevention is to maintain clean stalls, exercise and frequent cleaning of the feet, ideally daily. It is treated by eliminating the cause, and removing degenerated frog tissue. The foot should be cleaned, and the sulci of the frog packed with cotton soaked in 10 to 15% sodium sulfapyridine solution daily until the infection is controlled.

Thumps: See "**Synchronous Diaphragmatic Flutter**" in Chapter 11.

Tibia: The major bone of the leg between the stifle and the hock (Fig. 6–5).

Timed-feeders: A feed container that allows the food it contains to become available to the animal at the specific times for which it has been set, e.g., On Time Feeders (Specialty Fabrication, Wichita, Kansas, 67214).

Tocopherol: A compound that has vitamin E activity. See Chapter 2.

Tongue displacement: A vice in which the horse repeatedly forces the tongue over the bit or sticks it out the side of the mouth for periods of time. See "Oral Vices" in Chapter 20.

Total Digestible Nutrients (TDN): A term which indicates the energy density of a feedstuff. It is the sum of the percent of digestible fat times 2.25, digestible protein, and digestible carbohydrate (NFE and fiber) present in the feed. One pound of TDN is equal to approximately 2000 kcalories of digestible energy, and 1 kg about 4400 kcalories.

Toxoid: See **vaccine.**

Trace mineral: A mineral required by animals in their diet in very small amounts (in parts per million parts of diet, ppm, or mg/kg of diet or less). See Chapter 2.

Tracheotomy: Trachea is the windpipe from the larynx (voice box) to where it splits into bronchi in the lungs, and -otomy meaning to cut. Thus, a tracheotomy is the formation of an artificial opening into the trachea.

Transferrin: The protein which transports iron in the blood.

Trichostrongylus: See "Hairworms" in Chapter 9.

Triglycerides: A fat or oil, which is composed of glycerol with a fatty acid, which is a long chain of carbon atoms, attached to each of glycerol's 3 carbon atoms.

Trot: See **gaits.**

Trypsin: An enzyme secreted by the pancreas into the small intestine which digests protein. Some oilseeds, beans and peas contain substances which inhibit its activity causing a decrease in protein digestion which may result in a decreased growth rate of young animals.

Tuber or tuberous: A short, thickened, fleshy potato-like root, usually an underground stem with numerous eyes or nodes.

Tushes: See **canine teeth.**

Tusks: See **canine teeth.**

Twenty-eight hour law: The law in the United States that prohibits transporting livestock for a period longer than 28 consecutive hours without unloading, feeding, watering and resting for at least 5 consecutive hours before resuming transportation. On request of the livestock owner, the period can be extended to 36 hours.

Twitch: 1) a muscle spasm. 2) A handle with a rope or chain loop on one end. The loop of the twitch is placed around the upper lip of the horse. It is tightened by twisting the handle, decreasing the circumference of the loop around the lip. The squeezing of the lip is thought to stimulate the release of endorphins which calm most horses. The calming effect usually occurs for only a short period of time. An occasional horse may fight the twitch and become more fractious. If this response occurs, the horse should not be twitched.

Tying-up syndrome: Muscle spasms that occur after a period of prolonged or hard physical activity due to a depletion of the energy necessary for muscle relaxation (Table 11-6).

U

Umbel: A flat or rounded flower cluster in which the stalks radiate from a common point like an umbrella.

Umbilicus (umbilical stump): The 1 to 2 inch (2 to 5 cm) stump on the newborn's abdomen that, prior to birth, was attached to the placenta. Most of the young animal's nourishment prior to birth is passed to it from the mother through the umbilicus. Following birth, bacteria may gain access to the body via the umbilical stump. These bacteria may be carried by the blood causing septicemia, or may localize in the lung, resulting in pneumonia; in the brain, frequently resulting in death; or most commonly, in the joints, resulting in infected, swollen joints, and lameness. To prevent this, it should be cared for as described in Chapter 14.

Unsound: Any deviation from normal structure or function which interferes with normal use of the animal.

Unthrifty: In nutrition it means an animal with a poor, unhealthy appearance, or an animal that does poorly, i.e., grows slowly or has little vigor or vitality.

Urachus: Tube connecting the fetal bladder via the umbilical cord to the placenta. It normally closes at birth. If it remains open, urine will dribble from the umbilical cord. It may require cauterization to close it. See "Umbilical Care" in Chapter 14.

Urea: Consists chemically of two molecules of ammonia attached to one molecule of carbon monoxide (NH_2-CO-NH_2). It is produced in the liver and excreted primarily in the urine, and is the major means of the body's excreting nitrogen. Nitrogen is produced from the breakdown of body or dietary protein. Some urea produced by ruminants goes into the rumen (urea may also be fed to ruminants). In the rumen, urea is broken down to carbon dioxide and ammonia. Bacteria in the rumen utilize the ammonia to produce protein. The animal is able to digest and absorb this protein as it passes through the digestive tract. However, little is utilized by horses and horses are quite resistant to excess urea consumption and toxicosis. See "Non-Protein Nitrogen for Horses" in Chapter 1.

Uremia: Ur- indicating urine, and -emia in the blood; thus uremia indicating the presence of excess waste products normally excreted in the urine accumulating in the blood. Because most of the waste products are the nitrogenous compounds creatinine and urea, uremia is also referred to as azotemia. Azo- meaning the presence of a nitrogen group. Uremia occurs because body waste products cannot be excreted as rapidly as they are produced, generally because of decreased kidney function, obstruction to urine excretion, or a ruptured bladder.

Urticaria: See **hives** and **protein bumps** (Fig. 1-5).

V

Vaccinate (Inoculate): The administration of a vaccine to an animal. Depending on the vaccine, it may be given in a number of different ways, such as orally, or sprayed into the nostrils, or injected into the muscle, vein, skin, or under the skin (subcutaneously).

Vaccine: A preparation containing a virus, bacteria, or other infectious organism or toxin given to an animal to stimulate it to produce antibodies (immunoglobulins) and thus an immunity against that organism or toxin, and therefore, prevent the disease caused by that organism or toxin. When a vaccine contains a toxin, it is called a toxoid. The toxoid stimulates the animal to produce antibodies, called antitoxins, against the toxin.

Valence: The combining power of molecules, e.g., antigen and antibody, or number of positive or negative charges on an atom or ion.

Valgus: An abnormal deviation of a joint toward the midline, e.g., knock-knees. Opposite to varus in which the deviation is away from the midline.

Varus: An abnormal deviation of a joint away from the midline, e.g., bow legged at the knees or fetlocks. Opposite to valgus in which the deviation is toward the midline.

Vein: A thin walled tube that carries blood from all parts of the body to the heart. The blood in a vein is normally low in oxygen because it has diffused out of the blood into the tissue. This gives it a dark red color, whereas the blood in an artery is normally bright red because it is saturated with oxygen which it has picked up in its passage through the lungs. Veins are much closer to the body surface than are arteries. The blood in a vein is under little pressure, so that if a vein is cut, blood does not spurt out as it does when an artery is cut.

Vesicle or vesicular: A small sac or blister containing liquid.

Vertebrae: Bones making up the spinal column or back bone through which the spinal cord runs.

Vice: An undesirable or useless behavior that becomes a persistent, repetitive bad habit. Also referred to as a stereotypic behavior. See Chapter 20 for different types, causes, effects, and prevention of common vices in horses.

Villi: Small, threadlike, vascular processes or protrusions. They greatly increase the surface area from which they protrude, thus increasing the absorptive and/or secretory capacity that can occur at that surface. Those on the luminal surface of the intestine are necessary for absorption; which if decreased, such as due to inflammation, diarrhea occurs.

VFA or Volatile Fatty Acids: See **fatty acids.**

Vitamins: Organic (carbon-containing) compounds needed in minute amounts for normal body function, but which do not supply energy and are not a part of body structure. Some are produced in the horse's body (vitamins C and D), some are produced by micro-organisms in the intestinal tract (all of the B-vitamins and vitamin K), and some are supplied entirely by the diet (vitamins A and E). See Chapter 3.

W

Wafers: In nutrition wafers refer to hay pressed into a wafer or cube form. They are generally 1 to 2 inches (3 to 5 cm) in size (Fig. 4-5).

Walleye: A white eye; usually functions normally.

Water bag amniotic sac: The translucent innermost membranous sac in the uterus of the pregnant animal that contains fluid and the fetus.

Weaving: A vice in which the horse rhythmically shifts its weight from one forefoot to the other while swinging its head. It may occur in conjunction with head-nodding. See "Escape Vices" in Chapter 20.

Weed: A plant whose virtues have not yet been discovered—Ralph Waldo Emerson.

Wind puff (wind gall): Swelling of the synovial membrane lining a joint or tendon sheath that does not cause lameness. Most often on the fetlock, pastern or above the knee. The swelling usually occurs as a result of heavy work.

Wind sucker: A mare that, particularly when running, aspirates air, and usually also fecal material, into the vagina. This results in inflammation of the vagina and sometimes of the uterus. It is corrected by surgically suturing the upper portion of the lips of the vulva together. This is called a Caslick's operation. See "Prebreeding Examination of Mares" in Chapter 13. A horse that cribs or chews wood is also sometimes referred to as a wind sucker (Fig. 20-1).

Winking: In regard to a mare, winking indicates rhythmic opening and closing of the labia. It frequently is accompanied by frequent urination and a mating stance. This may occur when mares in heat are teased or are near a stallion or gelding.

Whey: What remains after most protein has been removed from milk. It contains primarily lactose or milk sugar.

Whistler: A horse that makes a whistling noise on inspiration. See **roaring.**

Whorled: A circle of three or more leaves or branches at a node or the stem.

Wobbler (Wobbler's syndrome): Incoordination of the back legs generally occurring in the growing horse, and resulting from damage to the spinal cord of the neck which may be caused by injury, protozoan infection, or nutritionally-induced osteoarthritis and osteochondritis of the vertebrae, which is generally associated with rapid growth. The nutritional inducements most commonly incriminated are feeding of excess grain, or inadequate calcium or phosphorus (see Chapter 16). It may also be due to a vitamin E deficiency or responsive to vitamin E administration. See "Equine Degenerative Myeloencephalopathy" in Chapter 2.

Wolf teeth: First premolars which are tight against the front of first major cheek teeth (second premolars) and are only 1/2 to 3/4 inch (1 to 2 cm) long. They are usually present only on top but occasionally lower ones are also present. They erupt during the first 6 months of life and are often shed at the same time as the first major cheek teeth (2 1/2 years of age); if not, they should be removed. See Chapter 9.

Wood chewing: Chewing of wood by the horse, generally as a result of boredom, from habit, or because the horse likes its taste. Not known to be due to a nutritional deficiency or imbalance. Most horses do not swallow the wood. Should not be confused with cribbing or wind sucking (Fig. 20-1).

Woods lamp or light: A lamp that gives off black light (long-wave ultraviolet light at 365 nm). It is used to examine feed to determine if it contains aflatoxin-producing mold. See "Field Mycotoxin Assays" in Chapter 19.

Worms: With respect to horses worms refers to worms and botfly larvae in the horse's stomach and intestines. Worming an animal means treating the animal to remove these worms. Blood worms are adult large strongyles. See Chapter 9.

Wort: The soluble fraction derived from mash (germinated cereal grain kernels and hops) to which yeast is added to produce alcohol.

X

X-rays: See **radiographs.**

EQUINE NUTRITIONAL REQUIREMENTS, FEED COMPOSITION, AND CONVERSION FACTORS

EQUINE NUTRITIONAL REQUIREMENTS TABLES

Appendix Table 1. Dietary Energy, Protein, Calcium, and Phosphorus Recommended in the Horse's Diet Dry Matter and Expected Amount of Air-Dry Feed Consumed

Appendix Table 2. Mineral Minimum and Upper Safe Concentrations Recommended in the Horse's Diet as Compared to Those Present in Feeds

Appendix Table 3. Vitamin Minimum and Upper Safe Concentrations Recommended in the Horse's Diet as Compared to Those Present in Feeds

Appendix Table 4. Daily Digestible Energy, Protein, Calcium, Phosphorus, and Vitamin A Recommended for Horses

Appendix Table 4-200. Daily Nutrient Requirements of Ponies (440 lb, or 200 kg, mature weight)

Appendix Table 4-400. Daily Nutrient Requirements of Horses (880 lb, or 400 kg, mature weight)

Appendix Table 4-500. Daily Nutrient Requirements of Horses (1100 lb, or 500 kg, mature weight)

Appendix Table 4-600. Daily Nutrient Requirements of Horses (1320 lb, or 600 kg, mature weight)

Appendix Table 4-700. Daily Nutrient Requirements of Horses (1540 lb, or 700 kg, mature weight)

Appendix Table 4-800. Daily Nutrient Requirements of Horses (1760 lb, or 800 kg, mature weight)

Appendix Table 4-900. Daily Nutrient Requirements of Horses (1980 lb, or 900 kb, mature weight)

Appendix Table 5. Digestible Energy Requirements for Physical Activity

FEED TABLES

Appendix Table 6. Nutrient Content of Horse Feeds

Appendix Table 7. Mineral Supplements Composition

Appendix Table 8. Feeds — Weight/Unit Volume

MISCELLANEOUS TABLES

Appendix Table 9. Conversion Factors

Appendix Table 10. Symbols, Weights, and Valences of Common Elements

APPENDIX TABLE 1
Dietary Energy, Protein, Calcium, and Phosphorus Recommended in the Horse's Diet Dry Matter and Expected Amount of Air-Dry Feed Consumed

Class of Horse	Digestible Energy-Mcal/lb (kg)	Max Grain in Diet–%	Crude Protein–%	Calcium–%	Phosphorus–%	Expected Feed Eaten–% of Body Wt/Day
Mature horses						
Maintenance	0.9 (2.0)	50	8	0.25	0.20	1.5–2.0
Working horses						
Light work[a]	1.15 (2.45)	50	10	0.3	0.25	1.5–2.5
Moderate work[a]	1.2 (2.65)	50	10.5	0.3	0.25	1.75–2.5
Intense work[a]	1.3 (2.85)	65	11.5	0.35	0.25	2.0–3.0
Stallions in breeding season	1.1 (2.4)	50	10	0.3	0.25	1.5–2.5
Pregnant mares						
First 9 months	0.9 (2.0)	50	8	0.25	0.20	1.5–2.0
9th & 10th months	1.0 (2.25)	50	10	0.5	0.35	1.5–2.0
11th month	1.1 (2.4)	50	11	0.5	0.35	1.5–2.0
Lactating mares						
First 3 months	1.2 (2.6)	50	13	0.5	0.35	2.5–3.0
3rd month on	1.1 (2.45)	50	11	0.35	0.25	2.0–2.5
Growing horses						
Nursing foal at 2 to 4 months, needs above milk	1.5–1.7 (3.3–3.8)	70	16	0.9[b]	0.6[b]	0.5–0.75[c]
Weanling at 4 months	1.3 (2.9)	70	14.5	0.8[b]	0.5[b]	2.5–3.5
Weanling at 6 months	1.3 (2.9)	70	14.5	0.7[b]	0.4[b]	2.5–3.5
Yearlings at 12 months	1.25 (2.8)	60	12.5	0.5[b]	0.3[b]	2.0–3.0
Long yearling at 18 months	1.2 (2.65)	50	12	0.4[b]	0.25[b]	2.0–2.75
Two-year-old at 24 months	1.15 (2.5)	50	11	0.35	0.20	2.0–2.5

[a] Examples are: light work = Western and English pleasure riding, bridle path riding, and equitation; moderate work = ranch work, roping, cutting, barrel racing, and jumping; intense work = race training and polo.
[b] Amounts of calcium and phosphorus are about 15% more than recommended by the National Research Council (NRC) because the amount necessary to maximize bone strength and ash content is higher than that required to maximize growth rate, and because the incidence of developmental orthopedic diseases has been reported to be lower with higher amounts.
[c] Amount recommended of creep feed consisting entirely of a grain-mix.

APPENDIX TABLE 2
Mineral Minimum and Upper Safe Concentrations Recommended in the Horse's Diet as Compared to Those Present in Feeds

Mineral	Amount in Total Diet Dry Matter		Amount Commonly Present in Dry Matter of		
	Minimum	Upper Safe	Alfalfa	Grasses	Grains
Major minerals–%:					
Calcium	0.8 to 0.3[a]	2[b]	0.8–2.0	0.2–0.5	0.02–0.10
Phosphorus	0.5 to 0.2[c]	1[d]	0.1–0.45	0.1–0.4	0.25–0.35
Sodium	0.1[e]	3[f]	0.03–0.25	0.01–0.25	0.01–0.1
Potassium	0.4[g]		1–4	0.5–3.5	0.2–0.7
Magnesium	0.1		0.15–0.6	0.05–0.5	0.1–0.2
Sulfur	0.15	1.25	0.2–0.5	0.1–0.35	0.1–0.25
Trace minerals–ppm (mg/kg):					
Selenium	0.1 & 0.2[h]	2–5	0.02–0.9	0.02–0.2	0.01–0.5
Iodine	0.1	5	0.1–0.2		0.05–0.15
Copper	7 or 25[i]	800	2–30	0.5–30	4–11
Zinc	15, 40 or 60[j]	500[k]	2–50	2–50	10–50
Manganese	20[l]	1000	5–50	5–60	10–50[m]
Iron	50	2000[n]	30–1200	30–300	20–110
Cobalt	0.05	10	0.1–0.6	0.1–0.6	0.05–0.25
Molybdenum	0.1	20	0.2–8[o]	0.1–4[o]	0.5–1.5
Aluminum	—	1500	< 50[p]	< 50[p]	
Fluoride		40	2–16[q]	2–16[q]	1–3
Lead		30			

[a] 0.8, 0.7, 0.5, and 0.4% at 4, 6, 12, and 18 mo of age, respectively; 0.5% for mares 3 mo before and after foaling; and 0.3% for other horses. The amounts for young horses are 15 to 20% higher than the minimum recommended by the National Research Council (NRC) because of studies suggesting higher amounts may increase bone strength and ash content and decrease developmental orthopedic diseases.

[b] In addition, calcium should not be more than 3 times the amount of phosphorus in the growing horse's diet or 6 times that in the mature horse's diet.

[c] 0.5, 0.4, 0.3, and 0.25% at 4, 6, 12, and 18 mo of age, respectively; 0.3% for mares 3 mo before and after foaling; and 0.2% for other horses. The amounts for young horses are 15 to 20% higher than the minimum recommended by the National Research Council (NRC) because of studies suggesting higher levels may increase bone strength and ash content, and decrease developmental orthopedic diseases.

[d] In addition, never more phosphorus than the amount of calcium.

[e] As sodium chloride (common salt). Increase to 0.3% if frequent sweating occurs.

[f] If sufficient non-saline-containing water is always easily available, much higher levels of sodium are not harmful, but they will limit the amount of that feed consumed.

[g] Increase to 0.6% in high energy-dense diets for horses with frequent excessive sweating.

[h] 0.2 ppm selenium is recommended in the last trimester of pregnancy, during lactation, for the foal, and for the horse in use and training for athletic performance.

[i] 7 ppm copper is recommended for mature horses, although no detrimental effects were observed in ponies fed 3.5 ppm, and the National Research Council (NRC) recommends 10 ppm for all mature and growing horses. However, 25 ppm is recommended for rapid growth from 2 to 10 mo of age, and 50 ppm is recommended in creep feeds because of studies suggesting that lower concentrations, while not affecting growth rate, may result in developmental orthopedic diseases, and therefore these higher levels may be beneficial in decreasing the risk of these diseases without any risk of harm.

[j] The National Research Council (NRC) recommends 40 ppm for all horses, based on studies showing that 4 ppm is inadequate and that 40 ppm is adequate. However, 17 ppm has been shown to be adequate during pregnancy and lactation. In addition, horse feeds frequently contain as low as 15 ppm zinc, and a naturally occurring zinc deficiency has not been reported in mature horses, nor has any benefit from adding additional zinc to their diet. Thus, 15 ppm appears to be adequate for mature horses. Although 40 ppm or even less is probably adequate for the young horse, some studies suggest that higher levels may decrease the incidence of cartilage defects and developmental orthopedic diseases. Because of this, 60 ppm is recommended for foals and 40 ppm for yearlings.

[k] Although levels of 9000 ppm zinc may be required to cause zinc toxicosis, levels as low as 500 ppm in the young horse's diet may result in developmental orthopedic diseases.

[l] The amount of manganese required isn't known. A deficiency from inadequate dietary manganese hasn't been reported or known to occur in horses. It is not uncommon for their feeds to contain less than 20 ppm. Thus, it would seem that 20 ppm is adequate, although the National Research Council (NRC) recommends twice this amount based upon data from other species.

[m] Except corn, which contains 3–9 ppm manganese.

[n] Much lower concentrations of iron are toxic to neonatal foals, with 8 mg/kg body wt (which is equivalent to 250 to 300 ppm or mg of iron/kg of total diet dry matter) causing death in 1-day-old foals and non-fatal illness in 3-day-old foals.

[o] Levels as high as 231 ppm have been reported in plants growing on soils industrially contaminated with molybdenum or containing naturally high levels of molybdenum.

[p] On high-aluminum acidic soils, forage may contain as much as 2500 ppm aluminum.

[q] May be higher if contaminated by fluoride-bearing dusts, fumes, or water.

APPENDIX TABLE 3

Vitamin Minimum and Upper Safe Concentrations Recommended in the Horse's Diet as Compared to Those Present in Feeds

Vitamin	Amount/kg[a] in Total Diet Dry Matter			Amount/kg[a] Commonly Present in Dry Matter of Average- or Better-Quality Feeds				
	Minimum for		Upper Safe Level[b]	Growing Forage	Alfalfa Hay	Grass Hay	Cereal Grains	Brewers' Yeast
	Maintenance	Other						
A-1000 IU	2	3	16	100–200[c]	5–75[c]	4–24[c]	1[c]	
D-IU	300[d]	800[d]	2200	200	2000	2000		
E-IU	50	100	1000	100–450[e]	10–80[e]	10–60[e]	5–30[e]	2–2.5[d]
K-mg	[f]	[g]						
Thiamin (B_1)-mg	3	5			3–4[h]		4–7	50–140
Riboflavin (B_2)-mg	2	2			5–20[h]		1–3	20–50
Niacin-mg					15–60[h]		15–60[i]	400–550
Pantothenate-mg					10–40[h]		5–30[j]	40–130
Pyridoxine (B_6)-mg					3–9[h]		3–8	30–50
Biotin-mg					0.1–0.7[h]		0.1–0.4	1–1.3
Folacin-mg				1.5–5	0.5–1	0.5–1	0.3–0.6	8–13
B_{12}-μg					11[h]		< 1	0.8–1.4
Choline-g					1–2[h]		0.5–1.2	3.5–4.8

[a] For the amount/lb divide the value given by 2.2. For the amount in parts per million (ppm) it is the same as that given in mg/kg, i.e., ppm = mg/kg. For conversion to other units see Appendix Table 9.

[b] The upper safe level is less than the amount above which toxicosis occurs. It is an amount that with prolonged continuous consumption would not be expected to cause any clinically or laboratory detectable alteration that if continued might lead to a detrimental effect.

[c] As beta-carotene with 1 mg = 400 IU of vitamin A. Beta-carotene, and therefore plants high in it, does not cause vitamin A toxicosis. Toxicosis is caused only by preformed vitamin A.

[d] Amount recommended for horses not exposed to sunlight. None is needed by those exposed to several hours of sunlight daily.

[e] Primarily as alpha-tocopherol with 1 mg = 1.49 IU of vitamin E. In 40 hays from various states, 50% contained less than 50 IU/kg and 15% over 80 IU/kg.

[f] A blank indicates there is no known requirement or upper safe level known.

[g] Natural forms of vitamin K (K_1 and K_2) are nontoxic. In contrast, parenteral administration of 2 to 8 mg of vitamin K_3 (menadione)/kg (1 to 3.6 mg/lb) of body wt may cause acute renal failure.

[h] Amount of most B vitamins are similar in different types of forages.

[i] Niacin in cereal grains is bound and may be unavailable for horses as it has been found to be for other animals.

[j] 30 in oats, 5 to 15 in other cereal grains.

APPENDIX TABLE 4
Daily Digestible Energy, Protein, Calcium, Phosphorus, and Vitamin A Recommended for Horses

Class of Horse	Daily Gain % of BW/d	Digestible Energy Mcal/horse/d	Crude Protein g/d	Calcium g/d	Phosphorus = g/d Ca ×	Vit A = IU × kg BW[a]
Mature Horse						
Maintenance for 500 kg (1100 lb) horse		16.4[b]	656[c]	20[d]	0.75	30
Working horses		Maintenance ×	Maintenance ×	Mcal DE/d ×		
Light work[e]		1.25	1.25	1.22	0.75	45
Moderate work[e]		1.50	1.50	1.22	0.75	45
Intensive work[e]		2.00	2.00	1.22	0.75	45
Stallions in breeding season		Maintenance ×	Maintenance ×	Mcal DE/d ×		
		1.25	1.25	1.22	0.75	45
Pregnant mares						
First 9 months same as Maintenance		Maintenance ×	Maintenance ×	Mcal DE/d ×		
9th month		1.11	1.22	1.9	0.75	60
10th month		1.13	1.24	1.9	0.75	60
11th month		1.20	1.32	1.9	0.75	60
Lactating mares		Maintenance ×	Maintenance ×	Maintenance ×		
First 3 months		1.8	2.3[f]	2.8	0.65	60
3rd month on		1.5	1.7[f]	1.8	0.65	60
Growing Horse		Mcal/100 kg BW[a]	Mcal DE/d ×	Mcal DE/d ×		
Weanling @ 4 months = 36 to 39% of expected mature wt[g]	0.5	8.5[h]	50	2.3	0.55	45
Weanling @ months = 44 to 47% of expected mature wt[g]						
Moderate growth	0.3	7	50	1.9	0.55	45
Rapid growth	0.4	8	50	2.0	0.55	45
Yearling @ 12 months = 63 to 67% of expected mature wt[g]						
Moderate growth	0.15	6	45	1.5	0.55	45
Rapid growth	0.20	6.7	45	1.6	0.55	45
Long yearling @ 18 months = 78 to 85% of expected mature wt[g]						
Not in training	0.1	5	42.5	1.35	0.55	45
In training	0.1	6.7	42.5	1.8	0.55	45
2-yr-old @ 24 months = 87 to 92% of expected mature wt[g]						
Not in training	0.04–0.06	4.2	42.5	1.25	0.55	45
In training	0.04–0.06	5.9	42.5	1.7	0.55	45

[a] BW = kg body weight (lbs ÷ 2.2)

[b] ± 3.0 Mcal/100 kg (220 lbs) of body weight above or below 500 kg (1100 lbs) up to 600 kg (1320 lbs), then 1.9, 1.6 and 1.2 Mcal for each successive 100 kg (220 lbs) of body weight above 600 kg (1320 lbs), e.g., a 900-kg (1980-lb) horse needs 16.4 + 3.0 + 1.9 + 1.6 + 1.2 = 24.1 Mcal/day.

[c] ± 120 g protein/100 kg (220 lbs) of body weight above or below 500 kg (1100 lbs) up to 600 kg (1320 lbs), then 76, 64, and 48 g for each successive 100 kg (220 lbs) of body weight above 600 kg (1320 lbs), e.g., a 900-kg (1980-lb) horse needs 656 + 120 + 76 + 64 + 48 = 964 g protein/day.

[d] ± 4 g calcium/100 kg (220 lbs) of body weight above or below 500 kg (1100 lbs).

[e] Examples are: light work = Western and English pleasure riding, bridle path riding, and equitation; moderate work = ranch work, roping, cutting, barrel racing, and jumping; and intense work = race training and polo.

[f] Protein needs are 2.6 and 1.9 times maintenance for lactating mares weighing 800 kg (1760 lbs) or more.

[g] See Table 15–2 for further information on expected size and growth rate of young horses.

[h] 9.5 Mcal/100 kg (220 lb) body wt for ponies (200 to 300 kg or 440 to 660 lb expected mature wt).

APPENDIX TABLE 4–200
Daily Nutrient Requirements of Ponies (440 lb, or 200 kg, mature weight)

Animal	Weight (kg)	Daily Gain (kg)	DE (Mcal)	Crude Protein (g)	Lysine (g)	Calcium (g)	Phosphorus (g)	Magnesium (g)	Potassium (g)	Vitamin A (1000 IU)
Mature Horses										
Maintenance	200		7.4	296	10	8	6	3.0	10.0	6
Stallions	200		9.3	370	13	11	8	4.3	14.1	9
(breeding season)										
Pregnant mares										
9 months	200		8.2	361	13	16	12	3.9	13.1	12
10 months			8.4	368	13	16	12	4.0	13.4	12
11 months			8.9	391	14	17	13	4.3	14.2	12
Lactating mares										
Foaling to 3 months	200		13.7	688	24	27	18	4.8	21.2	12
3 months to weaning	200		12.2	528	18	18	11	3.7	14.8	12
Working horses										
Light work[a]	200		9.3	370	13	11	8	4.3	14.1	9
Moderate work[b]	200		11.1	444	16	14	10	5.1	16.9	9
Intense work[c]	200		14.8	592	21	18	13	6.8	22.5	9
Growing Horses										
Weanling, 4 months	75	0.40	7.3	365	15	16	9	1.6	5.0	3
Weanling, 6 months										
Moderate growth	95	0.30	7.6	378	16	13	7	1.8	5.7	4
Rapid growth	95	0.40	8.7	433	18	17	9	1.9	6.0	4
Yearling, 12 months										
Moderate growth	140	0.20	8.7	392	17	12	7	2.4	7.6	6
Rapid growth	140	0.30	10.3	462	19	15	8	2.5	7.9	6
Long yearling, 18 months										
Not in training	170	0.10	8.3	375	16	10	6	2.7	8.8	8
In training	170	0.10	11.6	522	22	14	8	3.7	12.2	8
Two-year-old, 24 months										
Not in training	185	0.05	7.9	337	13	9	5	2.8	9.4	8
In training	185	0.05	11.4	485	19	13	7	4.1	13.5	8

APPENDIX TABLE 4–400
Daily Nutrient Requirements of Horses (880 lb, or 400 kg, mature weight)

Animal	Weight (kg)	Daily Gain (kg)	DE (Mcal)	Crude Protein (g)	Lysine (g)	Calcium (g)	Phosphorus (g)	Magnesium (g)	Potassium (g)	Vitamin A (1000 IU)
Mature Horses										
Maintenance	400		13.4	536	19	16	11	6.0	20.0	12
Stallions	400		16.8	670	23	20	15	7.7	25.5	18
(breeding season)										
Pregnant mares										
9 months	400		14.9	654	23	28	21	7.1	23.8	24
10 months			15.1	666	23	29	21	7.3	24.2	24
11 months			16.1	708	25	31	23	7.7	25.7	24
Lactating mares										
Foaling to 3 months	400		22.9	1,141	40	45	29	8.7	36.8	24
3 months to weaning	400		19.7	839	29	29	18	6.9	26.4	24
Working horses										
Light work[a]	400		16.8	670	23	20	15	7.7	25.5	18
Moderate work[b]	400		20.1	804	28	25	17	9.2	30.6	18
Intense work[c]	400		26.8	1,072	38	33	23	12.3	40.7	18
Growing Horses										
Weanling, 4 months	145	0.85	13.5	675	28	33	18	3.2	9.8	7
Weanling, 6 months										
Moderate growth	180	0.55	12.9	643	27	25	14	3.4	10.7	8
Rapid growth	180	0.70	14.5	725	30	30	16	3.6	11.1	8
Yearling, 12 months										
Moderate growth	265	0.40	15.6	700	30	23	13	4.5	14.5	12
Rapid growth	265	0.50	17.1	770	33	27	15	4.6	14.8	12
Long yearling, 18 months										
Not in training	330	0.25	15.9	716	30	21	12	5.3	17.3	15
In training	330	0.25	21.6	970	41	29	16	7.1	23.4	15
Two-year-old, 24 months										
Not in training	365	0.15	15.3	650	26	19	11	5.7	18.7	16
In training	365	0.15	21.5	913	37	27	15	7.9	26.2	16

APPENDIX TABLE 4–500
Daily Nutrient Requirements of Horses (1100 lb, or 500 kg, mature weight)

Animal	Weight (kg)	Daily Gain (kg)	DE (Mcal)	Crude Protein (g)	Lysine (g)	Calcium (g)	Phosphorus (g)	Magnesium (g)	Potassium (g)	Vitamin A (1000 IU)
Mature Horses										
Maintenance	500		16.4	656	23	20	14	7.5	25.0	15
Stallions	500		20.5	820	29	25	18	9.4	31.2	22
(breeding season)										
Pregnant mares										
9 months	500		18.2	801	28	35	26	8.7	29.1	30
10 months			18.5	815	29	35	26	8.9	29.7	30
11 months			19.7	866	30	37	28	9.4	31.5	30
Lactating mares										
Foaling to 3 months	500		28.3	1,427	50	56	36	10.9	46.0	30
3 months to weaning	500		24.3	1,048	37	36	22	8.6	33.0	30
Working horses										
Light work[a]	500		20.5	820	29	25	18	9.4	31.2	22
Moderate work[b]	500		24.6	984	34	30	21	11.3	37.4	22
Intense work[c]	500		32.8	1,312	46	40	29	15.1	49.9	22
Growing Horses										
Weanling, 4 months	175	0.85	14.4	720	30	34	19	3.7	11.3	8
Weanling, 6 months										
Moderate growth	215	0.65	15.0	750	32	29	16	4.0	12.7	10
Rapid growth	215	0.85	17.2	860	36	36	20	4.3	13.3	10
Yearling, 12 months										
Moderate growth	325	0.50	18.9	851	36	29	16	5.5	17.8	15
Rapid growth	325	0.65	21.3	956	40	34	19	5.7	18.2	15
Long yearling, 18 months										
Not in training	400	0.35	19.8	893	38	27	15	6.4	21.1	18
In training	400	0.35	26.5	1,195	50	36	20	8.6	28.2	18
Two-year-old, 24 months										
Not in training	450	0.20	18.8	800	32	24	13	7.0	23.1	20
In training	450	0.20	26.3	1,117	45	34	19	9.8	32.2	20

APPENDIX TABLE 4–600
Daily Nutrient Requirements of Horses (1320 lb, or 600 kg, mature weight)

Animal	Weight (kg)	Daily Gain (kg)	DE (Mcal)	Crude Protein (g)	Lysine (g)	Calcium (g)	Phosphorus (g)	Magnesium (g)	Potassium (g)	Vitamin A (1000 IU)
Mature Horses										
Maintenance	600		19.4	776	27	24	17	9.0	30.0	18
Stallions	600		24.3	970	34	30	21	11.2	36.9	27
(breeding season)										
Pregnant mares										
9 months	600		21.5	947	33	41	30	10.3	34.5	36
10 months			21.9	965	34	42	31	10.5	35.1	36
11 months			23.3	1,024	36	44	33	11.2	37.2	36
Lactating mares										
Foaling to 3 months	600		33.7	1,711	60	67	43	13.1	55.2	36
3 months to weaning	600		28.9	1,258	44	43	27	10.4	39.6	36
Working horses										
Light work[a]	600		24.3	970	34	30	21	11.2	36.9	27
Moderate work[b]	600		29.1	1,164	41	36	25	13.4	44.2	27
Intense work[c]	600		38.8	1,552	54	47	34	17.8	59.0	27
Growing Horses										
Weanling, 4 months	200	1.00	16.5	825	35	40	22	4.3	13.0	9
Weanling, 6 months										
Moderate growth	245	0.75	17.0	850	36	34	19	4.6	14.5	11
Rapid growth	245	0.95	19.2	960	40	40	22	4.9	15.1	11
Yearling, 12 months										
Moderate growth	375	0.65	22.7	1,023	43	36	20	6.4	20.7	17
Rapid growth	375	0.80	25.1	1,127	48	41	22	6.6	21.2	17
Long yearling, 18 months										
Not in training	475	0.45	23.9	1,077	45	33	18	7.7	25.1	21
In training	475	0.45	32.0	1,429	60	44	24	10.2	33.3	21
Two-year-old, 24 months										
Not in training	540	0.30	23.5	998	40	31	17	8.5	27.9	24
In training	540	0.30	32.3	1,372	55	43	24	11.6	38.4	24

APPENDIX TABLE 4–700
Daily Nutrient Requirements of Horses (1540 lb, or 700 kg, mature weight)

Animal	Weight (kg)	Daily Gain (kg)	DE (Mcal)	Crude Protein (g)	Lysine (g)	Calcium (g)	Phosphorus (g)	Magnesium (g)	Potassium (g)	Vitamin A (1000 IU)
Mature Horses										
Maintenance	700		21.3	851	30	28	20	10.5	35.0	21
Stallions	700		26.6	1,064	37	32	23	12.2	40.4	32
(breeding season)										
Pregnant mares										
9 months	700		23.6	1,039	36	45	33	11.3	37.8	42
10 months			24.0	1,058	37	46	34	11.5	38.5	42
11 months			25.5	1,124	39	49	35	12.3	40.9	42
Lactating mares										
Foaling to 3 months	700		37.9	1,997	70	78	51	15.2	64.4	42
3 months to weaning	700		32.4	1,468	51	50	31	12.1	46.2	42
Working horses										
Light work[a]	700		26.6	1,064	37	32	23	12.2	40.4	32
Moderate work[b]	700		31.9	1,277	45	39	28	14.7	48.5	32
Intense work[c]	700		42.6	1,702	60	52	37	19.6	64.7	
Growing Horses										
Weanling, 4 months	225	1.10	19.7[d]	986	41	44	25	4.8	14.6	10
Weanling, 6 months										
Moderate growth	275	0.80	20.0[d]	1,001	42	37	20	5.1	16.2	12
Rapid growth	275	1.00	22.2[d]	1,111	47	43	24	5.4	16.8	12
Yearling, 12 months										
Moderate growth	420	0.70	26.1[d]	1,176	50	39	22	7.2	23.1	19
Rapid growth	420	0.85	28.5[d]	1,281	54	44	24	7.4	23.6	19
Long yearling, 18 months										
Not in training	525	0.50	27.0	1,215	51	37	20	8.5	27.8	24
In training	525	0.50	36.0	1,615	68	49	27	11.3	36.9	24
Two-year-old, 24 months										
Not in training	600	0.35	26.3	1,117	45	35	19	9.4	31.1	27
In training	600	0.35	36.0	1,529	61	48	27	12.9	42.5	27

APPENDIX TABLE 4–800
Daily Nutrient Requirements of Horses (1760 lb, or 800 kg, mature weight)

Animal	Weight (kg)	Daily Gain (kg)	DE (Mcal)	Crude Protein (g)	Lysine (g)	Calcium (g)	Phosphorus (g)	Magnesium (g)	Potassium (g)	Vitamin A (1000 IU)
Mature Horses										
Maintenance	800		22.9	914	32	32	22	12.0	40.0	24
Stallions	800		28.6	1,143	40	35	25	13.1	43.4	36
(breeding season)										
Pregnant mares										
9 months	800		25.4	1,116	39	48	36	12.2	40.6	48
10 months			25.8	1,137	40	49	36	12.4	41.3	48
11 months			27.4	1,207	42	52	39	13.2	43.9	48
Lactating mares										
Foaling to 3 months	800		41.9	2,282	81	90	58	17.4	73.6	48
3 months to weaning	800		35.5	1,678	60	58	36	13.8	52.8	48
Working horses										
Light work[a]	800		28.6	1,143	40	35	25	13.1	43.4	36
Moderate work[b]	800		34.3	1,372	48	42	30	15.8	52.1	36
Intense work[c]	800		45.7	1,829	64	56	40	21.0	69.5	36
Growing Horses										
Weanling, 4 months	250	1.20	21.4[d]	1,070	45	48	27	5.3	16.1	11
Weanling, 6 months										
Moderate growth	305	0.90	22.0[d]	1,100	46	41	23	5.7	18.0	14
Rapid growth	305	1.10	24.2[d]	1,210	51	47	26	6.0	18.6	14
Yearling, 12 months										
Moderate growth	460	0.80	28.7[d]	1,291	55	44	24	7.9	25.4	21
Rapid growth	460	0.95	31.0[d]	1,396	59	49	27	8.1	25.9	21
Long yearling, 18 months										
Not in training	590	0.60	30.2	1,361	57	43	24	9.6	31.3	27
In training	590	0.60	39.8	1,793	76	56	31	12.6	41.2	27
Two-year-old, 24 months										
Not in training	675	0.40	28.7	1,220	49	40	22	10.6	35.0	30
In training	675	0.40	39.1	1,662	66	54	30	14.5	47.6	30

APPENDIX TABLE 4–900
Daily Nutrient Requirements of Horses (1980 lb, or 900 kg, mature weight)

Animal	Weight (kg)	Daily Gain (kg)	DE (Mcal)	Crude Protein (g)	Lysine (g)	Calcium (g)	Phosphorus (g)	Magnesium (g)	Potassium (g)	Vitamin A (1000 IU)
Mature Horses										
Maintenance	900		24.1	966	34	36	25	13.5	45.0	27
Stallions (breeding season)	900		30.2	1,207	42	37	26	13.9	45.9	40
Pregnant mares										
9 months	900		26.8	1,179	41	51	38	12.9	42.9	54
10 months			27.3	1,200	42	52	38	13.1	43.6	54
11 months			29.0	1,275	45	55	41	13.9	46.3	54
Lactating mares										
Foaling to 3 months	900		45.5	2,567	89	101	65	19.6	82.8	54
3 months to weaning	900		38.4	1,887	66	65	40	15.5	59.4	54
Working horses										
Light work[a]	900		30.2	1,207	42	37	26	13.9	45.9	40
Moderate work[b]	900		36.2	1,448	51	44	32	16.7	55.0	40
Intense work[c]	900		48.3	1,931	68	59	42	22.2	73.4	40
Growing Horses										
Weanling, 4 months	275	1.30	23.1[d]	1,154	48	53	29	5.8	17.7	12
Weanling, 6 months										
Moderate growth	335	0.95	23.4[d]	1,171	49	44	24	6.2	19.6	15
Rapid growth	335	1.15	25.6[d]	1,281	54	50	28	6.5	20.2	15
Yearling, 12 months										
Moderate growth	500	0.90	31.2[d]	1,404	59	49	27	8.6	27.7	22
Rapid growth	500	1.05	33.5[d]	1,509	64	54	30	8.8	28.2	22
Long yearling, 18 months										
Not in training	665	0.70	33.6	1,510	64	49	27	10.9	35.4	30
In training	665	0.70	43.9	1,975	83	64	35	14.2	46.2	30
Two-year-old, 24 months										
Not in training	760	0.45	31.1	1,322	53	45	25	12.0	39.4	34
In training	760	0.45	42.2	1,795	72	61	34	16.2	53.4	34

NOTE: Mares should gain weight during late gestation to compensate for tissue deposition. However, nutrient requirements are based on maintenance body weight.
[a] Examples are horses used in Western and English pleasure riding, bridle path hack, equitation, etc.
[b] Examples are horses used in ranch work, roping, cutting, barrel racing, jumping, etc.
[c] Examples are horses in race training, polo, etc.
[d] These values may be too high, as in one study 6- to 8-mo-old weanlings with an expected mature weight of 1540 lb (700 kg), consuming 17 Mcal/day, gained 2.5 lb/day (1.15 kg/d) and those 10- to 12-mo old consuming 25 Mcal/day gained 3.06 lb/day (1.39 kg/d).

APPENDIX TABLE 5
Digestible Energy Requirements for Physical Activity (Above That Needed at Rest)[a]

Physical Activity	Slow Walk	Fast Walk	Slow Trot	Endurance Racing Med. Trot/Slow Lope	Endurance Racing Fast Trot/Lope	Cantering, Galloping, Jumping	Strenuous Effort—Polo, Running
Speed							
meters/min	60	100	200	250	300	350–400	500–1000
miles/hr	2.2	3.7	7.5	9.3	11.2	13–15	19–37
Min:sec/mile	27:00	16:00	8:00	6:30	5:20	4–4:40	1:35–3:10
Mcal DE/Hr/100 kg (220 lb) total wt	0.17	0.25	0.6	1.0	1.3	2.0	3.9

[a] These requirements are up to 40% higher for horses in poor physical condition and the shorter the duration of the activity. For example, in one study the Mcal/hr/100 kg needed to gallop at 440 m (481 yds)/min for 2.8 km (1.75 miles) was 10.1 for unconditioned horses; after conditioning, the need was reduced to 7.3 for 2.8 km (1.75 miles) and 4.2 for 11.2 km (7 miles).

Requirements for Thoroughbreds and Standardbreds in intense race training and/or use are higher than would be determined from the values in this table, plus those for maintenance (Appendix Table 4). Thoroughbred race horses in training in the United States may need 32 to 37 Mcal DE/day. It's reported that in Britain during intense training and/or racing, as high as 50 Mcal/day is fed, while during early training 38 Mcal/day is fed. The lower requirement for horses in the United States is due to their lesser work per day compared to what is required of horses in Britain. In Standardbreds the daily requirement for training is about 37 Mcal/day.

Example calculation of energy needs: A 500-kg (1100-lb) horse carrying 80 kg (175 lb) at a slow trot for 3 hr daily would need (580 kg) × (0.6 Mcal/hr/100 kg body wt from this table) × (3 hr) = 10.4 Mcal for physical activity plus 16.4 Mcal for maintenance (Appendix Table 4–500) for a total of 26.8 Mcal/day. The amount of feed necessary to provide this amount of digestible energy would be 26.8 Mcal ÷ the Mcal provided by the feed consumed; e.g., 13.4 kg (29.5 lb) of full-bloom alfalfa hay [26.8 Mcal ÷ (2.2 Mcal/kg DM × 0.91 DM from Appendix Table 6)] = 13.4 kg as fed. An alternative would be to continue feeding the amount of feed that has been fed for maintenance and feed grain for the physical activity. If corn was fed, about 3 kg (6.7 lb) would be needed, [10.4 Mcal needed for physical activity as determined from this table) ÷ (3.85 Mcal/kg DM × 0.88 DM from Appendix Table 6) = 3.07 kg as fed].

APPENDIX TABLE 6
Nutrient Content of Horse Feeds[aa]

Feed	Dry Matter (DM)–%	Dig. Energy Mcal/lb (kg) DM	% in Feed Dry Matter				
			Crude Protein	Crude Fiber	Acid Detergent Fiber	Calcium	Phosphorus
Alfalfa (lucerne)–*Medicago sativa*							
grazed, late vegetative	23	1.3 (2.9)	22	24	24	1.7	0.3
grazed, full bloom	24	1.0 (2.3)	19	30	36	1.2	0.25
hay, early bloom	90	1.1 (2.5)	20	23	32	1.4	0.3
hay, full bloom	91	1.0 (2.2)	17	30	39	1.2	0.25
meal, dehydrated 17%	92	1.1 (2.4)	19	26	34	1.5	0.25
meal, dehydrated 15%	90	1.0 (2.2)	17	29	38	1.4	0.25
Almond Hulls	90	1.1 (2.4)	4–6	11–12		0.23	0.11
Apple Pomace–*Malus* spp.	90	1.3 (2.8)	5	10–16	20–26	0.1	0.15
Barley–*Hordeum vulgare*							
grain	89	1.67 (3.7)[a]	13	6	8	0.05	0.38
hay	88	0.92 (2.0)	9	27	–	0.24	0.28
straw	91	0.73 (1.6)	4	41.5	49	0.30	0.07
Beet, sugar–*Beta vulgaris altissima*							
pulp, dehydrated	91	1.2 (2.6)	10	20	27.5	0.7	0.1
Bran–see wheat or rice							
Brewers' Grains	92	1.2 (2.7)	25–28	15	24	0.33	0.55
Canola (double low rapeseed)–*Brassica napus* and *B. campestris*							
seeds, nonextracted	90	1.6 (3.6)	20	6	–	0.38	0.75
seed, meal	90	1.4 (3.1)	35–44	10–13	17	0.8	0.40
Carrots–*Daucus* spp.	12	1.7 (3.8)	10	9.5	11	0.40	0.35
Cereal Grains–see also specific grain							
grazed, early, vegetative	16–34	1.3 (2.9)	16–32	17–25	–	0.3–0.5	0.25–0.45
hays	89	0.9 (1.95)	9	30	40	0.15–0.3	0.2–0.3
straw	92	0.7 (1.5)	3–4.5	40–42	49	0.15–0.3	0.05–0.10
Citrus–Grapefruit, lemon, or orange							
pomace	91	1.3 (2.3)	6.5–9	10–16	20–26	0.7–2	0.12–0.2
Clovers							
grazed, early veg[b]	19–26	1.45 (3.2)	22	–	20	1–2	0.2–0.35
grazed, early bloom[b]	19–26	1.14 (2.5)	21–26	14–23	21–35	1–2	0.2–0.35
grazed, late bloom[b]	19–26	1.0 (2.25)	14.5	26	35	1–2	0.25–0.35
hay, *Trifolium* spp.[c]	89	0.85–1 (1.9–2.2)	14–22	21–31	32–36	1–2	0.23–0.33
hay, Alyce	90	0.83 (1.83)	12	40	–		
hay, sweet	89	0.88 (1.93)	14	36	–	1.3	0.25
Coconut–*Cocos nucifera*							
copra meal	92	1.3 (2.8)	23	15	–	0.2	0.65
Corn (Maize)–*Zea mays*							
grain	88	1.7 (3.85)[a]	8–10	2.5	4	0.05	0.3
cobs, ground	90	0.62 (1.36)	3	35	40	0.12	0.04
ears only	86	1.5 (3.3)	9	9.5	11	0.07	0.27
fodder (includes ears)	81	0.94 (2.06)	7–9	25–32	25–32	0.50	0.25
stover (no ears)	88	0.8 (1.7)	4–7	35–38	50–56	0.50	0.10
silage	25–35	1.22 (2.68)	8	24	28	0.3	0.23
gluten meal	91	1.4 (3.0)	47	5	–	0.16	0.5
Cottonseed–*Gossypium* spp.							
meal–41%	91	1.4 (3.0)	45	13	19	0.18	1.2
seeds, nonextracted	92	1.7 (3.7)	24	18–20		0.15	0.7
hulls	90	0.6 (1.3)	4	47	59	0.15	0.2
Distillers'							
grain	94	1.2 (2.6)	29–34	12–13	–	0.1–0.15	0.3–0.6
solubles	92	1.4 (3.1)	22–30	5–6	–	0.3–0.4	1.3–1.4
Emmer–*Triticum dicoccum*							
grain	91	1.2 (2.7)[a]	11–12	9–10	–	0.06	0.40
Fat, animal	99	3.6 (7.94)	0	0	0	0	0
Fish Meal							
anchovy	92	1.36 (3.0)	65–75	1	–	4.0	2.7
menhaden	92	1.4 (3.1)	60–70	1	–	5.6	3.2
white	92	1.5 (3.3)	60–70	1	–	8	3.9
Flax (Linseed)–*Linum usitatissimum*							
meal–37%	92	1.4 (3.0)	40	9	–	0.4	0.9
seeds	94	1.6 (3.6)	23	6.5	–	0.25	0.6

Fruit–see apple or citrus (grapefruit, orange, and lemon)
Gluten Meal–see corn and wheat
Grains–see brewers', distillers', cereal grain, hay and straw, and specific grain

(continued)

APPENDIX TABLE 6
Nutrient Content of Horse Feeds[aa]–(Continued)

Feed	Dry Matter (DM)–%	Dig. Energy Mcal/lb (kg) DM	% in Feed Dry Matter				
			Crude Protein	Crude Fiber	Acid Detergent Fiber	Calcium	Phosphorus
Grasses[d]							
grazed, growing[e]	27 (23–31)	0.9–1.1 (2.0–2.4)	11 (9–13)	31.5 (28–34)	33 (31–37)	0.35 (0.25–0.45)	0.28 (0.22–0.3)
grazed, growing[f]	27 (23–31)	0.95–1.15 (2.1–2.5)	18 (15–21)	23 (21–25)	34 (31–37)	0.5 (0.35–0.65)	0.4 (0.33–0.45)
grazed, mature[g]	40–55	0.7–0.8 (1.6–1.8)	6–10	30–35	–	0.2–0.3	0.15–0.25
hay, early growth[g]	90.5 (86–95)	0.8–1 (1.8–2.2)	11 (8–12)	32 (31–34)	38 (35–41)	0.45 (0.3–0.6)	0.26 (0.2–0.35)
hay, late growth[g]	90.5 (86–95)	0.7–0.9 (1.5–2.0)	7.7 (6–9)	33 (31–35)	40 (36–45)	0.3 (0.25–0.4)	0.22 (0.15–0.3)
Hulls–see specific type							
Lespedeza–Lespedeza striata							
grazed, late vegetative	25	1.0 (2.2)	16	24	–	1.2	0.28
hay, midbloom	91	0.95 (2.1)	10–13	28–30	–	1.2	0.2–0.35
Linseed–see Flax							
Lucerne–see Alfalfa							
Lupine–Sweet Yellow–Lupinus spp.							
seeds	89	1.7 (3.7)	45	16	–	0.26	0.44
hay	90	1.2 (2.7)	20	25	–	1–2	0.25
Maize–see corn							
Manure, poultry, no litter	90	1.0 (2.3)	25–28	10–16	–	6–9	2–3
Milk							
cows, skimmed	94	1.7 (3.8)	35.6	0.3	–	1.36	1.1
cows, whole	96	2.55 (5.6)	25–27	0.2	–	0.95	0.76
horse, fresh–see Table 15–4							
Millet–Setaria spp. or Panicum miliaceum (Broomcorn).							
grain	90	1.5 (3.3)[a]	11–14	6–9	–	0.06	0.3
Millet Pearl–Pennisetum glaucum							
grazed	21	0.77 (1.7)	10	31	–		
hay	87	0.7 (1.5)	8	37	–	0.3	0.2
Milo–see sorghum							
Molasses							
sugar beet	78	1.55 (3.4)	2–6[h]	0–0.5	0	0.15	0.03
sugar cane	74	1.6 (3.5)	2–6[h]	0–0.5	0	0.9–2	0.1–0.3
sugar cane, dehydrated	94	1.55 (3.4)	2–6[h]	5–10		0.9–2	0.1–0.3
Oats–Avena sativa							
grain, regular	90	1.45 (3.2)[a]	10–13	11–12	16	0.1	0.35
grain, heavy	90	1.55 (3.4)[a]	14	12	–	0.06	0.35
grain, hulless (groats)	90	1.85 (4.1)[a]	18	3	–	0.01	0.47
hay	91	0.87 (1.92)	9.5	32	38	0.3	0.25
hulls	92	0.7 (1.5)	4–6	33–36	40–44	0.15	0.1
straw	92	0.74 (1.62)	4.4	40	48	0.23	0.06
Oil, vegetable	100	4.08 (9.00)	0	0	0	0	0
Peas, Pisum spp.							
seeds	89	1.57 (3.45)	26	6	9	0.14	0.46
Peanut–Arachis hypogaea							
hay	91	0.87 (1.91)	11	33	41	1.23	0.16
hull (pods)	91	0.44 (0.97)	8	63	69	0.26	0.07
seed meal–47%	92	1.5 (3.25)	53	8.5	–	0.3	0.65
Potatoes, Irish–Solanum tuberosum							
tubers, fresh	22	1.5 (3.3)	9.5	2.5–3	–	0.04	0.24
tubers, dehydrated	91	1.5 (3.3)	8.7	2	–	0.07	0.21
peelings, fresh	23	1.55 (3.4)	8.9	3	–	0.14	0.19
cannery residue, wet	12	1.4 (3.1)	9.5	14	–	0.33	0.67
cannery residue, dehydrated	89	1.7 (3.8)	8	6.5	–	0.10	0.28
Rice–Oryza sativa							
grain, ground	89	1.75 (3.8)	7–9	7–9	–	0.07	0.36
bran	91	1.3 (2.9)	14	13	20	0.1	1.5–1.7
hulls	92	0.24 (0.5)	3	43	72	0.12	0.07
mill run	92	0.3 (0.68)	7	31.5	–	0.17	0.50
Rye–Secale cereale							
grain	88	1.75 (3.85)[a]	14	2.5	4	0.07	0.36
Safflower–Carthamus tinctorius							
seeds	93	1.5 (3.3)	19.5	31	–	0.25	0.75
seed meal–42%	90	1.2 (2.7)	49	9	–	0.3	1.8

(continued)

APPENDIX TABLE 6
Nutrient Content of Horse Feeds[aa]–(Continued)

Feed	Dry Matter (DM)–%	Dig. Energy Mcal/lb (kg) DM	% in Feed Dry Matter				
			Crude Protein	Crude Fiber	Acid Detergent Fiber	Calcium	Phosphorus
Silage–see corn or sorghum							
Sorghum (milo)–*Sorghum vulgare* and *S. bicolor*							
grain	90	1.6 (3.55)[a]	12.7	2.8	9.3	0.04	0.36
fodder	87	0.83 (1.83)	8.5	28		0.7	0.2
silage	25–35	0.8 (1.75)	8–10	24–28	21–27	0.7	0.2
stover, no grain	85	0.75 (1.64)	5	33		0.5	0.1
Soybean–*Glycine max*							
meal–44%	89	1.6 (3.5)	50	7	10	0.4	0.7
seeds, nonextracted	90	1.6 (3.5)	33–43	4–6	6–8	0.2–0.3	0.6–0.8
hulls, seed coats	90	0.85 (1.85)	11–13	36–45	46–54	0.4–0.7	0.15–0.2
Spelt–*Triticum spelta*							
grain	90	1.5 (3.3)[a]	13	10	–	0.13	0.42
Straw–see cereal grains and specific grain							
Sunflower–*Helianthus annuus*							
seeds, with hulls	94	1.4 (3.1)	18	31	–	0.18	0.56
seed meal–44%	93	1.25 (2.8)	50	12	–	0.45	1.0
hulls	92	0.9 (2.0)	4–6	43–51	–	0.38	0.13
Trefoil, birdsfoot–*Lotus corniculatus*							
grazed	19	1.0 (2.2)	21	21	–	1.7	0.25
hay	91	1.0 (2.2)	16	32	36	1.5	0.2
Triticale–*Triticale hexaloide*							
grain	91	1.7 (3.75)[a]	16.5	4	–	0.06	0.33
Wheat–*Triticum aestivum*							
grain, soft red or white	90	1.75 (3.85)[a]	11–12	2–3	3	0.06	0.35
grain, hard red	88	1.75 (3.85)[a]	14–17	2–3	4	0.05	0.42
bran	89	1.5 (3.3)	16–17	10–12	13–15	0.14	1.27
gluten	89	1.5 (3.2)	56	6.7	–	0.2	0.6
grazed, early, vegetative	22	1.3 (2.9)	27–33	17	28	0.4	0.4
hay	89	0.86 (1.9)	8.5	29	41	0.15	0.20
mill run	90	1.57 (3.5)	17	9	11	0.1	1.1
straw	91	0.74 (1.6)	3.5	42	55	0.17	0.05
Whey							
cows	93	1.84 (4.06)	14	0.2	0	0.9	0.8
cows, low lactose	94	1.64 (3.6)	17	0.2	0	1.5	1.1
Yeast, Brewers'–*Saccharomyces*						–	
cerevisiae	93	1.5 (3.3)	47–51	3–7		0.15	1.47
Yeast, Torula–*Torulopsis utilis*	93	1.5 (3.3)	52.5	2.5	–	0.63	1.8

[aa] The nutrient content of cereal grains and protein supplements varies little from the values given. However, that for forages varies widely. The amount of each nutrient given may vary more than twofold in the same type of forage. Thus, the values given are approximations only and, particularly for forages, should be determined by laboratory analysis of the actual feed being used.

[a] For horses these values for oats, corn (maize), barley, and probably spelt and emmer are not affected by processing (rolling, cracking, crimping, flaking, pelleting, etc.), whereas for sorghum grain (milo), wheat, rye, and probably millet and triticale, they are increased 10 to 15% by processing.

[b] Ladino (*Trifolium repens*) and red (*Trifolium pratence*).

[c] Alsike, crimson, Egyptian, ladino, Persian, red, and white clovers.

[d] All values given are the mean (range), except for digestible energy which is the range in Mcal/lb (Mcal/kg).

[e] Combined values for the following grasses, for which no difference was found between their reported nutrient contents: Bahia grass (*Paspalpum notatum*), coastal Bermuda grass (*Cynodon dactylon*), intermountain meadow plants (USA), orchardgrass (*Dactylis glomerata*), pangola grass (*Digitaria decumbens*), midwest prairie plants (prairie hay, USA), redtop (*Agrostis alba*), sorghum or Johnsongrass (*Sorghum halipence*) and timothy (*Phleum pratense*).

[f] Combined values for the following grasses for which no difference was found between their reported nutrient contents: Smooth bromegrass (*Bromus inermis*), reed canarygrass (*Phalaris arundinacea*), tall fescue-Kentucky 31 (*Festuca arundinacea*), Italian ryegrass (*Lolium multiflorum*) and crested wheatgrass (*Agropyron desertorum*).

[g] No difference was found between values reported for the different species of grasses listed in footnotes e and f when they were mature or for their hays, and, therefore, all values for these different species were combined. In addition, there was no difference between early- or mid-growth hays (2 to 4 weeks growth, early bloom, or vegetative versus 4 to 6 weeks' growth or mid-bloom) and, therefore, these values are combined and given as early growth, which were different from late growth hay (6 to 8 weeks' growth, full or late bloom, or mature).

[h] Much of the nitrogen in molasses is nonprotein, which is of little benefit or harm to horses. The value given, 2 to 6%, is for true crude protein, thus excluding nonprotein nitrogen.

APPENDIX TABLE 7
Mineral Supplements Composition[a]

Mineral Supplement	% of Mineral in Supplement as Fed[b] (For symbols of minerals, see Appendix Table 10.)				
Calcium & Phosphorus (Ca & P)	*Ca*	*P*	*Mg*	*S*	
Bone ash, charcoal, black, or char	30	14	0.6		
Bone meal, steamed	30–32	12–14	0.3	2.5	
Phosphate, dicalcium (dical)	21–22	18–20	0.6	1.1	
, monodicalcium	16	22	0.6	1.2	
, soft rock (colloidal clay)	17	9	0.4		
, curaco	34	14	0.8		
, rock	32–36	13–18	0.4		
Calcium (Ca)	*Ca*		*Mg*	*S*	
Calcium carbonate	38–39		0–0.05		
Calcium sulfate dihydrate (gypsum) ($CaSO_4 \cdot 2H_2O$)	22–23			18	
Limestone, calcitic, ground	34		2.1	0.04	
, dolmitic or magnesium	22		10		
Oyster shells, ground	38		0.3		
Slaked lime ($Ca(OH)_2$) (not a feed supp.)	54				
Dolime ($Ca(OH)_2$—$Mg(OH)_2$) (not a feed supp.)	30		18		
Phosphorus (P)		*P*	*Na*	*S*	
Phosphate, mono- or disodium (monophos)		22	16.2		
, diammonium		20–23			
, sodium tripoly (polyphosphate)		24	30		
Phosphoric Acid[b]		24		1.2	
Cobalt (Co)	*Co*				
Cobalt carbonate	46				
Copper (Cu)	*Cu*			*S*	
Copper sulfate, pentahydrate ($CuSO_4 \cdot 5H_2O$)	25.4			12.8	
Iodine (I)	*I*	*Na*	*Cl*		
Ethylenediamine dihydroiodide (EDDI)	79				
Iodized salt	0.007	39	60		
Iron (Fe)	*Fe*			*S*	
Ferrous sulfate, heptahydrate	21.4			12.1	
Magnesium (Mg)[c]	*Ca*	*P*	*Mg*	*S*	*K*
Magnesium carbonate (magnesite)	0.02		12–30[c]		
Magnesium hydroxide (milk of magnesia or brucite)			40		
Magnesium oxide[c]	0–3		51–59		
Magnesium phosphate		13	24		
Magnesium sulfate, monohydrate (Epsom salts) (kieserite)			16.5	22	
, heptahydrate			9.5	12.5	
Mica (Mg, Fe, and K silicate)			8		
Potassium magnesium sulfate (langbeinite)[c]			11.6	22.3	18.5
Manganese (Mn)	*Mn*				
Manganous carbonate	46				
Manganous oxide	77				
Potassium (K)	*K*	*Cl*	*Na*	*S*	*I*
Lite salt (equal parts KCl and NaCl)	25	54	20		
Potassium, bicarbonate	39				
, chloride (sodium-free salt)	50–52	47–48	1		
, iodide	21				68
, sulfate	41			17	
Selenium (Se)	*Se*		*Na*		
Sodium selenite (Na_2SeO_3)	45.6		26.6		
Sodium (Na)		*Cl*	*Na*		
Sodium bicarbonate (baking soda)			27		
Sodium chloride (salt)		60	39		
Trace-mineralized salt: typically is 98% salt, 0.35% Zn, 0.28% Mn, 0.175% Fe, 0.035% Cu, 0.007% Co, and 0.007% I					
Zinc (Zn)	*Zn*			*S*	
Zinc oxide	78				
Zinc sulfate, monohydrate	36			17.5	

[a] Most of the mineral supplements listed can be obtained at feed stores, but may be called by different names. For example, mono- or disodium phosphate and tripolyphosphate in some areas are called XP-4 and in others Sweet P, and monodicalcium phosphate is sometimes called biophos. In addition to the minerals shown here, there are numerous commercially available mineral mixes that contain two or more of these minerals mixed together in varying amounts, often along with various vitamins, proteins, molasses, and/or other substances. Thus, when trying to find a particular mineral supplement, rather than asking for one by the names given here, which may or may not be recognized, it is often better to ask for what they have that contains the specific mineral(s) wanted and what amount of these and other ingredients it contains. You may then want to evaluate the cost of it and other sources for the mineral(s) wanted as described in Chapter 7, and whether any additional substances it may contain are likely to be of benefit or of harm in considering its purchase and use. An extensive list of sources for obtaining not only minerals but most additives, supplements, and microingredients for animal diets is published yearly by Feed Management, Watt Publ., Mount Morris, IL, Tel. (815) 734-4171; most recently in volume 44, pages 6 to 31, Sept. 1993 issue.

[b] All contain 0 to 3% moisture except phosphoric acid, which contains 25% moisture.

[c] Magnesium oxide followed by potassium magnesium sulfate are the most prevalent feed-grade magnesium sources. Although magnesite contains 30.5% magnesium, its bioavailability is low and often a synthetic hydrated form of magnesium carbonate is used which contains 12% magnesium.

APPENDIX TABLE 8
Feeds—Weight/Unit Volume[a]

Feed (as fed)	lbs/qt	kg/L
Alfalfa meal	0.6	0.29
Barley, whole	1.5	0.72
, ground	1.2	0.58
Beet, pulp dried	0.6	0.29
Bran, wheat	0.5	0.24
, rice	0.7–0.8	0.34–0.4
Brewers' grain (dried)	0.6	0.29
Corn (maize), grain, whole	1.75	0.83
, cracked	1.6	0.72
, ear, husked	1.9	0.90
, ear, meal	1.4	0.67
Cottonseed, meal	1.5	0.72
, hulls, ground	0.37	0.18
, hulls, pelleted	1.2	0.56
Distillers' grains, dried	0.6	0.29
Emmer	1.1	0.5
Fat, animal	1.8	0.86
Fish meal	1.0	0.48
Gluten feed	1.3	0.62
Linseed meal	1.0	0.48
Milo (grain sorghum)	1.7	0.80
Millet	1.5	0.7
Molasses	3.0	1.4
Oats, regular, whole	0.85	0.41
, heavy, whole	1.0	0.48
, dehulled, whole	1.4	0.67
, ground	0.72 × unground value	0.72 × unground value
Oil, vegetable	1.9	0.92
Rice, ground	1.2	0.58
, hulls, ground	0.67	0.32
Rye, whole	1.7	0.8
, ground	1.5	0.70
Sorghum grain, whole (milo)	1.7	0.80
Soybean, meal	1.8	0.85
, whole	1.6	0.77
, hulls, ground	0.9	0.4
Spelt, whole	1.1	0.5
Triticale, whole	1.25	0.6
Wheat, whole	1.8	0.86
, ground	1.55	0.74
, mids	0.70	0.34

Forages (as fed)	cu ft/ton	cu meters/metric ton
Hay, baled	200–360	6–11
, cubed	60–70	2
, loose	450–600	14–19
Straw, baled	400–500	12.5–15.5
, chopped	250–350	8–11
, loose	675–1000	21–31

Minerals (as fed)	oz wt/teaspoon	oz wt/oz vol	grams/teaspoon
Most	0.11 to 0.18	0.63 to 1.04	3 to 5

[a] The true value for a specified feed may vary as much as 35% above or below the values given. An accurate value may be obtained only by weighing a volume of the actual feed fed.

APPENDIX TABLE 9
Conversion Factors[a]

To Change Value From	To	Multiply Value By
Area		
acres	sq ft	43,560 sq ft/a
acres	sq rods	160 sq rods/a
acres	sq rood	4 sq rood/a
rood	sq rod	40 sq rod/rood
section	acres	640 a/sec
section	sq miles	1 sq mi/sec
township	section	36 sec/ts
hectare	acres	2.471 a/ha
hectare	are	100 a/ha
are	centare	100 ca/a
centare	sq meters	1 sq m/ca
sq cm	sq inches	0.155 sq in/sq cm
sq meter	sq feet	10.76 sq ft/sq m
sq meter	sq yards	1.196 sq yd/sq m
sq meter	sq rods	0.0395 sq r/sq m
sq km	sq miles	0.386 sq mi/sq km
sq km	hectare	100 ha/sq km
Concentration Units		
g/kg	%	0.1 %/gpkg
kg/L	lb/bu	77.7 lbpbu/kgpL
kg/L	lb/qt	2.086 lbpqt/kgpL
lb/bu	kg/kl	1.287 kgpkl/lbpbu
lb/bu	lb/qt	0.02685 lbpqt/lbpbu
lb/short ton	kg/metric ton	0.5 kgpmt/lbpst
mg/g	mg/lb	453.6 mgplb/mgpg
mg/g	%	0.1 %/mgpg
mg/kg or L	%	0.0001 %/mgpkg
mg/lb	g/short ton	2 gpst/mgplb
mg %	mg/dl	1 mgpdl/mg%
%	g/short ton	9,072 gpst/%
%	lb/gal	0.0835 lbpgal/%
%	mg %	1,000 mg%/%
%	oz/gal	1.28 ozpgal/%
ppm	g/short ton	0.9072 gpst/ppm
ppm	mg/g	0.001 mgpg/ppm
ppm	mg/kg or L	1 mgpkg/ppm
ppm	ug/g or ml	1 μgpg/ppm
ppm	%	0.0001 ppm/%
ppm	ppb	1,000 ppb/ppm
μg/kg	μg/lb	0.4536 μgplb/μgpkg
cu meter/m ton	cu ft/short ton	32 ft³pst/m³mt
Concentration in Fluids		
		Don't Multiply, Instead
mg	mmole	mg ÷ Molecular Wt
mmole	mg	mM × Molecular Wt
mequivalence	mM	mEq ÷ Valence
mM	mEq	mM × Valence
mM	mosmole	1 mOsm/mM

Mol Wt of cpd = Sum of Mol Wt of all elements in that compound.
Mol Wt and Valence of an element = see Appendix Table 10.
Elements in a cpd = chemical formula for that cpd in, e.g., Chemistry Physics Handbook.

To Determine:
% of an element in a pure compound = (Mol Wt of element ÷ Mol Wt of cpd) 100.
% of an element in a nonpure compound = (% in pure cpd) × (1 − contaminate fraction).

Example:
% Ca in pure $CaCO_3$ = (Mol Wt Ca from App. Table 10) ÷ (Mol Wt $CaCO_3$ from App.
  Table 10) × 100 = [(40) ÷ (40 + 12 + 16 × 3)] × 100 = [(40) ÷ (100)] × 100 =
  40%
% Ca in $CaCO_3$ containing 2% moisture = (40%) × (1 − 0.02) = 40 × 0.98 = 39.2%

Energy		Multiply Value By
Calorie	nutritional	
	calorie	1 n.cal/Cal
kcal	Calorie	1 Cal/kcal
kcal	BTU	3.968 BTU/kcal
kcal	kjoule	4.1855 kj/kcal
kcal/kg	kcal/lb	0.4536 kcalplb/kcalpkg
Mcal	kcal	1000 kcal/Mcal
Therm	Mcal	1 Mcal/Therm
TDN lbs	kcal	2000 kcal/lb TDN
TDN kgs	kcal	4409 kcal/kg TDN
Starch Equiv. lb	kcal	2305 kcal/lb SE
Starch Equiv. kg	kcal	5082 kcal/kg SE
Length		
chain	feet	66 ft/ch
chain	rod	4 r/ch
fathoms	feet	6.08 ft/fa
feet	cm	30.48 cm/ft
furlong	meters	200 m/fu
furlong	poles	40 p/fu
furlong	rods	40 r/fu
furlong	lengths	5 l/fu
furlong	mile	$\frac{1}{8}$ mi/fu
furlong	yards	220 yd/fu
hands	inches	4 in/hand
inch	cm	2.54 cm/in
kilometers	miles	0.6214 mi/km

To Change Value From	To	Multiply Value By
Length (continued)		
leagues	miles	3 mi/league
link	inches	7.92 in/link
meters	feet	3.281 ft/m
meters	inches	39.37 in/m
meters	yard	1.0936 yd/m
miles	feet	5280 ft/mi
miles nautical	miles land	1.152 l mi/n mi
rod, pole or perch	feet	16.5 ft/rod
rod	links	25 link/rod
rod	yards	5.5 yd/rod
span	miles	9 mi/span
Metric Unit Prefixes		
micro-unit	unit	$1{,}000{,}000 = 10^6$
kilo-unit	unit	$1{,}000 = 10^3$
hecto-unit	unit	$100 = 10^2$
deca-unit	unit	$10 = 10^1$
unit	unit	$1 = 10^0$
deci-unit	unit	$0.1 = 10^{-1}$
centi-unit	unit	$0.01 = 10^{-2}$
mili-unit	unit	$0.001 = 10^{-3}$
micro-unit	unit	$0.000001 = 10^{-6}$
gamma-unit	unit	$0.000001 = 10^{-6}$
milli micro-unit	unit	$0.000000001 = 10^{-9}$
nano-unit	unit	$0.000000001 = 10^{-9}$
pico-unit	unit	$0.000000000001 = 10^{-12}$
Metabolites & Nutrients		
Glucose: mM/L	mg/dl	18 mgpdl/mMpL
Lactate: mM/L	mg/dl	8.9 mgpdl/mMpL
Urea: mM/L	mg/dl	6 mgpdl/mMpL
Vitamins:		
A: μM/L	μg/dl	28 μgpdl/μMpL
D: nM/L	ng/dl	0.39 ngpdl/nMpL
25-OH-D: nM/L	ng/dl	0.40 ngpdl/nMpL
1,25(OH)₂D: pM/L	pg/dl	0.42 pgpdl/pMpL
B₆: μM	mg	0.17 mg/μM
Folacin: μM/L	ng/ml	0.44 ngpml/nMpL
Vitamin C (Ascorbic		
Acid): μM/L	μg/ml	0.0182 μgpml/μMpL
mg beta-carotene	IU vit A for horse	400 IU/mg
Nitrate nitrogen (NO_3-N)	nitrate (NO_3)	4.4 NO_3/NO_3-N
Potassium nitrate (KNO_3)	nitrate (NO_3)	0.6 NO_3/KNO_3
Sodium nitrate ($NaNO_3$)	nitrate (NO_3)	0.7 NO_3/$NaNO_3$
Speed or Velocity		
knots/hr	land mi/hr	1.15 mph/knph
knots/hr	nautical mi/hr	1 nmph/knph
miles/hr	ft/min	88 fpm/mph
miles/hr	kilometers/hr	1.61 kph/mph
miles/hr	meters/min	26.82 mpm/mph
		Don't Multiply, Instead
miles/hr	min/mile	60 ÷ # of mph
min/mile	miles/hr	60 ÷ # min/mi
sec/mile	miles/hr	3600 ÷ # of sec/mi
Temperature		Don't Multiply, Instead
Fahrenheit	Centigrade or Celsius	5/9 (°F − 32) = °C
Centigrade or Celsius	Fahrenheit	9/5 (C° + 32) = °F
Volume		Multiply Value By
acre feet	gallons	325,900 gal/a-ft
barrels	gallons	31.5 gal/bbl
board foot	cubic inches	144 cu in/bft
bushels	cu feet	1.25 cu ft/bu
bushels	gallons	9.31 gal/bu
bushels	hectoliters	0.3524 hl/bu
bushels	peck	4 peck/bu
cord	cu feet	128 cu ft/cord
cu feet	gallon	7.48 gal/cu ft
cu feet	pounds water	62.4 lb/cu ft
cu inch	ml or cc	16.387 ml/cu in
cu meter	cu yard	1.308 cu yd/cu m
cup	oz	8 oz/cup
gallon, Imperial	gallon, USA	1.2 US gal/Imp gal
gallon	cu in	231 cu in/gal
gallon	pounds water	8.35 lb/gal
gallon	quarts	4 qt/gal
gill	pint	0.25 pt/gill
hogshead	barrel	2 bbl/hhd
liter	cu in	61.023 cu in/L
liter	gallon	0.2642 gal/L
liter	quart	1.057 qt/L
ounce	milliters	29.57 ml/oz
peck	quart	8 qt/peck
pint	cup	2 cup/pt
pint	milliter	473 ml/pt
pint	ounce	16 oz/pt
quart	liter	0.9464 L/qt
qt	pint	2 pt/qt
tablespoon	teaspoon	3 tsp/Tbs
teaspoon	milliter	5 ml/tsp

(continued)

(continued)

APPENDIX TABLE 9
Conversion Factors[a]–(continued)

To Change Value From	To	Multiply Value By
Weight		
dram	gram	1.77 g/dram
kilogram	pounds	2.2046 lb/kg
grain	mg	64.8 mg/grain
ounce	gram	28.35 g/oz
pounds	gram	453.6 g/lb
pounds	kilogram	0.4536 kg/lb
ton, long	pounds	2,200 lbs/T
ton, long	metric ton	1 m ton/T
ton, long	kilogram	1000 kg/T
ton, short	pounds	2,000 lbs/T
ton, short	metric ton	0.9072 m ton/T

[a] For the opposite conversion, divide by the number given in the Table instead of multiplying by it; i.e., if a value is in the units listed in this Table under "To," to determine the equivalent amount in units listed under "To Change Value From," divide the value by the number given in this Table instead of multiplying by it. For example: there are 2268 grams and you want to know the equivalent amount in pounds. As given in the Table, to change a value from pounds to grams, you multiply the number of pounds by 453.6 g/lb. Thus, to change 2268 g to pounds, you would divide 2268 g by 453.6 g/lb to determine that 2268 g is equal to 5 lbs. The best way to ensure that a conversion is done correctly is to use all units, with units being divided by similar units canceling each other out, just as a number divided by the same number cancels each other out. If this is done and the units remaining are those wanted, you know the conversion was made correctly as shown in the example below in converting 2268 g to pounds.

$$(2268 \text{ g}) \times \left(\frac{\text{lb}}{453.6 \text{ g}}\right) = 5 \text{ lb and thus you know } 2268 \text{ g} = 5 \text{ lb}$$

If the following was done instead, since the units remaining are not pounds as wanted, you know the conversion wasn't done correctly and instead of multiplying you must divide 2268 g by 453.6 g/lb.

$$(2268 \text{ g}) \times \left(\frac{453.6 \text{ g}}{\text{lb}}\right) = 1,028,764.8 \text{ g squared/lb}$$

Always using units in this manner is extremely helpful in preventing errors and in assisting one in knowing how to do a problem or make a conversion correctly.

APPENDIX TABLE 10
Molecular (Atomic) Weights and Valences of Common Elements

Element	Symbol	Usual Valence	Weight
Aluminum	Al	3	27
Barium	Ba	2	137.4
Calcium	Ca	2	40.1
Carbon	C	4	12
Chloride	Cl	1	35.5
Cobalt	Co	2	58.9
Copper	Cu	1,2	63.5
Fluorine	F	1	19
Hydrogen	H	1	1
Iodine	I	1	126.9
Iron	Fe	2,3	55.85
Lead	Pb	4	207.2
Magnesium	Mg	2	24.3
Manganese	Mn	1	54.9
Molybdenum	Mo	4,6	95.95
Nitrogen	N	3,5	14
Oxygen	O	2	16
Phosphorus	P	3,5	31
Potassium	K	1	39.1
Selenium	Se	2,4,6	79
Silicon	Si	4	28.1
Sodium	Na	1	23
Sulfur	S	2,6	32.1
Zinc	Zn	2	65.4

Index

Page numbers in *italics* indicate figures; those followed by "t" indicate tables.

Abdominal pain, exercise-induced, 215
Abortion
 inducement of, 239-240
 placenta and, 262
Acclimatization, heat stroke and, 210-211
Acer rubrum, 331, *331*
Acid
 amino, 12
  sulfur in, 28
 ascorbic, 59-61
 fatty, 18
 grain and, 80
 linoleic, 18
 pangamic, 196
Acid detergent fiber, in hay, 70, 380
Acid treatment, for mycotoxins, 351-352
Acid-base balance, 200
Acidified calf milk replacer, 275
Acidifier, urinary calculi and, 297
Acidosis, cecal, 75
Acid-treated feed, 80-81
Aconite, 341, *341*
Aconitum columbianum, 341, *341*
Acroptilon repens, *318*, 318-319
Additive in feed, 99-102. *See also* Supplement
Adenoma, pituitary, 191
Adenosine triphosphate, 193-195
Aerobic capacity, training and, 204
Aerobic exercise, 203
Aerobic metabolism, 194, 380
Aerophagia, with cribbing, 373-375
Aesculin, 302-303
Aesculus spp., 302-303, *304*
Aflatoxin, 349t, 360
 test kits for, 351t
Age
 of breeding stallion, 225
 estimation of, by teeth, 177-178, *178*, 178t
 for fitness training, 204-205
 size of horse and, 266t
Aged horse, feeding of, 191-192
Aggression
 as behavior problem, 376-378
 maternal, 248-249
Agropyron spp., 109
Air travel, stress of, 219
Airway, exercise-induced pulmonary hemorrhage and, 208-210
Alfalfa, 63-65
 for aged horse, 192
 blister beetle poisoning and, 365
 developmental orthopedic disorder and, 287
 nutrient content of, 71t, 419t
 pasture planted with, 108
 pellets of, *66*, 66-67
 planting of, 111
 tying-up syndrome and, 214
 weaning on, 123-128
Algae
 single-celled protein and, 89
 in water, 7

Alkali disease
 locoweed causing, 317
 selenium excess causing, 329
Alkali treatment, for mycotoxins, 351-352
Alkalinizing salt, for potassium-induced periodic paralysis, 299
Alkaloid
 larkspur, 340-341
 pyrrolizidine, 310-313, *310-313*
 taxine, 343-344
Alkalosis, 200, 380
Allergy
 diet-induced, 15-16, *16*
 photodermatitis and, 308-310, *309*, 309t, *310*
 respiratory, 291
 to vaccine, 166-167
Allium spp., 330-331
Almond hulls, 98
d-Alpha-tocopherol, 30
Alsike clover, 108, 314, 419t
Aluminum, phosphorus and, 25
Alveolus, dental, 23
Amelanchier alnifolia, 334, *335*
American Forage and Grasslands Council, 69-70
Amino acid, 12, 380
 growth and, 13-14
 sulfur in, 28
Ammonia
 liver disease and, 296
 ventilation of stable and, 182-183
Amniotic fluid, 245, 380
Amphetamine, 196
Amprolium, 53
Amsinckia intermedia, *312*
Amylase
 carbohydrates broken down by, 16
 fiber and, 17-18
Anabolic steroid
 for appetite stimulation, 290
 breeding stallion and, 225
Anaerobic capacity, training and, 203, 380
Analysis, nutrient, 112-137. *See also* Diet evaluation
Androgens, breeding stallion and, 225
Anemia
 infections, 175
 lead poisoning and, 364
 parasite induced, 167t, 168t
 plants inducing, 330-332, 331t, *332*, *333*
 vitamin B and, 44-45
Anger, signs of, 153
Angular leg deformity, 279-281
 management of, 288
Anhidrosis, exercise-induced, 211
Anoplocephala spp., 158-159
Anthrax, 175
Antibiotics
 for diarrhea, 293
 as feed additive, 101
 for foal, 253
 ionophore poisoning and, 361
 for strangles, 174

427

Antibody. *See also* immunoglobulin, 393
  encephalomyelitis, 170
  foal and, 254-256
  Potomac fever and, 174-175
Antifungal agent, 101-102
Antioxidant
  as feed additive, 102
  vitamin C as, 59
  vitamin E as, 30
Appaloosa, 297
Appetite
  hot weather and, 190
  potassium deficiency and, 27
Apple, thorn, 307-308
Arrow grass, 335, 336
Artemisia spp., 314-316, 315t, *316*
Artery, rupture of, during foaling, 273
Arthritis, 191
  juvenile, 281
Artificial insemination, 237, 238
  semen collection for, 226
Ascarid, *156*, 156-157
Asclepias spp., 337, *337*, 337t, *338*
Ascorbic acid, 59-61
Ascorbyl palmitate, 61
Aspartate aminotransferase, 207-208
Aspiration pneumonia, in foal, 249
Aster falcatus, white prairie, 326, *327*
Astragalus nisulcatus, 325-326, *326*
Astragalus spp., 300, *316*, 316-317, *317*
  teratogenicity of, 317, 333
Athletic performance, 193-223
  developmental orthopedic disease and, 277
  diets and supplements for, 195-198
  diseases due to, 208-215, 209t
  energy production and utilization for, 193-195, 194t
  feeding and supplements before, 198-199
  fitness evaluation for, 205-208, 207t
  fitness training for, 202-205
  injury due to, 215-218
  management summary for, 218-220
  selection of horse for, 220t, 220-222
  water and electrolytes for, 199-202
  weight loss from, 200t
Atriplex spp., 328, *328*
Avermectin
  effectiveness of, 159-160
  in seasonal deworming program, 161
Avidin, 56
Avocado poisoning, 344
Awn, grass, 301
Azalea, *305*
Azoturia, exertional, 211-213

Bacteria, in water, 7-8
Bag, feed, *150*
Bahigrasses, 109, 419t
Bale of hay, 65, 67
Balking, 378-379
Bark floor, 182
Barley, 75
  cost determinations for, 142
  foxtail, 301, *301*
  nutrient content of, 71t, 419t
Barn, 181-182. *See also* Stall
  ventilation of, 182-184, 382
Bastard strangles, 173, 174
Beans
  castor, 307
  field, 88
  as protein supplement, 87-88
Beard tongue, 328, *329*
Bedding
  eating of, 375-376
  in foaling stall, 243

storage of, 183
types of, 184, 185t
Beetle, blister, 364-366
Behavior
  after foaling, 246-248
  of gelding, 226
  grazing, 103-104
  imprint training and, 251-252
  problems of, 370-379
    escape vices and, 371-372
    flight or fight vices and, 376-379
    oral vices and, 372-376
Benzimidazole, 160t
Bermuda grass, 109, 420t
Bermudagrass staggers, 357
Beta-carotene, 45-47, 382
Bicarbonate, exertional myopathy and, 212-213
Big-head, 382
Bindweed toxicity, 303, *304*
Bioflavanoid
  athletic performance and, 196
  as feed additive, 102
Biotin, 56
  hoof and, 179
  hoof defects and, 291
Birds foot trefoil, 108
Be-still tree, 338
Bit teeth, 177
Biting, 377
  crib, 373-374
Black walnut, 322-323, *323*
Bladder
  sorghum poisoning and, 321
  stone in, 296-297
Blanketing, for cold weather, 188
Bleeding
  bioflavinoids and, 102
  exercise-induced pulmonary, 208-210, 382
  iron deficiency and, 38
  vitamin C and, 60
Blind staggers
  locoweed causing, 317
  selenium causing, 329
Blindness, vitamin A and, 48
Blisters, plants causing, 301
Blister beetle poisoning, 364-366
Blood. *See also* Bleeding
  anemia-inducing plants and, 330-332, *331*, 331t, *332*
  blister beetle poisoning and, 365
  in semen, 225
  vitamin A toxicosis in, 48
  vitamin K and, 50-51
Blood doping, 198-199, 382
Blood test for potassium-induced periodic paralysis, 298
Blood worm, 155, *156*
Blue flax, 335, *335*
Bluegrass, 109-110
Blue-green algae, 7
Body weight. *See* Weight
Bog spavin, 281
Bolting, 372, 378, 382
Bonding by foal and mare, 247
Bone. *See also* Orthopedic disorder, developmental
  calcitonin and, 24-25
  calcium deficiency and, 23
  developmental orthopedic disease and, 277
  exercise-induced injury to, 217-218
  fluorosis affecting, 40
  growth plate of
    enlargement of, 277, 279, *279*
    management of disorders of, 288
    trauma to, 284
  iodine imbalance, 34
  phosphorus deficiency and, 25
  vitamin A and, 48
  vitamin C, 59-60

vitamin D and, 49
  zinc and, 37
Bone cyst, 281, 282
Boot, injury prevention and, 216
Bot fly, *157*, 157-158, 382
  control program for, 163
  deworming program for, 161
Bottle, nursing, 275
Botulism, forage, 361-363
Botulism vaccine
  for broodmare, 229
  for growing horse, 272
Bovine colostrum, 257-258
Bowed tendon, 216-217
  exercise-induced, 216-217
Bracken fern, 320-321
Bran, as by-product feed, 94-95
Breeding, 224-241. *See also* Reproduction
Breeding stallion, 224-227
Brewer's grains, 87, 419t
Brewer's yeast, 87
  nutrient content of, 421t
Bristle grass, 301
Brome grass, 109, 419t
Bromus inermis, 109
Bronchodilator, 209
Broodmare, 229-241. *See also* Reproduction, broodmare care in
Broom weed, 326, *327*
Bruising, during foaling, 263
Bucked shins, 217, 383
Bucket feeding of orphan foal, 275-276
Buckeye, *304*
  toxicity of, 302-303
Buckwheat, 309-310, *310*
Budsage, 314
Buffer, as digestion enhancer, 100
Buffering, of blood, 198-199
Burdocks, 301
Burning of energy, 8-9
Burrow weed, 320
Bushel, weight of, 78t
Buttercups, *301*, 306, *306*
Buttress Foot, 383
By-product feed, 94-99, 96t

Cabbage, skunk, 332
Calcinosis, plant-induced, 324
Calcitonin, calcium excess and, 24-25
Calcitrol, 48-49
Calcium
  athletic performance and, 200
  developmental orthopedic disorder and, 286, 287
  feed analysis and, 114-115, 117, 419-421t
    for lactating mare, 133-136
    for weanling, 124-133
  for growing horse, 265t
  imbalance of, 20-25, 21t-23t, *24*
  kidney failure and, 296
  in milk, 270, 270t
  in pasture forage, 104t
  plant-induced calcinosis and, 324
  predicting foaling time and, 244
  reproduction and, 234t
  as supplement, 82, 422
  synchronous diaphragmatic flutter and, 213
  tying-up syndrome and, 213-214
  urinary calculi and, 297
  vitamin D toxicosis and, 50
Calculus
  bladder, 296-297
  intestinal, 294-295
Calf milk replacer, acidified, 275
Calorie, definition of, 9, 384
Camas, death, 344, *344*
Cambendazole, 160t
Canine teeth, 177, 384
Canola, 86-87, 419, 419t

Cantharidin, 365
Cap, dental, 177
Carbohydrate
  energy conversion and, 8-9
  food deprivation and, 10
  types and utilization of, 16-18
Carbon, in plants, 8
Carbon dioxide, 8
Carbon disulfide, 160t
Cardiac disease, 297
Cardiac glycoside-induced sudden death, 337-340
Cardiovascular system
  athletic performance and, 221-222
  training and, 203, 204
Caries, dental, 177, 384
Carnitine, 196
Carpal bone fracture, 218
Carpitis, 218, 384
Cartilage
  angular leg deformity and, 279-281
  developmental orthopedic disease and, 277
  joint damage and, 281-282
Caslick's operation, 237, 384
Cassia occidentalis, 323-324
Caster oil plant, *306*, 306-307
Castration, 226
Catilleja spp., 328, *328*
Caudal thigh-muscle injury, 216
Cecal acidosis, corn and, 75
Cecal fluid, diarrhea and, 293, 384
Cellulose, definition of, 385
Centaurea spp., *318*, 318-319
Central nervous system
  equine encephalomyelitis and, 169-171
  equine herpes virus and, 172
  lead poisoning and, 363
  liver disease and, 295-296
  plants toxic to, 314t, *314-322*, 314-322
Cereal grains, 70-79, 71t, *73*, *74*, 78t
  characteristics of, 71-72
  developmental orthopedic disorder and, 286-287
  nutrient content of, 71t, 419t
  pasture planted with, 108
  processing of, 76-77, *77*
  protein supplement of, 82-83, 84t-85t, 85-89
  quality of, 77-78
  storage of, 78-79, *79*
  types of, 72-76, *73*, *74*
Cervical star, 262
Cervical vertebra, 277, 279, *279*, *280*
Cestrum diurnum, 324
Cestrum spp., 307-308
Chelating agent
  as digestion enhancer, 100
  as feed supplement, 82
Chewing
  tail or mane, 67, 375
  wood, 372-373
    forage feeding to combat, 147
    pellets or cubes as only forage and, 67
Chick peas, 88
Chickling vetch, 88
Chigger, 168t
Chimney, 183
Chips, wood, as bedding, 184
Chloride
  deficiency of, 27
  in water, 7
Chokecherry, western, 335, *336*
Choline, 58-59
Chopped hay, 66
Chronic obstructive pulmonary disease, 291-292, *292*
  ventilation of stable and, 183
Chute, nurse mare, *273*
Cicer arietinum, 88
Cicuta spp., *342*, 342-343, *343*
Cicutoxin, 343

Citrinin, 348
Citrus bioflavinoid, 102
Claviceps spp., 355–356
Clippings, lawn grass, 99
Clostridium botulinum, 361–363
Clostridium botulinum vaccine, 272
Clostridium perfringens vaccine, 229
Clotting factors, vitamin K and, 51
Clover
    nutrient content of, 419t
    overseeding of grass pasture with, 110
    pasture planted with, 108
    spoiled, 331–332, *332*, 349t
    vitamin K and, 51
Coat, anhidrosis and, 211
Cobalamin, 57–58
Cobalt, 422
    dietary, 21t, 39
    in milk, 269
Coffee weed, 323–324
Coffin joint, flexor deformity of, 282
Cold
    anhidrosis and, 211
    feeding during, 187–188
    tolerance of, 183–184
Cold processing of grain, 76
Colic
    exercise-induced, 215
    in foal, 260–261
    foaling and, 263
    plants inducing, 302–308, 303t, *304–308*
    sand induced, 293
Coliform bacteria, in water, 8
Colitis, ehrlichial, 174–175
Collar, electric shock
    for aggressive behavior, 377
    for wind sucking and cribbing, 375
Colon, removal of, 295
Colostrum, 254–256, 255t, 385
Commercial feed, additives to, 62–63
Commercial grain mix, custom mix versus, 137
Commercial milk replacer, 274t, 274–275
Commercial supplement, inadequate, 81–82
Communication, 152–154
Complete feed, 91–94, 385
Compression, wobblers syndrome and, 279
Computer program, for diet analysis, 123
Conception
    beta-carotene and, 47
    diagnosis of, 238–239
Concrete floor, 182
Condensed molasses solubles, 98
Conditioner, hair, 180
Conditioning for athletic performance, 202–205
Condyle, bone stress injury and, 217–218
Congenital disorder
    angular leg deformity as, 280
    flexor deformity as, 282
    locoweed causing, 317
Coniine, 341–342
Conium maculatum
    sudden death caused by, *341*, 341–342, *342*
    teratogenicity of, 333–334
Contamination
    fluorosis caused by, 40
    parasite control and, 162
    of water, 7–8
Continual deworming program, 161–162
Contraction, of flexor tendon, 282–283
Convection, heat loss by, 199
Conversion, of energy, 8–9
Conversion tables, 424t–425t
Convolvulus arvensis, 303, *304*
Cooling
    after athletic performance, 219–220
    evaporative, 199

    heat stroke and, 210–211
    post-exercise exhaustion and, 214–215
Copper, 422
    developmental orthopedic disorder and, 286
    for growing horse, 265t
    imbalance of, 21t, 35–36
    in milk, 270, 270t
    in pasture forage, 104t
Copulation, 225–226
Cord
    spinal, wobblers syndrome and, 279
    umbilical, 246
        care of, 249–251
Corn, 74–75
    cost determinations for, 142, 143
    moldy corn disease and, 349t, 357–360
    nutrient content of, 71t, 419t
    oats versus, 72
Corn stover, as bedding, 184
Corpus luteum
    estrous cycle and, 236
    vitamin A and, 46
Corticosteroid, for appetite stimulation, 290
Cost of feeding, 138–144, *139*
Cottonseeds
    cost of, 142
    nutrient content of, 419t
    poisoning from, 366–368
    as supplement, 83, 85
Cough
    chronic obstructive pulmonary disease and, 291
    exercise-induced pulmonary hemorrhage and, 208
Cowpeas, 88
Cow's milk, 274, 274t
Cracking, of cereal grain, 77
Cramps, exercise-induced, 213–214
Creatinine phosphokinase, 207–208
Cretinism, 386
Creep feeder, for foal, 268–269
Creeping indigo, *313*, 313–314
Crib wetting, 372
Cribbing, 373–375
Crimping of grains, 77, *77*
Crimson clover, 108
Crofton weed, 320
Crotalaria spectabilis, 312, *312*
Croup muscle, exercise-induced injury to, 216
Crowding behavior, 377
Crown vetch, 108–109
Crude protein, 12–13
    in hay, 70
Crushed grain, 77
Cubed, hay, *66*, 67, 386
Culicoides spp., 159
Culture, yeast, 100–101
Cums, malt, 87
Cupola, 183
Curbed hocks, 262, 386
Custom grain mix, 137
Cuttings, hay, 67–68, 68t
Cyanide
    absorption of, 85
    pasture grass and, 110
    reproductive effects of, 234t
    sorghum and, 321
    sudden death from, 334t, 334–337, *335*, *336*
Cyanthostome, 155–156
Cynoglossum officinale, 311, *311*
Cyst, bone, 281

Dactylis glomerata, 109
D-alpha-tocopherol, 30
Dam. *See* Mare
Day-blooming jessamine, 324

Death. *See also* Poisoning
  botulism causing, 362
  exercise-induced pulmonary hemorrhage and, 208
  of foal, 262
  gossypol poisoning and, 367
  ionophore antibiotic causing, 361
  overweight and, 12
  plants causing, 334t, 334-344, *335-344*, 337t
Death camas, 344, *344*
Deciduous teeth, 178t
Deep digital flexor tendon deformity, 283
Deficiency, nutritional. *See* Nutritional deficiency
Deformity
  angular leg, 279-281
    management of, 288
  flexor
    acquired, 282-283
    congenital, 282
    in foal, 261
Degenerative disease, 32-33
Dehy pellet, *66*, 66-67, 387
Dehydration
  athletic performance and, 200
  diarrhea in foal and, 260
  post-exercise exhaustion and, 214-215
  signs of, 6-7
Demineralization
  calcium deficiency and, 23
  phosphorus deficiency and, 25
Demodex spp., 168t
Dental care, for aged horse, 192
Dental disorder, 175-178, *176, 178*, 178t
Dental Star, 387
Deprivation, food, 10
Dermatophytosis, *166*, 168t. *See also* Ringworm
Desensitization
  of foal, 251-252
  for heaves, 292
Detergent fiber in hay, 70
Developmental orthopedic disease, 277-288. *See also* Orthopedic
    disease, developmental
Dew poisoning, 314
Deworming, 159-162, 160t
  of broodmare, 229-230
  of growing horse, 272
Diaphragmatic flutter, synchronous, 213
Diarrhea
  in foal, 259t, 259-261
  plants inducing, 302-308, 303t, *304-308*
  sand-induced, 293-294
Dicoumarol
  in sweet clover, 332, 348
  vitamin K and, 51
Dictyocaulus arnfieldi, 159
Diet evaluation. *See also* Feed; Feeding; Nutrient
  information needed for, 113-122
    amount of feed needed as, 118-122, *119, 120*, 121t
    nutrient content of feed as, 114-118, *115, 116*
    nutrients needed as, 113-114
  need for, 112-113
  preparation of grain mix and, 136-137
  procedure for, 122-136
  for weanling
    on alfalfa, 128-133
    on pasture, 123-128
Diet-induced allergy, 15-16, *16*
Digestibility, starch, 72
Digestion, additives to enhance, 100
Digit grass, 109, 419t
Digital flexor tendon deformity, 283
Digitalis purpurea, 337-338, *339*
Digoxin, 339
1,25-Dihydroxyvitamin D_2, 49
Dilantin, 213
Dimethyl sulfone, 196

Disease, 289-299. *See also* Infection
  chronic obstructive pulmonary, 291-292, *292*
  diarrhea and, 293-294
  in foal, 258
  heart, 297
  hoof defect and, 290-291
  inadequate feed consumption with, 289-290
  intestinal
    calculi and, 294-295
    impaction and, 294
    removal or dysfunction, 295
  liver, 295-296
  potassium-induced periodic paralysis and, 297-299
  rectal/vaginal, 295
  renal, 296
  urinary tract, 296-297
Disinfection, of foaling stall, 243
Distemper, *173*, 173-174
Distiller's grains, 87, 419t
Diuretic
  heart disease and, 297
  potassium deficiency and, 27
DMG, 196
DMSO, 196
DNA blood test, 298
Dominance hierarchy, 152-153
  feeding and, 153-154
Door of stall, 181
Doping, blood, 199
Dormer, 183
Draft horse
  competition training for, 203
  energy needed by, 10
  as nurse mare, 273
Draschia spp., 158
Dried beet pulp, 98-99, 419t
Dried brewer's yeast, 87, 421t
Dried hay, 65
Dried milk products, 88, 420t
Dried poultry manure, 89, 420t
Drooling, plants inducing, 301
Dropped fetlock, in foal, 261-262
Drug
  for aggressive behavior, 377
  athletic performance and, 196
Dry coat, 211
Dry feed
  maximum daily intake, 10
  water needed with, 4
Dry matter
  broodmare, 231t
  for idle, worked and aged horses, 187t
Dry matter fraction, in feed analysis, 117-118
  for lactating mare, 134-136
  for weanling, 124-134
Drying, of grain, 76

Eating of feces, 375-376
Ectoparasites, 164-165
Edema, allergy causing, 16
EDTI, 34, 422t
Eggs, parasitic, *156*, 163
Ehrlichiosis, monocytic, 174-175
Ejaculation, 225
Elderberry, 335, *336*
Electric shock collar
  for aggressive behavior, 377
  for cribbing and wind sucking, 375
Electric wire fence, 184-185
Electrolytes
  athletic performance and, 195, 198-202
  synchronous diaphragmatic flutter and, 213
  tying-up syndrome and, 213-214
ELEM, moldy corn disease and, 358

Embryo
  mare's diet and, 230
  transfer of, 237
  twin, abortion of, 240
Emmer, 76, 419t
Encephalomalacia, nigropallidal, 318
Encephalomyelitis, equine, 169–171
Endurance activity
  definition of, 193
  heart size and, 221–222
  hematocrit and, 205–206
  training for, 219, 220
  water and electrolytes and, 201
Enema, for meconium impaction, 253
Energy
  for athletic performance, 193–195, 194t, 196
  cold weather and, 188
  deficiency of, 10–11
  developmental orthopedic disorder and, 287
  in diet evaluation, 122
  dietary, 8–12, 9, 11t
  excess, 11–12
    developmental orthopedic disorder and, 285
  fat supplements and, 90
  feed analysis and, 115
    for weanling, 125
  hot weather and, 190
  kidney failure and, 296
  need for, 9–10, 411t
  pregnancy and, 232–233
  sources and use of, 8–9
  for working horse, 186
Enhancer, digestion, 100
Ensiling of grain, 79–80
Enterolith, 294–295
Environment
  parasite control and, 162
  respiratory disorder and, 292
Enzyme
  as digestion enhancer, 100
  fitness indicated by, 207–208
  in flaxseed, 85
  in horsetail, 319
  as mold inhibitor, 102
Epididymis, testosterone and, 226
Epiphysitis, 277, 279, 279, 280, 388. See also Orthopedic disease, developmental
Equal-moisture basis, 117
Equine encephalomyelitis, 169–171
Equine ergotism, 355–356
Equine infectious anemia, 175
Equine influenza, 171
Equine monocytic ehrlichiosis, 174–175
Equine viral arteritis, 172
Equisteum arvense, 319
Ergocalciferol, 48
Ergot poisoning, 349t
Eruption bump, 177
Escape vice, 371–372
Estrogen, pregnancy diagnosis by, 239
Estrogen poisoning, 349t
Estrous cycle, 235–237, 236
Ethylene diaminedihydroiodide, 34, 422t
Ethoxyquin, 29
Eupatorium rugosum, 320, 320
Eupatorium urticaefolium, 300
European hemlock
  sudden death caused by, 341, 341–342, 342
  teratogenicity of, 333–334
Evaporative cooling, 199
Exercise. See also Athletic performance
  of breeding stallion, 224
  developmental orthopedic disorder and, 287–288
  for growing horse, 271–272
  growth plate trauma and, 284
  weight reduction and, 12

Exercise-induced disease, 208–215, 209t
  pulmonary hemorrhage as, 208–210
  synchronous diaphragmatic flutter as, 213
  tying-up as, 213–214
Exertion, types of, 193
Exhaustion, exercise-induced, 214–215
External parasites, 164–165, 167t–168t, 169t
Extruded grain mix, 92–94
Extrusion, vitamin stability during, 45t
Eye
  stomachworms and, 158
  vitamin A and, 46, 47, 48
Eyelid edema, allergy-induced, 16

Fagopyrum escultentum, 309–310, 310
Fang teeth, 177
Fartlek training, 204
Fast-twitch muscle fibers, 194–195
Fat, dietary, 18. See also Obesity
  athletic performance and, 194–195, 197–198, 218
  broodmare and, 235
  energy conversion and, 8–9
  excess energy stored as, 11–12
  food deprivation and, 10
  hot weather and, 190
  liver disease and, 296
  selenium/vitamin E deficiency and, 31–32
  supplements, 89–91, 90t, 419t
Fat necrosis syndrome, 353–354
Fatigue
  athletic performance and, 195
  exercise-induced, 214–215
Fat-soluble vitamins, 30–31
Fatty acid, dietary, 18
Fear, 376
Febantel, 160t
Fecal flotation for parasite detection, 162, 163
Fecal water, hay pellets and, 67
Feces
  eating of, 375–376
  of foal
    first, 247, 252–253
    orphaned, 276
  meconium, 247
Feed, 3–18. See also Feeding; Feed-related poisoning
  antibiotic additives in, 101
  bolting of, 372
  complete, 91–94
  cost of, 138–144, 139
  determining amount needed, 120–122
  energy from, 8–12, 9, 11t
  harvested, 62–102
    additives in, 99–102
    by-product, 94–99, 96t
    cereal grains as, 70–79, 71t, 73, 74, 78t
    fat and oil supplements in, 89–91, 90t
    grain mixes and, 91–94, 92t, 93t, 94t
    hay and, 63–66, 63–70, 64t, 65t, 70t
    high-moisture, 79–81
    protein supplements in, 82–83, 84t–85t, 85–89
    vitamin-mineral supplements in, 81–82
  inadequate consumption of, 289–290
  nutrient requirements for, 411t–418t
  nutrients in, 112–137, 419t–421t. See also Diet evaluation; Nutrient
  protein and, 12–16, 14t, 15, 16
  samples of, for mycotoxin testing, 350
  water and, 3–4, 4t, 6, 6–8, 7t, 8t
  weight per volume of, 423t
Feeder
  creep, for foal, 268–269
  types of, 148
Feeding
  of aged horse, 191–192
  angular leg deformity and, 279
  athletic performance and, 195–198, 218, 220

of breeding stallion, 224
of broodmare, *230*, 230t, 230-232, 231t, *232*
change of diet and, 154
in cold weather, 187-189, 188t, 189t
developmental orthopedic disorder and, 285-287
diarrhea in foal and, 260
exertional myopathy and, 212
of forage, 147-149, *148*
frequency of, 150-151
of grain, *149*, 149-150, *150*
group socialization and, 152-154
of growing horse, 264-270, 265t, 266t, 267t, *269, 270*, 270t
in hot weather, 189-191
of ill horse, 289-299. *See also* Disease
for maintenance or work, 186-187
monitoring of health status and, 151-152
orthopedic disorder and, 284
rhabdomyolysis and, 212
selenium excess treatment and, 330
skin and, 180
water and, 3-4, 4t, *6*, 6-8, 7t, 8t, 147
wood chewing and, 373
Feed-related poisoning, 346-369
blister beetle, *364*, 364-366
botulism, 361-363
clinical signs of, 3347t
gossypol, 366-368
ionophore antibiotic, 361
lead, *363*-364
mycotoxin, 346-361. *See also* Mycotoxin poisoning
nitrate, 368-369
Femoral fracture, during foaling, 273
Fenbendazole, 160t
Fencing, 184-185
Ferritin, 39
Fertility. *See also* Reproduction
of breeding stallion, 224-225
gossypol poisoning and, 367
masturbation and, 227
vitamin C and, 60
Fertilization, of pasture, 106-107, 107t
Fescue
fungus in, reproductive effects of, 234t
for pasture, 109
nutrients, contents of, 419t
Fescue poisoning, 349t, 352-355
Fetal fluid, 246
Fetal membrane, 249
Fetlock
bone cyst in, 282
developmental orthopedic disease and, 277
dropped, 261-262
flexor deformity of, 283
osteochondritis dissecans of, 281
Fetterbush, *305*
Fetus
equine herpes virus in, 172
fluoride affecting, 40
viability of, 238-239
Fever
Potomac horse, 174-175
shipping, *173*, 173-174
Fiber
cold weather and, 189
dietary, 17
diarrhea and, 293
feed analyzed for, 115
hay quality and, 69-70
hot weather and, 190
muscle, 194-195, 222
in feeds, 73-74, 94t, 419t-421t
Fiddleneck, 312, *312*, 312
Field beans, 88
Field bindweed, 303, *304*
First law of thermodynamics, 8
First premolar, 177

Fish meal, 89
nutrient content of, 419t
Fitness for athletic performance, 202-205
evaluation of, 205-208, 207t
Flavoring agents in feed, 100
Flax
nutrient content of, 419t
wild blue, 335, *335*
Flaxseed, 85-86, 419t
Flea, 167t
Fleet enema, for meconium impaction, 253
Flexor deformity, 282-283
in foal, 261-262
management of, 288
Flight or fight vices, 376-379
Floating of teeth, 177
Floor of stall, 181-182
Fluid
cecal, 293
fetal, 246
uterine, foal-heat breeding and, 238
Fluid therapy
for exercise-induced colic, 215
post-exercise exhaustion and, 214
Fluoride, 21t, 39-41
Fluorosis, 40
Flutter, synchronous diaphragmatic, 213
Fly
bot, *157*, 157-158
types of, 167t
Foal. *See also* Foaling
antibiotic and nutrient supplements for, 253
behavior of, 246-248
botulism in, 362
care of, 249-262, 250t
dental, 176
deworming program for, 161, 163-164
imprint training and, 251-252
respiratory assistance and, 249, 251t
supplements for, 253
umbilical cord and, 249-251
copper imbalance affecting, 36
eating of feces by, 375-376
exercise for, 271-272
feeding of, 264-276, 265t, 266t, 267t, *269, 270*, 270t
fescue poisoning and, 353, 354
growth promotants for, 271
illness in, 258-262
immunity of, 254-258, 255t, 256t
iodine imbalance affecting, 34
iron deficiency in, 38
lead poisoning and, 364
orphaned, feeding of, 272-276
protein deficiency in, 113
record keeping about, 180
selenium deficiency in, 233
stool passage of, 252-253
vaccination and parasite control in, 272
vitamin A and, 47-48
vitamin E deficiency in, 31-33
zinc recommendations for, 37
Foal-heat breeding, 238
Foaling
fescue poisoning and, 353, 354
induction of, 244-245
injury during, 262-263
length of pregnancy and, 242-243
mare's weight after, 231
predicting time of, 243-244, 244t
preparations for, 242-243
stages of, 245-246
Folacin, 56-57, 413t
Follicle-stimulating hormone, 236
Foot, fescue, 353
Foot care, *178*, 178-179
Foot injury, exercise-induced, 216

Forage
  for aged horse, 192
  athletic performance and, 198, 219
  beta-carotene in, 47
  botulism from, 361-363
  for broodmare, 232
  developmental orthopedic disorder and, 286
  feeding practices for, 147-148, *148*
  fescue poisoning and, 352-355
  fluorosis and, 40
  harvested, 62-102. *See also* Harvested feed
  lead-contaminated, 364
  for maintenance or work, 186-187
  nutrient content of, 114-118, 419t-421t
  pasture and, 103-111. *See also* Pasture
  protein supplement of, 82-83, 84t-85t, 85-89
  selenium in, 29-30
  thiamin and, 53, 413t
  for thin, weak horse, 11
  vitamin A in, 46
  vitamin E in, 30
  weaning and, 271
  for weanling, 124
  weight of, 423
Formaldehyde, for disinfecting foaling stall, 243
Formulation of diet, 112-137. *See also* Diet evaluation
Foxglove, 337-338, *339*
Foxtail barley, 301, *301*
Foxtail millet, 110
Fracture
  calcium deficiency and, 23
  pelvic, during foaling, 273
  stress, 218
Freezing behavior, 378-379
Frightened horse, 153
Fringed sage, 314
Frozen colostrum bank, 257
Fruit, 99
Fumonisin mycotoxin, 357-360
Fungus
  heaves caused by, 291-292
  mycotoxin poisoning and, 346-361. *See also* Mycotoxin poisoning
  reproductive effects of, 234t
  Rhizoctonia leguminocola, 301
Furosemide
  athletic performance and, 196
  exercise-induced pulmonary hemorrhage and, 209
  potassium deficiency and, 27
  synchronous diaphragmatic flutter and, 213
Fusarioum mold, 357-360

Gait
  athletic performance and, 222
  exertional myopathy and, 212
Gambels oak, *304*
Gamma hydroxybutyrate, 196
Gamma oryzanol, 196
Gamma-glutamyltransferase, 205
Gamma-glutamyltranspeptidase, 208
Gastric ulcer
  diarrhea in foal and, 260
  in foal, 260-261
Gastrointestinal system
  athletic performance and, 201
  diarrhea and, 293-294
  exercise-induced colic and, 215
  food deprivation and, 11
  illustration of, *5*
  impaction of, 294
    meconium, 252-253
  intestinal calculus and, 294-295
  parasites of, 155-156
  plants affecting, 302-308, 303t, *304-308*
Gastrophilus spp., *157*, 157-158

Gelding, 226
Genetic disorder
  developmental orthopedic, 284-285
  potassium-induced periodic paralysis as, 297
  wind sucking as, 374
German millet, 110
Gestation, 242. *See also* Foaling; Pregnancy
Giardia, in water, 8
Girth, weight determination from, 119, *121*
Girth-itch, *166*, 168t
Gluten, 87, 419t, 423t
  kidney failure and, 296
Glycogen
  athletic performance and, 194-195
    fat supplement and, 197-198
  exertional myopathy and, 212
  training and, 202
Glycoside
  cyanogenic, 336-337
  flaxseeds and, 85
Gnat, 167t
Goat's milk, 274, 274t
Goiter, 34, *34*, 391
Golden weed, 326
Gonadotropin, 239, 391
Goose grass, 335, *336*
Gossypol poisoning, 366-368
Grain
  athletic performance and, 198, 218
  brewer's, 87, 419t
  for broodmare, 231
  cereal, 70-79, 71t, *73*, *74*, 78t
    nutrient content of, 71t, 419t-421t
    processing of, 76-77, *77*
    protein supplement of, 82-83, 84t-85t, 85-89
    quality of, 77-78
    storage of, 78-79, *79*
    types of, 72-76, *73*, *74*
  cost determinations for, 142-144
  developmental orthopedic disorder and, 286-287
  enteroliths and, 295
  exertional myopathy and, 212
  feeding of, *149*, 149-150, *150*
  for growing horse, 264-265
  milk replacer and, 276
  nutrient content of, 419t
  for physical activity, 187t
  for thin, weak horse, 11
  vitamins in, 43, 413t
    vitamin D toxicosis and, 50
  weaning and, 271
Grain mix, 91-94
  additives to, 62-63
  for growing horse, 264-265
  preparation of, 136-137
Grain protein supplement, 87
Grain sorghum, 75
Grain sorghum hybrid, *322*
Grass
  blister beetle poisoning and, 366
  for broodmare, 232
  cereal grains and, 70. *See also* Grain, cereal
  developmental orthopedic disorder and, 286, 287
  fescue poisoning and, 352-355
  for ill horse, 290
  Johnson, *321*, 321-322
  Klein, 314
  for lactating mare, 133-136
  lawn grass clippings and, 99
  nitrogen for, 107
  nutrient content of, 71t, 420t
  in pasture, 103
  pasture management and, 105
  pasture planted with, 109

salivation caused by, 301
snake, 319, *319*
sorghum. *See* Sorghum
Sudan, 321-322, *322*
Grass hay, *63*, 65, *65*
    for lactating mare, 134-136
Grass peas, 88
Grass staggers, 349t
    mycotoxin poisoning and, 356-357
Grazing, rotational, 105-106, *106*
Grazing behavior, 103-104
Grease heel, 178, *178*
Grindelia spp., 326-327, *327*
Grinding of grain, 76-77
Grooming of foal, 246-247, 248
Group socialization, 152-154
Growing horse, 264-276
    feeding of, 264-270, 265t, 266t, 267t, *269*, *270*, 270t
    growth promotant for, 271-272
    nutrient requirements of, 411t, 414t-418t
    orphaned or early-weaned, 272
    parasite control in, 272
    vaccination for, 272
    weaning of, 270-271
Growth
    beta-carotene and, 46
    hoof, 179
    orthopedic disorder caused by, 283-284
    protein needs for, 13
    thiamin deficiency and, 53
    vitamin B$_{12}$ and, 58
Growth hormone, 271
Growth plate
    enlargement of, 277, 279, *279*
        management of, 288
    trauma to, 284
Growth promotant, 271
Grub, 167t
GTT. *See* Gamma-glutamyltransferase; Gamma-glutamyltranspeptidase
Gumweed, 326-327, *327*
Guterrezia sarothrae, 326, *327*

Habronema spp., 158
Hair coat
    care of, 179-180
    cold weather and, 188, 188t
    selenium excess and, 329, *329*
Hairworm, 158
Halogeton, 302
Halter, on foal, 252
Hand mating, 237-238
Handling of foal, 251
Haplopappus engelmannii, 326
Harvested feed, 62-102. *See also* Feed, harvested
Hay, *63-66*, 63-70, 64t, 65t, 70t
    for aged horse, 192
    blister beetle poisoning and, 365, 366
    for broodmare, 232
    cuttings of, 67-68, 68t
    determining amount needed, 120-122
    diet evaluation and, for lactating mare, 134-136
    feeding of, 149
    fescue poisoning and, 354
    forms of, 65-67, *66*
    least-cost determination for, 140, 141-144
    nutrients in, 114-118, *115*, 419t-421t
    quality of, 68-69, *69*
    storage of, 183
    types of, 63-65, *64*, 64t
    vitamin D in, 49
Haylage, 79-80
Health problem, 289-299. *See also* Disease
Health record, 180
Heart, 221
Heart disease, 297

Heart rate
    fitness and, 205, 206-207
    post-exercise exhaustion and, 214
    training and, 204, 219
Heat
    anhidrosis and, 211
    athletic performance and, 199-200, 220
    corn and, 74
    for exercise-induced injury, 215-216
    foal-heat breeding and, 238
    mare in, 235-237
    oxidation producing, 9
    water loss and, 4, 6
Heat stroke, exercise-induced, 210-211
Heated barn, ventilation of, 183
Heating
    feed, 17, 392
    for mycotoxins, 351-352
Heave line, 291, *292*, 392
Heaves, 291-292, *292*, 392
Heavy oats, 73-74
Heel, grease, 178, *178*, 391
Hematinic, 196, 392
Hematocrit
    fitness evaluation and, 205-206
    iron and, 39
Hemicellulose, 17-18
Hemlock
    sudden death caused by, *341*, 341-342, *342*
    teratogenicity of, 333-334
    water, *342*, 342-343, *343*
Hemoglobin, iron and, 39
Hemolytic uterus in foals, 392
Hemorrhage
    bioflavinoids and, 102
    exercise-induced pulmonary, 208-210
    iron deficiency and, 38
    vitamin C and, 60
Hepatic disease, 295-296
    plants inducing, 309t, *310-313*, 310-314, 313t
Heredity, 220
Hernia, in foal, 261, 393
Herpes virus, 171-172
Hierarchy, dominance, 152-154
    feeding and, 153-154
High-moisture feed, 79-81
Hock
    angular leg deformity and, 281
    bone cyst in, 282
    curbed, in foal, 262
    developmental orthopedic disease and, 277
    joint cartilage damage in, 281
Hoof
    angular leg deformity and, 281
    defects of, 290-291
    disorders of, *178*, 178-179
    exercise-induced injury to, 216
    flexor deformity and, 282
    selenium excess and, 329-330, *330*
    shoeing of, 179
Hordenine, 357
Hordeum jubatum, 301
Hordeum vulgare, 75
Hormone
    estrous cycle and, 236, 237
    follicle-stimulating, 236
    growth, 271
    inadequate energy intake and, 10
    luteinizing, 236
    parathyroid, 23
    thyroid, 33-35
    thyroid-stimulating, 33
Horse chestnut, *304*
    diarrhea caused by, 302-303
Horsehage, 80

Horserush, 319, *319*
Horsetail, 319, *319*
Hot feed, corn as, 74
Hot weather, 189-191
Hounds tongue, 311, *311*
Housing, 180-184
Hulls, 96-98, 420t, 423t
    oat, 73-74
Humidity, 220
Hydrophilic mucilloid, psyllium, 293
Hymen, 237
Hypericin, 309
Hypericum perforatum, 309
Hyperlipidemia
    in broodmare, 235
    food deprivation and, 10
Hyperparathyroidism, calcium and, 23, *24*
Hyperthyroidism, 34-35
Hypocalcemic tetany, exercise-induced, 213-214
Hypothyroidism, 34-35

Illness, 289-299. *See also* Disease
Immunity, for foal, *254*, 254-258
Immunoglobulin
    for foal, 254-256, 255t, 256t
    weaning and, 270-271
Immunotherapy, for heaves, 292
Impaction, intestinal, 294
    meconium, 252-253
Imprint training of foal, 251-252
Indian paintbrush, 328, *328*
Indian peas, 88
Indigo, *313*, 313-314
Indolizidine alkaloid, 317
Indospicine, 313-314
Induction
    of estrous cycle, 237
    of foaling, 244-245
Infection
    anthrax, 175
    equine encephalomyelitis, 169-171
    equine infectious anemia, 175
    equine viral arteritis, 172
    foal's immunity and, 254-258
    influenza, 171, 393
    parasitic, 155-165. *See also* Parasite
    Potomac horse fever, 174-175
    rhinopneumonitis and, 171-172
    for strangles, 173-174
    tetanus, 168-169
    umbilical, 250-251
    vaccination program for, 165-168
        for broodmare, 229
    viral arteritis and, 172
    water contamination causing, 7-8
    wobblers syndrome caused by, 279
Infertility
    gossypol poisoning and, 367
    masturbation and, 227
    vitamin C and, 60
Influenza, equine, 171, 393
    vaccine for, 272
Infusion, uterine, abortion via, 240
Injury
    athletic, 215-218
    to mare, during foaling, 262-263
Inoculant, intestinal, for foal, 253
Inoculation, soil, 111
Inosine, 196
Insect
    blister beetle poisoning and, 364-366
    grain and, 78
    parasites, 164-165
Insecticide, for parasites, 165

Insemination, artificial, 226
Internal parasite, 155-165. *See also* Parasite
    growing horse and, 272
Interval deworming program, 161
Interval training, 204, 394
Interval weaning, 271
Intestinal disorder. *See* Gastrointestinal system
Intestinal inoculant, for foal, 253
Intrinsic factor, 58
Intromission, 225
Iodine, 422
    imbalance of, 21t, 33-35, *34*
        in broodmare, 233
    in salt, 26
Ionophore antibiotic poisoning, 361
Ipratropium, 209
Iron
    gossypol poisoning and, 367
    imbalance of, 21t, 38-39
    in pasture forage, 104t
    toxicity of, for foal, 253
    in water, 7
Irritation, as vaccine reaction, 167-168
Ivermectin
    dosage of, 160t
    for stomachworms, 158
Ixodes dammini, 164

Jessamine
    day-blooming wild, 324
    toxicity of, 307-308
Jibbing, 378-379, 394
Jimmy weed, 320
Jimson weed, 307, *307*
Johnson grass, *321*, 321-322
    cyanide poisoning from, 335
    for pasture, 110
    pasture planted with, 108
Joint
    cartilage damage to, 281-282
    flexor deformity and, 282-283
Joule, definition of, 394
Juglans nigra, 322-323, *323*
Jumping, training for, 203
Juvenile arthritis, 281

Kalmia latifolia, 304, *305*
Kentucky bluegrass, 109-110, 420t
Keratin, selenium excess and, 329
Kicking, 371-372, 377
Kidney beans, 88
Kidney failure, 296
Kidney toxicosis, 349t
Kink in tail, 153
Klamath weed, 309
Klein grass, 314, 420t
    for pasture, 109
Knee
    angular leg deformity and, 280-281
    bone cyst in, 282
    bone fracture of, 218
    of foal, 262

Laceration, rectal or vaginal, 295
Lactate
    exercise and, 205
    fitness indicated by, 207, 207t
Lactate dehydrogenase, 207-208
Lactation
    diet evaluation for, 133-136
    feeding during, 230-231, 232
    nutrition effects on, 234
    protein needs for, 13

Lactose, digestion of, 16
Ladino clover
    overseeding of grass pasture with, 110
    pasture planted with, 108
Lameness
    athletic performance and, 195
    calcium deficiency and, 23
    developmental orthopedic disorder causing, 277-287. *See also*
        Orthopedic disorder, developmental
    exercise-induced, 215-218
    plants inducing, 322-330, *323-330*, 325t
Large intestine, removal of, 295
Larkspur poisoning, *340*, 340-341
Laryngeal neuropathy, 221
Lasalocid poisoning, 361
Laser, for exercise-induced injury, 216
Lasix, potassium deficiency and, 27
Lathryrogens, 88
Lathyrus sativus, 88
Lawn grass clippings, 99
Laxative, for meconium impaction, 253
Lead poisoning
    botulism versus, 362
    causes and treatment of, 363-364
Least-cost feed, 140-144
Lecithin, 58-59
Lectins, 88
Leg
    angular deformity of, 279-281
        management of, 288
    of foal, abnormality of, 261
    growth plate enlargement in, 277, 279, *279, 280*
    wobblers syndrome and, 279
Leg wrap, for flexor deformity, 282
Legume
    fungal infection of, 301
    locoweed as, *316*, 316-317, *317*
    overseeding of grass pasture with, 110
    pasture planted with, 108
    planting of, 111
    as protein supplement, 87-88
Legume hay, *63*, 63-65
    grades of, 70t
Lespedeza, 420t
    pasture planted with, 108-109
Lethal white foal syndrome, 252
Leucothoe spp., *305*
Libido, of breeding stallion, 224
Lice, 167t
Life span of horse, 191
Ligament injury, 216-217
Light
    need for, 181
    photodermatitis and, 308-310, *309*, 309t, *310*
Lignin, 17
Liming of foaling stall, 243
Line, heave, 291, *292*
Linoleic acid, 18
Linseed meal, 85-86, 420t, 423t
Linum spp., *335, 335*
Lipid. *See* Fat
Lite salt, 201
    post-exercise exhaustion and, 214
Live yeast culture
    athletic performance and, 196, 218
    for growing horse, 271
Liver
    copper metabolism by, 35
    folate and, 57
    vitamin A and, 46
Liver disease, 295-296
    photodermatitis with, 308-309
    plants inducing, 309t, *310-313*, 310-314, 313t
Liver enzyme, 208
Lockjaw, 168-169

Locold, 316
Locoweed, 300, *316*, 316-317, *317*
    teratogenicity of, 317, 333
Lolium spp., 110
Long, slow distance training, 203, 218
Lotus corniculatus, 108
Low-sodium salt, 201
Lucerne hay. *See* Alfalfa
Lucky nut tree, 338
Lunging aggression, 377
Lungworm, 159
Lupine, nutrient content of, 420t
Lupine poisoning, 348
Luteinizing hormone, 236
Lycopersicon spp., 307-308
Lyme disease, 164
Lyonia spp., *305*
Lysine
    growth and, 14, 14t
    in pasture forage, 104t

Maggot, 167t
Magnesium, 422
    in colostrum, 244
    imbalance of, 21t, 27-28
    reproduction and, 234t
    in water, 7
Maize, 74-75. *See also* Corn
    nutrient content of, 71t, 419t
Male teeth, 177
Maleberry, *305*
Malt sprouts, 87
Mammary gland, induced foaling and, 245
Mammary secretion, foaling time and, 244
Management practices, 155-185
    dental, 78, 175-178, *176*, 178t
    disease control, 165-175. *See also* Infection
    fencing and, 184-185
    foot care, *178*, 178-179
    housing and, 180-184, *182*, 185t
    parasite control, 155-165. *See also* Parasite
    record keeping and, 180
    skin and hair-coat care, 179-180
Mane chewing, 375
Manganese, 422
    imbalance of, 21t, 37-38
    in milk, 269
    in pasture forage, 104t
    reproduction and, 233
Manure
    nutrient content of, 421t
    poultry, 89, 420t
Mare
    abortion inducement, 239-240
    aggression of, 248-249
    athletic performance of, 222
    breeding of, 229-241. *See also* Foaling; Reproduction
    colostrum of, 254-256
    foal and, 246-248
    lactating
        diet evaluation for, 133-136
        milk production by, 234-235
    weaning and, 270-271
Marestail, 319
Massage, for exercise-induced injury, 216
Masturbation, in stallion, 226-227
Matchweed, 326, *327*
Maternal aggression, 248-249
Maturity, 191-192
    size of horse at, 266t
Meal, oilseeds, 82-83
Mechanical by injurious plants, 302t
Meconium, 247, 252-253
Medial septum, persistent, 237
Medicago sativa. *See* Alfalfa

Medroxyprogesterone, 377
Melilotus officinalis, *331*, 331-332
Melilotus spp., 108
Membrane
 fetal, 249
 of foal, 247
Merckoquant Total Water Hardness Test Strip, 244
Mesh fence, 184
Mesquite, 302
Metamucil, 293
Methionine, 58
Methyl sulfonyl methane, 196
Middle distance activity, 193
 heart size and, 221-222
 training for, 203, 218
Midge
 Onchocerca cervicales transmitted by, 159
 types of, 167t
Milk
 diarrhea in foal and, 260
 dried, 88
 induced foaling and, 245
 nutritional value of, 267-268
 for orphaned foal, 274-276
 protein content of, 13
 replacers, 274t, 274-275, 276
Milk production
 diet for, 230-231
 nutrition effects on, 234
Milkvetch, 316-318
 two-grooved, 325-326, *326*
Milkweed poisoning, 337, *337*, 337t, *338*
Millet, 76
 nutrient content of, 71t, 420t
 for pasture, 110
Milo, 75, *322*, 420t
Mineral
 broodmare and, 232, 233
 calcium, 20-25, 21t, 22t, 23t, *24*
 cobalt, 21t, 39
 copper, 21t, 35-36
 developmental orthopedic disorder and, 285-286
 in diet evaluation, 122
 dietary, 19-41
 feed analysis for, 116
 feed supplements of, 82
 imbalance of, 21t, 27
 iodine, 21t, 33-35, *34*
 iron, 21t, 38-39
 least-cost determination for, 141
 magnesium, 21t, 27-28
 manganese, 21t, 37-38
 molybdenum, 21t, 36
 potassium, 21t, 27
 recommended amounts of, 412t
 selenium, 21t, 28-33. *See also* Selenium
 sodium chloride, 21t, 25-27
 sulfur, 21t, 28
 vitamin E, 21t, 30-33
 zinc, 21t, 36-37
Mineral supplement
 composition of, 422t
 variation in consumption of, 113
Miserotoxin, 317
Mite, types of, 168t
Mix, grain, 91-94
 additives to, 62-63
 for growing horse, 264-265
 preparation of, 136-137
Moisture
 feed analyzed for, 114-115
 of grains, 79
 in hay, 65

Molasses, 98
 nutrient content of, 420t
 for weanling, 125, 126
Mold
 in cereal grain, 77-78
 in corn, 74
 in hay, *70*
 inhibitors of, 101-102
 mycotoxins poisoning and, 346-361. *See also* Mycotoxin poisoning
Moldy corn disease, 357-360
 causes and effects of, 349t
 grass staggers and, 356
Molybdenum
 copper absorption and, 35
 imbalance of, 21t, 36
 in milk, 269
Monensin poisoning, 361
Monitoring, of heart rate, 206-207
Monkshood poisoning, 341, *341*
Monocytic ehrlichiosis, 174-175
Monosaccharide, in diet, 16-17
Monoterpene, 315
Morning glory, toxicity of, 303, *304*
Mortality. *See* Death
Moss, peat, as bedding, 184
Mountain laurel, 304, *305*
Mountain pieris, *305*
Mounting of mare, 225
Mouth, sore, 176
Moxidectin, 160t
Mucilloid, psyllium hydrophilic, 293
Muscle
 athletic performance and, 194t, 194-195, 222
  exertional myopathy and, 211-213
  training and, 203
 exercise-induced injury to, 216
 food deprivation effect on, 11
 plants affecting, 322-330, *323-330*, 325t
 potassium-induced periodic paralysis and, 297-299
 selenium/vitamin E deficiency and, 31
 sodium chloride deficiency and, 27
 vitamin E deficiency and, 31
Muscle enzyme, 208
Mutilation, self, 378
Mycotoxin poisoning, 346-361, 396
 aflatoxin, 360
 diagnosis of, 348, 349t, 350
 ergotism and, 355-356
 feed sampling for, 350
 fescue poisoning and, 352-355
 field assays in, 350-351
 grass staggers and, 356-357
 moldy corn disease and, 357-360
 rhizoctonia leguminicola and, 301
 stachybotryotoxicosis and, 360-361
 treating feeds for, 351-352
Myeloencephalopathy, degenerative, 32-33
Myopathy
 exertional, 211-213
 selenium/vitamin E deficiency causing, 31

Nadrolone, 196
Narasin poisoning, 361
Navicular disease, 397
Near infrared reflectance spectroscopy, 116-117
Necrosis, fat, 353-354
Neonatal care, 249-262. *See also* Foal, care of
Nerium oleander, 338, *339*
Nervous system
 equine encephalomyelitis and, 169-171
 equine herpes virus and, 172
 lead poisoning and, 363
 liver disease and, 295-296

plants toxic to, 314t, *314-322*, 314-322
synchronous diaphragmatic flutter and, 213
Neuropathy, laryngeal, 221
Neurotoxic plant, 314t, *314-322*, 314-322
moldy corn disease and, 357-360
Neutral detergent fiber, in hay, 70
Neutralizer, as digestion enhancer, 100
Niacin, 54-55, 413t
Nicotinamide, 54
Nicotinic acid, 54
Night-blooming jessamine, 324
Nightshade, 307-308
Nigropallidal encephalomalacia, 318
Nitrate, in water, 7
Nitrate poisoning, 368-369
Nitrogen
nonprotein, 14
for pasture, 107
in plants, 8
in protein, *116*
Nitrogen free extract, 116, 397
Nitroglycoside, 317
Nitrotoxin, 317-318
Nomogram for weight estimation, *119*
Nonbiological bedding, 184
Nonprotein nitrogen, 14, 397
Nonstabled foal, rate of maturing of, 272
Nurse mare, *273*, 273-274
Nursing, 247
aggression during, 248
colostrum and, 254-256, 255t
passive immunity and, 256-258
Nursing bottle, 275
Nursing foal, feeding of, 267-268
Nutrient. *See also* Feed; Feeding; Mineral; Nutritional deficiency; Vitamin
for aged horse, 192
classes of, 3, 4t
cold weather and, 187-189
deficiency of, 4t
developmental orthopedic disorder and, 285-286
diet evaluation and, 112-137. *See also* Diet evaluation; Feed
energy from, 8-12, *9*, 11t
in feeds, 419t-421t
for foal, 253
in grain mix, 92t
in hay, 64t, 68-69, 419t-421t
hoof defects and, 290-291
hoof growth and, 179
inadequate consumption of, 289-290
necessary, 113-114
of pasture forage, 103, 104t
requirements for, 411t-418t
total digestible, 9
Nutritional deficiency
calcium, 22-24
choline, 59
folate, 57
iron, 38
lactation affected by, 234
magnesium, 27-28
manganese, 37-38
potassium, 27
selenium, 29, 31-33
in foal, 233
sodium chloride, 27
sulfur, 28
thiamin, 53
vitamin, 42
C, 59-60
D, 49
E, 31-33
water and electrolyte, 200-202
Nutritional status, 151-152

Oak toxicity, 303-304
Oats, *73*, 73-74, 77
corn and sorghum versus, 72
cost determinations for, 142
nutrient content of, 71t, 420t
Obesity
in broodmare, 231
hot weather and, 190
mortality risk of, 12
overfeeding causing, 152
physical activity and, 12
pregnancy and, 232-233
Obstruction
gastrointestinal, in foal, 261
intestinal, 294-295
Obstructive pulmonary disease, chronic, 291-292, *292*
OCD. *See* Osteochondritis dissecans
Ochoratoxin A, 348
Octacossanol, 196
Oil
in diet, 18
skin, 179-180
Oil supplement, 89-91, 90t, 420t
Oilseed, 82-83
Oleander, 338, *339*
Onchocerca cervicales, 159
Onion poisoning, 330-331
Open knees, 277, *280*
Open-front shed, 180-181
Oral disorder, 175-178, *176*, *178*, 178t
Oral vice, 372-376
Orchard grass, 109, 420t
Organic minerals, 82. *See also* Mineral
Organophosphate, for deworming, 160t
Orphaned foal, feeding of, 272-276, *273*
Orthopedic disease, developmental, 277-288
angular leg deformities in, *279*, 279-381, *280*
causes and effects of, *278*
contracted flexor tendons in, 282-283, *283*
copper affecting, 37-38
genetics of, 284-285
growth plate enlargement in, 277, 279
improper feeding and, 265
joint cartilage damage in, 281-282
management of, 287-288
milk composition and, 270
nutritional causes of, 285-287
rapid growth causing, 283-284
trauma causing, 284
wobblers syndrome and, 279
Oryza sativa, 76
Osselets, 398
Osteochondritis dissecans, 281-282
Overfeeding, 152. *See also* Obesity
Overgrazing, of pasture, 105
Overheated feed, 17
Overseeding of grass pasture, 110
Overtraining, 205
Overuse injury, 205
Overweight horse. *See* Obesity
Ovulation, 235-237
twinning and, 240
Oxalate
calcium binding with, 22
calcium deficiency and, 24
Oxfendazole, 160t
Oxibendazole, 160t
Oxidation
energy conversion by, 8-9
selenium and, 28
Oxygen
athletic ability and, 221
athletic performance and, 193-195
loss of fitness and, 205

Oxytropis, 316
Oxytropis spp., 300
Oxyuris equi, 158

Pain
  bone stress injury causing, 217
  eating as cause of, 290
  exercise-induced abdominal, 215
  exertional myopathy and, 212
  flexor deformity causing, 283
Palpation, pregnancy diagnosis by, 239
Pandiculation, by foal, 247–248
Pangamic acid, 196
Panting, heat stroke and, 210
Pantothenic acid, 55, 413t
Paper, as bedding, 184
Paralysis, potassium-induced periodic, 297–299
Parascaris equorum, 156, 156–157
Parasite
  bots as, 157, 157–158
  control of
    deworming methods for, 159–162
    environmental, 162, 162
    monitoring of, 162–163
    program for, 163–164
  diarrhea and, 294
    in foal, 260
  external, 164–165, 167t–168t, 169t
  growing horse and, 272
  hairworms as, 158
  internal, 155–165
  lungworms as, 159
  pinworms as, 158
  stomachworms as, 158
  strongyles as
    large, 155
    small, 155–157, 156
  tapeworms as, 158–159
  threadworms as, 158
Parathyroid hormone, 23, 24
Parrot mouth, 176
Paspalum staggers, 356–357
Passive immunity, 256–258
Pasture, 103–111
  for broodmare, 232
  diet evaluation and
    for lactating mare, 133–134
    for weanling, 123–128
  fertilization of, 106–107, 107t
  fescue poisoning and, 352–355
  foaling in, 242–243
  grazing behavior in, 103–104
  grazing management and, 104–106, 106, 107t
  growing horse and, 267
  lead-contaminated, 364
  nutrient content of, 114–118
  parasite control and, 162
  planting of, 107–111
  purpose and benefit of, 103
  toxic plants in, 301. See also Poisonous plant
  weed control in, 107
Pasture breeding of mare, 237
Pasture weaning, 271
Pawing, 371–372
Peanut, nutrient content of, 420t
Peanut hulls, as bedding, 184
Peanut meal, 86
Pearl millet, 110, 420t
Peas, as protein supplement, 87–88, 420t
Peat moss, as bedding, 184
Pecking order, 152–153
Peer group of foals, 248

Pellet
  for aged horse, 192
  hay, 66–67
  milk replacer, 276
Pelleted grain mix, 92–94
Pelleting, vitamin stability during, 45t
Pelvic fracture, during foaling, 273
Pennisetum spp., 110
Penstemon spp, 328, 329
Perennial plant, 108
Perennial ryegrass staggers, 356–357
Perforated ulcer, in foal, 261
Performance weight, optimal, 151–152
Perinatal death, 262
Perineal tear, during foaling, 263
Periodic paralysis, potassium-induced, 297–299
Periodontal disease, 177
Peroxide, vitamin E and, 29
Pesticide, for external parasites, 164
Phalaris staggers, 357
Phenolic disinfectant, 243
Phenothiazine, 160t
Phenytoin, exertional myopathy and, 213
Phomopsis leptostomiformis, 348
Phosphorus
  for broodmare, 232
  deficiency of, 113
  developmental orthopedic disorder and, 286, 287
  feed analysis and, 114–115
    for lactating mare, 133–136
    for weanling, 124–133
  for growing horse, 265t
  imbalance of, 20–25, 21t, 22t, 23t, 24
  kidney failure and, 296
  in milk, 270, 270t
  in pasture forage, 104t
  as supplement, 422
  vitamin D toxicosis and, 50
Photodermatitis, plants inducing, 308–310, 308–310
Photosynthesis, 8
Phylloerythrin, 308–309
Physical activity, grain needed for, 187t
Physitis, 277, 279, 279, 280
Phytolacca americana, 304, 306, 306
Pieris spp., 305
Pigment
  fagopyrim, 309–310
  gossypol poisoning and, 366
  hypericin, 309
  selenium/vitamin E deficiency and, 32
Pinworm, 158
Piperazine, 160t
Piperidine alkaloid, 341–342
Pisum spp., 88
Pituitary adenoma, 191
Placenta, 245, 246
  retained, 262
Plank of fence, 185
Plant
  energy from, 8
  fluoride in, 39
  poisonous, 300–345. See also Poisonous plant
Planting of pasture, 107–111
Plasma chloride, 200
Plasma enzyme, 207–208
Plasma lactate concentration, 207, 207t
Plate, growth, 277, 279, 279
Play, by foal, 247, 248
Plumbism, 363–364
Pneumonia
  aspiration, in foal, 249
  foal, 258–259
Poa pratensis, 109–110
Pod grass, 335, 336

Poison hemlock, *341*, 341–342, *342*
　teratogenicity of, 333–334
Poisoning. *See also* Poisonous plant
　by algae, 7
　feed-related
　　blister beetle, *364*, 364–366
　　botulism, 361–363
　　clinical signs of, 347t
　　gossypol, 366–368
　　ionophore antibiotic, 361
　　lead, 363–364
　　mycotoxin, 346–361. *See also* Mycotoxin poisoning
　　nitrate, 368–369
　plant, 300–345
Poisonous plant
　anemia-inducing, 330–332, 331t, *332*, *333*
　colic or diarrhea from, 302–308, 303t, *304–308*
　lameness-inducing, 322–330, *323–330*, 325t
　liver disease from, *310–313*, 310–314, 313t
　mechanical injury from, 302t
　neurotoxic, 314t, *314–322*, 314–322
　photodermatitis-inducing, 308–310, *308–310*
　salivation-inducing, *301*, 301–302
　selenium excess caused by, 325t, *325–330*, 325–330
　sudden death caused by, 334t, 334–344, *335–344*, 337t
　teratogenic, 332–334, *333*, 333t
Pokeweed, 304, 306, *306*
Polymer fence, 185
Pony, vitamin A toxicosis in, 48
Post, fence, 185
Post-exercise exhaustion, 214–215
Potassium, 422
　athletic performance and, 200, 201
　heart disease and, 297
　in water, 7
Potassium-induced periodic paralysis, 297–299
Potato
　as feed, 99
　nutrient content of, 420t
　toxicity of, 307–308
Potomac horse fever, 174–175
Poultry manure, 89, 420t
Prebreeding examination
　of mare, 237
　of stallion, 224–225
Pregnancy. *See also* Foaling
　abortion inducement and, 239–240
　breeding methods and, 237–238
　diagnosis of, 238–239
　energy needs during, 10
　equine herpes virus in, 172
　estrous cycle and, 235–237, *236*
　feeding during, *230*, 230t, 230–232, 231t, *232*
　fescue poisoning and, 353, 354
　lead poisoning and, 364
　length of, 242–243
　milk production and, 234–235
　nutritional effects on, 232–233
　parasite control during, 229–230
　prebreeding examination and, 237
　protein needs during, 13
　teratogenic plants and, 317, 332–334, *333*, 333t
　twin, 240–241
　vitamin A and, 46
Premature birth, 242
Premature separation of placenta, 262
Premolar, 177
Presentation of foal, 245–246
Prince's plume, 326, *327*
Probiotics, 100–101
　for athletic performance, 196
　for growing horse, 271
Progesterone
　for aggressive behavior, 377
　pregnancy diagnosis by, 239

Prognathism, 176
Prolapse, uterine or rectal, 273
Prostaglandins
　for abortion inducement, 239–240
　estrous cycle and, 236
Protease inhibitor, 88
Protein, 12–16
　allergy to, 15–16, *16*
　athletic performance and, 196–197, 218
　for broodmare, 232–233
　deficiency of, 14–15, *15*
　　signs of, 113
　developmental orthopedic disorder and, 285–286, 287
　in diet evaluation, 122
　energy conversion and, 8–9
　excess of, 15
　feed analysis and, 114–115
　　for growing horse, 265t
　　for lactating mare, 133–136
　　for weanling, 124–133
　hay quality and, 69
　hot weather and, 190
　kidney failure and, 296
　liver disease and, 296
　for maintenance and work, 186–187
　in milk replacer, 275
　nitrogen versus nonnitrogen, *116*
　in pasture forage, 104t
　single-cell, 89
Protein supplement, 82–83, 84t–85t, 85–89
　animal-source, 88–89
　variation in consumption of, 113
Protoanemonin, 306
Proximate analysis of feed, 116, 400
Prunus virginiana, 335, *336*
Psyllium hydrophilic mucilloid, 293
Pteridium aquilinum, 320–321
Pulling competition, 203
Pulmonary disease, chronic obstructive, 291–292, *292*
Pulmonary hemorrhage, bioflavinoid and, 102
Pulp
　fruit, 99
　sugar beet, 98–99, 419t
Pulse proteins, as protein supplement, 87–88
PVC fence, 185
Pyrantel
　in continual deworming program, 161–162
　dosage of, 160t
Pyridoxine, 55–56, 413t
Pyrrolizidine alkaloid poisoning, 310–313, *310–313*
Pyruvate, 321

Quarter Horse
　muscle fibers in, 222
　potassium-induced periodic paralysis in, 297
Quaternary ammonium compound, 243
Quercus spp., 303–304, *304*

Rabies, botulism difference, 362
Rabies, 174–175
Race horse. *See also* Athletic performance
　developmental orthopedic disease in, 277
　fat supplements for, 197
　vitamin B₁₂ for, 58
Radiographic evaluation of
　angular leg deformity, 280
　of developmental orthopedic disease, 277
Ragwort, Ridell and Tansy, 311
Rail fence, 185
Rancidity of feed, 18
Ranunculus spp., 306, *306*
Rapeseed, 86
Rapid growth, 283–284

Rattlebox, *312*, 312
Rearing, behavioral problems, 377
Record keeping, 180
Recovery from training workout, 203
Rectal examination
 of broodmare, 237
  pregnancy diagnosis by, 239
Rectal prolapse from foaling, 273
Rectal/vaginal surgery, 295
Rectal temperature. *See* Temperature
Recurrent laryngeal neuropathy, 221
Red blood cells, doping with, 199
Red clover, overseeding with, 110
Red maple poisoning, 331, *331*
Reflex, laryngeal, 221
Rejection of foal, 249
Renal clearance ratio, 401
Renal disease
 feeding and care of horse with, 296
 toxicosis and, 349t
 vitamin K, 52
Replacer, milk, 274t, 274-275, 276
Reproduction
 beta-carotene and, 46-47
 breeding stallion and, 224-227
 broodmare care in, 229-241
  abortion inducement and, 239-240
  after foaling, 262
  behavior of, 246-248, 247t
  breeding methods and, 237-238
  estrous cycle and, 235-237, *236*
  feeding and, *230*, 230t, 230-232, 231t, *232*
  foaling and, 242-246. *See also* Foal
  gestation period and, 242
  induced foaling and, 244-245
  injury during foaling and, 262-263
  maternal aggression and, 248-249
  nutritional effects on, 232-233
  parasite control and, 163, 229-230
  prebreeding examination and, 237
  prediction of foaling time and, 243-244, 244t
  pregnancy diagnosis and, 238-239
  preparation for foaling and, 242-243
  twinning and, 240-241
 gossypol effects on, 367
 record keeping for, 180
 selenium/vitamin E deficiency and, 31
 vitamin E and, 33
Resinweed, 326-327, *327*
Resistance, to dewormer, 159
Respiratory assistance for foal, 249
Respiratory system
 chronic obstructive pulmonary disease and, 183, 291-292, *292*
 exercise-induced pulmonary hemorrhage and, 208-210
 fitness evaluation and, 205
 of foal, 249
  pneumonia and, 258-259
 infection of
  influenza, 171
  rhinopneumonitis, 171-172
Rest
 loss of fitness with, 205
 for tendon injury, 217
Resuscitation of foal, 249
Retina, vitamin A and, 46
Rhabdomyolysis
 acute, 211-213
 slow-onset, 213-214
Rhinopneumonitis, 171-172, 401
Rhinopneumonitis vaccine
 for broodmare, 229
 for growing horse, 272
Rhizoctonia leguminocola, 301
Rhododendron catawbiense, *305*

Riboflavin, 54, 413t
Rice, 76
 nutrient content of, 71t, 420t
Richweed, 320, *320*
Ricin, 307
Ricinus communis, *306*, 306-307, *307*
Ridell's ragwort, 311
Ringworm, *166*, 168t
Rodac plate, 243
Rodent, grains and, 78
Rolled oats, 77
Roof, of stable, 183
Rotational grazing, 105-106, *106*, 107t
Roundworm, *156*, 156-157
Rubber floor, 182
Rubber nylon fence, 185
Rupture, uterine, during foaling, 263
Russian knapweed, *318*, 318-319
Rye, 76
 nutrient content of, 71t, 420t
 triticale and, 76
Rye grass, 110, 420t
Rye grass staggers, 356-357

Sac, water, premature placental separation, 262
Safflower, nutrient content of, 420t
Sagebrush, 314-316, 315t, *316*
St. John's wort, 309
Salinomycin poisoning, 361
Salivation-inducing plants, *301*, 301-302
Salmonella, in water, 8
Salt
 athletic performance and, 201, 220
 dietary, 25-27
 for growing horse, 264
 heart disease and, 297
 iodine in, 33
 post-exercise exhaustion and, 214
 for potassium-induced periodic paralysis, 299
 urinary calculi and, 297
Saltbush, 328, *328*
Sambucus spp., 335, *336*
Sample, feed
 for diet evaluation, 114, *115*
 for mycotoxin testing, 350
Sand
 as bedding, 184
 diarrhea or colic caused by, 293-294
 for stall floor, 182
Sand sage, 314
Saskatoon berry, 334, *335*
Sataria spp., 76
Scours, 259t, 259-261
Scrotum of breeding stallion, 225, 226
Scurvy, vitamin C and, 60
Season, breeding
 estrous cycle and, 235-237, *236*
 stallion and, 226
Seasonal deworming program, 161
Seaweed, iodine in, 33
Sebum, 179-180
Secale cereale, 76
Secretion, foaling time and, 243
Seed, fescue, 355
Selenium
 for athletic performance, 196
 broodmare and, 233
 excess of, 324-330
  diagnosis of, 330
  effects of, 328-330
  plants causing, 325t, *325-328*, 325-328
  treatment of, 330
 for growing horse, 264

hoof defects and, 290
imbalance of, 21t, 28–33
in milk, 270, 270t
Self-mutilation, 378
Semen evaluation of breeding stallion, 224–225
Senecio spp., 310–313, *310–313*
Senna, coffee, 323–324
Septum, medial, persistent, 237
Serviceberry, 334, *335*
Setaria spp., 301
Sex, 222
Sexual behavior
    of breeding stallion, 224–225
    of mare, 235–238
Shaker foal syndrome, 362
    vaccination for, 272
Shampooing, 180
Shavings, wood, as bedding, 184
Shed, open-front, 180–181
Shin, bucked, 217
Shipping fever, *173*, 173–174
Shock, rhabdomyolysis and, 212
Shock collar, electric
    for aggressive behavior, 377
    for cribbing and wind sucking, 375
Shoeing, 179
    exercise-induced injury and, 216
Shoulder, osteochondritis dissecans of, 281
Shying, 378
Sickle hocks, 281, 403
Silage, 79–80
    nutrient content of, 114–118, 421t
Silicon, zeolite and, 99–100
Single-cell protein, 89
Skeletal disease, vitamin D and, 49
Skin
    care of, 179–180
    pesticide affecting, 165
    photodermatitis and, 308–310, *309*, 309t, *310*
    stomachworms and, 158
    thyroid disorder and, 35
Skunk cabbage, 332
Slavramine, 301
Sleep, by foal, 247
Sleeping sickness, 169–171, 403
Slobbering disease, 349t
Slow-onset rhabdomyolysis, 213–214
Slow-twitch muscle fibers, 194–195
Small intestine, removal of, 295
Smell, nurse mare and, 273
Snake grass, 319, *319*
Snake weed, 326, *327*
Snakeroot, white, 300, 320, *320*
Sodium, 422
    heart disease and, 297
    in water, 7
Sodium bicarbonate
    athletic performance and, 198, 219
    exertional myopathy and, 212–213
Sodium chloride. *See also* Salt
    dietary, 25–27
    imbalance of, 21t, 25–27
    post–exercise exhaustion and, 214
Sofcheck Water Hardness Test Strip, 244
Soil, selenium in, 29–30
Soil preparation for pasture, 110–111
Solanaceae, 307–308
Solanine toxin, 307–308
Solid food, for foal, 267–270
Sore, summer, 158
Sorghum, 75
    nutrient content of, 421t
    oats versus, 72
    for pasture, 108, 110

poisoning from, 321–322, *322*
    cyanide, 335
Sounds, 153
Sour horse, 191
Soybean hulls, 97
Soybean meal
    cost determinations for, 142
    nutrient content of, 71t, 421t
    as supplement, 83
    for weanling, 125
Spaying, 222
Spectroscopy, 116–117
Spelt, 76
    nutrient content of, 71t, 421t
Sperm
    evaluation of, 224–225
    season of year and, 226
Spinal cord, wobblers syndrome and, 279
Spirurids, 158
Splint bone, fracture of, 218
Split estrus, 236
Spoiled sweet clover, 331–332, *332*
Spore, fungal, heaves caused by, 291–292
Spotted hemlock
    sudden death caused by, *341*, 341–342, *342*
    teratogenicity of, 333–334
Sprint, 193
    interval training and, 204
    training for, 203
Stabled foal, rate of maturing of, 272
Stachybotryotoxicosis, 349t, 360–361
Staggers
    blind
        locoweed causing, 317
        selenium causing, 329
    grass, 349t, 356–357
Stall, 181–182
    escape behavior and, 371–372
    foaling in, 243
Stallion
    breeding of, 224–227
    equine viral arteritis in, 172
    rejection of, 235
Standing, by foal, 247
Stanleya pinnata, 326, *327*
Star, cervical, 262
Starch, dietary, 16–18
    digestibility of, 72
Starvation, 10, 289
Steatitis, 31
Steroid
    for appetite stimulation, 290
    breeding stallion and, 225
Stiffness, 212
Stillbirth, 262
Stomachworm, 158
Stone
    bladder, 296–297
    intestinal, 294–295
Stool. *See* Feces
Storage
    of grains, 78–79
    of hay, 65t, 65–66, *69*
Stover, 95–96
    as bedding, 184
Strain
    exercise-induced, 216
    in growing horse, 271–272
Strangles, *173*, 173–174, 405
Strangles vaccine, 272
Straw, 95–96
    as bedding, 184
Stress injury, to bone, 217–218
Stretching, by foal, 247–248
Striking, 377

Stroke, heat, 210–211
Strongyles, 155–156
    deworming program for, 159, 161
    diarrhea in foal and, 260
Strongyloides westeri, 158
Struvite stone, 294
Succinylcholine, for aggressive behavior, 377
Sucking, wind, 374–375
Suction, of foal's airway, 249
Sudan grass, 321–322, *322*
    cyanide poisoning from, 335
    for pasture, 110
    pasture planted with, 108
Sudden death
    gossypol poisoning and, 367
    plants causing, 334t, 334–344, *335–344*, 337t
Sudex, 110
Sugar, types of, 16–18
Sugar beet pulp, 98–99
Sugar cane residue, as bedding, 184
Sulfate, in water, 7
Sulfur
    imbalance of, 21t, 28
    in milk, 270t
Summer slump, 353
Summer sore, 158
Summer syndrome, fescue poisoning and, 353
Sunflower, nutrient content of, 421t
Sunflower hulls, 97–98
Sunflower seed meal, 86
Sunlight
    photodermatitis and, 308–310, *309*, 309t, *310*
    vitamin D and, 48–49
Superoxide dismutase, 196
Superoxide scavenger, 37
Supplement
    for athletic performance, 195–198
    biotin, for hoof defects, 291
    fat and oil, 89–91, 90t
    for foal, 253
    kidney failure and, 296
    least-cost determination for, 141
    variation in consumption of, 113
    vitamin-mineral, 44–45, 45t, 81–82
Supplementation, vitamin C, 60–61
Surgery, for osteochondritis dissecans, 282
Suspensory ligament, injury to, 217
Swainsonine, 317
Sweating
    anhidrosis and, 211
    athletic performance and, 199–202
    fatigue and, 195
    potassium and, 27
    water lost by, 4, 6
Sweet clover
    pasture planted with, 108
    spoiled, 331–332, *332*, 349t
        vitamin K and, 51
Sweet peas, 88
Swelling of joint, 281
    of knee, in foal, 262
Synchronous diaphragmatic flutter, 213
Synthetic bedding, 184

Tail, hair lose from, 329
Tail, kink in, 153
Tail chewing, 375
    pellets or cubes as only forage and, 67
Tall fescue
    fescue poisoning and, 352–355
    for pasture, 109
Tan bark floor, 182
Tannin, 304
Tapeworm, 158–159
Tarweed, 312

Taste preference, change in, 113
Taxine, 343–344
Tear
    during foaling, 263
    muscle, exercise-induced, 216
Teasing, 235
Teeth, 175–178, *176*, *178*, 178t
    age estimation by, 177–178, *178*, 178t
    of aged horse, 192
    calcium deficiency and, 23
    fluorosis affecting, 40
Temperature
    blister beetle poisoning and, 365
    cold weather and, 187–189, 188t
    foaling time and, 243, 244
    post-exercise exhaustion and, 214
    water loss and, 4, 6
Temporary teeth, 177
Tendinitis
    calcium deficiency and, 23
    exercise-induced, 216–217
Tendon
    exercise-induced injury to, 216–217
    flexor, in foal, 261–262
Teratogenic plant, 332–334, *333*, 333t
    locoweed as, 317
Testicle
    of breeding stallion, 225
    retained, in gelding, 226
Testosterone
    breeding stallion and, 225
    gelding and, 226
Tetanus, 168–169, 406
    botulism versus, 362
Tetanus toxoid, 229
Tetany
    exercise-induced, 213–214
    magnesium deficiency causing, 28
Thermodynamics, first law of, 8
Thiabendazole, 160t
Thiamin, 52–54, 413t
    bracken fern and, 320, 321
Thiaminase, 320
Thiomolybdate, 36
Thistle, yellow star, *318*, 318–319
Thorn apple, 307–308
Thoroughbred
    developmental orthopedic disease in, 277
    as nurse mare, 273–274
Threadworm, 158
Throat, narrow, 221
Thrush, of foot, 178, 406
Thumps, 213
Thyroid
    exertional myopathy and, 212–213
    iodine and, 33–35, *34*
Thyroid-stimulating hormone, 33
Tick
    control of, 164
    paralysis, 359t
    types of, 168t
Timothy, 65, *65*, 110
Tissue bedding, 184
Titret Calcium Hardness Test Kit, 244
d-alpha-Tocopherol, 30
Togavirus, 172
Tomato, toxicity of, 307–308
Tongue displacement, 372
Tooth, 175–178, *176*, *178*, 178t
    age estimation by, 177–178, *178*, 178t
    of aged horse, 192
    calcium deficiency and, 23
    fluorosis affecting, 40
Total digestible nutrients, 9, 407
Total dissolved solids, in water, 7

Toxicity
    of nonprotein nitrogen, 14
    of pesticide, 165
    of plants, 300-345. *See also* Poisonous plant
    of water, 7
Toxicosis
    choline, 59
    cobalt, 39
    cyanide. *See* Cyanide
    fescue, 352-355
    iodine, 33, 35
        in foal, 233
    iron, 39
    nitrate, water causing, 7
    selenium, 29-30, 32
    sodium chloride, 26
    thiamin, 53-54
    vitamin A, 48
    vitamin C, 61
    vitamin D, 49-50
    vitamin D-like, 324
    vitamin K, 52
Toxin
    in blister beetle, 365
    in horse chestnut, 302-303
Toxoid. *See also* Vaccine
    botulism, 229
    tetanus, 229
Trace minerals. *See* Minerals
Trace-mineralized salt, 26
    for broodmare, 233
    for growing horse, 264
Training
    for athletic performance, 202-205
    of growing horse, 271-272
    imprint, of foal, 251-252
    of orphan foal, 276
    pregnancy after leaving, 233
Transfusion, blood doping and, 199
Transport
    of pregnant mare, 234
    stress of, 219
Trauma
    angular leg deformity and, 279-280
    athletic injury and, 215-218
    orthopedic disorder caused by, 284
    plants causing, 302t
    wobblers syndrome and, 279
Travel. *See* Transport
Tremetol, 320
Trichostrongylus axei, 158
Trichothecenes, 348
Trifoil, nutrient content of, 421t
Trifolium hybridum, 314
Triglochin spp., 335
Triglyceride, 18
Trimming of hoof, 179
Triticale, 76
    nutrient content of, 71t, 421t
Triticum aestivum, 75-76
    pasture planted with, 108
Tryptophan-niacin conversion, 54
Tube feeding, liver disease and, 296
Tumor, aging and, 191
Turpentine weed, 326, *327*
Tushes, 177
Tusk, 177
Twinning, 240
Two-grooved milkvetch, 325-326, *326*
Tying-up syndrome, 213-214

Udder, induced foaling and, 245
Ulcer, in foal, 260-261

Ultrasound
    for exercise-induced injury, 216
    pregnancy diagnosis by, 239
    twinning and, 240
Ultraviolet radiation, vitamin D and, 48-49
Umbilical cord, 246
    care of, 249-251
Underfeeding, causes of, 152
United States Department of Agriculture, 69-70
Unsaturated fatty acid, 18
Urea
    dietary, 14
    kidney failure and, 296
Urinary calculi, 296-297
Urine
    blister beetle poisoning and, 365
    sorghum poisoning and, 321
Urticaria, diet-induced, 16, *16*
Uterine contractions in foaling, 245
Uterine fluid, foal-heat breeding and, 238
Uterine lavage, abortion via, 240
Uterine prolapse, 273
Uterine tear, during foaling, 263

Vaccination, 165-175
    for anthrax, 175
    of broodmare, 229-230
    for equine encephalomyelitis, 169-171
    for equine herpes virus, 172
    for equine viral arteritis, 172
    of growing horse, 272
    for influenza, 171
    for Potomac horse fever, 175
    for strangles, 173, 174
    for tetanus, 168-169
Vacuum packing of grain, 80
Vagina
    prebreeding examination of, 237
    surgery on, 295
Vegetables, as feed, 99
Ventilation of stable, 182-184
Veratrum spp., 332, *333*
Vertebra
    growth plate enlargement in, 277, 279, *279*, *280*
    wobblers syndrome and, 279
Vetch
    chickling, 88
    pasture planted with, 108
Vice, 370-379. *See also* Behavior
Vicia faba, 88
Vigna sinensis, 88
Vinegar, for intestinal stones, 295
Viral infection
    arteritis caused by, 172
    equine encephalomyelitis and, 169-171
    equine influenza and, 171
    rhinopneumonitis and, 171-172
Vitamin, 42-61
    A, 45-48, *47*
        for foal, 253
        reproduction and, 233
    for athletic performance, 196
    B, for appetite stimulation, 290
    B_1, 52-54
    B_2, 54
    B_6, 55-56
    B_{12}, 57-58
    biotin, 56
    broodmare and, 233
    C, 59-61
    characteristics and functions of, 43t
    choline, 58-59
    cobalamin, 57-58
    D, 48-50

Vitamin (Continued)
  diet evaluation for, 114, 122
  E, reproduction and, 233
  feed analysis for, 116
  folacin, 56-57
  general information about, 42-45
  K, 50-52
  kidney failure and, 296
  niacin, 54-55
  pantothenic acid, 55
  pyridoxine, 55-56
  recommended amounts of, 413t
  stability of, 44t, 45t
  supplements of, 81-82, 413t
    variation in consumption of, 113
Vitamin D-like toxicosis, 324

Wafer, hay, 66-67
Walking by foal, 247
Warfarin, vitamin K and, 51
Waste, feed, minimizing, 144
Water, 3-4, 6-8
  athletic performance and, 195, 198, 199-202, 220
  cold weather and, 189
  contaminants of, 7-8, 8t
  deficiency of, 4t, 6-7
  in diet evaluation, 122
  exertional myopathy and, 212
  flavoring of, 219
  for foal, 269
  guide for suitability of, 7t
  heart disease and, 297
  intake management of, 147
  need for, 3-4
  for pasture, 111
  post-exercise exhaustion and, 214
  quality of, 7-8
  sodium chloride excess and, 26-27
  synchronous diaphragmatic flutter and, 213
Water hemlock, 342, 342-343, 343
Water sac
  breaking of, 245
  premature placental separation and, 262
Waterer, 6
Weakness
  food deprivation and, 11
  plants causing, 322-330, 323-330, 325t
Weaning
  aggression during, 248
  feeding during, 270-271
Weanling
  diet evaluation for
    on alfalfa, 128-133
    on pasture, 123-128
  feeding of, 265-267
Weather
  cold, 187-189, 188t
  hot, 189-191
Weed. See also Plant
  Burrow weed and, 320
  coffee, 323-324
  control of, in pasture, 107, 111
  Jimmy, 320
  jimson, 307, 307
  klamath, 309
  Klein, 109, 314
  locoweed and, 316, 316-317, 317
  pokeweed, 304, 306, 306
  richweed and, 320, 320
  Russian knapweed and, 318, 318-319
  tarweed and, 312
Weende analysis of feeds, 116
Weight
  of aged horse, 192
  athletic performance and, 200

  of broodmare, 232-233
  of feed, 423t
    per bushel, 78t
  fitness indicated by, 206
  measurement of, 118-120, 119, 121
  optimal, 151-152
  during pregnancy, 231
  reduction of, 12
Western chokecherry, 335, 336
Western false hellebore, 332
Wheat, 75-76
  nutrient content of, 71t, 421t
  pasture planted with, 108
  triticale and, 76
Wheat grass, 109, 420t
Whey, nutrient content of, 421t
White clover, 108
White muscle disease, 31-32
White prairie aster, 326, 327
White snakeroot, 300, 320, 320
White sweet clover, spoiled, 331-332
Wild blue flax, 335, 335
Wild onion poisoning, 330-331
Willow-leafed jessamine, 324
Wind chill, 189t
Wind sucking, 237, 374-375, 408
Winter wheat grazing, 108
Wire fence, 184-185
Wobblers syndrome, 32-33, 279, 408
Wolf teeth, 177, 408
Wood chewing, 372-373
  forage feeding to combat, 147
  pellets or cubes as only forage and, 67
Wood shavings, as bedding, 184
Wooden fence, 185
Woody aster, 326, 326
Work
  energy needs for, 10
  water loss and, 4, 6
Working horse, feeding of, 186-187
Workout for athletic performance, 202-205
Worm, parasitic, 155-165
  deworming and, 159-162, 160t
    of broodmare, 229-230
    of growing horse, 272
Wrap, leg, for flexor deformity, 282

Xylorrbiza glabriuscula, 326

Yearling, feeding of, 265
Yeast
  brewer's, 87
  nutrient content of, 413t, 421t
  single-celled protein and, 89
Yeast culture, 100-101
  athletic performance and, 196, 218
  for growing horse, 271
Yellow oleander, 338
Yellow star thistle, 318, 318-319
Yellow sweet clover, spoiled, 331-332, 332
Yew poisoning, 343-344
Young horse, 264-276. See also Growing horse

Zea mays, 74-75, 419t
Zearalenone, 348
Zeolite, 99-101
Zigadenus venenosus, 344, 344
Zinc, 422
  developmental orthopedic disorder and, 286
  for growing horse, 265t
  imbalance of, 21t, 36-37
  in milk, 270, 270t
  in pasture forage, 104t, 412t
  vitamin E and, 29